Fetal Cardiology

AF757822

John Simpson • Vita Zidere
Owen I. Miller
Editors

Fetal Cardiology

A Practical Approach to Diagnosis and Management

Springer

Editors
John Simpson
Evelina London Children's Hospital
Guy's and St Thomas'
NHS Foundation Trust
London
UK

Vita Zidere
Evelina London Children's Hospital
Guy's and St Thomas'
NHS Foundation Trust
London
UK

King's College Hospital
NHS Foundation Trust
London
UK

Owen I. Miller
Evelina London Children's Hospital
Guy's and St Thomas'
NHS Foundation Trust
London
UK

ISBN 978-3-030-08460-8 ISBN 978-3-319-77461-9 (eBook)
https://doi.org/10.1007/978-3-319-77461-9

© Springer International Publishing AG, part of Springer Nature 2018
Softcover re-print of the Hardcover 1st edition 2018
This work is subject to copyright. All rights are reserved by the Publisher, whether the whole or part of the material is concerned, specifically the rights of translation, reprinting, reuse of illustrations, recitation, broadcasting, reproduction on microfilms or in any other physical way, and transmission or information storage and retrieval, electronic adaptation, computer software, or by similar or dissimilar methodology now known or hereafter developed.
The use of general descriptive names, registered names, trademarks, service marks, etc. in this publication does not imply, even in the absence of a specific statement, that such names are exempt from the relevant protective laws and regulations and therefore free for general use.
The publisher, the authors and the editors are safe to assume that the advice and information in this book are believed to be true and accurate at the date of publication. Neither the publisher nor the authors or the editors give a warranty, express or implied, with respect to the material contained herein or for any errors or omissions that may have been made. The publisher remains neutral with regard to jurisdictional claims in published maps and institutional affiliations.

This Springer imprint is published by the registered company Springer Nature Switzerland AG
The registered company address is: Gewerbestrasse 11, 6330 Cham, Switzerland

Foreword

This book represents a major collaborative effort between experts in fetal cardiology, fetal medicine and genetics from recognised centres of excellence in the UK. It provides a plethora of images and videos and extensive description of the essential views for examination of the anatomy and function of the fetal heart and features of the major types of congenital heart defects.

In the case of heart defects, the reader will gain a clear understanding of the diagnosis and the need to search for other abnormalities by detailed ultrasound examination. Invasive testing, examination of cell-free DNA in maternal blood, parental counselling and postnatal care are also discussed. To date, fetal cardiac imaging has been almost exclusively the preserve of ultrasound. This book includes the latest advances in fetal cardiac MRI to investigate anatomic abnormalities and assessment of blood flow.

The book provides essential reading for experts in fetal medicine and paediatric cardiology but also for obstetricians, sonographers and midwives because fetal echocardiography and the diagnosis and management of fetal heart abnormalities constitute an integral part of prenatal care.

Kypros Nicolaides

Acknowledgements

The contribution of all members of the fetal cardiology team at Evelina London Children's Hospital and King's College Hospital to diagnosis and management is acknowledged. Pioneers in fetal cardiology from our centre, including Professor Lindsey Allan, Professor Gurleen Sharland and the late Dr. Ian Huggon, are thanked for their inspirational teaching and commitment.

Thanks to my wife Sahar and my children Angus and Alexandra for their support and for putting up with me during the writing of this book.

John Simpson

I would like to thank my parents Gunta and Andris for all their love and support at every stage of my career.

Vita Zidere

I acknowledge the support of my wife Vanda, and of my children Hamish, Maddy and Angus, whilst putting together this book.

Owen I. Miller

Contents

Abbreviations

A	Atrium
Ao	Aorta
ALSA	Aberrant left subclavian artery
ARSA	Aberrant right subclavian artery
AVSD	Atrioventricular septal defect
bpm	Beats per minute
CAT	Common arterial trunk
CHD	Congenital heart disease
CoA	Coarctation of the aorta
CPAM	Congenital pulmonary airway malformation
CTR	Cardio-thoracic ratio
D	Duct (arterial)
DILV	Double inlet left ventricle
DORV	Double outlet right ventricle
HLH	Hypoplastic left heart
IA	Innominate artery
IVC	Inferior vena cava
L	Left
LA	Left atrium
LCA	Left carotid artery
LPA	Left pulmonary artery
LSA	Left subclavian artery
LV	Left ventricle
LVOT	Left outflow tract
MAPCAS	Major aortopulmonary collateral arteries
MV	Mitral valve
O	Oesophagus
PA	Pulmonary artery
PAIVS	Pulmonary atresia with intact ventricular septum
PLSVC	Persistent left superior vena cava
PV	Pulmonary vein
R	Right
RA	Right atrium
RCA	Right carotid artery

RVOT	Right ventricular outflow tract
RPA	Right pulmonary artery branch
RSA	Right subclavian artery
RV	Right ventricle
STIC	Spatio-temporal image correlation
SVC	Superior caval vein
T	Trachea
TAPVC	Total anomalous pulmonary venous connection
TGA	Transposition of the great arteries
TR	Tricuspid regurgitation
ToF	Tetralogy of Fallot
TV	Tricuspid valve
V	Ventricle
VSD	Ventricular septal defect

List of Videos

The videos can be viewed and downloaded from http://extras.springer.com.

Video 4.4	Left ventricular outflow tract view with red signal showing normal velocity anterograde flow across the aortic valve. Orientation: spine to right of screen, left ventricle inferior
Video 4.5	Right ventricular outflow tract/pulmonary artery view. Left panel shows 2D greyscale, right panel shows simultaneous Color Flow Doppler. Initially showing main pulmonary artery with normal anterograde flow, sweeping slightly more superiorly the branch pulmonary arteries clearly seen. Orientation: spine to left of screen, right side uppermost
Video 4.6	Three vessel view. Orientation: spine lowermost on screen, fetal left on right side of screen. The three vessels; the superior caval vein is seen in cross section as a dark circle, next the aorta and then pulmonary artery are seen forming a V-shape with apex to the (fetal) left of spine. Color Flow Doppler shows anterograde flow with uniform velocity, in both aorta and pulmonary artery
Video 4.7	Three vessel view. Orientation: spine lowermost on screen, fetal left on right side of screen. There is forward flow in the aorta but proximal pulmonary artery shows (red) retrograde Color Flow Doppler as supply comes from arterial duct due to pulmonary valve atresia
Video 4.8	Sagittal aortic arch view. Orientation; spine uppermost, cephalad to left of screen, caudal to right of screen. Three major aorto-pulmonary collateral arteries are seen arising from thoracic descending aorta, in this case due to pulmonary atresia
Video 5.1	Normal four-chamber view of the heart. There is dynamic function of both the left and right ventricles with complete opening of the tricuspid and mitral valves during diastole
Video 5.2	Four-chamber view with color flow Doppler showing inflow to both Ventricles (red) and flow out of the left ventricle (blue). There is no mitral or tricuspid valve regurgitation
Video 5.3	The heart is enlarged and the left ventricle contracts particularly poorly. There is significant mitral and tricuspid valve regurgitation shown by the blue jets
Video 5.4	The ultrasound cursor is placed at 90° to the plane of the ventricular septum. This permits visualisation of the motion of both the left and right ventricular free walls on the M-mode trace on the right. The image can be frozen and the end-diastolic and systolic dimensions of the ventricles can be measured to compute the fractional shortening
Video 5.5	Four-chamber view of the fetal heart. The green lines mark the epicardial and endocardial surfaces of the myocardium which is tracked through the cardiac cycle to allow computation of longitudinal strain (myocardial deformation)
Video 5.6	The heart is enlarged. There is prominent flow through the left pulmonary veins (shown in red) due to the presence of a large pulmonary arteriovenous malformation. This leads to volume loading of the heart accounting for its enlargement

defect. Color flow Doppler demonstrates antegrade flow within the large artery (aorta) and in the much smaller one (pulmonary artery), which arises from the anterior right ventricle and crosses over the first one. This constellation of findings in this 13 week fetus is consistent with tetralogy of Fallot

Video 6.7 This first trimester image demonstrates left aortic arch and an aberrant right subclavian artery arising from the descending aorta behind the trachea and below the transverse aortic arch and heading towards the right shoulder

Video 7.1 The four-chamber view demonstrates cardiomegaly in this example of critical aortic stenosis. A dilated, echogenic and non-apex forming left ventricle is seen. The left atrium appears dilated due to mitral regurgitation and a restrictive atrial septum which are confirmed on color flow Doppler

Video 7.2 The fetal heart is displaced into the right chest and the cardiothoracic ratio is decreased due to congenital diaphragmatic hernia

Video 7.3 A large perimembranous ventricular septal defect with inlet extension is seen in an apical four-chamber view in this fetus. There is the loss of off-setting of the atrioventricular valves. However, this is not an atrioventricular septal defect as there two separate atrioventricular valves and the primum atrial septum is present

Video 7.4a A moderate mid-muscular ventricular septal defect with a bidirectional flow pattern seen on color flow Doppler

Video 7.4b In this case a small mid-muscular ventricular septal defect seen on color flow Doppler in the four-chamber view on the right panel. Note that there is no obvious defect seen on 2D greyscale, left sided panel

Video 7.5a A transverse sweep from abdomen to great arteries is demonstrated in this video. Cross-section of the abdomen confirms normal situs. The loss of "off-setting" and straight atrioventricular valves in ventricular systole is indicative of a complete atrioventricular septal defect. The great artery connections and transverse aortic arch are normal

Video 7.5b Another example of a complete atrioventricular septal defect is seen in this video. Normal cardiac situs and normal great artery connections are also confirmed

Video 7.5c A large atrioventricular septal defect is seen in this four-chamber view

Video 7.5d This early fetal heart examination demonstrates loss of off-setting due to an atrioventricular septal defect

Video 7.6 In the sagittal plane the short axis view of the left ventricle and the right ventricle are obtained. The right ventricle is anterior just below the sternum and the left ventricle is located more posteriorly. There is the appearance of a common atrioventricular valve which spans across the ventricular septum in a case of atrioventricular septal defect

artery appears smaller than the aorta but with forward flow across the valve and the arterial duct

Video 7.23 The four-chamber view demonstrates an example of tricuspid valve dysplasia. The tricuspid valve appears thickened but not displaced. There is marked cardiomegaly due to severe enlargement of the right atrium caused by tricuspid regurgitation

Video 7.24 In this video an apical four-chamber view demonstrates atrioventricular discordance. The pulmonary venous chamber (left atrium) is anterior to the spine. This connects to a ventricle with a moderator band at the apex. There is reversed off-setting of the atrioventricular valves. The left-sided atrioventricular valve arises closer to the apex indicating that this is the tricuspid valve. This indicates the morphological right ventricle is on the left side. The right-sided ventricle is smooth walled indicative of a morphological left ventricle. These features are consistent with atrioventricular discordance

Video 7.25 The outflow tract assessment reveals that the pulmonary artery arises from the morphological left ventricle and is seen first on sweeping cranially. The aorta arises anterior and to the left of the pulmonary artery from the morphologic right ventricle

Video 7.26 There is reversed flow in the aortic arch during diastole. This is seen in cases of fetal growth restriction due to the 'brain sparing effect'

Video 8.1 Normal four-chamber view in fetus with transposition of the great arteries

Video 8.2 Sonographic sweep showing the branching pulmonary artery arising from the left ventricle. On sweeping more cranially, the aorta can be seen to arise from the right ventricle. The normal 3VT appearance is not evident

Video 8.3 In this video, the branching PA is seen more posteriorly followed by visualisation of the aorta more anteriorly as the ultrasound probe is angulated superiorly

Video 8.4 Sonographic sweep utilising color Flow Doppler to illustrate the pulmonary artery arising from the LV and, more cranially, the aorta arising from the RV

Video 8.5 Parallel arrangement of the great arteries with the aorta anterior is evident in this video. There is loss of the normal "crossing" pattern of the great arteries

Video 8.6 This is a sagittal projection of transposition of the great arteries. The arteries arise in parallel from the heart with the aorta anterior. Note that the aortic arch is superior to the ductal arch and that the plan of the two arches is similar so that they my both be seen in the same sonographic cut, in contrast to the normal heart

Video 8.7 A large perimembranous VSD is clearly evident on the four-chamber view in this fetus with TGA

Video 8.8 In this video the left panel show that the great arteries arise in parallel but that the pulmonary artery is significantly smaller

Organisation of Screening for Congenital Heart Disease

1

John Simpson

Abstract

Prenatal diagnosis of congenital heart disease is associated with improved survival and reduced morbidity for some forms of critical congenital heart disease (CHD). Most population screening is based on detection of affected fetuses by incorporation of cardiac views in the midtrimester anomaly scan. This is further refined by first trimester screening by methods such as nuchal translucency (NT) thickness to detect fetuses at high risk for CHD who then undergo more detailed assessment. Pregnancies with historic or maternal risk factors CHD such as family history of CHD or maternal diabetes mellitus are typically offered specialist fetal echocardiography rather than relying solely on the midtrimester anomaly scan. Published recommendations have established not only cardiac referral indications but also optimal screening views with a relatively high degree of consistency between published standards. Following a prenatal diagnosis of CHD, a multidisciplinary team is required to provide appropriate diagnostic and prognostic information, investigation for associated abnormalities, parental support and co-ordination of care pathways.

Keywords

Prenatal diagnosis · Screening · Congenital heart disease · Nuchal translucency · Anomaly scan · Referral indications · Low risk population · High risk population · Scan · Echocardiogram · Fetal heart

Background

Congenital heart disease (CHD) is the commonest group of congenital malformations with an incidence of 8 per 1000 livebirths of whom around half will require surgery or catheter intervention in infancy. Cardiovascular disease accounts for half of deaths due to malformations in infancy emphasising that CHD is not only relatively common but also an important cause of mortality and morbidity. Due to the nature of the fetal circulation, the majority of fetuses with CHD will not show signs of cardiac failure during fetal life so the detection of affected fetuses largely relies on recognition of abnormal sonographic appearances. For example, in hypoplastic left heart syndrome, the right ventricle can support the systemic arterial circulation due to blood flow though the arterial duct to the systemic circulation. At the outset, it might be questioned why screening for CHD would be advocated at all. Firstly, there is evidence that for certain cardiac lesions, including hypoplastic left heart, transposition of the great arteries, pulmonary atresia and coarctation of the aorta, prenatal diagnosis has a positive impact on postnatal

J. Simpson
Evelina London Children's Hospital, Guy's and St Thomas' NHS Foundation Trust, London, UK
e-mail: john.simpson@gstt.nhs.uk

© Springer International Publishing AG, part of Springer Nature 2018
J. Simpson et al. (eds.), *Fetal Cardiology*, https://doi.org/10.1007/978-3-319-77461-9_1

outcome with a reduction in either mortality or improved condition at presentation (Holland et al. 2015). Secondly, detection of CHD may lead to the detection or other structural fetal anomalies or karyotypic abnormalities. Commoner examples of this include the detection of trisomy 21 following diagnosis of a complete atrioventricular septal defect (AVSD) or a 22q11 deletion following detection of tetralogy of Fallot. Thirdly, prenatal detection affords parents the time to understand the nature of the CHD, interventions required (with their associated risks) and longer term prognosis. Depending on the severity of the lesion, gestational age and legal framework, the parents may also have the option of termination of pregnancy. Finally, in selected fetuses, notably those with arrhythmias or critical obstruction to the left or right ventricular outflow tract, prenatal diagnosis may permit prenatal drug therapy or cardiac intervention respectively (Araujo Júnior et al. 2016).

The approach to identification of CHD can broadly be subdivided into "low risk" and "high risk" pregnancies depending on whether or not there are any specific risk factors for CHD. The approach in the low risk population differs from the high risk population (Fig. 1.1).

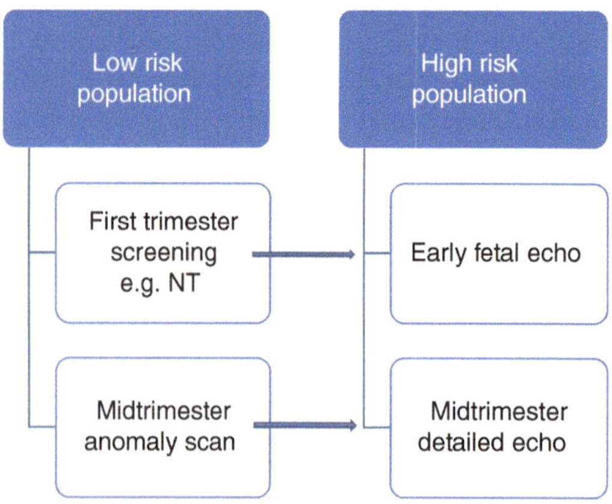

Fig. 1.1 Organisation of screening. This flow chart gives an overview of the type of pathways for the "low risk" versus "high risk" population. In the absence of risk factors, the pregnancy is assessed by first trimester screening and then by the midtrimester anomaly scan. If abnormal screening results or sonographic findings are identified then pregnancies move to the "high risk" pathway (horizontal arrows). Abbreviations: *NT* nuchal translucency thickness, *echo* echocardiography

The Low Risk Population

In the low risk population, fetuses are assessed by techniques which are applied to the whole population. The most common approach is to include selected cardiac views into "routine" midtrimester anomaly scans so that those who deviate from normality may be referred for comprehensive assessment. The exact screening approach adopted will vary from country to country but most international bodies and screening programmes advocate a series of transverse sonographic cuts of the fetal thorax into standard views to gauge normality of the heart position, rhythm, four chamber view, outflow tracts and aortic/ductal arch (Allan et al. 2004; The International Society of Ultrasound in Obstetrics 2013; Donofrio et al. 2014).

Individual centres have reported excellent results of screening for congenital heart disease and all data confirms an improved diagnostic yield when views of the outflow tracts are included in addition to the four chamber view. There is, however, likely to be a publication bias for results reported from single centres—few centres will actively seek to publish poor results. The effectiveness of screening for CHD at a national or regional level shows a high variability between countries, regions and hospitals suggesting that a uniform screening standard is hard to achieve. As an example, United Kingdom data from the 1990s showed an overall detection of serious CHD of 24% with far better detection of lesions with an abnormal four chamber view compared to lesions which depended on extended views of the outflow tracts for their detection (Bull 1999). There are a large number of factors which could impact on variation of prenatal detection of CHD including training and experience of sonographers, equipment factors, time allocation for scans and different scan protocols.

Some countries, including the United Kingdom, have adopted national standards for imaging of the fetal heart during midtrimester anomaly scans with the aim of improving prenatal detection rates and reducing regional variation. The introduction of first-trimester ultrasound scans is also having an impact on assessment of the low risk population. Measurement of nuchal translucency (NT) thickness was introduced to refine and improve prenatal diagnosis of trisomy 21 but it is now well-recognised that NT has an association with CHD which is independent of the fetal karyotype. Furthermore, the NT thickness correlates with the incidence of CHD. Published data has suggested that NT screening may detect 20–45% of CHD depending on the NT threshold adopted (95th versus 99th percentile) (Sotiriadis et al. 2013) hence this technique has helped to identify a group who should undergo detailed fetal echocardiography. In addition to measurement of NT, some groups have further refined the technique by assessment of tricuspid regurgitation (TR) and/or ductus venosus flow patterns in the first trimester. Tricuspid regurgitation is assessed by pulsed wave Doppler and CHD risk increased if TR is present. Those fetuses who demonstrate reversal of flow in the ductus venosus coincident with atrial contraction have been reported to have an increased risk of CHD but the effectiveness as a screening tool remains a topic of debate (Prats et al. 2012).

High-Risk Population

Some groups of fetuses are at high risk of CHD because of either fetal, maternal or familial factors. Given the background live-born incidence of CHD of around 0.8%, consideration needs to be given to the fetal risk which should lead to referral for detailed assessment of the fetal heart. In practice, most accept a risk of more than about 2–3% as a reasonable threshold to prompt such referral (Donofrio et al. 2014). This is by no means uniform and will depend on local facilities/resources and availability of expert opinion. Accepted risk factors for CHD are shown in Table 1.1 and discussed in more detail below.

Table 1.1 Indications for detailed fetal echocardiography

Historic indications
• Family history of congenital heart disease
– Maternal or paternal CHD
– Sibling CHD
Fetal indications
• Suspected CHD on anomaly scan
• Fetal arrhythmias e.g. fetal tachycardia, bradycardia
• Increased NT
– >99th percentile ≥ 3.5 mm
– >95th percentile ≥ 2.2.–2.6 mm according to CRL
• Extra-cardiac abnormality e.g. congenital diaphragmatic hernia, exomphalos, duodenal atresia, cystic hygroma
• Abnormal loading conditions
– Agenesis of ductus venosus, fetal anemia, fetal tumors with large vascular supply e.g. sacrococcygeal teratoma, arteriovenous malformations
• Fetal hydrops
• Abnormal fetal karyotype e.g. Trisomy 21/18/13/XO
• Monochorionic pregnancy
– Risk of cardiac abnormality
– Twin-Twin transfusion syndrome
Maternal indications
• Maternal drugs
– Use of prostaglandin synthetase inhibitors e.g. ibuprofen
– Teratogenicity e.g. lithium or anticonvulsants
• Diabetes Mellitus or other metabolic conditions e.g. phenylketonuria
• Maternal Infection e.g. parvovirus
• Maternal antibody status/connective tissue disease e.g. positive anti-Ro, anti-La antibodies
• Assisted conception/in vitro fertilization

Family History of Congenital Heart Disease

In pregnancies where a first degree relative of the fetus is affected with CHD (mother/father/sibling of the fetus) it is widely accepted that this constitutes an indication for detailed fetal echocardiography. It should be emphasised that the risk of recurrence should take account of all information relating to the index case. For example, if a previous pregnancy has been complicated by Trisomy 21 and an atrioventricular septal defect, the recurrence risk is that of Trisomy 21, not the cardiac lesion. In many cases, the exact cause of CHD in the index case cannot be identified and in this setting an empiric recurrence risk is usually quoted. Maternal CHD is an accepted risk factor for CHD in the fetus. The exact incidence in the offspring of affected mothers depends on the type of CHD but can be up to 8% (Burn et al. 1998). Paternal CHD is also an accepted indication for fetal cardiac assessment with a recurrence risk which was observed to be similar to the sibling recurrence risk at around 2–3% (Gill et al. 2003). Previous work has reported that far fewer fetuses with paternal CHD are referred than maternal, suggesting that a history of CHD in the father is not always elicited (Gill et al. 2003). Some groups of lesions may have a higher recurrence risk including left heart obstructive lesions e.g. hypoplastic left heart syndrome and laterality disturbance e.g. isomerism of the atrial appendages.

Fetal Risk Factors

Suspected Congenital Heart Disease

Of any indication to assess the fetal heart in detail, suspected CHD has the highest yield of affected cases. In our own series, 50% of cases referred because of a suspected cardiac abnormality are diagnosed with CHD following detailed fetal echocardiography.

Nuchal Translucency

Initial reports suggested that the majority of CHD could be detected by using the 95th percentile of NT as a threshold for detailed fetal echocardiography (Hyett et al. 1999). This has major logistic implications because this would require 5% of the pregnant population to undergo detailed assessment which may not be universally achievable. In current practice most units use a higher threshold of 3.5 mm (99th percentile) for referral for detailed fetal echocardiography but there remains considerable regional and international variation, driven by logistic factors and cost-effectiveness. Among fetuses with an NT >99th percentile (3.5 mm), the absolute incidence of CHD is 6–7%, but this is a continuum with a higher incidence as the NT thickness increases. A recent meta-analysis reported that 44% of fetuses with CHD and a normal karyotype had an NT >95th percentile, and 20% had NT >99th percentile (Sotiriadis et al. 2013).

Extra-Cardiac Abnormality

Some extra-cardiac abnormalities are associated with CHD, meriting detailed assessment. These abnormalities include exomphalos, diaphragmatic hernia and cleft lip/palate.

Fetal Hydrops

Fetal hydrops may be due to underlying structural congenital heart disease or cardiac arrhythmia. In hydrops of cardiac aetiology the fetal heart is typically enlarged.

Fetal Arrhythmias

Fetal tachycardia (>200 beats per minute) and persistent fetal bradycardia (<100 beats per minute) are indications for detailed fetal echocardiography.

Abnormal Fetal Karyotype

Fetuses with abnormal karyotype, including major aneuploidies are at increased risk for CHD. Referrals for this indication have traditionally been made after chorionic villous sampling or amniocentesis, but recently a much larger uptake of non-invasive prenatal testing (NIPT) has emerged. This technique evaluates placental cell-free DNA in the maternal blood. This is being used for the detection of aneuploidies as well as sex chromosome disorders. Some NIPT has been extended to other microdeletion syndromes e.g. 22q11 deletion.

Monochorionic Pregnancy

Monochorionic twin pregnancies are known to be at increased risk of structural heart disease and also twin–twin transfusion syndrome. Twin-twin transfusion syndrome characteristically leads to pulmonary valve/subpulmonary obstruction in the recipient twin. An increased incidence of coarctation of the aorta in the donor twin has also been described.

Maternal Indications for Detailed Fetal Echocardiography

Maternal Drugs

Prostaglandin synthetase inhibitors e.g. ibuprofen may cause constriction of the arterial duct. Other drugs such as lithium or anticonvulsants have been associated with structural heart disease.

Diabetes Mellitus

Maternal diabetes mellitus is an indication for detailed fetal echocardiography because of an increased risk of structural heart disease (3% in our series) or of late development of myocardial hypertrophy, particularly if glycaemic control is poor. Other metabolic conditions, notably maternal phenylketonuria has also been associated with CHD.

Maternal Infection

Maternal infection may constitute a referral indication if the infection is known to have a potential effect on cardiac development or to affect cardiac function. Parvovirus and Coxsackie virus may both cause fetal myocarditis and Parvovirus may induce fetal anaemia leading to circulatory overload and fetal hydrops.

Maternal Antibody Status/Connective Tissue Disease

Mothers who are known to carry anti-Ro and/or anti-La antibodies are at risk for development of fetal heart block. Such antibodies may rarely cause fetal cardiomyopathy even in the absence of rhythm disturbance.

Assisted Conception

There appears to be an increased risk of CHD associated with in vitro fertilisation (IVF) including intracytoplasmic sperm injection (ICSI). The recommendations in this regard are conflicting and confounding variables such as multiple pregnancies, maternal age and the underlying reason for infertility complicate interpretation. IVF is included as a referral indication for fetal echocardiography by some bodies including the American Society of Echocardiography and American Heart Association (Rychik 2004; Donofrio et al. 2014).

Pathways for Assessment of Low Risk and High Risk Populations

The precise pathways for the "low risk" and "high risk" populations are shown diagrammatically in Fig. 1.1. The low risk population typically undergoes screening in the first trimester which will vary between countries and regions. First trimester screening may include serum screening for trisomy 21 and measurement of NT which may itself be refined by additional assessment of tricuspid valve regurgitation and/or ductus venosus flow patterns. Abnormal screening results at this point may generate indications for the offer of invasive prenatal testing for karyotypic abnormalities and for detailed fetal echocardiography. The timing of fetal echocardiography in this setting will be determined by the nature of the findings and local facilities for early fetal echocardiography. If screening results in the first trimester do not cause concern then the heart will be assessed as part of the midtrimester anomaly scan according to institutional protocol or other standards. Further detailed assessment of the fetal heart is not normally undertaken if the findings are within normal limits at that time of the midtrimester anomaly scan. If a cardiac abnormality or other fetal abnormality associated with CHD is identified at the midtrimester anomaly scan then detailed fetal echocardiography is undertaken at that point to confirm or refute the presence of CHD. Thus, there is a potential for horizontal movement between the two pathways at any stage of pregnancy.

In the high risk population, if there is a major historic risk factor, for example a previous baby with severe CHD or a severe elevation of NT, fetal echocardiography may be undertaken as early as 12–14 weeks gestational age to assess the main cardiac structures. At our unit, early fetal echocardiography will be offered if NT is >3.5 mm (99th percentile), if there is a previous history of severe CHD or if there is suspicion of underlying CHD at the time of the first trimester scan. Even if the initial fetal echocardiographic findings are normal in the first trimester, the fetal echocardiogram will still be repeated in the midtrimester when a more comprehensive cardiac assessment can be achieved.

Management Following Prenatal Diagnosis of Congenital Heart Disease

If CHD is identified before birth then parents should receive information and support about the condition and prognosis of their baby, as well as potential associations. This may involve multiple disciplines including fetal medicine, geneticists, neonatologists, nurse specialists and midwives. Different facets of such management are covered in more detail in other chapters of this book. For parents who elect to continue pregnancy, tailored care is required which will include discussion of site and mode of delivery and an understanding of the likely initial and longer term postnatal management. If parents elect to terminate the pregnancy, ongoing support will also be required which will include the offer to discuss other results, such as the results of post-mortem examination (Fig. 1.2).

Efficacy and Cost-Effectiveness of Prenatal Screening for CHD

For any prenatal screening test, including prenatal detection of CHD, the means of applying this in clinical practice is important both with respect to the effectiveness of the screening test in terms of prenatal detection rate, but also in terms of cost effectiveness. Data on cost effectiveness is relatively scarce but recent reports have demonstrated cost effectiveness by reduced cost of transport of new-born infants to tertiary cardiac centres if the CHD was recognised before birth (Jegatheeswaran et al. 2011). Other work has modelled the costs associated with different screening strategies and referral patterns and concluded that screening by four-chamber view and outflow tracts followed by referral to fetal cardiology following suspicion of congenital heart disease represented the most cost-

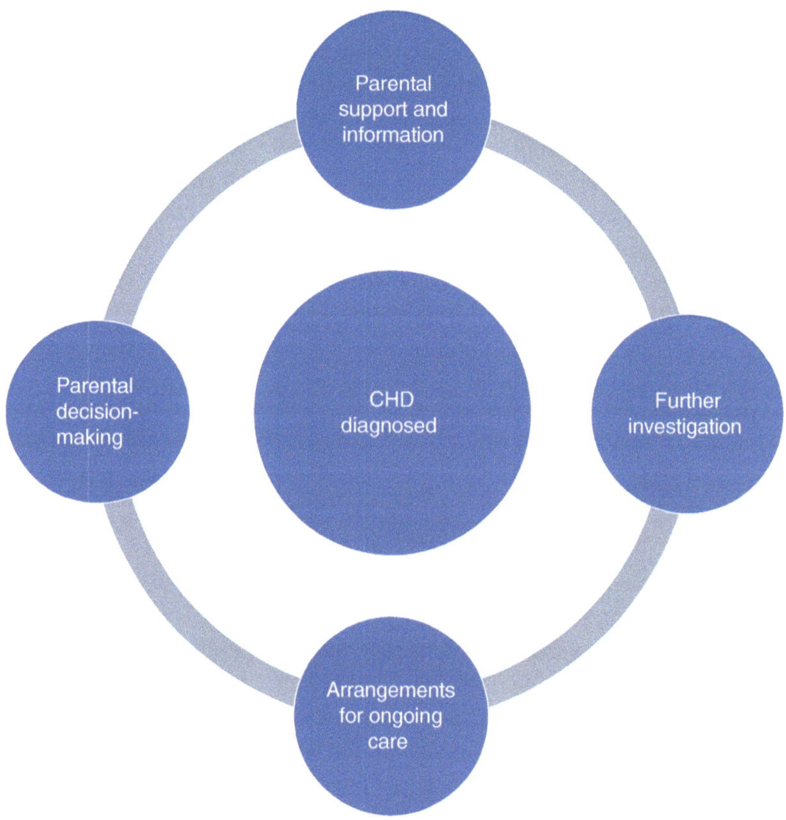

Fig. 1.2 Management pathways following prenatal diagnosis of congenital heart disease. This figure shows the type of approach taken after a prenatal diagnosis of CHD which includes provision of information, involvement of subspecialities for further investigation through to planning of ongoing care. This is a multidisciplinary challenge to optimise care. Abbreviations: *CHD* congenital heart disease

effective model (Pinto et al. 2014). A high cost was associated with the addition of NT screening but in many developed countries NT is already established to identify fetuses at high risk for trisomy unrelated to its application to detection of CHD.

Most published work relates to organisation of screening for CHD in the developed world where access to high level care and appropriate specialists it taken for granted. Situations where resources are limited, including in the developing world, pose challenges. Data from India has reported that, among parents of children with CHD, only 2.2% of families were aware of fetal echocardiography (Warrier et al. 2012). Furthermore in settings with limited resources there may be a lack of facilities for ongoing management of CHD and treatment may have major financial implications for families.

A further consideration with respect to the place of prenatal diagnosis of CHD is the introduction of pulse oximetry screening of new-born infants to detect subnormal oxygen saturations or a difference in pre and post-ductal saturations. This form of postnatal screening has not been uniformly introduced but might be considered to weaken the argument for prenatal screening by reducing the time taken to suspect CHD postnatally. However, prenatal diagnosis of CHD allows time for full counselling about prognosis and identification of associated anomalies when parents have options including continuing or terminating pregnancy. Currently, prenatal screening for CHD and postnatal pulse oximetry are emerging as complementary techniques to optimise the diagnosis and treatment of infants with CHD.

References

Allan L, Dangel J, Fesslova V, et al. Recommendations for the practice of fetal cardiology in Europe. Cardiol Young. 2004;14:109–14.

Araujo Júnior E, Tonni G, Chung M, et al. Perinatal outcomes and intrauterine complications following fetal intervention for congenital heart disease: systematic review and meta-analysis of observational studies. Ultrasound Obstet Gynecol. 2016;48:426–33.

Bull C. Current and potential impact of fetal diagnosis on prevalence and spectrum of serious congenital heart disease at term in the UK. Lancet. 1999;354:1242–7.

Burn J, Brennan P, Little J, et al. Recurrence risks in offspring of adults with major heart defects: results from first cohort of British collaborative study. Lancet. 1998;351:311–6.

Donofrio MT, Moon-Grady AJ, Hornberger LK, et al. Diagnosis and treatment of fetal cardiac disease: a scientific statement from the American Heart Association. Circulation. 2014;129:2183–242.

Gill HK, Splitt M, Sharland GK, Simpson JM. Patterns of recurrence of congenital heart disease: an analysis of 6,640 consecutive pregnancies evaluated by detailed fetal echocardiography. J Am Coll Cardiol. 2003;42:923–9.

Holland BJ, Myers JA, Woods CR. Prenatal diagnosis of critical congenital heart disease reduces risk of death from cardiovascular compromise prior to planned neonatal cardiac surgery: a meta-analysis. Ultrasound Obstet Gynecol. 2015;45:631–8.

Hyett J, Perdu M, Sharland G, et al. Using fetal nuchal translucency to screen for major congenital cardiac defects at 10-14 weeks of gestation: population based cohort study. BMJ. 1999;318:81–5.

Jegatheeswaran A, Oliveira C, Batsos C, et al. Costs of prenatal detection of congenital heart disease. Am J Cardiol. 2011;108:1808–14.

Pinto NM, Nelson R, Puchalski M, et al. Cost-effectiveness of prenatal screening strategies for congenital heart disease. Ultrasound Obstet Gynecol. 2014;44:50–7.

Prats P, Ferrer Q, Comas C, Rodríguez I. Is the addition of the ductus venosus useful when screening for aneuploidy and congenital heart disease in fetuses with normal nuchal translucency? Fetal Diagn Ther. 2012;32:138–43.

Rychik J, Ayres N, Cuneo B, Gotteiner N, Hornberger L, Spevak PJ, Van Der Veld M. American Society of Echocardiography guidelines and standards for performance of the fetal echocardiogram. J Am Soc Echocardiogr. 2004;17(7):803–10.

Sotiriadis A, Papatheodorou S, Eleftheriades M, Makrydimas G. Nuchal translucency and major congenital heart defects in fetuses with normal karyotype: a meta-analysis. Ultrasound Obstet Gynecol. 2013;42:383–9.

The International Society of Ultrasound in Obstetrics. ISUOG Practice Guidelines (updated): sonographic screening examination of the fetal heart. Ultrasound Obstet Gynecol. 2013;41:348–59.

Warrier D, Saraf R, Maheshwari S, et al. Awareness of fetal echo in Indian scenario. Ann Pediatr Cardiol. 2012;5:156–9.

Screening Views of the Fetal Heart

2

Lindsey E. Hunter

Abstract

International guidelines have been published describing standard screening views of the fetal heart ensuring a systematic approach is undertaken by all practitioners involved in the prenatal detection of major congenital heart disease (CHD).

This systematic approach involves a series of transverse cuts in a caudal to cranial direction including the cardiac situs, four chamber view, left ventricular outflow tract, right ventricular outflow tract, three vessel view (3VV) and finally the three vessel and trachea (3VT) view. This approach aims to increase the prenatal detection of major forms of CHD using a system which can be incorporated into fetal anomaly screening programs.

Keywords

Fetus · Fetal heart · Screening · Prenatal diagnosis · Four chamber view · Left ventricular outflow tract · Right ventricular outflow tract · Three vessel view

Electronic Supplementary Material The online version of this chapter (https://doi.org/10.1007/978-3-319-77461-9_2) contains supplementary material, which is available to authorized users.

L. E. Hunter
Royal Hospital for Children, Glasgow, UK
e-mail: lindsey.hunter@ggc.scot.nhs.uk

Introduction

Congenital heart disease (CHD) is the most common congenital anomaly to affect the fetus and neonate, with an incidence of around 8 per 1000 live births of which half are severe enough to require surgical or catheter intervention. Prenatal screening relies on detailed sonographic examination of the fetal heart, normally undertaken between 18 and 22 weeks gestation in 'low risk' pregnancies. Detailed fetal echocardiography is indicated in 'high risk' pregnancies when the fetus has a significantly increased risk of developing CHD.

The objective of prenatal cardiac screening is to identify severe or critical CHD early in pregnancy. Studies have suggested assessment of the four chamber view alone may detect over 50% of major CHD, but addition of the outflow tract views has been reported to increase the detection of CHD in excess of 90%, however population based studies typically fall short of such projections. Detection of CHD in the second trimester allows optimal time for detailed discussion with the family, parental choice, prenatal intervention if indicated, appropriate timing and location of delivery and the provision of a neonatal cardiac management plan. Conversely, normal screening views exclude most forms of CHD.

© Springer International Publishing AG, part of Springer Nature 2018

J. Simpson et al. (eds.), *Fetal Cardiology*, https://doi.org/10.1007/978-3-319-77461-9_2

Recommended Approach

International guidelines have been published to provide a consensus and systematic approach for assessing the fetal heart by screening sonographers, fetal medicine specialists and paediatric cardiologists (Yagel et al. 2001; Allan et al. 2004; Rychik et al. 2004; Carvalho et al. 2013; Fetal Echocardiography Task Force 2011; Fetal Anomaly Screening Programme 2017). To ensure the highest diagnostic accuracy, a systematic approach should be taken when assessing the morphological connections of the fetal heart. Traditionally the fetal heart is examined in a series of transverse slices: cardiac situs; four chamber view; left ventricular outflow tract (LVOT); right ventricular outflow tract (RVOT); three vessel view (3VV) and three vessel and trachea view (3VT). This systematic approach has been recommended by most guidelines for screening for congenital heart disease. The four chamber view can be used as a starting reference point and used to orientate the inexperienced echocardiographer. In the transverse plane a single rib should be visualised encircling the fetal thorax to ensure images are not taken 'off axis'. An 'off axis' view can lead to misinterpretation and risk an abnormality be suspected within a normal heart or, alternatively, an abnormality being overlooked. Additional views of the normal fetal heart are covered in Chap. 3 of this book.

Furthermore, as the fetal heart structures are small and fast moving it is essential to optimise image acquisition. The choice of ultrasound probe may alter both with gestational age and maternal habitus. Higher frequency probes provide better image resolution but poorer tissue penetration, thus lower frequency probes may be beneficial during a third trimester scan or if there is a raised maternal body mass index. To maximum the frame rate, the region of interest (ROI) around the fetal thorax should be adjusted by narrowing the sector width, optimising the depth and aligning the ultrasound focus appropriately. The dynamic range and image persistence is reduced to produce an image which is higher contrast than standard settings with crisp views of fast moving structures such as heart valves. Most obstetric ultrasound systems have a designated fetal heart preset which should be used to optimise image quality initially, with fine adjustments according to operator preference. The optimisation of colour flow Doppler is covered in detail in Chap. 4 and some screening recommendations do not specify the use of this modality. Colour persistence is typically reduced for cardiac views with colour scale adjusted according to the anticipated flow velocities in the chambers or vessels studied.

Summary of Views

Fetal Orientation

Before examining the intra-cardiac structures it is essential to determine the fetal orientation within the maternal abdomen. A transverse cut is obtained through the fetal abdomen and the transducer tilted anteriorly and posteriorly confirming fetal position e.g. cephalic, breech or transverse (Video 2.1).

Using this information and the location of the fetal spine, the left and right side of the fetus will be determined. The fetal stomach and cardiac apex should lie on the same side, on the left of the fetus. At the outset, it is important to determine that the cardiac apex and the fetal stomach are truly on the left. Both heart and stomach could be on the right with mirror-image arrangement of the heart and internal organs (situs inversus). The heart and stomach should never appear on opposite sides. Once established, the relative position of the cardiac apex and stomach allows the fetal echocardiographer to remain orientated to the fetal left and right, even if there are multiple fetal movements during the course of the examination.

Although the images presented in this chapter suggest a series of isolated views, the heart is best assessed by including sweeps of the transducer cranially starting with views just below the level of the four chamber view. This incorporates visualisation of the key views of the heart including (from caudal to cranial) arrangement of the abdominal vessels and stomach, four chamber view, left ventricular outflow tract, right ventricular outflow tract and three vessel or three vessel trachea view. Each of these five sets of projections have their own characteristics and checklist which will be addressed in turn. In a fetus with optimal views, it may be possible to incorporate all anatomic views in a single sweep but more commonly views from slightly different sonographic projections will be required. This will also be discussed. The appearances at different levels in a fetus with a constant orientation are illustrated in Figs. 2.1, 2.2, 2.3, 2.4 and 2.5 and Videos 2.2, 2.3, 2.4, 2.5 and 2.6. Additional views will be included where necessary to show the advantages and limitations of some sonographic projections.

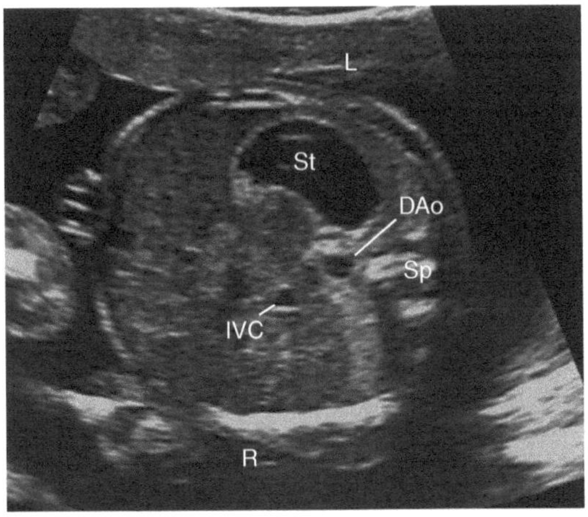

Fig. 2.1 Normal cardiac situs. The descending aorta lies anteriorly and to the left of the fetal spine. The IVC lies anterior and to the right of the descending aorta. Abbreviations: *St* stomach, *DAo* descending aorta, *Sp* spine, *IVC* inferior vena cava

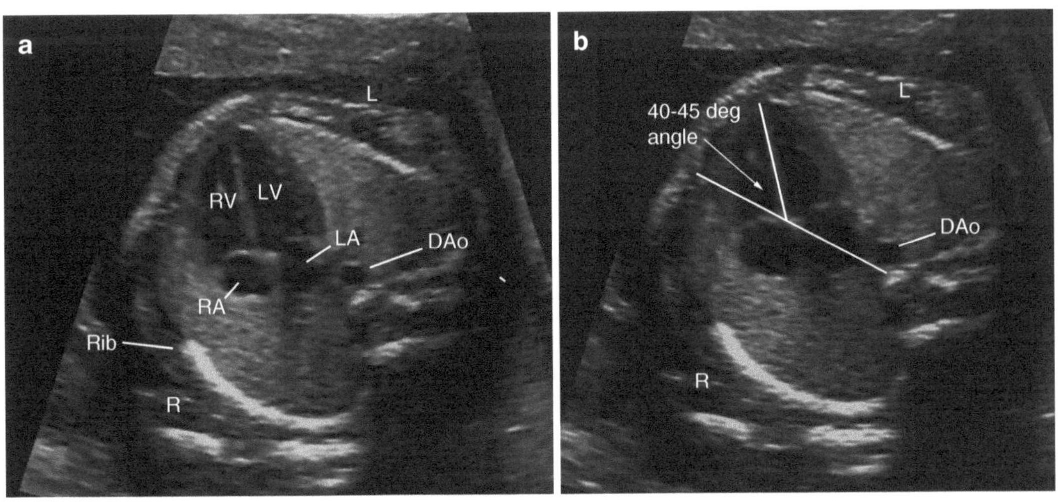

Fig. 2.2 (**a**) Normal four chamber view. There is a single rib around the fetal thorax. The heart occupies around one third of the area of the thorax and there is a balanced size of the left and right atriums and ventricles. (**b**) Normal cardiac axis. A line can be drawn from the spine through the crux of the heart, with another following the plane of the ventricular septum. The angle between these lines is normally 40–45°. Abbreviations: *LV* left ventricle, *RV* right ventricle, *LA* left atrium, *RA* right atrium, *DAo* descending aorta

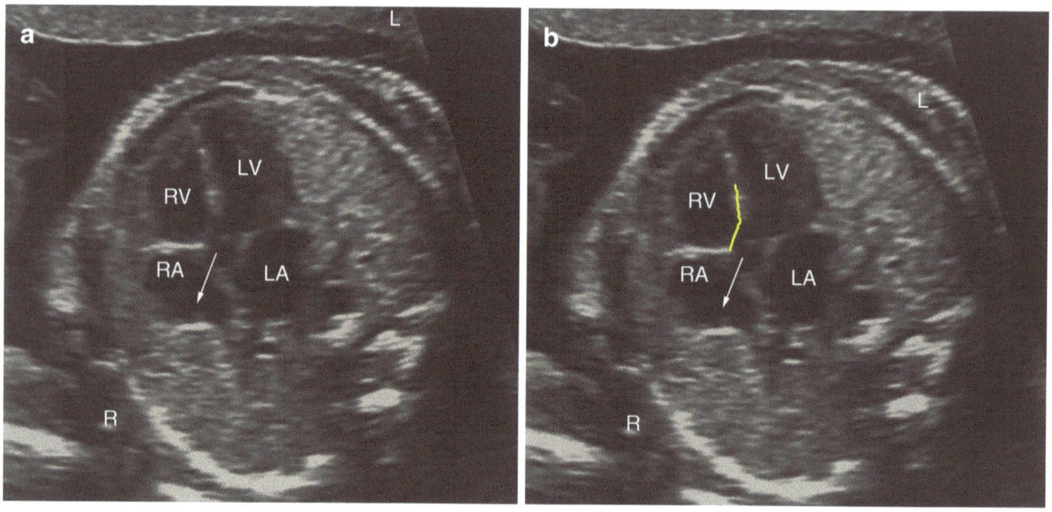

Fig. 2.3 (**a**) Normal LVOT view. The LVOT arises in continuity with the interventricular septum, and is directed towards the right shoulder of the fetus (arrow). (**b**) Continuity of the anterior wall of the aorta and interventricular septum, demonstrated by the yellow line. Abbreviations: *LV* left ventricle, *RV* right ventricle, *RA* right atrium, *LA* left atrium

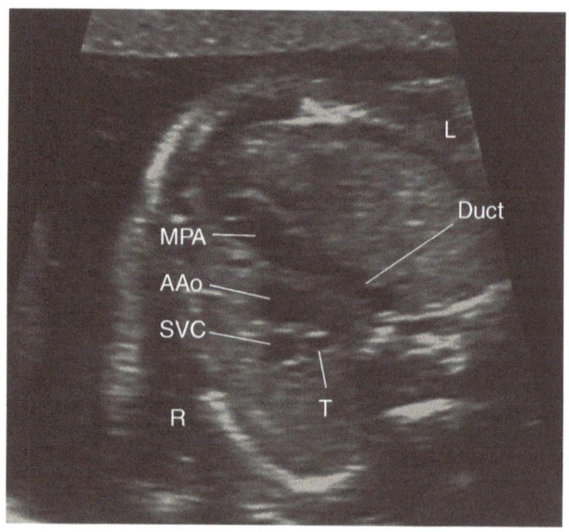

Fig. 2.4 Normal right ventricular outflow tract. The RVOT has a direct antero-posterior orientation. The main pulmonary artery (MPA) continues posteriorly towards the spine as the arterial duct. The aorta is seen in cross-section just to the right of the MPA and the superior vena cava to the right of the aorta. The trachea is seen more posteriorly with characteristic bright “cuff”. Depending on the level of the plane, the branch pulmonary arteries may or may not be seen arising from the MPA. Abbreviations: *MPA* main pulmonary artery, *AAo* ascending aorta, *SVC* superior vena cava, *T* trachea

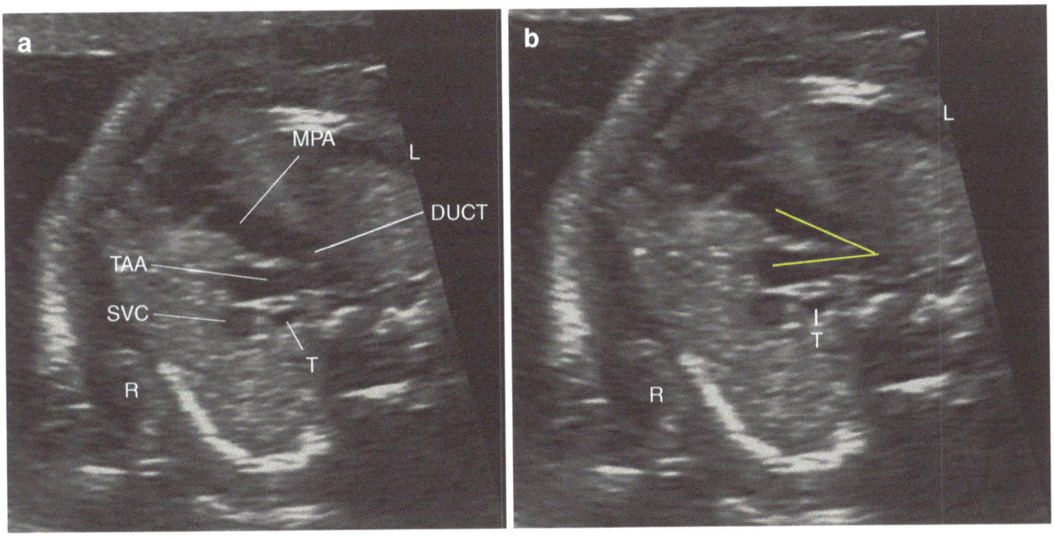

Fig. 2.5 (**a**, **b**) Three vessel trachea view. (**a**) This view is slightly superior to the view of the right ventricular outflow tract. The main pulmonary arteries continues posteriorly as the arterial duct where is meets the transverse aortic arch in a "V" shape. The size of the transverse aortic arch and arterial duct should be similar. The superior vena cava is seen in cross section to the right of the transverse aortic arch. The trachea is posterior to the transverse aortic arch and SVC and outside of the "V" formed by the aortic and ductal arches. (**b**) This image is identical to that in (**a**) but with yellow lines showing the V shape between the aortic and ductal arches. The most distal portion of the aortic arch is the aortic isthmus just prior to connection to the descending aorta. The trachea is normally to the right of this V shape and not between the arches. Abbreviations: *TAA* transverse aortic arch, *MPA* main pulmonary artery, *SVC* superior vena cava, *T* trachea

Normal Arrangement of the Abdominal Vessels (Abdominal Situs)

In the normal fetus, the stomach lies to the left. The descending aorta should be seen pulsating, positioned anterior and just to the left of the spine. The inferior vena cava (IVC) lies anterior and to the right of both the aorta and the spine (Fig. 2.1, Video 2.2). Hence, in the normal examination the IVC and descending aorta should be visualised on opposite sides of the spine. Table 2.1 provides a checklist of the most important features of the cardiac situs view.

Table 2.1 Cardiac situs

• Fetal stomach and cardiac apex on the left
• Inferior vena cava to the right of the spine
• Descending aorta to the left of the spine

Cardiac Size and Location in the Chest

The heart normally fills a third of the area of the fetal thorax (Fig. 2.2a, Video 2.3). This ratio can be calculated by measuring the area of the heart divided by the area of the thorax to produce the cardiothoracic ratio (CTR). An alternative method is to compare the circumference of the heart to the circumference of the thorax—this ratio of circumferences should be less than 50%. Within the fetal thorax the heart lies with the apex pointing anterior and to the left at a 40–45° angle from the midline (Fig. 2.2b). This axis is readily measured by drawing a line directly anterior from the spine through the crux of the heart. The angle of the ventricular septum as it intersects this line gives the cardiac angle. In some heart abnormalities the axis of the heart is rotated, so more detailed assessment of the heart is indicated in that setting. This method is also helpful to assess if the heart lies to the left or right of its normal position in the thorax. For example, a left sided diaphragmatic hernia may push the heart to the right of the thorax.

Four Chamber View

The four chamber view is a crucially important view of the heart in screening for CHD. The plane of the fetal ribs corresponds to the four chamber view. Thus, a well-orientated four chamber view of the fetal heart should include a single rib around the fetal thorax. This view is shown in Fig. 2.2a (Video 2.3). In this view, in the midtrimester, the left and right sided chambers of the fetal heart should be of similar size. In the third trimester, slight dominance of the right heart structures is often observed as a normal feature. The left atrium is the most posterior chamber in the fetal heart and lies just anterior to the fetal spine and descending aorta. The left atrium connects to the left ventricle via the mitral valve. The more anteriorly positioned right atrium connects to the right ventricle via the tricuspid valve. Thus, the left atrium is the most posterior cardiac chamber and the right ventricle is the most anterior which assists in rapidly identifying each of the chambers of the heart. The ventricular septum, 'primum' atrial septum and insertion of the mitral and tricuspid valves meet as the 'crux' of the heart. If images are of high quality, it can be appreciated that the mitral valve inserts into the ventricular septum slightly further from the apex of the heart than the tricuspid valve (Fig. 2.6a). This is known as differential insertion of the mitral and tricuspid valves, and is often referred to as offsetting of the atrioventricular valves. In some forms of congenital heart disease, for example some types of ventricular septal defect, differential insertion of these valves is lost. Both mitral and tricuspid valves should be observed to open freely and close completely through the cardiac cycle. The left and right ventricles have characteristic features other than their relative position. The left ventricle is smooth walled, and the mitral valve has no insertion into the ventricular septum. In contrast, the right ventricle has a more roughened 'trabeculated' appearance with pronounced region of trabeculated muscle (moderator band) towards the apex (Fig. 2.6b, Video 2.7). On detailed examination of the atrial septum, there should always be a tongue of tissue

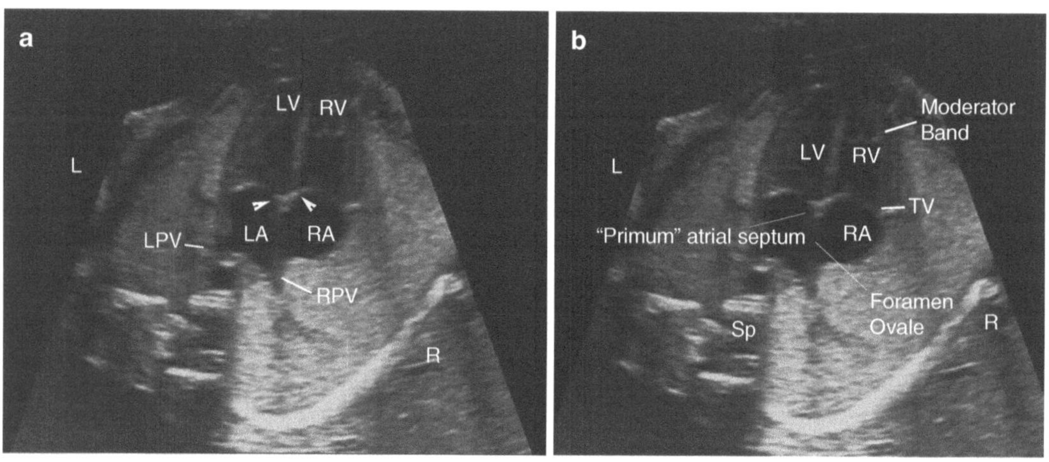

Fig. 2.6 (**a**) Differential insertion of the tricuspid and mitral valves. This four chamber view illustrates that the tricuspid valve (yellow arrow) inserts slightly further towards the apex of the heart than the mitral valve (white arrow). The connection of the right and left pulmonary veins to the back of the left atrium is well visualised in this example. (**b**) Additional features of the normal four chamber view. The apex of the right ventricle has a characteristic prominent region of trabeculation known as the moderator band which is helpful to identify the right ventricle. At the crux of the heart there should always be a piece of tissue, the primum atrial septum, visible on the atrial side of the crux. Abbreviations: *LV* left ventricle, *RV* right ventricle, *LA* left atrium, *RA* right atrium, *LPV* left pulmonary veins, *RPV* right pulmonary veins, *Sp* spine, *TV* tricuspid valve

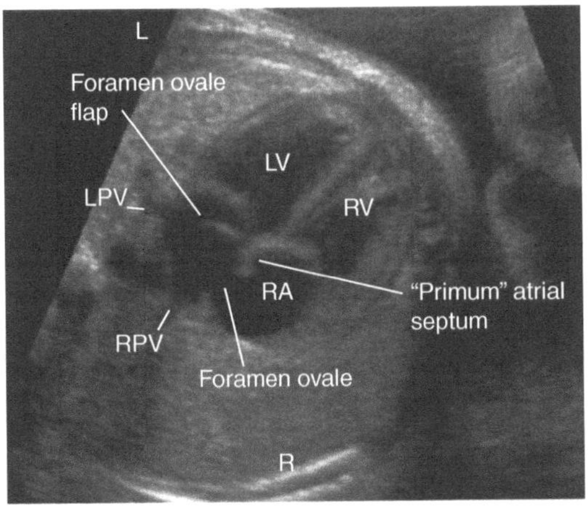

Fig. 2.7 Normal appearance of the atrial septum. This four chamber view illustrates normal features of the atrial septum. The primum atrial septum is well seen as well as the normal communication between the left and right atriums, the foramen ovale. The foramen ovale 'flap' is normally seen in the left atrium because blood normally passes right to left across the atrial septum. The left and right pulmonary veins are seen connecting to the left atrium. Abbreviations: *LPV* left pulmonary veins, *RPV* right pulmonary veins

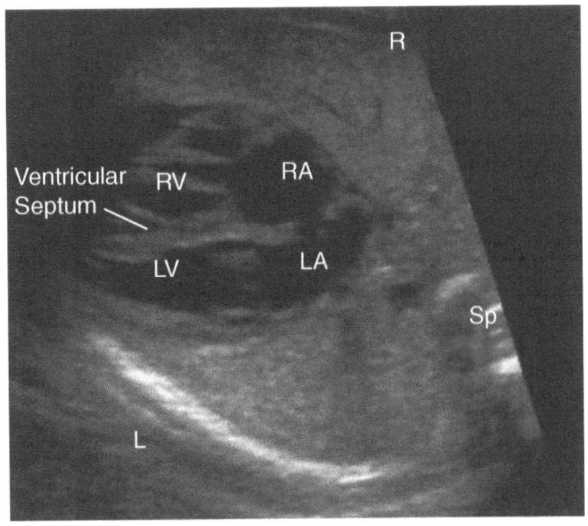

Fig. 2.8 Normal ventricular septum. This image shows how clearly the ventricular septum is seen when the ultrasound beam is orthogonal to the ventricular septum. The issue of 'drop out' of the ventricular septum is usually resolved if this sonographic projection can be achieved. In practice, multiple views of the ventricular septum are optimal. Abbreviations: *LV* left ventricle, *RV* right ventricle, *LA* left atrium, *RA* right atrium

on the atrial side of the crux of the heart. This is known as the primum atrial septum (Fig. 2.7, Video 2.7) which may be absent in some cardiac defects such as atrioventricular septal defects. Posterior and to the right of the primum septum, there is a normal communication between the left and right atriums known as the foramen ovale. Due to blood shunting right to left across the atrial septum during fetal life, the flap valve covering the foramen ovale is often easy to visualise within the left atrium and is a normal finding (Fig. 2.7, Video 2.7). The ventricular septum should be confirmed to be intact during screening views. Images where the ventricular septum is parallel to the plane of insonation (Fig. 2.2) will show the ventricular septum less well than when the plane of insonation is orthogonal to the ventricular septum (Fig. 2.8). Thus, in practice, different views of the ventricular septum may need to be obtained, particularly if there is a suspicion of a ventricular septal defect versus 'drop out' of the ventricular septum. This is a particular issue for the region of the ventricular septum where it becomes very thin (membranous) adjacent to the insertion of the mitral and tricuspid valves.

Table 2.2 Four chamber view checklist

• Four cardiac chambers – Two atriums and two ventricles
• Ventricles equal in size
• Atriums equal in size
• Two separate AV valve orifices
• Normal AV valve offset
• AV valves moving freely
• Moderator band towards right ventricular apex
• Ventricular and atrial septum complete
• Two ventricles contract equally
• Foramen ovale flap in the left atrium
• Heart occupies 1/3 of area of thorax
• Apex of the heart to the left

Many of the features of the four chamber view are easier to appreciate on moving rather than still images, and obtaining different projections of the fetal heart can assist in showing different facets of the normal anatomy. Most ultrasound systems include the ability to freeze images and allow the operator to scroll through images which assists in confirmation of normality. Table 2.2 provides a checklist of the most important features of the four chamber view assessment.

Left Ventricular Outflow Tract (LVOT)

The left ventricular outflow tract (LVOT) is visualised by tilting the transducer cranially from the four chamber view. The LVOT arises from the centre of the heart in continuity with the interventricular septum and courses towards the right shoulder (Fig. 2.3a, b, Video 2.5). The posterior aspect of the LVOT is in continuity with the anterior leaflet of the mitral valve. In the normal fetal heart an imaginary line can be drawn from the interventricular septum through the anterior wall of the LVOT and the aorta (Fig. 2.3b). It will assist to obtain views of the LVOT in different sonographic projections to optimise visualisation of this region. Images with the ultrasound beam near orthogonal to the ventricular septum and aorta are particularly helpful (Fig. 2.9). Discontinuity between the interventricular septum and LVOT is not normal and can be observed in different cardiac defects including tetralogy of Fallot or common arterial trunk. The aortic valve should be observed to open and close during the cardiac cycle. The valve leaflets should be thin and open freely with no evidence of dysplasia or restricted leaflet motion. A practical tip is that the leaflets of the aortic valve should normally 'disappear' as the ventricle contracts because the valve leaflets open fully against the wall of the aorta. It is important to note that only the aortic and mitral valve are visualised in the LVOT view, as the tricuspid valve lies inferiorly and the pulmonary valve superiorly.

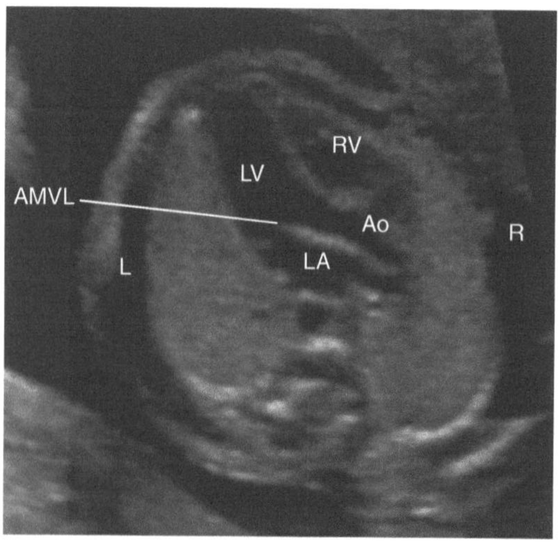

Fig. 2.9 Optimal view of left ventricular outflow tract. This sonographic projection of the LVOT is optimal to confirm the normal anatomy of this region. The ultrasound beam is near orthogonal to the LVOT. The ventricular septum is continuous with the anterior wall of the aorta and the anterior leaflet of the mitral valve is continuous with the posterior wall of the aorta. Abbreviations: *LV* left ventricle, *RV* right ventricle, *LA* left atrium, *Ao* aorta, *AMVL* anterior mitral valve leaflet

Table 2.3 Aorta/left ventricular outflow tract checklist

• LVOT arising from the centre of the heart directed to the right shoulder
• Ventricular septum continuous with anterior wall of the aorta
• Aortic valve opens freely

Table 2.3 provides a checklist of the most important features of the aorta/LVOT view assessment.

Right Ventricular Outflow Tract (RVOT)

Tilting the transducer cranially from the LVOT, the RVOT arises close to the anterior wall of the fetal thorax which courses directly back towards the spine as the main pulmonary artery which continues into the arterial duct (Fig. 2.4, Video 2.5). The pulmonary valve has thin leaflets that should open freely with no restriction. The aorta and pulmonary artery should be of a very similar diameter—any major discrepancy in the size of the great arteries should raise the suspicion of congenital heart disease. The defining characteristic of the main pulmonary artery is that it gives rise to the right and left branch pulmonary arteries. On tilting the transducer cranially from the four chamber view, if the sonographic plane is relatively superior, then the RVOT may be seen to continue into the arterial duct with no obvious branching (Fig. 2.4). The duct lies slightly superior to the left and right pulmonary arteries so that caudal angulation may be necessary to see the branch pulmonary arteries. When transverse sonographic cuts are used the arterial duct may be visualised along with one or other of the branch pulmonary arteries (Fig. 2.10a, b, Video 2.8). If a plane just below the arterial duct is insonated then the two branch pulmonary arteries may be visualised together (Fig. 2.10c, Video 2.9). Most importantly when tilting the transducer cranially, the

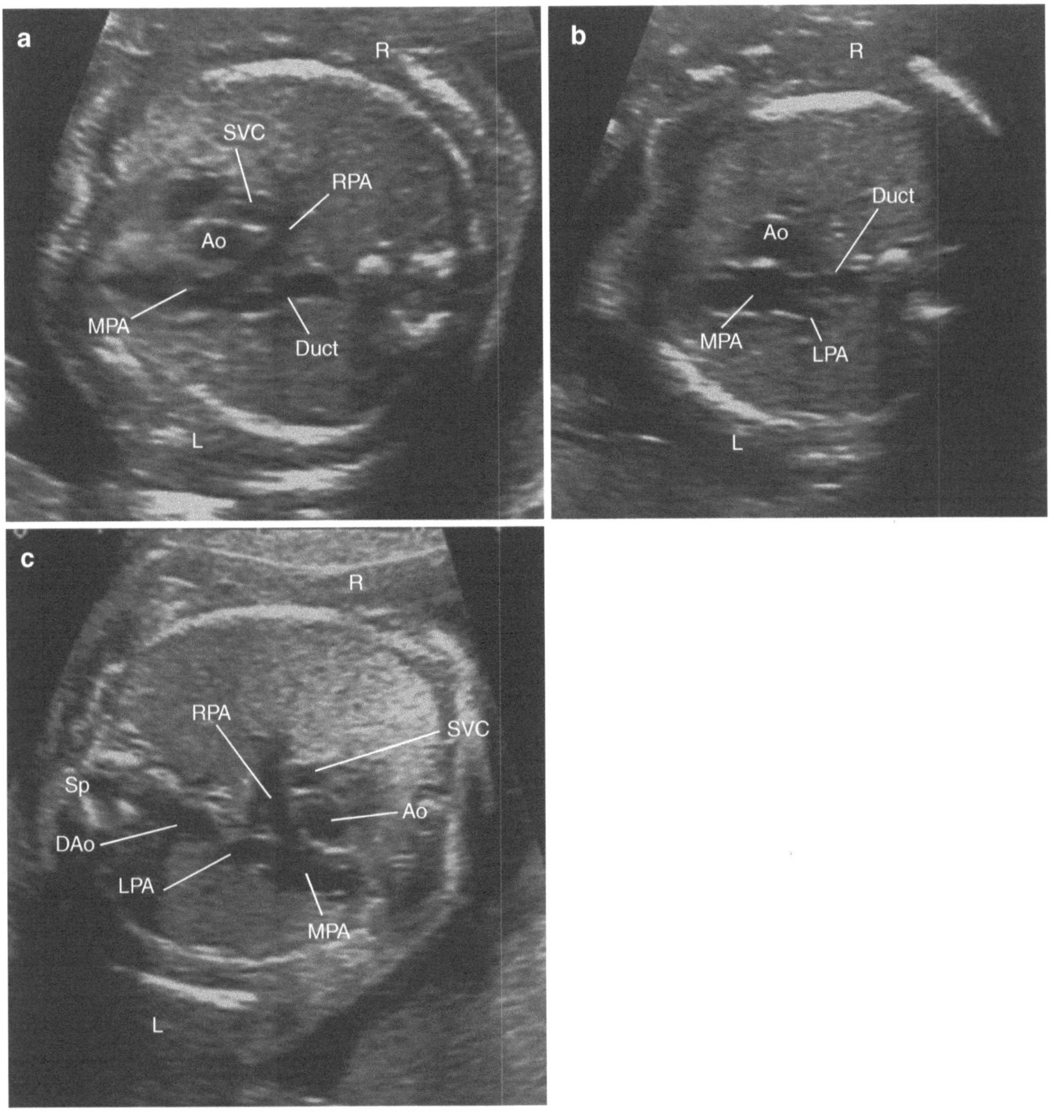

Fig. 2.10 (**a**–**c**) Normal branching of the main pulmonary artery. (**a**) This is a three vessel view cut at a plane where the main pulmonary artery can be seen to branch into the arterial duct and the right pulmonary artery. (**b**) This image shows the main pulmonary artery dividing into the arterial duct and the left pulmonary artery. In practice, very fine movements of angulation are necessary to define the branching pattern of the main pulmonary artery. (**c**) This image shows the bifurcation of the main pulmonary artery into the right and left pulmonary arteries just below the level of the arterial duct. Abbreviations: *MPA* main pulmonary artery, *LPA* left pulmonary artery, *RPA* right pulmonary artery, *Ao* aorta, *SVC* superior vena cava, *Sp* spine, *DAo* descending aorta

LVOT and RVOT are not visualised in the same transverse cut and are traditionally described as crossing each other: the aorta is directed towards the right shoulder and the pulmonary artery has an antero-posterior orientation. The appreciation of the different planes of the LVOT and RVOT is an important component of the normal examination. The 'sweep' from LVOT to RVOT by cranial angulation of the transducer is shown in Video 2.9.

Three Vessel View (3VV)

In the transverse plane of the upper mediastinum the three vessel view shows the main pulmonary artery coursing directly backwards towards the spine. The main pulmonary artery continues into the arterial duct which appears slightly narrower and continues posteriorly to meet the descending aorta. Adjacent to the pulmonary artery, the aortic arch and superior vena cava (SVC) are visualised in cross section. The normal sequence from left to right: pulmonary artery/duct; aorta; SVC (Fig. 2.4, Video 2.5). In the normal fetal heart the pulmonary artery is slightly larger than the aorta which in turn is slightly larger than the SVC. In summary, it is essential not only to examine the number of vessels present in the three vessel view, but the relative vessel size and the orientation of the vessels.

Table 2.4 provides a checklist of the most important features of the RVOT/3VV assessment.

Three Vessel and Trachea View (3VT View)

The three vessel and trachea (3VT) view is an extension of the three vessel view (3VV) in the upper mediastinum. In the transverse plane, tilting the transducer cranially from the 3VV, the transverse aortic arch curves towards the left fetal shoulder, permitting visualisation of the full length of the transverse aortic arch. In the normal fetal heart the aortic arch normally sweeps to the left of the trachea towards the descending aorta (Fig. 2.5a, Video 2.6). The ductal arch which is continuous with the main pulmonary artery continues in a straight line towards the fetal spine, meeting the aortic arch in a 'V' shape at the aortic isthmus (Fig. 2.5b, Video 2.6). It is important to visualise the full length of the aortic arch to the distal portion at the aortic isthmus (Fig. 2.5a, b). The relative size of the aortic and ductal arches should be compared. These vessels should appear of similar size. A significant discrepancy between the size of the aortic and ductal arch should raise the suspicion of a cardiac abnormality. Table 2.5 provides a checklist of the most important features of the 3VT assessment.

Table 2.4 Three vessel view checklist

• RVOT arises anteriorly and courses directly posteriorly
• The pulmonary valve opens freely
• The pulmonary artery is seen to bifurcate
• PA continues posteriorly as the duct towards the spine
• Ascending aorta is seen to the right of the pulmonary artery
• The aorta and pulmonary artery of similar size
• The superior vena cava to the right of the ascending aorta

Integration of Views

Although the key screening views have been presented separately in this chapter, in practice the sonographer will often sweep through the different views from situs views through to views of the upper mediastinum. Video 2.11 demonstrates a full echocardiographic sweep from the four chamber view to the 3VT view.

Limitations of Screening Views for Congenital Heart Disease

In most settings, screening views for CHD are undertaken in the context of an anomaly scan which is not restricted to cardiac assessment but includes overall assessment of the fetal anatomy and growth. There are variations in screening protocols between different regions which will impact on the detection of different forms of CHD. Some 'postnatal' cardiac lesions cannot be predicted from fetal screening, such as secundum atrial septal defects (the foramen ovale is normally open during fetal life) and persistence of patency of the arterial duct after birth. The quality of sonographic imaging will depend on ultrasound system quality, maternal habitus, fetal lie and other factors which may impact on the ability to visualise the fetal heart. Units will typically have policies in place to rescan fetuses where the fetal lie is suboptimal and precludes adequate imaging.

Some forms of congenital heart disease are notoriously difficult to detect, for example, anomalous drainage of the pulmonary veins, particularly if colour flow Doppler is not part of the

Table 2.5 Three vessel and trachea view checklist

• The transverse aorta and pulmonary artery meet as a V shape to the left of the trachea
• Ductal and aortic arch of similar size
• SVC seen in cross section to the right of the aorta

screening protocol. Small ventricular septal defects or defects in unusual locations within the ventricular septum may not be visualised even on high quality screening views. Other forms of congenital heart disease, including aortic valve stenosis, pulmonary valve stenosis, coarctation of the aorta and cardiomyopathies may progress with advancing gestational age so that abnormalities are not evident on screening views of the heart in the midtrimester. Thus, parental expectations need to be set appropriately with respect to the sonographic screening approach to CHD (Hunter and Simpson 2014).

Size of Different Cardiac Structures

During a screening examination, the requirement to measure different cardiac structures varies according to the guidelines followed. When assessing the size of cardiac structures such as the great arteries or the ventricles, it is important to understand what is normal for a fetus of a given size or gestational age. Clearly, as the baby grows, the heart will also become larger, thus the same range of normality cannot be used across all gestational ages or fetal sizes. One means of expressing the size of a cardiac structure relative to the normal range for size or gestation is by the use of "Z-scores" (Schneider et al. 2005; Pasquini et al. 2007; Chubb and Simpson 2012; Vigneswaran 2018). If a measurement is exactly on the mean (average) for size or gestational age then the Z score is zero. Negative values represent values below the population mean and conversely positive Z scores represent values above the mean. For example, if a measurement has a Z-score of +1.5, this indicates that the measurement is 1.5 standard deviations above normal. Fetal Z scores are an additional benefit to detailed 2D fetal echocardiography and allow the practitioner to monitor the growth of the cardiac structures. Z scores are limited by intra and inter observer variability but can be advantageous in aiding detailed fetal cardiac assessment by confirmation of normality or to risk stratification the prenatal and postnatal prognosis of CHD. Fetal Z scores are available for multiple cardiac structures. These are frequently built in to imaging archives or else available online, for example www.parameterz.com or by downloading Apps such as Cardio Z. Examples of the types of measurements for which Z-scores can be calculated are shown in Fig. 2.11a, b.

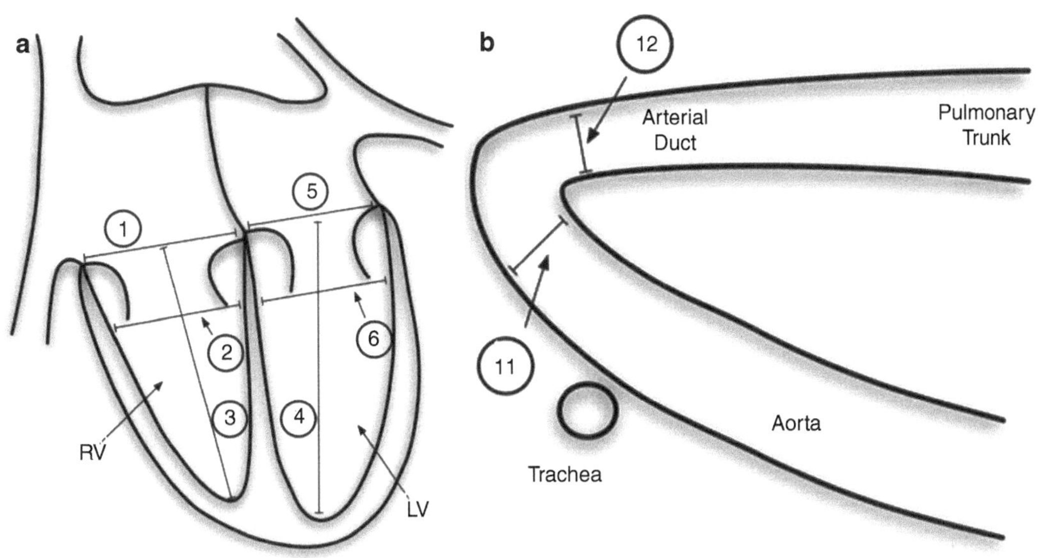

Fig. 2.11 (**a**, **b**) Measurement of fetal cardiac structures for the assessment of gestational z scores reproduced with permission from Cardio Z. (**a**) Four chamber view. 1—Tricuspid valve annulus; 2—Right ventricle diastolic diameter; 3—Right ventricle length; 4—Left ventricle length; 5—Mitral valve annulus; 6—Left ventricle diastolic diameter. (**b**) Three vessel tracheal view. 11—Aortic isthmus; 12—Distal arterial duct diameter. *RV* right ventricle, *MPA* main pulmonary artery, *PA* pulmonary artery, *RPA* right pulmonary artery

Additional Online Resources

An online tutorial produced by one of the authors of this book (Prof John Simpson) covers all of the key screening views including:

The four chamber view: https://www.youtube.com/watch?v=XTi_JtdnMJM

Left ventricular outflow tract: https://www.youtube.com/watch?v=jDl_XpGUJEU

Right ventricular outflow tract: https://www.youtube.com/watch?v=rW2r55AS3Xk

Three vessel view: https://www.youtube.com/watch?v=5arsJCjTqGg

The Fetal Medicine Foundation has an online cardiac course and other resources at: at https://fetalmedicine.org/fetal-echocardiography-1.

References

Allan L, Dangel J, Fesslova V, Marrek J, Mellander M, Oberhansli I, Oberhoffer R, Sharland G, Simpson J, Sonesson SE. Recommendations for the practice of fetal cardiology in Europe. Cardiol Young. 2004;14(1):109–14.

Carvalho JS, Allan LD, Chaoui R, Copel JA, Devore GR, Hecher K, Lee W, Munoz H, Paladini D, Tutschek B, Yagel S. ISUOG Practice Guidelines: sonographic screening examination of the fetal heart. Ultrasound Obstet Gynecol. 2013;41(3):348–59.

Chubb H, Simpson J. The use of z scores in paediatric cardiology. Ann Pediatr Cardiol. 2012;5(2):179–84.

Fetal Anomaly Screening Programme, United Kingdom. https://www.gov.uk/government/publications/fetal-anomaly-screening-programme-handbook. Accessed 29 July 2017.

Fetal Echocardiography Task Force. AIUM practice guideline for the performance of fetal echocardiography. J Ultrasound Med. 2011;30(1):127–36.

Hunter LE, Simpson JM. Prenatal screening for structural congenital heart disease. Nat Rev Cardiol. 2014;11(6):323–34.

Pasquini L, Mellander M, Seale A, Matsui H, Roughton M, Ho SY, Gardiner HM. Z scores of the fetal aortic isthmus and duct: an aid to assessing arch hypoplasia. Ultrasound Obstet Gynecol. 2007;29(6):628–33.

Rychik J, Ayres N, Cuneo B, Gotteiner N, Hornberger L, Spevak P, Van Der Vel M. American Society of Echocardiography guidelines and standards for performance of the fetal echocardiogram. J Am Soc Echocardiogr. 2004;17(7):803–10.

Schneider C, McCrindle BW, Carvalho JS, Hornberger LK, McCarthy KP, Daubeney PE. Development of Z-scores for fetal cardiac dimensions from echocardiography. Ultrasound Obstet Gynecol. 2005;26(6):599–605.

Vigneswaran TV, Akolekar R, Syngelaki A, Charakida M, Allan LD, Nicolaides KH, Zidere V, Simpson JM. Reference ranges for the size of the fetal cardiac outflow tracts from 13 to 36 weeks gestation: a single-center study of over 7000 cases. Circ Cardiovasc Imaging. 2018;11(7):e007575. https://doi.org/10.1161/CIRCIMAGING.118.007575.

Yagel S, Cohen SM, Achiron R. Examination of the fetal heart by five short axis views: a proposed screening method for comprehensive cardiac evaluation. Ultrasound Obstet Gynecol. 2001;17(5):367–9.

Extended Views of the Fetal Heart

3

Vita Zidere and John Simpson

Abstract

Extended views of the fetal heart are helpful additions to the standard screening views in advanced fetal cardiac assessment. These include additional transverse sweeps above the aortic arch and sagittal views of the fetal heart.

The transverse sweep above the aortic arch permits visualisation of the innominate vein and head and neck vessels. The systemic venous connections, aortic arch, ductal arch and short axis views of the atrioventricular valves can be visualised in sagittal views. The distinctive branching pattern of the head and neck vessels from the aortic arch can also be demonstrated.

Electronic Supplementary Material The online version of this chapter (https://doi.org/10.1007/978-3-319-77461-9_3) contains supplementary material, which is available to authorized users.

V. Zidere (✉)
Evelina London Children's Hospital, Guy's and St Thomas' NHS Foundation Trust, London, UK

King's College Hospital NHS Foundation Trust, London, UK
e-mail: vita.zidere@gstt.nhs.uk

J. Simpson
Evelina London Children's Hospital, Guy's and St Thomas' NHS Foundation Trust, London, UK
e-mail: john.simpson@gstt.nhs.uk

Keywords

Congenital heart disease · Fetal echocardiography · Sagittal view · Short axis · Ductal arch · Aortic arch · Subclavian artery · Ductus venosus

Introduction

Screening views of the fetal heart are visualised in a series of standard transverse views where important structures can be seen and in the vast majority of cases normality can be confirmed or an abnormality detected. These views include assessment of cardiac situs, four chamber view, outflow tracts, ductal and aortic arches, this is described in Chap. 2 (Allan et al. 2004; The American Institute of Ultrasound in Medicine 2013; The International Society of Ultrasound in Obstetrics 2013; Donofrio et al. 2014).

Further transverse sweeps above the aortic arch permit visualisation of the innominate vein draining into the superior vena cava and examination of the pattern of branching of the head and neck vessels from the aortic arch, to confirm origin of subclavian arteries in particular.

In a sagittal plane, the systemic venous connections to the right atrium can be seen in longitudinal cut. The ascending aorta and entire aortic arch with its distinctive branching pattern can be demonstrated. Similarly the ductal arch can also be cut in a sagittal fashion to show its characteristic morphology.

© Springer International Publishing AG, part of Springer Nature 2018
J. Simpson et al. (eds.), *Fetal Cardiology*, https://doi.org/10.1007/978-3-319-77461-9_3

Principally, the sagittal plane is obtained by rotating 90° clockwise from the transverse plane. Additional sagittal views of the fetal heart can add value to routine or advanced fetal cardiac investigation. Thus, the standard fetal cardiac sagittal planes are further discussed in more detail below.

Sagittal View of the Inferior Vena Cava and Superior Vena Cava

This plane, where the venous connections to the right atrium can be seen, is obtained by angling the probe to the fetal right from the sagittal view of the aortic arch view (Fig. 3.1).

Key Features

- Superior vena cava and inferior vena cava connections to the right atrium
- The superior vena cava and inferior vena cava should be of similar size

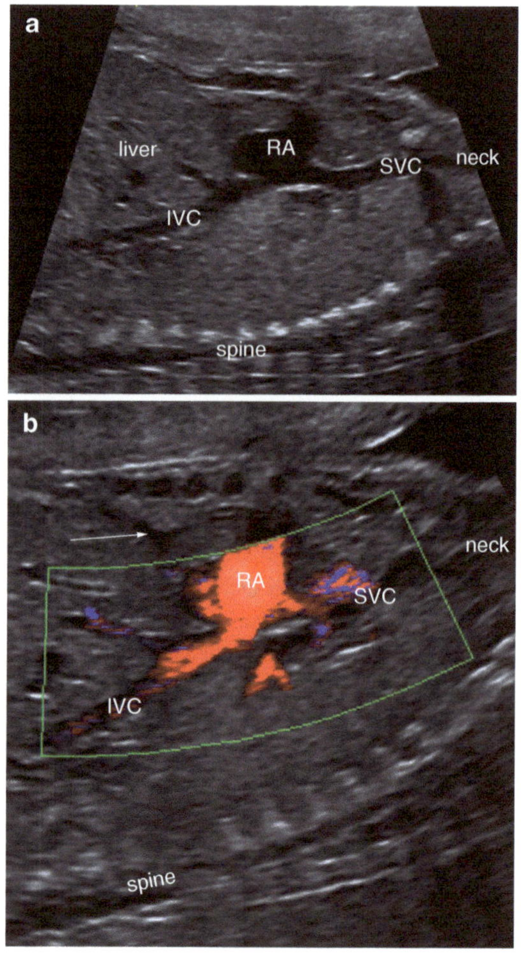

Fig. 3.1 (**a**) A longitudinal (sagittal) plane of the fetus showing the inferior vena cava and the superior vena cava draining into the right atrium. (**b**) Colour flow Doppler confirms a normal flow pattern, towards the fetal heart, in both the inferior vena cava and the superior vena cava

Sagittal View of the Ductal Arch

This view is obtained by angling the transduced in a directly antero-posterior cut plane. The arterial duct is demonstrated in long axis and the aorta is seen as a circular structure in short axis. The connection of the right atrium to the tricuspid valve and right ventricle to pulmonary artery can also be appreciated in this view (Fig. 3.2, Video 3.1).

Key Features

- The pulmonary valve lies anterior and cranial to the aortic valve which is seen in transverse cut
- The pulmonary artery branches into the arterial duct and the left pulmonary artery
- The arterial duct connects the main pulmonary artery to the descending aorta forming a ductal arch
- The tricuspid valve and pulmonary valve are patent
- The left atrium lies between the ascending and descending aorta
- The inferior vena cava connects to the right atrium

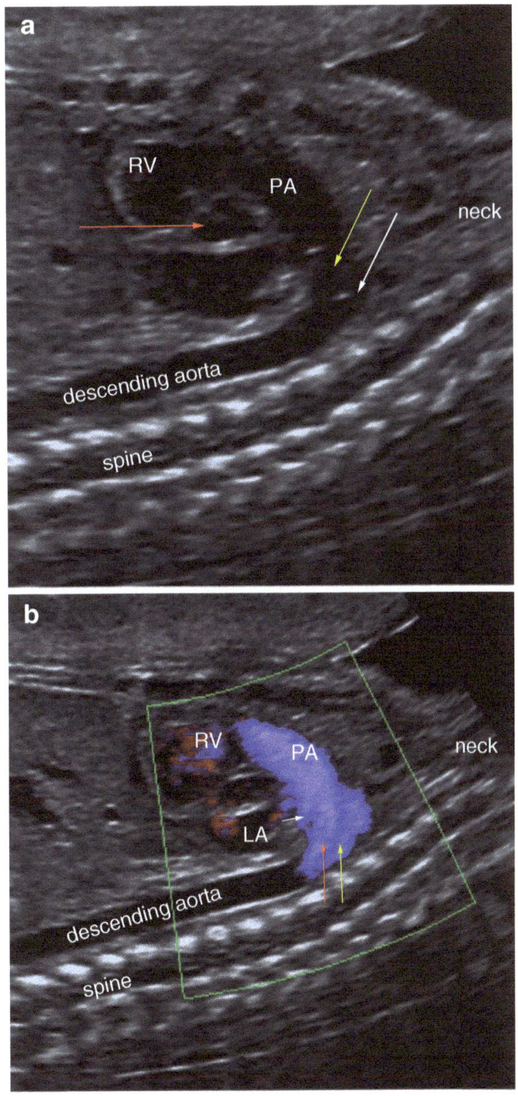

Fig. 3.2 (**a**) A longitudinal plane of the fetus demonstrates the pulmonary artery in continuity with the ductal arch (yellow arrow) connecting to the descending aorta. The distal part of the aortic arch, isthmus (white arrow), is seen in longitudinal cut as well. The aortic valve can be appreciated in short axis (red arrow). (**b**) In a longitudinal plane of the fetus both the ductal and distal aortic arches are seen. The antegrade flow throughout the pulmonary artery, left pulmonary artery (white arrow), and arterial duct (red arrow) and in the distal part of the aortic arch (yellow arrow) are demonstrated in this image

Sagittal View of the Aortic Arch

This plane is obtained by cutting the fetus with the ultrasound beam in the long axis with subtle transducer angulation from the right of the sternum anteriorly to the left of the spine posteriorly.

The aortic arch can be visualized in its entirety as well as its head and neck vessels. The right pulmonary artery is seen in short axis underneath the aortic arch. The atriums, atrial septum (Fig. 3.3, Videos 3.2a and 3.2b) and drainage of the inferior vena cava to the right atrium can also be seen.

Key Features

- The aorta arises in the center of the chest
- The aortic arch is seen as a continuation of the ascending aorta
- The aortic arch gives rise of head and neck vessels
- The right pulmonary artery lies below the arch and it is seen in transverse cut
- The left atrium lies between the ascending and descending aorta
- The patient foramen ovale is seen (flap lies in the left atrium)
- The inferior vena cava drains into the right atrium
- Left pulmonary veins entering the left atrium may be seen on colour flow Doppler

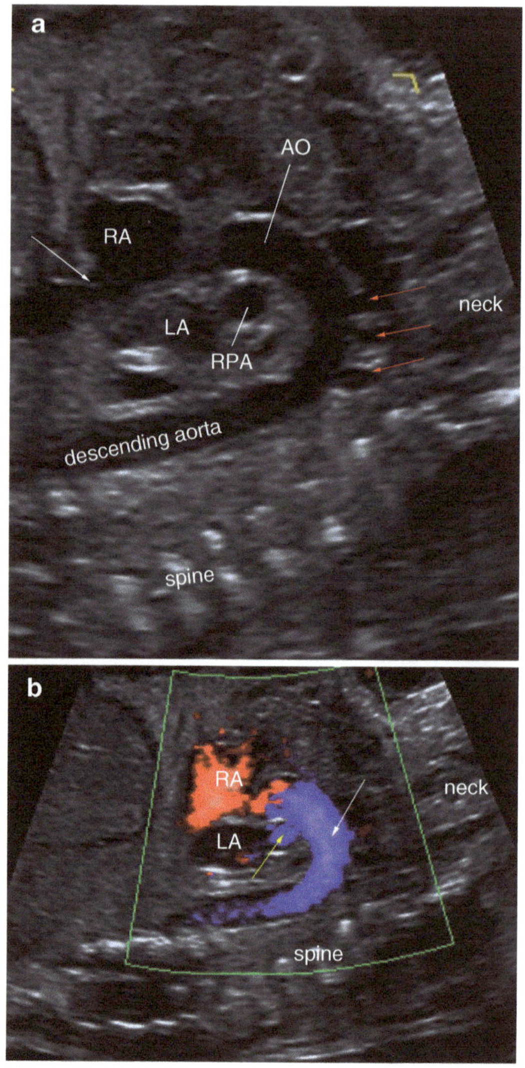

Fig. 3.3 (**a**) A longitudinal plane of the fetus demonstrates the aortic arch with the head and neck vessels (red arrows) and inferior vena cava (white arrow) draining into the right atrium also in longitudinal cut. (**b**) Colour Doppler confirms normal antegrade flow pattern within aortic (white arrow) and right pulmonary artery (yellow arrow)

Sagittal View of the Short Axis of the Right and Left Ventricles

The short axis of the right and left ventricles is seen when the ultrasound beam is directed parallel and to the left of the fetal sternum. In this view, the different shapes of the ventricles can be appreciated. The right ventricle is anterior and wraps around the posteriorly positioned left ventricle. The posteriorly located left ventricle is circular with two distinguishable papillary muscles and a bileaflet atrioventricular valve confirming a mitral valve and a morphological left ventricle. In addition, the portion of the right outflow tract arising from the anterior right ventricle can be seen (Fig. 3.4, Videos 3.3 and 3.4).

Note that additional use of colour Doppler in all longitudinal views should confirm an unaliased flow in the caval veins towards the right atrium and in the pulmonary veins towards the left atrium. Antegrade flow across both the pulmonary artery and aorta as well as in the arterial duct and aortic arch are also appreciated in this view. The reader is referred to online resources produced by the authors to supplement these images and videos (https://www.youtube.com/watch?v=K__UEZRV2N4).

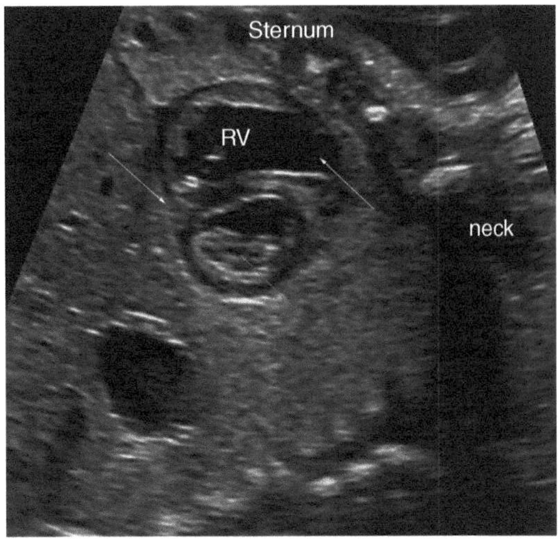

Fig. 3.4 In the sagittal plane the short axis view of the left ventricle and the right ventricle are obtained. The right ventricle is anterior just below the sternum and the left ventricle is located more posteriorly. The short axis view of the mitral valve (red arrow) shows both leaflets of the MV as well as the papillary muscles. The right ventricular outflow tract is visualised anteriorly and superiorly (yellow arrow) and the diaphragm more inferior (white arrow)

Subclavian Artery Assessment in Transverse Plane

Normally connected subclavian arteries can be seen just above the aortic arch on a sweep from transverse aortic arch towards the neck. (Borenstein et al. 2010). Though the head and neck vessels are usually well seen in longitudinal views, the actual anatomy of the right and left subclavian artery anatomy in the fetus is better assessed by colour flow Doppler in transverse view (Fig. 3.5). Pulsed Doppler can be used to confirm an arterial flow pattern to differentiate from venous flow.

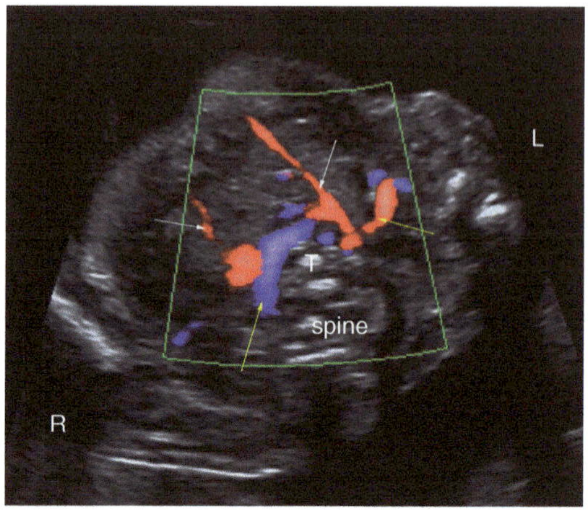

Fig. 3.5 The transverse cut of the upper thorax, just above the aortic arch, shows the subclavian arteries (yellow arrows) arising from the aortic arch in long axis in front of the trachea (T) on colour Doppler. The internal thoracic or internal mammary arteries (white arrows) are seen arising from the subclavian arteries near their origin and running towards the anterior chest wall

Assessment of the Ductus Venosus

The ductus venosus can be identified in right ventral mid-sagittal view of the fetus using conventional colour Doppler or power Doppler settings (Maiz et al. 2008). In the first trimester, newer Doppler techniques encode the blood pool (Fig. 3.6a) which makes it very easy to demonstrate the umbilical vein and ductus venous connection to the inferior vena cava. A ductus venosus waveform (Fig. 3.6b), which has a characteristic triphasic waveform, can be obtained by pulsed Doppler.

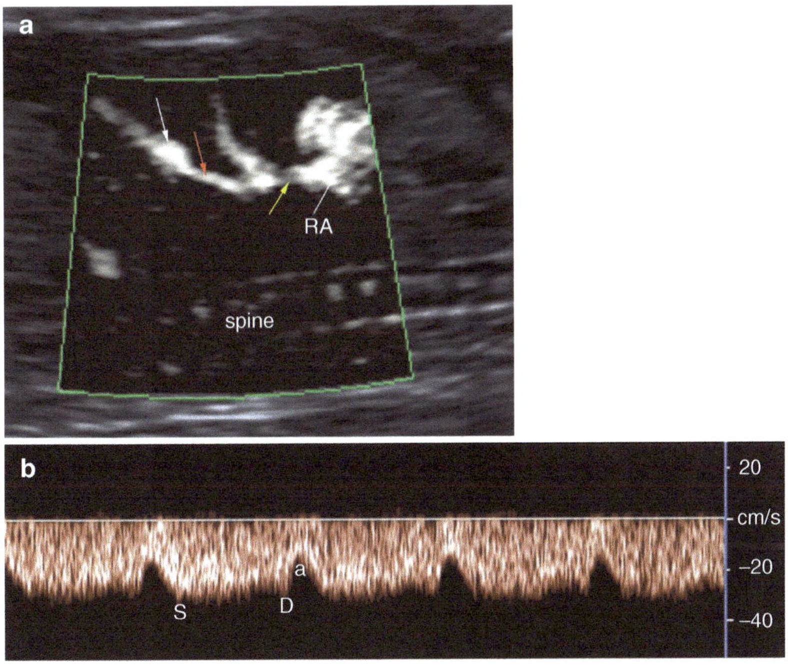

Fig. 3.6 (**a**) Imaging of the ductus venosus, inferior vena cava and right atrium obtained using superb micro-vascular imaging Doppler at first trimester. This demonstrates flow within an umbilical vein (white arrow) which continues into the smaller vessel, the ductus venosus (red arrow), and then to the IVC (yellow arrow) and right atrium. (**b**) This figure demonstrates the normal physiological flow pattern in the ductus venosus at 14 weeks' gestation. The "S" wave has the highest velocity and coincides with ventricular contraction. The "D" wave relates to early diastolic filling of the ventricles and the "a" wave, which has the lowest velocity, is due to atrial contraction

References

Allan L, Dangel J, Fesslova V, et al. Recommendations for the practice of fetal cardiology in Europe. Cardiol Young. 2004;14:109–14.

Borenstein M, Minekawa R, Zidere V, et al. Aberrant right-subclavian artery at 16 to 23 + 6 weeks of gestation: a marker for chromosomal abnormality. Ultrasound Obstet Gynecol. 2010;36(5):548–52. https://doi.org/10.1002/uog.7683.

Donofrio MT, Moon-Grady AJ, Hornberger LK, et al. Diagnosis and treatment of fetal cardiac disease: a scientific statement from the American Heart Association. Circulation. 2014;129(21):2183–242. https://doi.org/10.1161/01.cir.0000437597.44550.5d.

Maiz N, Plasencia W, Dagklis T, et al. Ductus venosus Doppler in fetuses with cardiac defects and increased nuchal translucency thickness. Ultrasound Obstet Gynecol. 2008;31(3):256–60. https://doi.org/10.1002/uog.5262.

The American Institute of Ultrasound in Medicine. AIUM practice guideline for the performance of fetal echocardiography. J Ultrasound Med. 2013;32(6):1067–82. https://doi.org/10.7863/ultra.32.6.1067.

The International Society of Ultrasound in Obstetrics. ISUOG Practice Guidelines (updated): sonographic screening examination of the fetal heart. Ultrasound Obstet Gynecol. 2013;41(3):348–59. https://doi.org/10.1002/uog.12403.

Use of Doppler Techniques in Fetal Echocardiography

4

Owen I. Miller

Abstract

Doppler techniques including Colour Flow Doppler, Spectral Doppler and more recently Tissue Doppler are fundamental to comprehensive fetal echocardiography. Meticulous attention to technique, including angle of insonation and correct Doppler settings will result in highly reproducible and accurate data. Incorrect transducer selection, poor angle of insonation and inappropriate gain or scale settings will result in poor quality and possible inaccurate data.

Keywords

Fetal · Heart · Doppler · Congenital heart · Echocardiography

Introduction

Fetal cardiac screening is predominantly concerned with establishing anatomical connections using 2D imaging to rule out structural abnormalities. However, once a cardiac abnormality is suspected, more detailed further analysis is required, including the use of Doppler echocardiography. Conventional Colour Flow Doppler and spectral Doppler will add value by describing movement within the blood pool, thus allowing assessment of the adequacy of inflows and outflow tracts, competency of valves and defining direction of blood flow at critical points in the fetal circulation.

Pulsed Doppler echocardiography has been clinically available for 40 years (Baker et al. 1977), followed soon after by Colour Flow imaging (Miyatake et al. 1984). All modern curved array obstetric and fetal cardiac ultrasound transducers include a facility for colour flow Doppler and Pulsed Wave (PW) spectral Doppler using standard Doppler ultrasound protocols. Pulsed Wave Doppler allows the operator to define a zone of interrogation (sample volume) and provide flow velocity data within that defined zone. The well-described limitations of PW Doppler including maximum velocity restrictions imposed by the Nyquist limit, do not routinely limit its usefulness in the fetal circulation due to the generally low blood flow velocity, but in selected cases where measurement of a high velocity signal is required then a Continuous Wave (CW) transducer should be used. Transducers incorporating CW Doppler are primarily designed for cardiovascular applications and therefore may have more limited performance for fetal heart examination, particularly regarding 2D image quality

Electronic Supplementary Material The online version of this chapter (https://doi.org/10.1007/978-3-319-77461-9_4) contains supplementary material, which is available to authorized users.

O. I. Miller
Evelina London Children's Hospital, Guy's and St Thomas' NHS Foundation Trust, London, UK
e-mail: owen.miller@gstt.nhs.uk

© Springer International Publishing AG, part of Springer Nature 2018

J. Simpson et al. (eds.), *Fetal Cardiology*, https://doi.org/10.1007/978-3-319-77461-9_4

compared to dedicated curved-array imaging transducers.

Both colour flow Doppler and spectral Doppler are angle-dependent modalities and the angle of insonation (θ) is critical when obtaining and interpreting the Doppler information. Unlike 2D greyscale (B-mode) imaging where the ideal insonation may be perpendicular to the structure of interest; spectral Doppler measurements or colour flow mapping should ideally be parallel to blood flow, either towards or away. Doppler shift is related to the cosine of the angle of insonation (cos θ) and angles greater than approximately 20–30° will be significantly inaccurate. When perpendicular (θ = 90°; Cos 90° = 0), so Doppler of flow moving perpendicular would not be registered.

Colour Flow Doppler

Colour Flow Doppler (CFD) superimposes Doppler-shift flow information on the 2D greyscale imaging; it is therefore important to optimise greyscale imaging before employing CFD; for example, over-gained greyscale will limit colour flow information.

CFD uses the convention of Blue-Away, Red-Towards (BART) to code movement either away or towards the transducer and depending on the manufacturer and machine settings various default colour maps are available to demonstrate the varying velocities within the colour box. Colour persistence should be minimised when assessing cardiac flows. Too high a persistence setting may impede interpretation of flow dynamics due to the relatively rapid movement of cardiac structures and blood flow when compared with extracardiac flows.

CFD is displayed within a region of interest (ROI) box; the ROI is in turn composed of numerous individual colour pixel units, each able to display its own velocity colour signal. Given that each ROI box will contain numerous pixel units, the wider the box, the greater the amount of information to process and hence the lower the temporal resolution. Ideally, the operator should use as narrow a colour box as possible but to include all structures of interest. For turbulent flow with varying velocities, the CFD will also display a range of colour shades. Conventionally, higher velocity is shown as a lighter shade and lower velocity a darker shade.

The user-selected colour maps are designed to enhance different flow profiles. There is no one correct colour map, rather each department may choose to define a preferred colour map thus potentially reducing interobserver variability when reviewing studies from different operators. More important than a chosen colour map, is an understanding of the limitations of CFD particularly in relation to velocity range, Nyquist limit and aliaising (see below).

CFD registers the Doppler shift from received echoes returning after striking moving blood (primarily erythrocytes). The Doppler shift derived will depend on multiple factors:

- The Pulse Repetition Frequency (PRF), which is the number of ultrasound pulses that occur per second and is determined by depth of image. As imaging depth increases the number of pulses returned decreases (PRF decreases). Therefore, it is important to set an imaging depth which is appropriate for CFD, avoiding excessive depth beyond the structure of interest as sampling in the far field will decrease PRF.
- The Nyquist limit is defined as half the PRF (i.e. PRF/2), hence a higher PRF will allow a higher Nyquist limit. Velocities above the Nyquist limit will not be registered accurately and will appear as turbulent flow when using CFD. In addition to adjusting the depth of the imaging (affects PRF), an appropriate Nyquist limit can be effected by Transducer (fundamental) frequency; a lower frequency transducer will induce less Doppler shift and therefore allow a higher Nyquist limit.

Optimising CFD

Blood flow within the fetal heart will have different velocities depending on site and gestation; e.g. pulmonary veins will have low velocity flow: <20 cm/s in second trimester, <40 cm/s at term (Lenz and Chaoui 2002). Normal outflow tract velocities are higher but still in the range 50–110 cm/s, also increasing normally towards term. As velocity beyond the Nyquist limit will be represented by "aliaising", it is important to optimise CFD to the flow being sampled. Aliaising can be avoided by:

- Selecting an appropriate transducer, as a lower (fundamental) frequency transducer will allow a higher Nyquist limit (see above)
- Optimise angle of insonation, as angles >30° will result in inaccurate CFD
- Imaging at less depth, thus increasing PRF
- Set scale to range of expected velocities, for expected low velocity flow e.g. pulmonary veins, set low velocity range; for outflow tracts, set higher velocity range.

Colour Doppler can be used at any stage in the comprehensive fetal echocardiogram, however, its overuse may mask abnormalities best seen on 2D (B-mode) imaging. Our practice is therefore to obtain comprehensive 2D greyscale dataset of video clips and still images, including all relevant structures and then either simultaneously (depending on fetal lie) or as a second series of video clips, obtain all CFD imaging or indeed a full video sweep from inlet to outlet (Video 4.1). Most modern ultrasound platforms have facility to simultaneously display grey scale and colour images side by side, which is very useful particularly in the mobile fetus (Fig. 4.1). This simultaneous display is achieved without loss of temporal or spatial resolution so can be employed without hesitation. The complete fetal echocardiogram should include CFD of all cardiac segments and should be considered an adjunct to confirm and add detail to what is already seen on 2D imaging, particularly where an abnormality is suspected. More recently, higher sensitivity colour Doppler designed to capture low flow has been available on some platforms and is ideal for lower velocity signals such as pulmonary veins and fetal septal defects. Although such low velocity CFD can confirm pulmonary venous connections; these connections are often already well seen with 2D grey-scale imaging (Fig. 4.2) (Video 4.2).

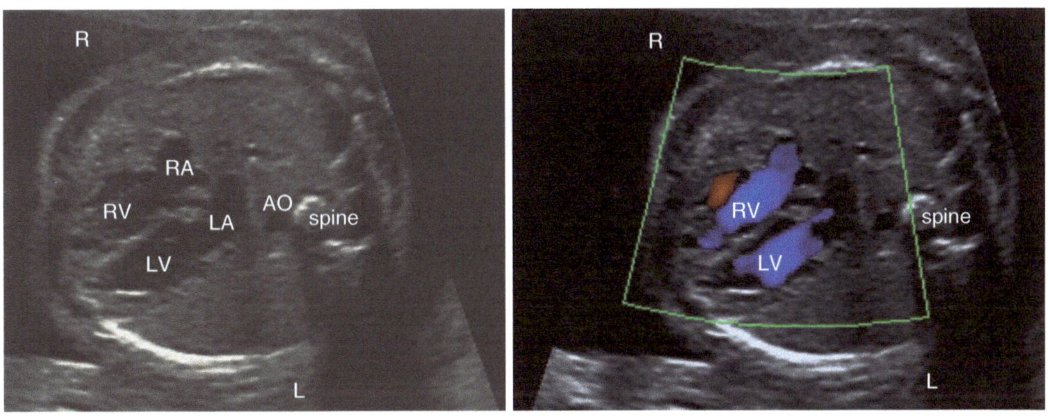

Fig. 4.1 Four chamber view with 2D grey scale in left panel and simultaneous Colour Flow Doppler in right panel, showing normal inflows across mitral and tricuspid valves. *R* right, *L* left, *RA* right atrium, *LA* left atrium, *RV* right ventricle, *LV* left ventricle, *AO* aorta

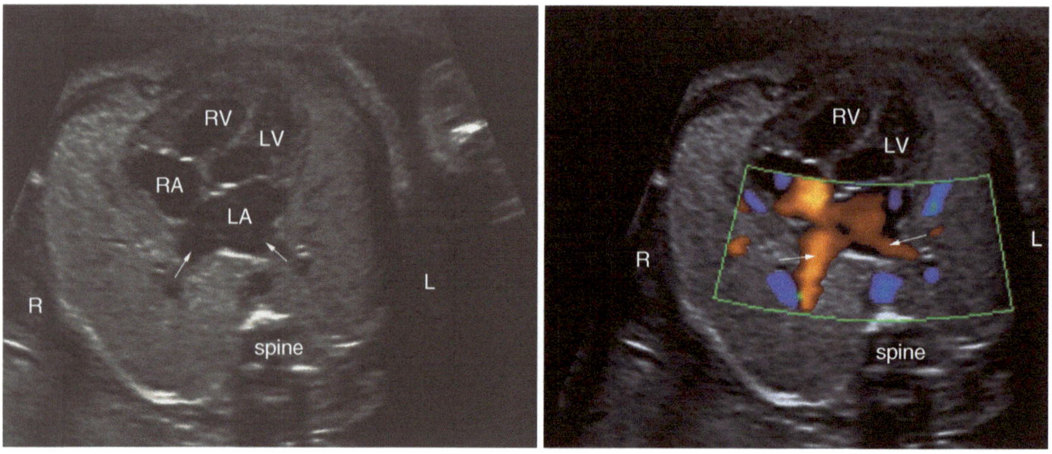

Fig. 4.2 Modified four chamber view, focussing on pulmonary veins, with 2D grey scale in left panel and simultaneous Colour Flow Doppler in right panel, *arrows* show right and left pulmonary veins. 2D grey scale confirms that pulmonary veins are already identifiable and right panel shows how Colour Flow Doppler adds further detail. *R* right, *L* left, *RA* right atrium, *LA* left atrium, *RV* right ventricle, *LV* left ventricle

Colour Flow Doppler of Specific Cardiac Structures

Interatrial Septum

The foramen ovale should be widely patent in the normal fetus with flow moving generally from right atrium to left atrium. This flow is usually at low velocity so settings should reflect this velocity range to demonstrate normality. Restrictive atrial communications are associated with adverse outcome in certain congenital heart lesions; for example, in ventriculo-arterial discordance (Transposition of the Great Arteries), patency of the foramen ovale is vital to ensure good mixing. A restrictive atrial communication in this setting is usually evident as a bulging atrial septum on 2D but also by a narrow colour jet. Equally worrying, reversed flow (left atrium to right atrium) may be seen in left heart obstruction such as mitral atresia and restriction of the foramen in this condition is associated with a poorer outcome (Vigneswaran et al. 2017).

AV Junction

The adequacy and morphology of the atrioventricular connections are enhanced by using CFD to document separate inflows, colour flow width and direction across left and right AV valves is well seen (Fig. 4.1). Mitral or Tricuspid regurgitation

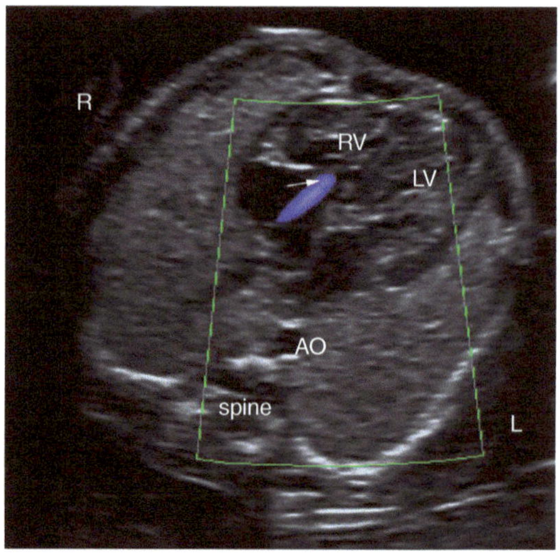

Fig. 4.3 Four chamber view, with Colour Flow Doppler showing Tricuspid Regurgitation jet (arrow). *R* right, *L* left, *RV* right ventricle, *LV* left ventricle, *AO* aorta

is easily demonstrated using CFD (Fig. 4.3) (Video 4.3). The jet of mitral or tricuspid regurgitation will be of higher velocity that the respective mitral or tricuspid inflow signal, so adjustment of velocity setting will be required to minimise aliaising.

Outflow Tracts

Visualising the left ventricular outflow tract (LVOT) (Fig. 4.4) and then right ventricular out-

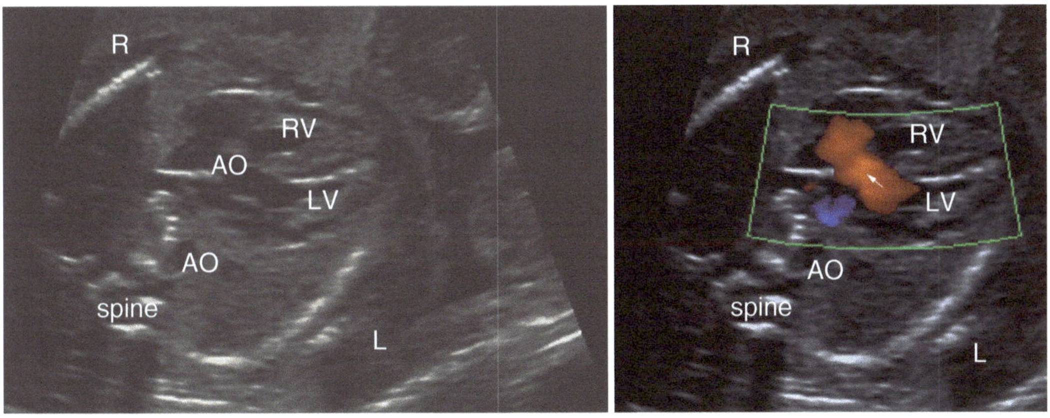

Fig. 4.4 Left ventricular outflow tract (LVOT) view, with simultaneous display of 2D grey scale and Colour Flow Doppler. Arrow (in right panel) shows uniform colour towards transducer in a normal LVOT. *R* right, *L* left, *RV* right ventricle, *LV* left ventricle, *AO* aorta

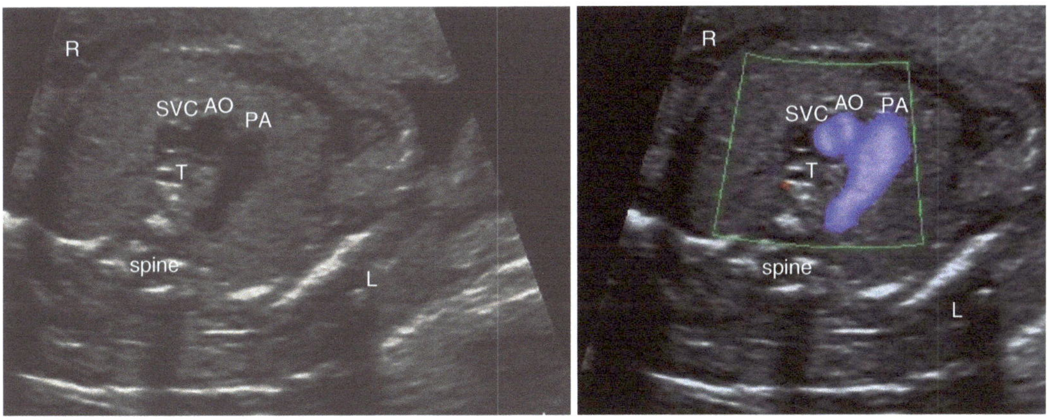

Fig. 4.5 Right ventricular outflow tract (RVOT) view, with simultaneous display of 2D grey scale and Colour Flow Doppler. Right panel shows uniform colour towards transducer in a normal pulmonary artery. *R* right, *L* left, *SVC* superior vena cava, *AO* aorta, *PA* pulmonary artery, *T* trachea

flow tracts (RVOT) (Fig. 4.5) is part of the standard data set.

CFD across the LVOT confirms the smooth transition from ventricle to aorta and the absence of turbulence suggests normal patency of the aortic valve (Video 4.4). LVOT velocity (50–110 cm/s) is expected to be higher that the mitral inflow velocity (10–40 cm/s), so Doppler velocity range will need to be set to reflect this expected range. Failure to increase Doppler velocity setting when moving from inflow to outflow may result in CFD aliaising.

Blood flow velocity across the RVOT is in a similar range to the LVOT and Doppler setting should reflect this. Following the main pulmonary artery more distally will confirm confluent branches (Video 4.5).

Three Vessel View

Colour flow can be applied to the segments of great arteries seen in the three-vessel view (3VV); the transverse aortic arch and the ductal continuation. CFD can confirm normal anterograde flow (Fig. 4.6) (Video 4.6) in both arches. Flow in the ductal arch normally has the highest velocity measured in the normal fetal heart.

In the presence of left heart obstruction, the 3VV may show reverse flow in the aortic arch (Fig. 4.7); or in the presence of right heart obstruction may show reverse flow from the duc-

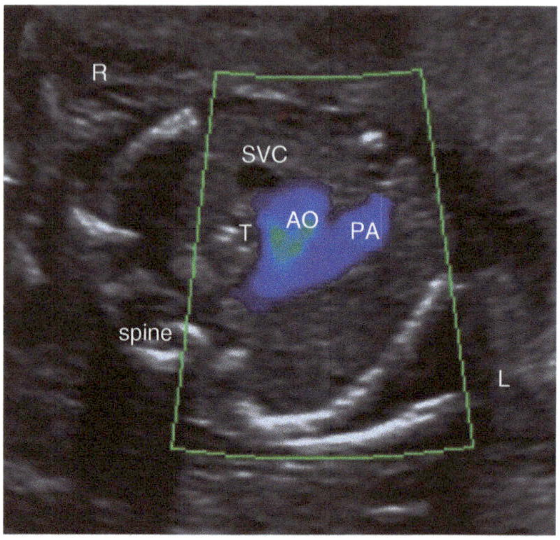

Fig. 4.6 Three Vessel View showing *Superior Vena Cava* to right, aorta and then pulmonary artery to left. Anterograde flow seen in both great arteries, no colour flow signal is seen in SVC as flow is perpendicular to transducer. *R* right, *L* left, *SVC* superior vena cava, *AO* aorta, *PA* pulmonary artery, *T* trachea

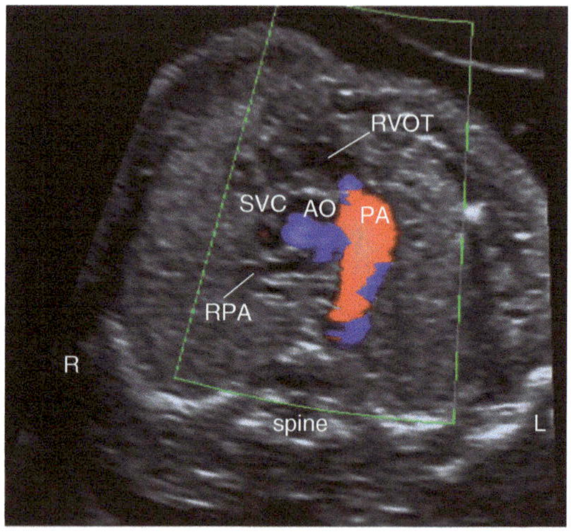

Fig. 4.8 RVOT view. Blue colour flow signal is anterograde in aorta. Red flow represents retrograde flow from the duct into the main pulmonary artery due to right heart obstruction, in this case pulmonary atresia. *R* right, *L* left, *RVOT* right ventricular outflow tract, *PA* pulmonary artery, *RPA* right pulmonary artery, *AO* aorta, *SVC* superior vena cava

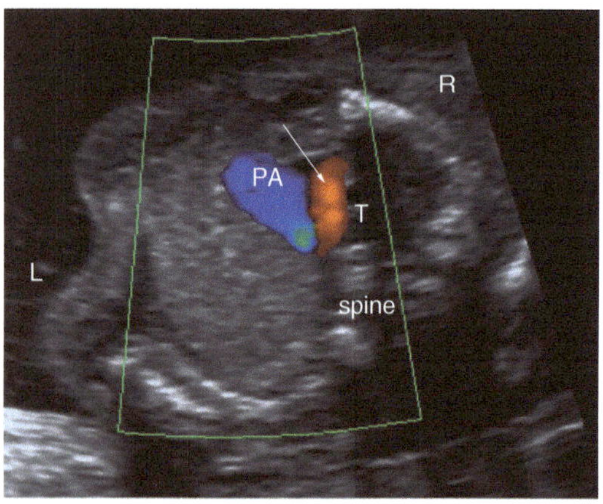

Fig. 4.7 Three Vessel View and Trachea. Blue colour flow signal is anterograde in pulmonary artery and duct. Arrow demonstrates retrograde (red) flow in transverse aortic arch due to left heart obstruction. *R* right, *L* left, *PA* pulmonary artery, *T* trachea

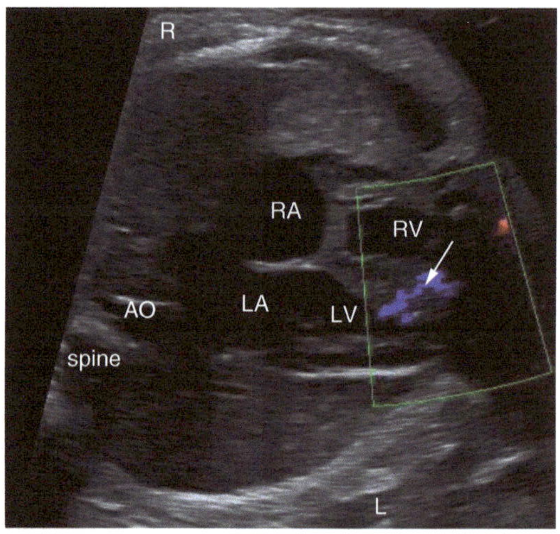

Fig. 4.9 Four chamber view with Colour Flow Doppler shows a moderate muscular ventricular septal defect (arrow) in apical ventricular septum. *R* right, *L* left, *RA* right atrium, *LA* left atrium, *RV* right ventricle, *LV* left ventricle

tal arch into the main pulmonary artery (Fig. 4.8) (Video 4.7).

Ventricular Septum

Ventricular septal defects may be seen using CFM, but due to the similar ventricular pressure, the velocity of any flow may be low velocity and due to high RV pressures in the fetus, CFD across a VSD is expected to be bidirectional. The use of a specific low flow modality or settings may enhance detection (Fig. 4.9).

Other Intracardiac Shunts

Abnormal intracardiac shunts are also best demonstrated using CFM. Rare ventriculo-atrial communications or aorto-ventricular tunnels can be confirmed. Coronary to cameral fistulae, often see in association with pulmonary atresia with intact ventricular septum (PA/IVS) are often only visible with careful application of CFD (Fig. 4.10) and spectral Doppler to confirm timing within cardiac cycle.

In Pulmonary Atresia with Ventricular Septal Defect (PA/VSD), pulmonary blood flow may be augmented by Major Aorto Pulmonary Collateral Arteries (MAPCAs). These can be notoriously difficult to image but may be see posteriorly between heart and descending aorta (Fig. 4.11) (Video 4.8).

Pulsed Wave (PW) Doppler

PW Doppler uses short bursts (pulse-echoes) of ultrasound, sent and received at a given repetition rate (Pulse Repetition Frequency). By sampling at a specific time interval, PW Doppler defines a "range gate" or "sample volume" within which the signals will be registered (D'Hooge and Mertens 2016). For the operator, this is a user-definable feature commonly call the "Gate width" or similar nomenclature. The gated timing of PW Doppler allows targeted interrogation of velocities within a narrow sample volume (Reeder et al. 1986). Each user should be familiar with how to set and adjust the range gate; using too large a gate will degrade the quality of the PW information and contain a greater spread of velocities; using too narrow a gate may mean that the area of interest moves in and out of range during the cardiac cycle. The velocity range measurable is limited by the Nyquist limit and PRF; signals beyond the Nyquist limit will be registered as aliasing. Unlike CFD where aliaising is displayed by a different/opposite colour, when using PW Doppler, aliaising is displayed on the spectrogram as signal which "wraps around" the maximum velocity and appear on the other side of the baseline. When using the common transducers found on most commercially available platforms, maximum velocities of up to 150–200 cm/s are measureable before aliaising occurs. This velocity envelope is sufficient for the great majority of routine measure-

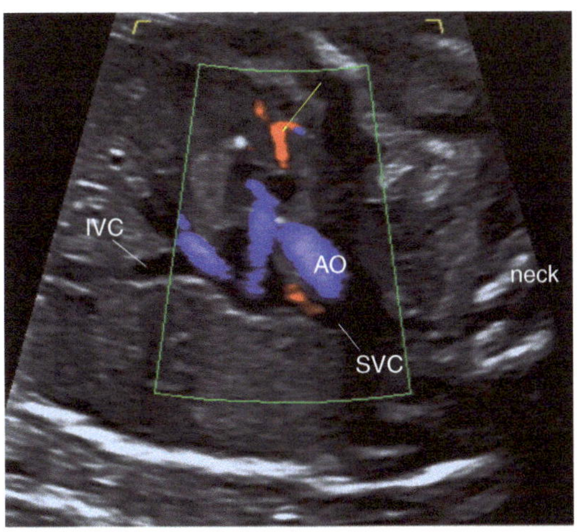

Fig. 4.10 Sagittal bicaval view, demonstrating normal systemic venous connections. Arrow points to a (red) colour flow signal representing a coronary to RV sinusoid associated in this case with pulmonary atresia-intact ventricular septum. *SVC* superior vena cava, *IVC* inferior vena cava, *AO* aorta

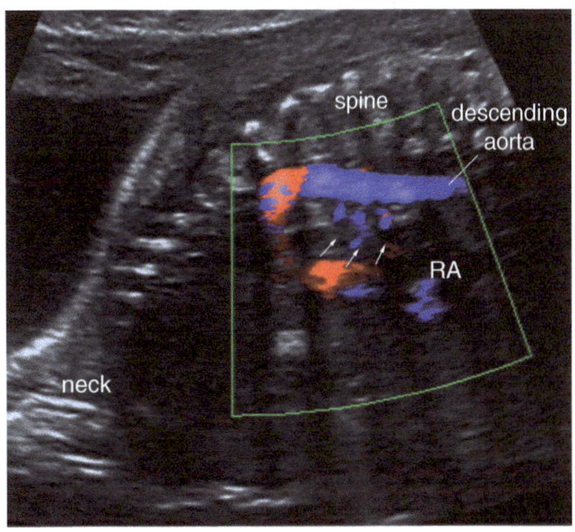

Fig. 4.11 Sagittal view, demonstrating the proximal descending aorta running across the top of the image. Arrows show blue flow (away from transducer) in three Major Aorto-Pulmonary Collateral Arteries (MAPCA), associated in this case with pulmonary atresia-ventricular septal defect. *RA* right atrium

ments including pulmonary veins, ventricular inlets, outlets and septal defects. For abnormalities showing velocity outside of this velocity range, a transducer with CW Doppler should be selected.

Pulse Wave Doppler of Specific Cardiac Structures

Pulmonary Veins

2D imaging and CFD will reliably demonstrate the pulmonary venous connection in most cases. Pulmonary venous inflow Doppler is however part of the standard fetal echocardiogram (Lee et al. 2008). The sample volume gate should be positioned where the pulmonary veins enters the left atrium. There is usually forward flow in systole and diastole, with cessation of flow or a small reversal of flow during atrial contraction in late diastole (Fig. 4.12).

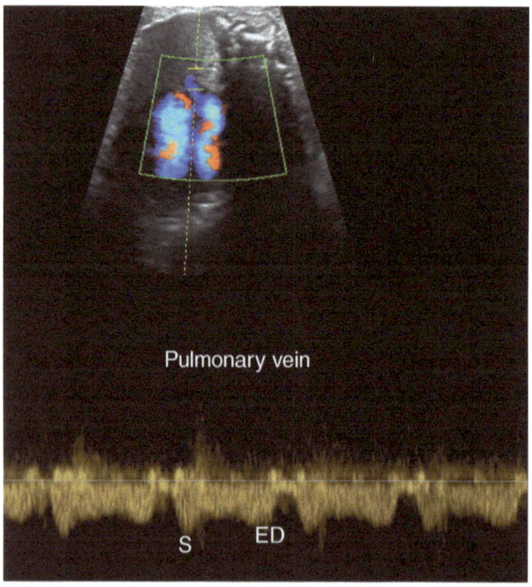

Fig. 4.12 Pulse Wave Doppler of a right pulmonary vein. Upper image shows cursor aligned with pulmonary vein flow and range gate within pulmonary vein. Lower image shows Doppler spectrogram with anterograde flow throughout the cardiac cycle from systole extending to end-diastole. *S* systole, *ED* end diastole

Velocities of flows in the systolic and diastolic peaks are similar

- 10 cm/s at 16 weeks' gestation
- 30–40 cm/s at term
- reversal "a" wave usually less than 10 cm/s.

Atria-Ventricular Connections

PW Doppler inflow velocities should be measured, ideally in the 4ChV, when an appropriate

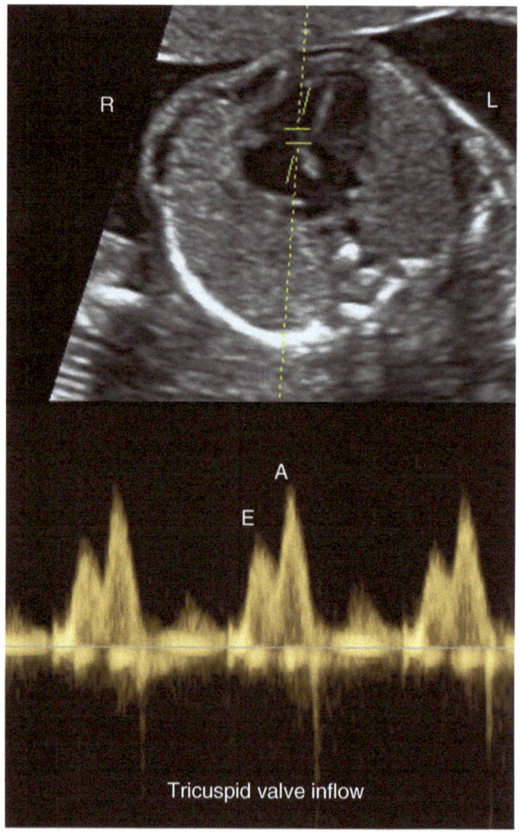

Fig. 4.13 Pulse Wave Doppler of normal tricuspid valve inflow in a fetus at 20 weeks gestation. Upper image shows cursor aligned with tricuspid inflow and range gate within the ventricle, just below tricuspid valve annulus. Lower image shows Doppler spectrogram with biphasic diastolic inflow signal made of early (E) wave and later atrial contraction (A) wave signals. The E wave is of lower velocity in the first and second trimester and increases to equal the A wave velocity towards term. *R* right, *L* left, *E* early inflow wave, *A* atrial contraction inflow signal

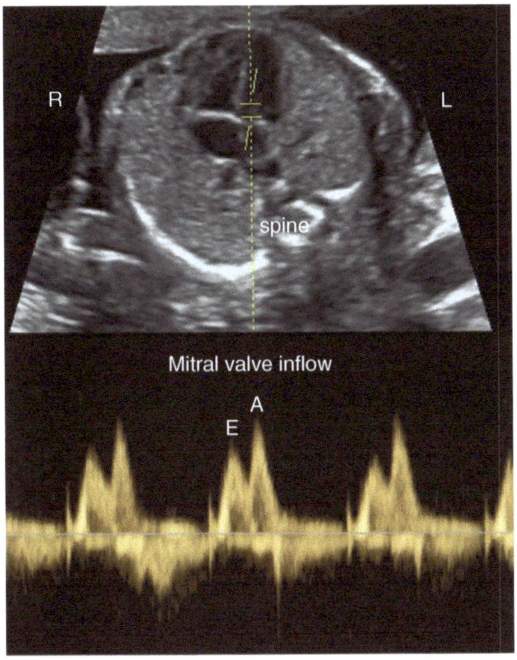

Fig. 4.14 Pulse Wave Doppler of normal mitral valve inflow in a fetus at 20 weeks gestation. Upper image shows cursor aligned with mitral inflow and range gate within the ventricle, just below mitral valve annulus. Lower image shows Doppler spectrogram with biphasic diastolic inflow signal made of early (E) wave and later atrial contraction (A) wave signals. The E wave is of lower velocity in the first and second trimester and increases to equal the A wave velocity towards term. *R* right, *L* left, *E* early inflow wave, *A* atrial contraction inflow signal

angle of insonation (<20–30°) is achievable. In the normal fetus, the TV inflow velocity (Fig. 4.13) is usually of higher velocity than that seen across the MV (Fig. 4.14) (Reed et al. 1986). The normal biphasic pattern with E and A waves is present after the eighth week of gestation (van Splunder et al. 1996) but the E/A ratio is usually <1 compared to the usual post-natal E/A ratio >1. The E wave is initially of lower velocity (15–30 cm/s) due to the reduced compliance of the fetal myocardium (Hernandez-Andrade et al. 2012), but increases throughout gestation to approach or equal the A wave velocity near term. The A wave has less variability, having an early gestation velocity starting

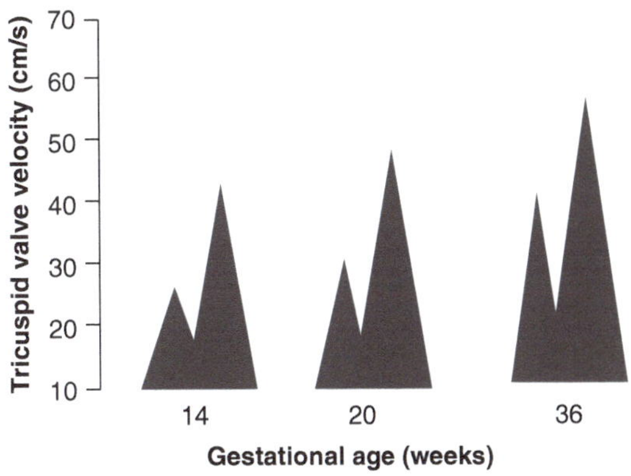

Fig. 4.15 Schematic representation of tricuspid inflow velocities at early, mid and late gestation, based on data from our unit. Although the A wave does increase during pregnancy, the E/A ratio increases at a greater rate

near 30 cm/s, increasing to 45–50 cm/s near term (Fig. 4.15).

Outflow Tracts

Both LVOT and RVOT Doppler velocities are usually obtainable by moving from four chamber view to the outflow tract views (de Carvalho et al. 2013), good technique is essential to minimise underestimation (see Table 4.1).

The peak velocity across the outflow tracts is highly reproducible and increases gradually with gestation and the normal values in the mid-trimester are 80–100 cm/s (Groenenberg et al. 1991) with the pulmonary artery velocity (Fig. 4.16) often marginally lower than the aortic velocity (Fig. 4.17). The arterial duct velocity in the normal fetus has the highest velocity (up to 150–160 cm/s) (Fig. 4.18). The outflow tract velocities are influenced by the downstream vascular resistance and alterations in Doppler velocities should be interpreted both with a view to any more proximal outflow tract obstruction but also changes to the distal vascular resistance.

A rare but important finding on ductal Doppler is a high velocity continuous flow suggestive of premature ductal constriction. This is invariably associated with RV dysfunction and requires urgent fetal medicine assessment and intervention.

Table 4.1 Technique to obtain optimal spectral Doppler

Sampling site	Position of cursor and range gate	Doppler settings	Comments
Inflows: mitral and tricuspid valves	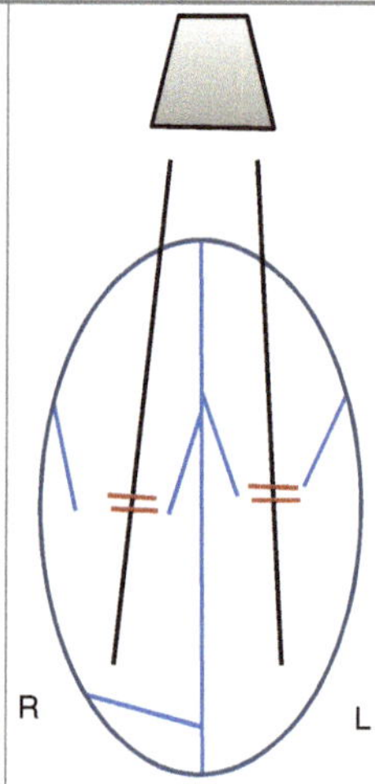	Gate width: 3 mm Velocity range: 10–40 cm/s	E wave initially lower in early gestation but increases to equal A wave near term
Left ventricular outflow tract spectral Doppler	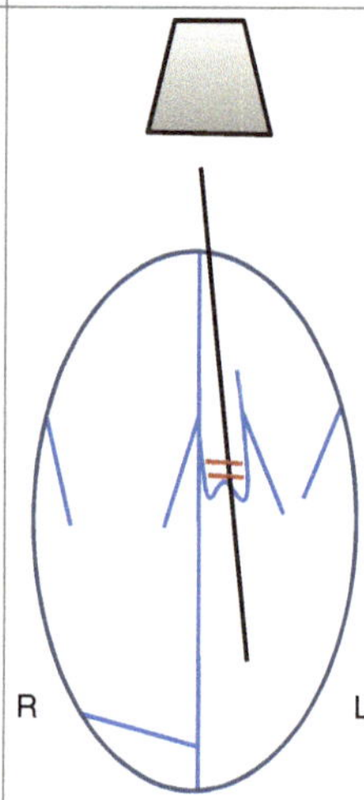	Gate width: 3 mm Velocity range: 50–110 cm/s	Single peak of forward flow in systole, with a short time to peak Peak velocity increases with gestation; 30–40 cm/s at 14 weeks, 100–120 cm/s near term
Right ventricular outflow tract spectral Doppler	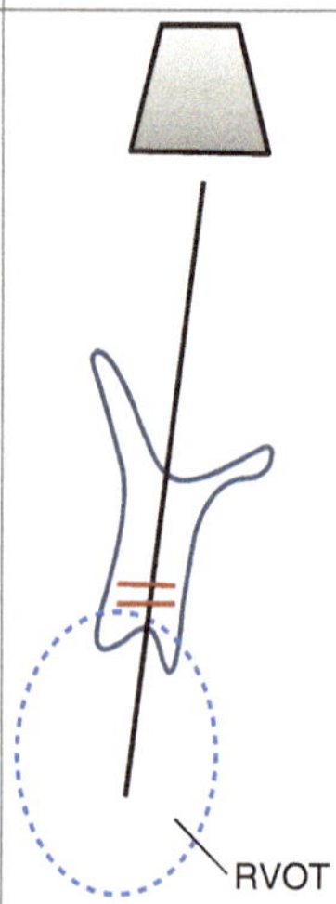	Gate width: 3 mm Velocity range: 50–110 cm/s	Peak velocity in the normal aorta often slightly higher than in the normal pulmonary artery

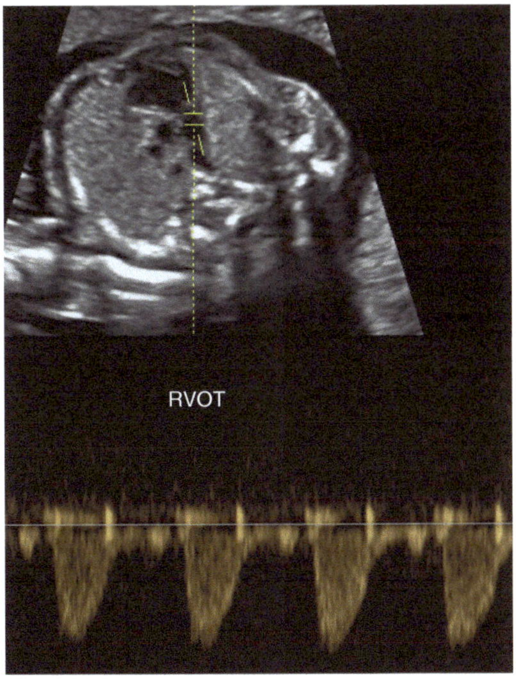

Fig. 4.16 Pulse Wave Doppler of normal pulmonary artery flow in a fetus at 20 weeks gestation. Upper image shows cursor aligned with pulmonary artery flow and range gate within the main pulmonary artery above the pulmonary valve. Lower image shows Doppler spectrogram with a dominant anterograde signal with a steep rise in early systolic velocity representing right ventricular ejection into a low compliance pulmonary circulation

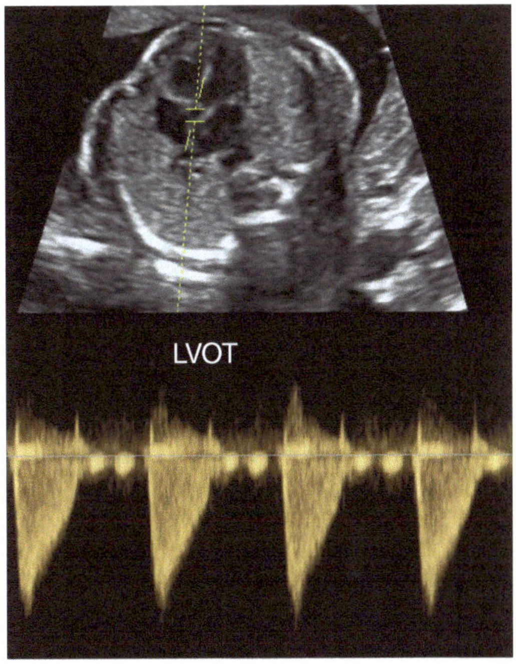

Fig. 4.17 Pulse Wave Doppler of normal aortic outflow in a fetus at 20 weeks gestation. Upper image shows cursor aligned with aortic flow and range gate within the ascending aorta above the aortic valve. Lower image shows Doppler spectrogram with a dominant anterograde signal with a steep rise in early systolic velocity

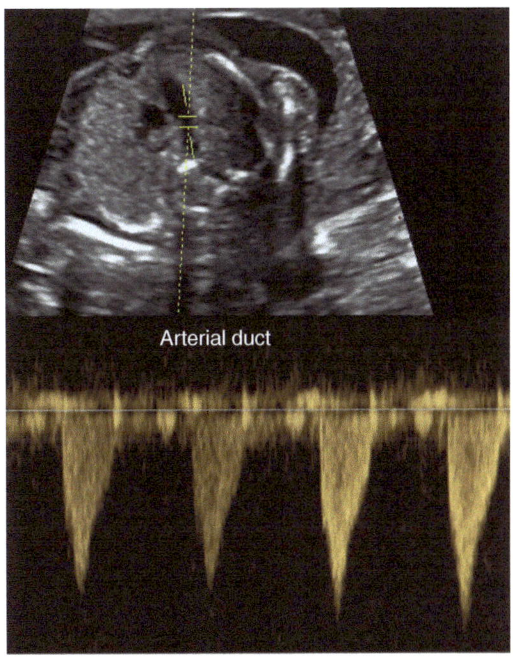

Fig. 4.18 Pulse Wave Doppler of normal flow in the arterial duct in a fetus at 20 weeks gestation. Upper image shows cursor aligned with ductal flow and range gate within the arterial duct beyond the pulmonary artery bifurcation. Lower image shows Doppler spectrogram with a dominant anterograde signal and a peak velocity higher than either pulmonary artery or aortic flow. The flow measured in the fetal arterial duct is commonly the highest velocity within the normal fetal circulation

Flow Reversal

Within the fetal spectrum of left heart hypoplasia/obstruction the flow in the proximal ascending aorta may be abnormal. Reversal of flow from ductus into ascending aorta may be see both on colour flow and confirmed with PW Doppler. There is usually a corresponding decrease in aortic calibre presenting as great artery disproportion.

Similar flow reversal may be see into a diminutive main pulmonary artery in cases of pulmonary atresia, where there is no effective forward flow from the ventricular mass and fetal pulmonary blood flow is derived from retrograde filling from the aorta via the arterial duct.

Continuous Wave Doppler

Continuous Wave (CW) Doppler registers all velocities along the line of insonation, CW is not limited by a Nyquist limit barrier and can therefore be used to measure high velocity signals. Such high velocity jets are unusual in the normal fetal heart and CW Doppler is not routinely available on usual obstetric/fetal cardiology (curved array) transducers.

Lesions associated with high velocity signals may include mitral and tricuspid regurgitation and rarely aortic or pulmonary valve stenosis, although other signs of pathology will usually coexist.

Continuous Wave Doppler is angle-dependent and the same caveats for PW technique, particularly regarding angle of insonation (θ), exist for CW Doppler.

Tissue Doppler Imaging and Speckle Tracking Echocardiography

Tissue Doppler and Deformation Imaging (Speckle Tracking) is being increasingly used in the assessment of fetal cardiac function (see Chap. 5).

References

Baker DW, Rubenstein SA, Lorch GS. Pulsed Doppler echocardiography: principles and applications. Am J Med. 1977;63:69–80.

D'Hooge J, Mertens LL. Ultrasound physics. In: Echocardiography in pediatric and congenital heart disease. 2nd ed. Chichester; 2016. p. 3–18.

de Carvalho JS, Allan LD, Chaoui R, Copel JA, DeVore GR. ISUOG Practice Guidelines (updated): sonographic screening examination of the fetal heart. Ultrasound Obstet Gynecol. 2013;41:348–59.

Groenenberg IA, Hop WC, Wladimiroff JW. Doppler flow velocity waveforms in the fetal cardiac outflow tract: reproducibility of waveform recording and analysis. Ultrasound Med Biol. 1991;17:583–7.

Hernandez-Andrade E, Benavides-Serralde JA, Cruz-Martinez R, Welsh A, Mancilla-Ramirez J. Evaluation of conventional Doppler fetal cardiac function parameters: E/A ratios, outflow tracts, and myocardial performance index. Fetal Diagn Ther. 2012;32(1–2):22–9.

Lee W, Allan L, Carvalho JS, Chaoui R, Copel J, Devore G, Hecher K, Munoz H, Nelson T, Paladini D, Yagel S. ISUOG consensus statement: what constitutes a fetal echocardiogram? Ultrasound Obstet Gynecol. 2008;32:239–42.

Lenz F, Chaoui R. Reference ranges for Doppler-assessed pulmonary venous blood flow velocities and pulsatility indices in normal human fetuses. Prenat Diagn. 2002;22:786–91.

Miyatake K, Mitsunori M, Kinoshita N, Izumi S, Owa M, Takao S, Sakakibara H, Nimura Y. Clinical applications of a new type of real-time two-dimensional Doppler flow imaging system. Am J Cardiol. 1984;54:857–68.

Reed KL, Meijboom EJ, Sahn DJ, Scagnelli SA, Valdes-Cruz LM, Shenker L. Cardiac Doppler flow velocities in human fetuses. Circulation. 1986;73:41–6.

Reeder GS, Currie PJ, Hagler DJ, Tajik AJ, Seward JB. Use of Doppler techniques (continuous-wave, pulsed-wave, and color flow imaging) in the noninvasive hemodynamic assessment of congenital heart disease. Mayo Clin Proc. 1986;61:725–44.

van Splunder P, Stijnen T, Wladimiroff JW. Fetal atrioventricular flow-velocity waveforms and their relation to arterial and venous flow-velocity waveforms at 8 to 20 weeks of gestation. Circulation. 1996;94:1372–8.

Vigneswaran TV, Zidere V, Miller OI, Simpson JM, Sharland GK. Usefulness of the prenatal echocardiogram in fetuses with isolated transposition of the great arteries to predict the need for balloon atrial septostomy. Am J Cardiol. 2017;119(9): 1463–7.

Fetal Cardiac Function

5

John Simpson

Abstract

Assessment of cardiac function in an integral part of the assessment of the fetal circulation. Cardiac dysfunction can be assessed by standard echocardiographic modalities including 2D, M-mode and Doppler echocardiography. Other techniques may enhance quantification of cardiac function, particularly in a research setting, including tissue Doppler, 3D echocardiography and speckle tracking. Most recently fetal cardiovascular magnetic resonance imaging (CMR) has been applied to the fetal circulation to measure regional blood flow. Accurate measurement of fetal cardiac function can enhance understanding of cardiac dysfunction in the context of structural defects, cardiomyopathies and abnormalities of fetal cardiac loading conditions.

Keywords

Cardiac function · Fetus · Doppler · M-mode · Tissue Doppler · 3D echocardiography

Electronic Supplementary Material The online version of this chapter (https://doi.org/10.1007/978-3-319-77461-9_5) contains supplementary material, which is available to authorized users.

J. Simpson
Evelina London Children's Hospital, Guy's and St Thomas' NHS Foundation Trust, London, UK
e-mail: john.simpson@gstt.nhs.uk

Introduction

This chapter aims to provide a core understanding of echocardiographic assessment of the function of the fetal heart. The focus will be on a practical approach to assessment of fetal cardiac function using standard techniques. Advanced modalities which can provide further insight into abnormal cardiac function will also be discussed. A detailed discussion of each and every scenario where assessment of cardiac function may be of assistance is beyond the scope of this chapter. The reader is referred to a number of reviews of the subject (Simpson 2004; Van Mieghem et al. 2009; Godfrey et al. 2012; Michelfelder et al. 2016).

The Fetal Circulation

The normal fetal circulation is fundamentally different from the postnatal circulation. The fetal and postnatal circulations are compared diagrammatically in Fig. 5.1 (Hunter and Simpson 2014). Differences between the prenatal and postnatal circulation include the presence of shunts at atrial level (foramen ovale) and between the great arteries (arterial duct), high pulmonary vascular resistance and a low systemic vascular resistance due to low resistance of both the cerebral and placental circulations. The effect of this is that pressures in the left and right heart circulations are similar dur-

© Springer International Publishing AG, part of Springer Nature 2018

J. Simpson et al. (eds.), *Fetal Cardiology*, https://doi.org/10.1007/978-3-319-77461-9_5

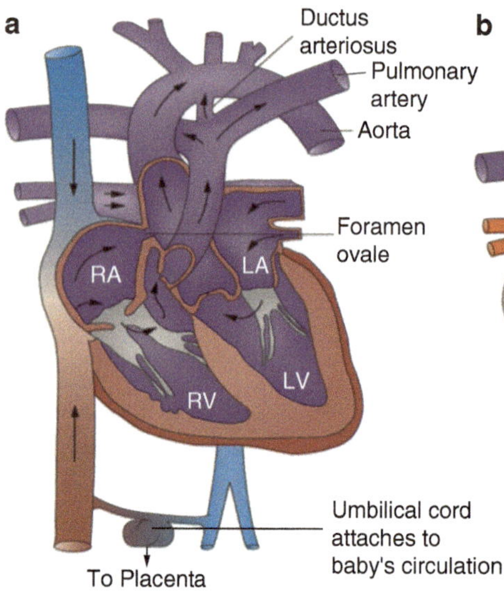

Fig. 5.1 Fetal and postnatal circulations. (**a**) Fetal circulation. Oxygenated blood from the placenta returns to the RA via the umbilical vein and ductus venosus. Blood passes from the RA to the LA via the patent foramen ovale. The second fetal shunt occurs between the main pulmonary artery and the descending aortic arch in the form of the arterial duct (ductus arteriosus). Fetal PVR is high compared with in the postnatal circulation. Therefore, most blood being pumped out of the RV passes through the arterial duct into the descending aorta. (**b**) Immediate postnatal circulation. Physiological adaptations that occur after birth result in a marked drop in PVR and an increase in the pulmonary venous return to the left atrium. This change results in functional closure of the foramen ovale. A postnatal increase in systemic vascular resistance and arterial pressure occurs, coupled with the fall in PVR. Consequently, blood flows from the aorta to the pulmonary circulation via the arterial duct until it constricts and finally closes after birth. (**c**) Normal postnatal circulation. Deoxygenated blood passing through the right-heart structures is completely separated from the oxygenated blood passing through the left-heart structures. The foramen ovale and arterial duct have closed, preventing shunting between the atria and the great arteries, respectively. Abbreviations: *LA* left atrium, *LV* left ventricle, *PVR* pulmonary vascular resistance, *RA* right atrium, *RV* right ventricle. (Reproduced with premission from Hunter and Simpson 2014)

ing fetal life. The systemic arterial pressure is lower during fetal life than postnatally, whereas the pulmonary artery pressure is higher during fetal life than after birth. During fetal life, the lungs are filled with fluid and pulmonary vascular resistance is high so that the vast majority of the right ventricular output reaches the systemic arterial circulation via the arterial duct. The fetal cardiac output, when indexed for body size is far higher during prenatal life than after birth, thus the fetal circulation represents a high flow/low pressure systemic arterial circulation. There is a significant increase in left and right ventricular systolic pressure with advancing gestational age.

With respect to flow distribution and oxygen delivery, the most oxygenated blood in the fetal circulation returns to the heart from the placenta via the umbilical vein and ductus venosus. This blood streams preferentially from the right atrium to the left atrium so that highly oxygenated blood reaches the fetal brain. The streaming of blood within the heart and extracardiac shunts are shown in detail in Fig. 5.2 (Kiserud and Acharya 2004).

A Practical Approach to Assessment of Fetal Cardiac Function

There are a large number of different indices of cardiac function which have been described. The approach outlined below is designed to be based on features which are visible on screening views of the fetal heart but which can be supplemented by ultrasound modalities fitted to virtually all

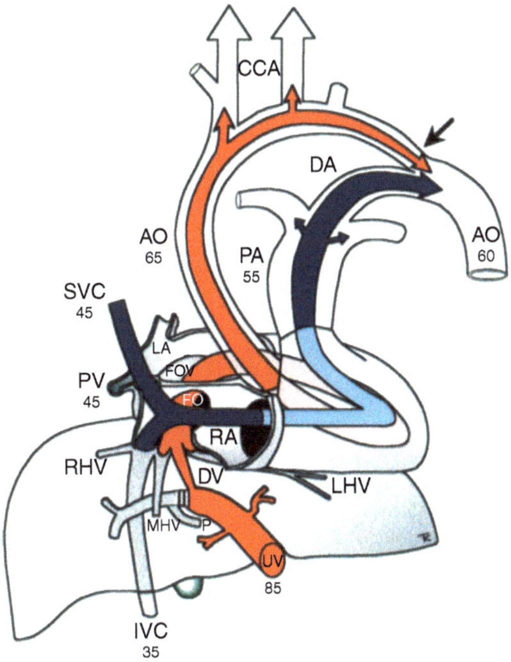

Fig. 5.2 Pathways of the fetal heart and representative oxygen saturation values (in numbers). The via sinistra (red) directs well oxygenated blood from the umbilical vein (UV) through the ductus venosus (DV) (or left half of the liver) across the inferior vena cava (IVC), through the foramen ovale (FO), left atrium (LA) and ventricle (LV) and up the ascending aorta (AO) to join the via dextra (blue) in the descending AO. Deoxygenated blood from the superior vena cava (SVC) and IVC forms the via dextra through the right atrium (RA) and ventricle (RV), pulmonary trunk (PA) and ductus arteriosus (DA). The isthmus aortae (arrow) and the section of the left portal vein between the main stem (P) and the DV (striped area) represent watershed areas during hemodynamic compromise. *CCA* common carotid arteries, *FOV* foramen ovale valve, *LHV* left hepatic vein, *MHV* medial hepatic vein, *PV* pulmonary vein, *RHV* right hepatic vein. (Reproduced with permission from Kiserud and Acharya 2004)

ultrasound systems used to assess the fetal heart. Later in this chapter other modalities will be described which can differ significantly according to the ultrasound system used.

Abnormal Features on the Four-Chamber View

The four-chamber view of the fetal heart is the usual starting point from which abnormal cardiac function should be suspected. This is supplemented in affected cases by more detailed quantification of systolic and diastolic function (Table 5.1).

1. Heart size: In the normal fetus, the fetal heart occupies around one third of the cross-sectional area of the fetal thorax in the four-chamber view (Fig. 5.3a, b, Videos 5.1 and 5.2). From invasive studies, the heart size correlates with venous filling pressures which increase as the heart fails. The size of the heart is most commonly expressed as a proportion of the size of the cross-section of the thorax (cardiothoracic ratio) either using the area of the heart related to the area of the thorax (heart normally one third of the area of the thorax) or a ratio of circumferences of the heart and thorax (the normal circumference ratio is 0.5 or less).
2. Subjective impression of ventricular function: The normal fetal heart is typically dynamic due to high volume flow coupled with low

Table 5.1 Core features of the four-chamber view in the setting of normal and abnormal cardiac function

Metric	Normal heart	Cardiac dysfunction
Heart size	1/3 of area of thorax	Heart >1/3 of area of thorax
Subjective assessment of function	Dynamic	Reduced
AV valve inflow (Doppler)	Biphasic	Monophasic
AV valve regurgitation colour flow Doppler	Mild TV regurgitation "physiological" in some fetuses	Mitral and/or tricuspid valve regurgitation
AV valve regurgitation pulsed Doppler	No AV valve regurgitation or mild TR only. TR not holosystolic on PW Doppler	Holosystolic MV and/or TV regurgitation
Associated features	None	Skin oedema, ascites, pleural effusion, pericardial effusion

Abbreviations: *AV* atrioventricular, *TV* tricuspid valve, *MV* mitral valve, *TR* tricuspid valve regurgitation, *PW* pulsed wave

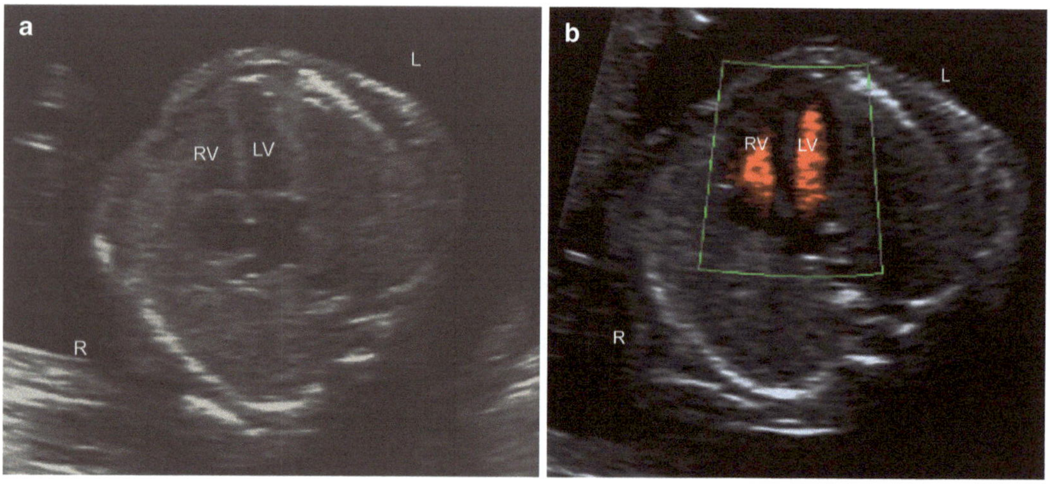

Fig. 5.3 (**a**, **b**) The left pane shows a normal four chamber view illustrating that the heart occupies around one third of the area of the thorax. The right pane confirms that equal sized colour flow Doppler jets enter the right and left ventricles of the heart

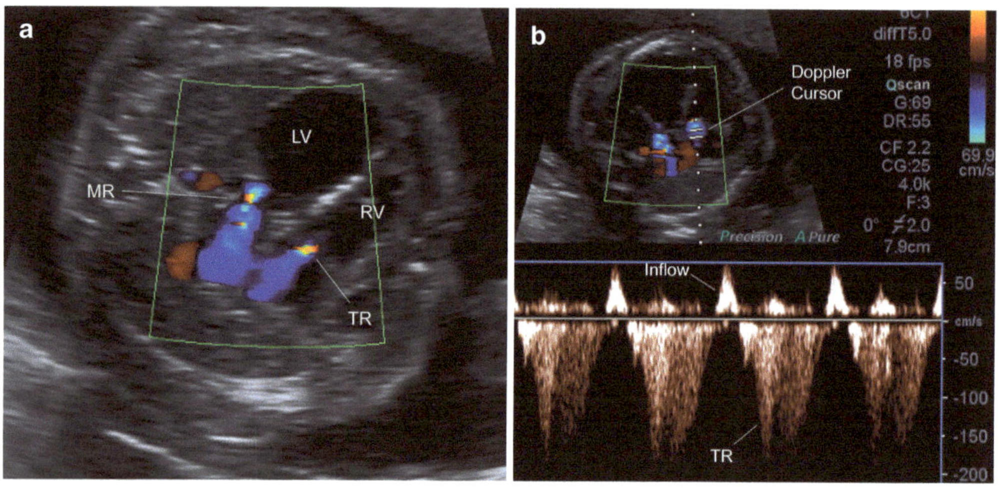

Fig. 5.4 (**a**, **b**) Mitral and tricuspid valve regurgitation. The pane on the left shows mitral and tricuspid valve regurgitation. Mild tricuspid valve regurgitation may be observed in the normal fetus. The right hand pane shows holosystolic tricuspid valve regurgitation and monophasic tricuspid valve inflow which is abnormal

resistance (Videos 5.1 and 5.2). This is a purely subjective measure but widely adopted in normal practice.

3. Supportive evidence of impairment of cardiac function: Fetal skin oedema, pleural effusions, pericardial effusions and ascites provide supporting evidence of cardiac failure, but may occur for a number of reasons and are not specific for fetal cardiac failure. Cardiac enlargement in association with these features is strongly associated with a cardiac cause.
4. Colour flow Doppler assists in demonstrating flow within the systemic and pulmonary veins, intracardiac flow and flow in the great arteries (Fig. 5.3a, b, Video 5.2). Mild tricuspid valve regurgitation is frequently observed in the normal midtrimester fetus, but moderate or severe tricuspid valve regurgitation is not a normal finding in the midtrimester. Mitral valve regurgitation is seldom observed in the normal fetus. Figure 5.4a, b shows abnormal mitral and tricuspid valve regurgitation

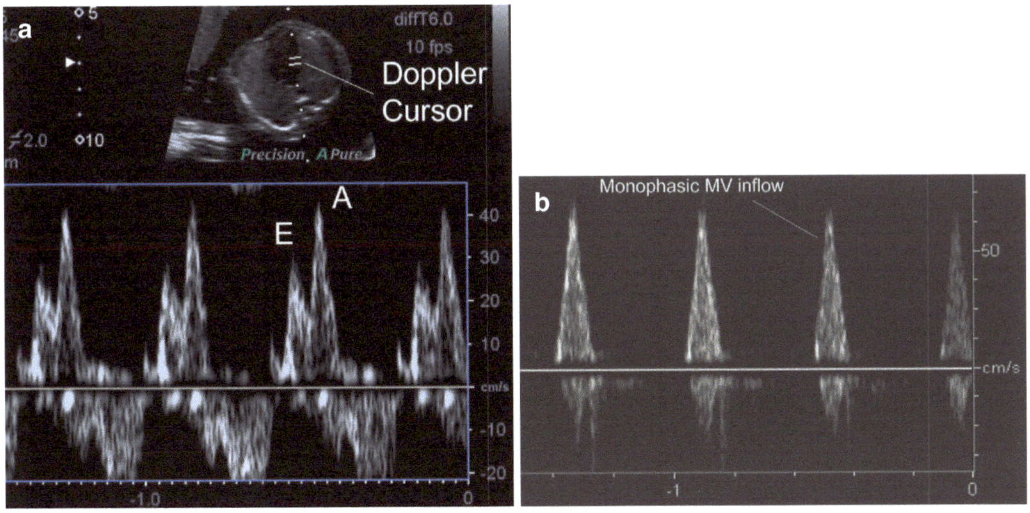

Fig. 5.5 (**a**, **b**) Normal and abnormal AV valve inflow pattern. The left pane shows a normal mitral valve inflow pattern which has early (E) and late (A) waves resulting in a biphasic inflow pattern. The E velocity increases with gestational age whilst the A wave velocity is more constant. In contrast, the right pane shows an abnormal inflow pattern related to ventricular diastolic dysfunction and/or systolic dysfunction. There is only a single peak of inflow to the ventricle with a shorter filling period than normal

accompanied by cardiac enlargement. Video 5.3 shows these features in real-time.

5. Pulsed Doppler interrogation of the atrioventricular valve inflow normally shows a biphasic inflow pattern. In the fetus with poor ventricular function the inflow time shortens and the inflow pattern becomes monophasic (Fig. 5.5a, b).

Indices of Cardiac Function

The approach described above assists in the differentiation of normal from abnormal cardiac function but does not permit quantification of the degree of abnormality. Nor does this approach differentiate function in terms of how the heart contracts and ejects blood (systolic cardiac function) versus filling properties of the heart (diastolic function). Thus, other methods are used to provide objective measurement which are outlined below.

Fractional Shortening

The fractional shortening of the LV or RV can be measured by M-mode or cross-sectional echocardiography. For the M-mode technique the cursor is placed orthogonal to the plane of the ventricular septum. This permits measurement of the dimension of the LV and RV cavities at end-diastole and end-systole (Fig. 5.6a, b, Video 5.4). From these measurements the fractional shortening can be measured according to the following equation.

$$\text{Fractional shortening}(\%) = \frac{\text{LV end} - \text{diastolic dimension} - \text{LV end} - \text{systolic dimension}}{\text{LV end} - \text{diastolic dimension}}$$

The normal range of fractional shortening by this method is 28–40% which is fairly constant across gestational ages. The M-mode method is limited by dependence on a particular fetal lie to achieve the optimal sonographic cut. Some ultrasound systems permit the alteration of the angle of the M-line to optimise the measurement. In contrast to the normal M-mode appearances shown in Fig. 5.6, an abnormal M-mode tracing of the left ventricle is illustrated in Fig. 5.7 where there is little or no contraction of the LV.

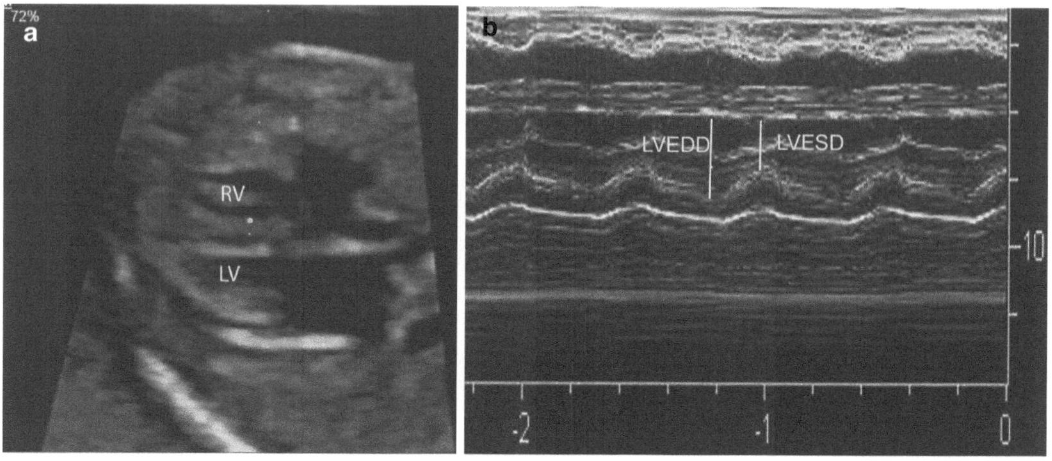

Fig. 5.6 (**a**, **b**) Normal M-mode orientation and M-mode trace. The left pane shows the cursor placed orthogonally across both the left and right ventricles. The cursor is placed at the tips of the atrioventricular valves. The M-mode tracing is shown in the right pane. The left ventricular end-diastolic dimension is measured at the largest diameter of the ventricle and systolic dimension at the minimum diameter. Abbreviations: *LVEDD* left ventricular end-diastolic dimension, *LVESD* left ventricular end-systolic dimension

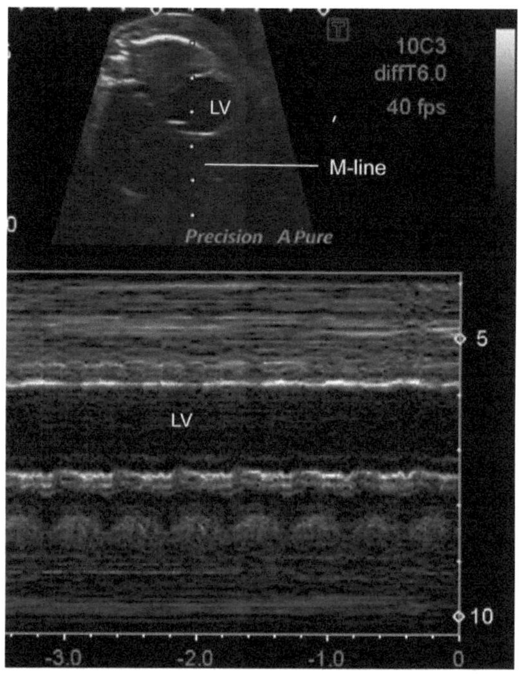

Fig. 5.7 Abnormal M-mode trace. In this abnormal tracing the M-line is placed across the left and right ventricles. There is virtually no contraction of the left ventricle

Ventricular Ejection Fraction

An alternative method for measuring ventricular systolic function is to planimeter the LV at end-diastole and end-systole. The volume of the ventricle is computed by dividing the ventricle into a number of discs (Fig. 5.8). Planimetry is performed at end-diastole and end-systole and ejection fraction is computed according to the formula:

$$\text{LV ejection fraction} = \frac{\text{LV end} - \text{diastolic volume} - \text{LV end} - \text{systolic volume}}{\text{LV end} - \text{diastolic volume}}$$

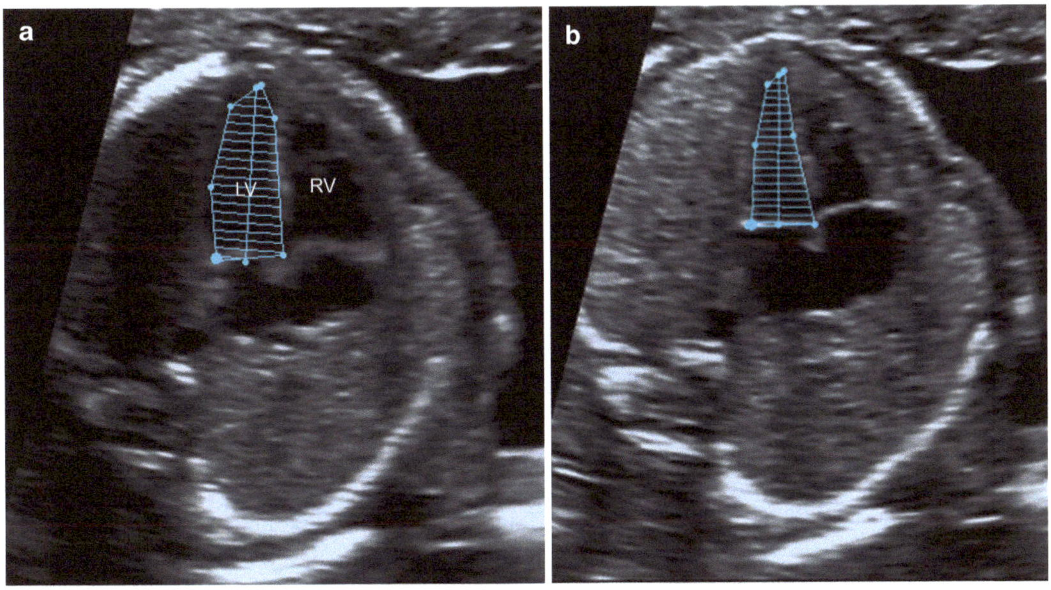

Fig. 5.8 (**a**, **b**) 2D echo assessment of LV ejection fraction. The left pane shows planimetry of the left ventricle at end-diastole which is then divided into equal sized "discs" in a semi-automated fashion. The ventricle is then measured at end-systole—if assumptions are made about the shape of the ventricle, its volume is computed at end-diastole and end-systole from which the LV ejection fraction is calculated

The normal range is 50–70%. Limitations of the technique are that it depends on good resolution of the endocardial border and that it makes geometric assumptions about the shape of the ventricle so that it can only be applied to the left ventricle and not to the right ventricle due to the complex geometric shape of the latter. The limitations with respect to the right ventricle may be overcome by the use of a 3D echocardiographic approach which is discussed later in this chapter.

Myocardial Performance Index

The M-mode and 2D planimetry methods outlined above, depend on measurement of the size of ventricular cavities to compute functional information. Thus, they depend on assumptions of ventricular shape and on the accuracy of point measurement or planimetry of the small chambers in the fetal heart.

Analysis of Doppler flow patterns has potential advantages in that they can be applied to both the left and right ventricles and are not dependent on a particular ventricular geometry. Furthermore, unlike the measurement of fractional shortening or ejection fraction, Doppler methods can provide information on both systolic and diastolic function. The myocardial performance index (MPI) or Tei index has been proposed as an index of global cardiac function because it contains measurement of both systolic and diastolic time intervals. The time intervals measured can be derived from either pulsed Doppler or tissue Doppler.

The MPI is calculated using the formula below:

$$\text{MPI} = \frac{\text{Isovolumic contraction time} + \text{Isovolumic relaxation time}}{\text{Ventricular ejection time}}$$

The index may be applied to both the right and left ventricles. For the left ventricle, if the Doppler cursor is placed between the mitral and aortic valves then both mitral inflow and aortic outflow can be visualised on the same trace (Fig. 5.9). For the right ventricle, calculation of the MPI using pulsed Doppler is more difficult because the right ventricular inflow and outflow cannot be visualised on the same trace. Thus, the inflow Doppler is used calculate the time between tricuspid valve closure and opening, and the right ventricular ejection time is calculated from the pulmonary valve Doppler. Thus, the MPI can be derived but is based on two separate Doppler traces. An alternative method is to use tissue Doppler echocardiography to calculate the MPI. The advantage of tissue Doppler is that the index can be derived on a single trace for both the right and left ventricles (Fig. 5.10). The disadvantage is that many ultrasound systems used for fetal cardiac assessment do not have this modality on cart. This technique is discussed in more detail later in this chapter. The myocardial performance index is independent of the morphology of the ventricle being studied, and is relatively easy to calculate. For time interval measurements it is not critically dependent on a particular angle of insonation. However, given that the index is derived from both systolic and diastolic parameters, the index will be impacted both by systolic and diastolic performance. Furthermore, there are concerns about reproducibility of the index and the normal ranges are not consistent between different groups of researchers (Maheshwari et al. 2015). This makes it difficult to compare results between different centres or different

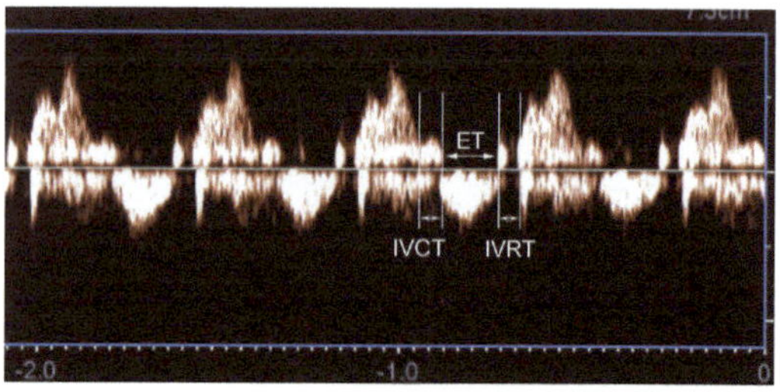

Fig. 5.9 Myocardial performance index. This figure shows the mitral inflow and aortic outflow patterns obtained with the Doppler cursor placed between the mitral and aortic valves. The E and A waves of the mitral valve inflow are shown as well as velocity of flow across the aortic valve. The measurement of the isovolumic contraction time (IVCT), ejection time (ET) and isovolumic relaxation time (IVRT) are illustrated. These three time intervals permit calculation of the myocardial performance index (IVCT + IVRT/ET). Abbreviations: *IVCT* isovolumic contraction time, *IVRT* isovolumic relaxation time, *ET* ejection time

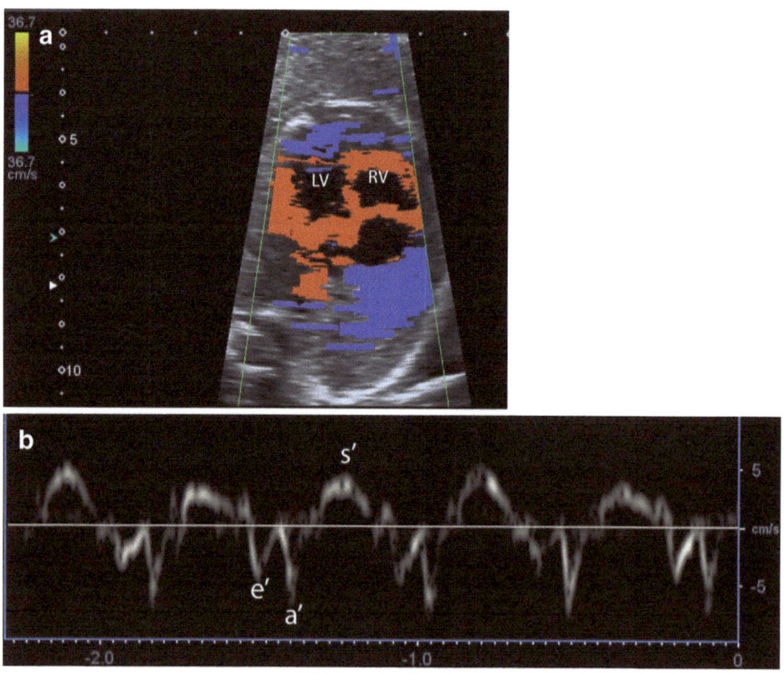

Fig. 5.10 (**a**, **b**) Tissue Doppler Imaging. Colour tissue Doppler (**a**) encodes the mean velocity of the myocardium. The myocardium appears coloured whereas the blood pool is black. Pulsed tissue Doppler imaging samples myocardial velocities at a given point. In the example in (**b**) (right pane), the cursor was placed at the mitral valve annulus. The s' velocity relates to ventricular contraction and the e' and a' waves relate to myocardial velocity during early diastole and late diastole respectively. The time intervals can be measured to calculate the myocardial performance index in an analogous manner to pulsed Doppler

observers. For the left ventricular MPI most studies report a normal range somewhere between 0.3 and 0.45 but with considerable variation between studies and gestation-related trends. To address issues of observer variability, automated means of calculating the MPI are being introduced.

Echocardiographic Assessment of Diastolic Function

The dominant modality for the assessment of diastolic function in the fetus is pulsed wave Doppler. This is most commonly applied at the level of the atrioventricular valves but is also extensively used to interrogate the pulmonary and systemic veins (caval veins, hepatic veins, ductus venosus and umbilical vein).

Atrioventricular valve inflow patterns are characterised by a biphasic flow pattern. A normal mitral valve inflow pattern is shown in Fig. 5.5a. In contrast to postnatal life the early E wave has a lower velocity than the A wave. With advancing gestational age the E wave becomes higher velocity and the A wave velocity changes less so that the E/A ratio increases with gestation. In the fetus with diastolic dysfunction the inflow time typically shortens and there is an abnormal monophasic inflow pattern (Fig. 5.5b).

The inferior vena cava is relatively difficult to interrogate because a number of different venous channels converge into this vein including the hepatic veins and the ductus venosus. For this reason, the hepatic veins and ductus venosus are more commonly assessed separately (Fig. 5.11a–d). The ductus venosus has typical systolic and diastolic peaks with a reduction in velocity coincident with atrial contraction. If there is diastolic dysfunction of the right ventricle and/or abnormal loading conditions of the right heart, reversal of flow in the ductus venosus coincident with atrial contraction may

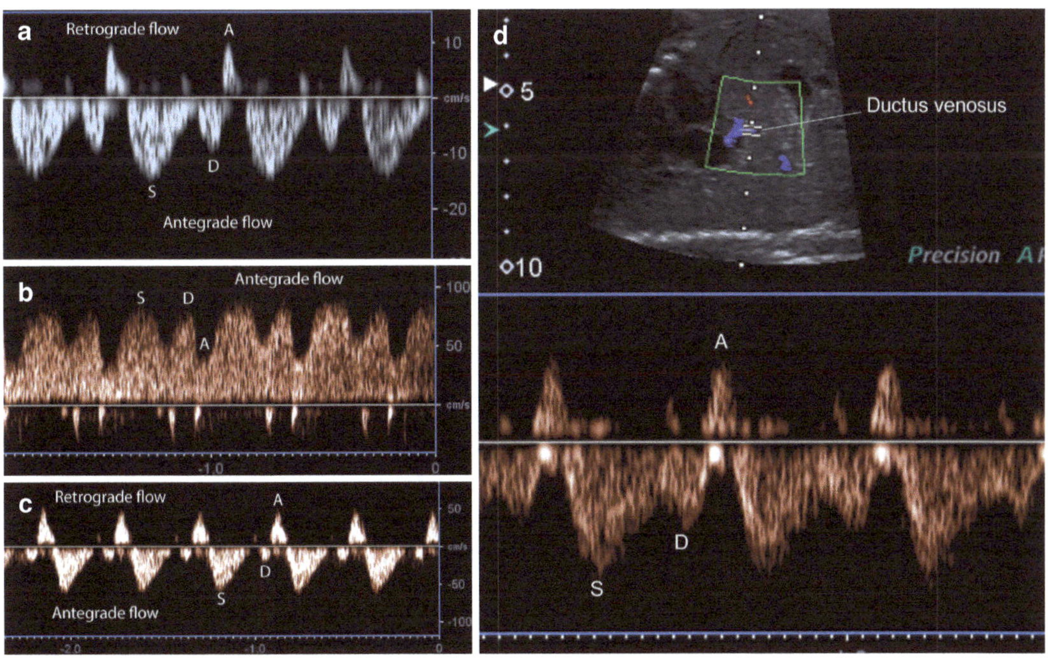

Fig. 5.11 (**a**, **b**) Doppler interrogation of normal hepatic vein and ductus venosus flow. In (**a**) the Doppler cursor has been placed in the hepatic veins. Flow into the right atrium is shown below the baseline and retrograde flow above. During ventricular systole there is flow into the right atrium but this flow reverses when the atrium contracts. Pane (**b**) shows normal flow in the ductus venosus which flows towards the heart during ventricular systole (S) and early diastole (D) with a reduced velocity of antegrade flow coincident with atrial contraction (A). (**c**, **d**) Doppler interrogation of abnormal hepatic venous (**c**) and ductus venosus flow (**d**). In the Doppler cursor has been placed in the hepatic veins. Flow into the right atrium is shown below the baseline and retrograde flow above. During ventricular systole there is flow into the right atrium but this flow reverses when the atrium contracts. The right pane shows flow in the ductus venosus which flows towards the heart during ventricular systole (S) and early diastole (D). There is reversal of flow when the atrium contracts (A)

Table 5.2 The cardiovascular profile score

Category	2 points	1 point	0 points
Hydrops	None	Ascites or pericardial or pleural effusion	Skin edema
Heart size (HA/CA)	>0.2 and ≤0.35	0.35–0.5	<0.2 or >0.5
Cardiac function	Normal MV and TV, biphasic diastolic filling, LV or RV SFs >0.28	Holosystolic TR or LV or RV SFs <0.28	Holosystolic MR or TR dP/dt < 400, monophasic diastolic filling
Arterial umbilical Doppler	Normal	AEDV	REDV
Venous Doppler	Normal	DV atrial reversal	UV pulsations

AEDV absent end-diastolic velocity, *DV* ductus venosus, *HA/CA* heart to chest area ratio, *LV* left ventricle, *MR* mitral valve regurgitation, *MV* mitral valve, *REDV* reversed end-diastolic velocity, *RV* right ventricle, *SF* ventricular shortening fraction, TR dP/dt change in pressure over time of TR jet, *TR* tricuspid valve regurgitation, *TV* tricuspid valve, *UV* umbilical vein. (Reproduced with permission from Wieczorek 2008)

occur (Fig. 5.11d). The hepatic veins may also be interrogated. These show flow towards the right atrium during ventricular systole and early diastole. If right atrial pressure is elevated then reversal of flow occurs with atrial contraction and becomes more pronounced as atrial pressure rises (Fig. 5.11c).

Integration of Different Techniques

One of the challenges in the assessment of fetal cardiac function is how information derived from M-mode, cross-sectional and Doppler imaging techniques can be integrated to give a composite score and whether such scoring is valid. One scoring system which has gained popularity is the cardiovascular profile score (Wieczorek et al. 2008) which gives a score of 0–2 for each of the following categories: presence of hydrops, heart size (cardiothoracic ratio), Doppler ventricular filling pattern/fractional shortening, umbilical arterial Doppler flow pattern and venous Doppler (Ductus venosus or umbilical vein). This leads to an overall score out of 10 with lower values indicating more severe ventricular dysfunction. The components of this score are illustrated in Table 5.2.

Advanced Echocardiographic Techniques for Evaluation of Cardiac Function

Three-Dimensional Imaging

3D echocardiography has been used to calculate right and left ventricular volumes, ejection fraction and cardiac output. There are two major techniques for acquisition of 3D data which are (1) spatio-temporal image correlation (STIC) (Simioni et al. 2011) and (2) real-time 3D echocardiography which utilises “matrix” transducers. STIC image acquisition involves a sweep of a cross-sectional ultrasound beam through the region of interest. The size of the acquired area and time to acquire the sweep (typically 5–15 s) is user-defined. Once the data has been acquired the STIC algorithm permits visualisation of a single cardiac cycle of 3D data which can be interrogated either through cross sectional slices or as a 3D rendered image. The exact configuration varies between manufacturers but includes generation of multiple slices which can be measured to calculate ventricular volumes, or else a semi-automated 3D “cast” of the ventricular cavity can be displayed along with the computed volume. It is important to recognise that the composite cardiac cycle displayed has never truly existed but is composed of multiple closely sequential 2D slices obtained at the time of STIC acquisition. A limitation of the technique includes the relatively long time to acquire the data so that fetal movement artefact remains a significant challenge. Real-time 3D echocardiography systems utilise “matrix” array transducers which consist of multiple rows of piezoelectric elements which send and receive simultaneously to produce a real-time 3D image of the region of interest. This technique can also be used to compute ventricular volumes and ejection fraction. Whatever technique is employed it is important to understand the difference in geometry of the left and right ventricles. The left ventricle has a cone shape which lends itself readily to 3D rendering and geometric assumptions. The same is not true of the right ventricle which has a more complex shape and effectively "wraps around" the left ventricle. In current practice, these techniques remain largely confined to a research setting rather than routine clinical practice.

Tissue Doppler Imaging

Tissue Doppler imaging (TDI) encodes velocity of motion of the myocardium rather than the blood pool (Fig. 5.10a, b). Myocardial motion can be interrogated using a sample volume placed in the myocardium in an analogous manner to than employed for pulsed wave Doppler interrogation of blood flow. This displays the myocardial velocity in early diastole (e'), late diastole (a') and systole (s') (Fig. 5.10b). An alternative is to employ colour encoded tissue Doppler which displays the mean velocity of the myocardium using a similar red/blue colour encoding as colour flow Doppler of blood flow (Fig. 5.10a) (Comas and Crispi 2012). Normal ranges are available for each of these techniques which change with advancing gestational age. It is important to recognise that pulsed and colour encoded tissue Doppler velocities cannot be used interchangeably because the pulsed Doppler technique measures peak velocity whereas the colour tissue Doppler encodes mean velocity. Advantages of the TDI technique include assessment of longitudinal function of the myocardium (from apex to base) which is a sensitive marker of myocardial function, and high sampling rate. Disadvantages include angle dependency of myocardial velocities so that use of the technique may be precluded by a difficult fetal lie where the Doppler cursor cannot be accurately aligned to the direction of myocardial motion. Interrogation of colour TDI is offline which increases the time for analysis and TDI may not be included with many ultrasound systems particularly for curvilinear probes used to image the fetal heart. In addition to measurement of myocardial velocity, TDI can be used instead of pulsed wave Doppler for the calculation of the myocardial performance index. The time intervals measures to compute this index include the ejection time (duration of the s' wave), isovolumic contraction time and isovolumic relaxation time in an analogous manner to the pulsed Doppler method. These time intervals are less angle dependent than measurement of velocities but can still be prone to observer error.

Speckle Tracking (2D Strain) Techniques

In recent years, there has been considerable interest in the application of speckle tracking techniques for the quantification of deformation of the fetal myocardium. These techniques track the unique speckle pattern of the myocardium on the standard greyscale images of the fetal heart (Germanakis and Gardiner 2012). This allows tracking of the change of the length of myocardium as it contracts during systole and relaxes during diastole. The application of this technique is illustrated in Fig. 5.12a, b (Video 5.5). The technique has the major advantage of being angle-independent and thus overcomes the challenge of a highly variable fetal position. Furthermore, analysis of the greyscale image of standard imaging planes using a semi-automated process means that operators do not require extensive training in data acquisition and post-processing is relatively rapid and repeatable. The major variable measured by the technique is myocardial strain. Strain is calculated by the following formula:

$$\text{Strain}(\%) = \frac{\text{Final length of myocardium} - \text{original length of myocardium} \times 100}{\text{Original length of myocardium}}$$

There are three types of strain including deformation from apex to base of the heart (longitudinal strain), change in thickness of the myocardium (radial strain) and deforma-

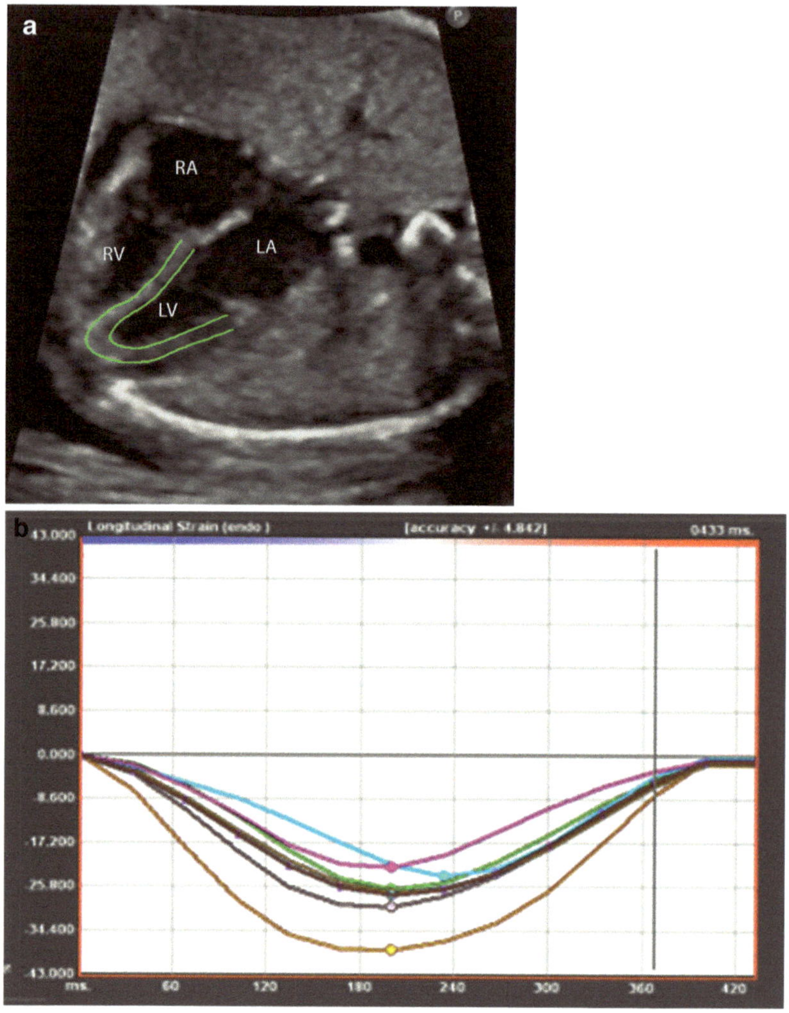

Fig. 5.12 (**a**, **b**) Speckle tracking (2D strain). The upper pane shows a four chamber view with the myocardium delineated by the green lines. The unique speckle pattern of the myocardium is tracked through the cardiac cycle so that the deformation of the myocardium is quantified. The pane below shows the longitudinal strain. By convention shortening of the myocardium is given a negative value. The colours represent the different segments of the myocardium so that regional as well as global information is provided

tion in a circumferential orientation (circumferential strain). For the most part, during fetal life, longitudinal strain is measured because it tends to become abnormal first and is therefore a sensitive marker of disease. Radial strain is difficult to measure because the fetal myocardium is so thin and it is difficult to consistently reproduce the same short axis cut plane to accurately measure circumferential strain. The disadvantages of the technique include variation between different ultrasound systems and debate about the potential impact of variables such as frame rate. The application of the technique is typically in specialist centres rather than routine sonographic assessment.

Measurement of Fetal Cardiac Output

The fundamental role of the fetal heart is to perfuse tissues to permit normal metabolism, growth and development. Measurement of cardiac output is fundamental to the assessment of the fetal circulation.

Echocardiographic Methods

Doppler echocardiography has been the most widely employed technique for the measurement of fetal cardiac output. Normal ranges for the right, left and combined ventricular outputs have been published. The technique involves pulsed Doppler interrogation of flow across the aortic or pulmonary valve. The Doppler trace is

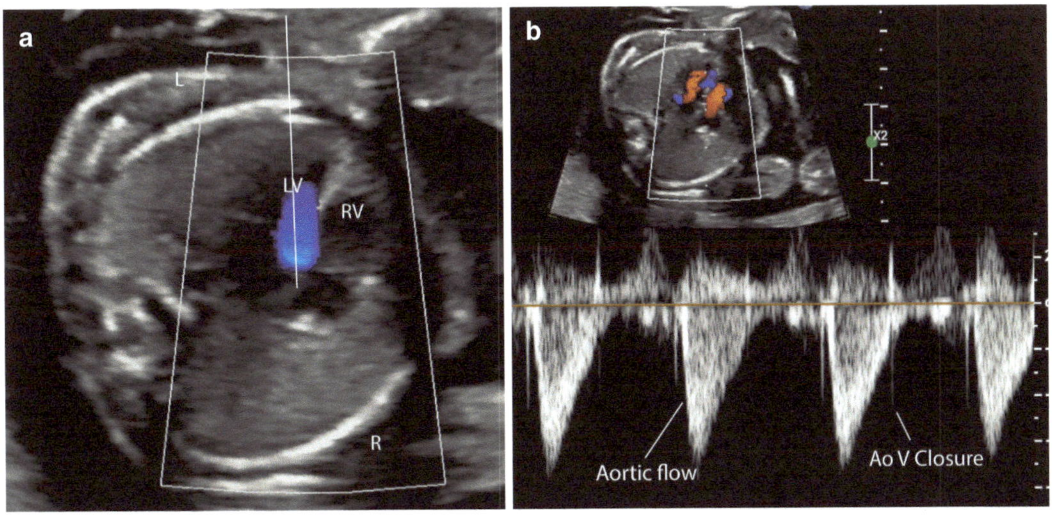

Fig. 5.13 (**a**, **b**) Doppler interrogation of aortic flow. In the left pane (**a**) the blue flow indicates flow in the left ventricular outflow tract directly away from the ultrasound probe. This is a good angle for Doppler assessment of flow. The right pane (**b**) shows pulsed Doppler of flow with the cursor placed just distal to the aortic valve. Correct placement is confirmed by the presence of aortic valve "clicks" as the aortic valve opens and closes

planimetered to calculate the velocity-time integral (stroke distance) (Fig. 5.13a, b). The diameter of the vessel through which the flow is occurring is measured so that the cross-sectional area of the vessel can be calculated.

The cardiac output is then calculated according to the formula:

$$CO = VTI \times (\pi r 2) \times HR$$

Abbreviations: CO—cardiac output, VTI—velocity time integral, r—radius of vessel, HR—heart rate.

Advantages of this method include its non-invasive nature but limitations include the need to align precisely to the direction of flow, the potential for measurement error of the vessel and assumption of laminar as opposed to turbulent flow. This means that relatively large measurement errors may occur in the estimation of cardiac output by this method.

An alternative to the measurement of flow by Doppler is to compute ventricular stroke volume by 2D or 3D echocardiography and then to multiply stroke volume by the fetal heart rate. When 2D echo is used, assumptions have to be made about the shape of the left or right ventricle which limits applicability (Fig. 5.8). 3D techniques can avoid some geometric assumptions but are not as widely used in current practice.

Fetal Cardiovascular Magnetic Resonance Imaging (CMR)

During postnatal life, CMR is the gold standard technique for measurement of ventricular volumes and flow through vessels. This is because the CMR technique allows complete visualisation of endocardial borders and a "slice by slice" means of interrogation can be used to calculate volumes independent of the shape of the ventricle. Furthermore, by precise alignment to the fetal vessels, flow in the major arteries and veins can be measured accurately. Many of the CMR sequences depend on the availability of an ECG signal to time acquisition of images (image gating) which is extremely difficult during fetal life. In very recent years, CMR has been used to calculate flow through the fetal heart in specialist centres. CMR permits accurate delineation of the size of the vessel and sampling of flow velocity though the vessel (Fig. 5.14). Normal values of right and left ventricular output by CMR during fetal life have been published as well as the methodology. In addition to calculation of blood flow,

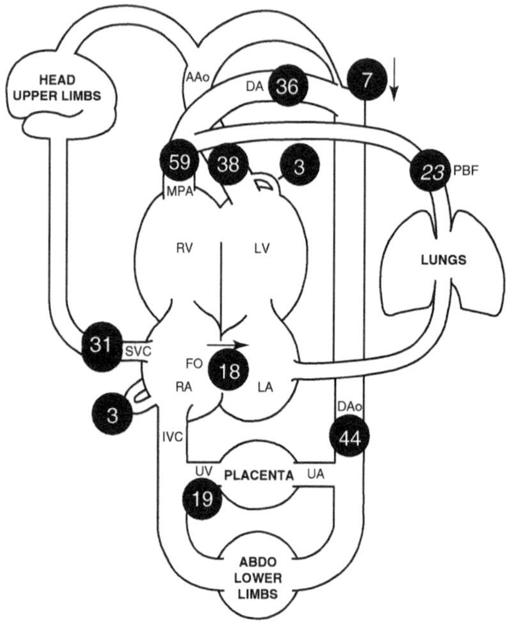

Fig. 5.14 Flow estimation by fetal cardiac magnetic resonance imaging. Phase contrast magnetic resonance imaging permits measurement of flow through the veins and arteries around the heart. This permits computation of flow volume and flow within and around the heart. This figure shows the percentage of the cardiac output passing through each region

CMR is now being employed to measure oxygen saturation non-invasively within the fetal circulation so that oxygen delivery and metabolism by different tissues can be quantified. Challenges in the use of MRI to evaluate the fetal heart include the temporal and spatial resolution of the technique, lack of an ECG signal to "gate" acquisitions and fetal motion. Currently, use of the technique is limited to specialist research centres. Nonetheless, rapid progress is being made in the application of this technique to the fetal heart which is discussed further in Chap. 11.

Management of Affected Cases

There are a huge number of fetal diseases which may impact on fetal cardiac function. A broad categorisation is shown in Table 5.3. A comprehensive discussion of the management of cases affected by functional impairment is beyond the scope of this book. The management of individual congenital heart lesions is covered in the relevant chapter and the impact of fetal arrhythmias on some aspects of functional assessment is covered in that chapter. In many instances, abnormal cardiac function may be secondary to an identifiable disease process, for example twin-twin transfusion syndrome. In such cases, treatment is generally targeted at the underlying cause. Abnormal loading conditions can cause cardiac enlargement and dysfunction. Figure 5.15 (Video 5.6) shows the increased pulmonary venous return cause by a pulmonary arteriovenous malformation.

Table 5.3 Disease states for which assessment of cardiac function is important

Congenital heart defects
Hearts which are functionally single ventricle e.g. hypoplastic left heart
Aortic valve stenosis, pulmonary valve stenosis
Absent pulmonary valve syndrome
Abdominal coarctation (rare)
Arrhythmias
Complete heart block
Tachycardias
Cardiomyopathy
Dilated cardiomyopathy
Primary heart muscle disease, inborn errors of metabolism, genetic
Non-compaction of the myocardium
Hypertrophic cardiomyopathy
Noonan syndrome, diabetes
Myocarditis
Viral myocarditis e.g. Coxsackie, Parvovirus
Abnormal loading conditions
Abnormal pressure load
Constriction of the arterial duct
Placental insufficiency
Abnormal volume loading
Fetal anaemia e.g. rhesus disease, Parvovirus infection
Volume loading
Sacrococcygeal teratoma or other tumours
Arteriovenous malformations
Agenesis of the ductus venosus
Twin-twin transfusion syndrome

Fetal dilated cardiomyopathy will typically express itself as a dilated, poorly contracting heart with atrioventricular valve regurgitation, monophasic inflow patterns and hydrops in the worst affected cases (Sivasankaran et al. 2005; Weber et al. 2014). Although fetal echocardiography shows the functional abnormality, identification of the underlying cause poses particular difficulties in diagnosis during fetal life. It is essential to exclude "pseudo cardiomyopathy" due to occult obstruction of ventricular outflow such as constriction of the arterial duct or post-ductal coarctation. Fetal anaemia should be investigated by middle cerebral artery Doppler +/− fetal blood sampling. Viral studies should be undertaken, particularly to exclude Parvovirus and Coxsackie virus infections. The family history is important as 10% of cases in the series from our centre were recurrences and should raise the possibility of an inborn error of metabolism or genetic abnormality including mitochondrial disorders. Many of these disorders may be difficult to investigate during fetal life because relevant samples of blood or tissue are difficult to obtain. The appearance of the myocardium should be carefully assessed. Deep crypts in the myocardium are diagnostic of noncompaction of the myocardium which may itself be familial (Fig. 5.16a, b, Videos 5.7 and 5.8). Parental investigation is indicated when this condition is diagnosed. There is a significant limit to the extent of investigation of inborn errors of metabolism which can be undertaken prior to birth (Sivasankaran et al. 2005; Weber et al. 2014). Some units will undertake targeted investigation based on fetal blood sampling but many will await postnatal investigation. Management of affected cases involves a multidisciplinary approach including fetal medicine specialists, clinical geneticists and specialists in metabolic disease. Careful planning is required for investigation in the neonatal period or post-mortem in the event of intra-uterine demise.

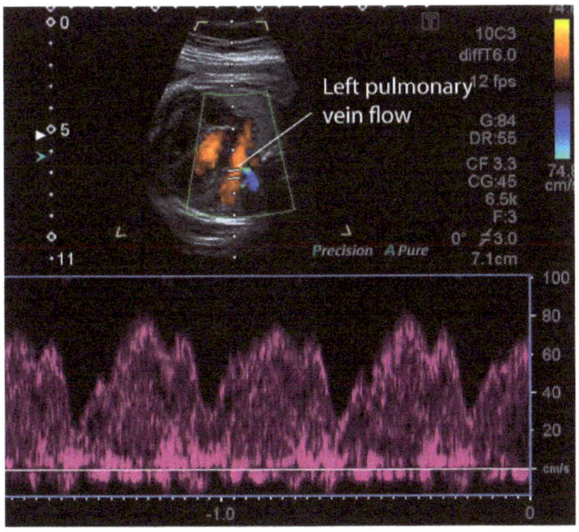

Fig. 5.15 This image shows the Doppler flow pattern in the left pulmonary veins of a fetus with a left sided pulmonary arteriovenous malformation. This caused significant cardiac enlargement. The flow velocities in the left pulmonary veins are higher than normal due to markedly increased left pulmonary venous return

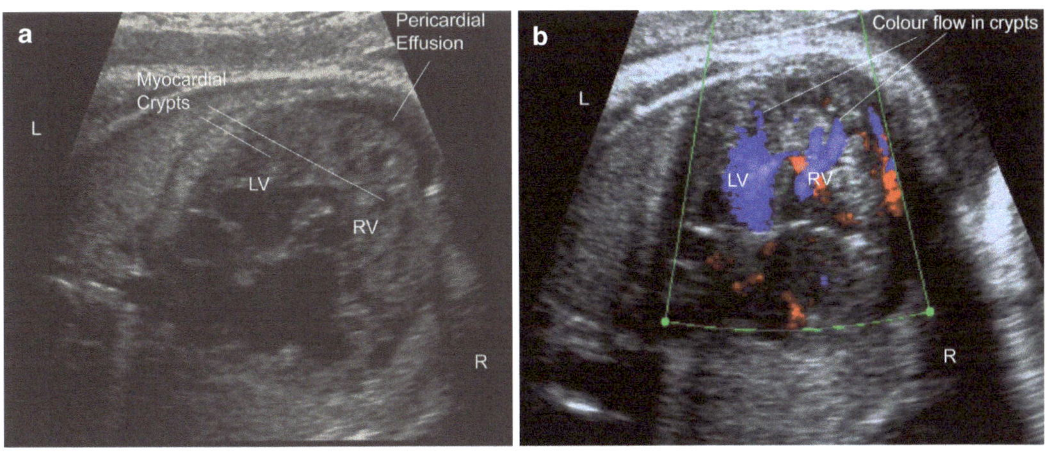

Fig. 5.16 (**a**, **b**) Noncompaction of the myocardium. The heart is enlarged. The left pane (**a**) shows deep trabeculations or "crypts" in the apical portion of the myocardium of both the left and right ventricle. There is a pericardial effusion around the apex of the heart. The right pane (**b**) shows colour flow entering the crypts in the left and right ventricular apex

References

Comas M, Crispi F. Assessment of fetal cardiac function using tissue Doppler techniques. Fetal Diagn Ther. 2012;32:30–8. https://doi.org/10.1159/000335028.

Germanakis I, Gardiner H. Assessment of fetal myocardial deformation using speckle tracking techniques. Fetal Diagn Ther. 2012;32:39–46. https://doi.org/10.1159/000330378.

Godfrey ME, Messing B, Cohen SM, Valsky DV, Yagel S. Functional assessment of the fetal heart: a review. Ultrasound Obstet Gynecol. 2012;39:131–44. https://doi.org/10.1002/uog.9064.

Hunter LE, Simpson JM. Prenatal screening for structural congenital heart disease. Nat Rev Cardiol. 2014;11:323–34. https://doi.org/10.1038/nrcardio.2014.34.

Kiserud T, Acharya G. The fetal circulation. Prenat Diagn. 2004;24:1049–59. https://doi.org/10.1002/pd.1062.

Maheshwari P, Henry A, Welsh AW. The fetal modified myocardial performance index: is automation the future? Biomed Res Int. 2015;2015:1–9. https://doi.org/10.1155/2015/215910.

Michelfelder E, Allen C, Urbinelli L. Evaluation and management of fetal cardiac function and heart failure. Curr Treat Options Cardiovasc Med. 2016;18:55. https://doi.org/10.1007/s11936-016-0477-3.

Simioni C, Nardozza LMM, Araujo Júnior E, Rolo LC, Zamith M, Caetano AC, Moron AF. Heart stroke volume, cardiac output, and ejection fraction in 265 normal fetus in the second half of gestation assessed by 4D ultrasound using spatio-temporal image correlation. J Matern Fetal Neonatal Med. 2011;24:1159–67. https://doi.org/10.3109/14767058.2010.545921.

Simpson J. Echocardiographic evaluation of cardiac function in the fetus. Prenat Diagn. 2004;24:1081–91. https://doi.org/10.1002/pd.1065.

Sivasankaran S, Sharland GK, Simpson JM. Dilated cardiomyopathy presenting during fetal life. Cardiol Young. 2005;15:409–16. https://doi.org/10.1017/S1047951105000855.

Van Mieghem T, DeKoninck P, Steenhaut P, Deprest J. Methods for prenatal assessment of fetal cardiac function. Prenat Diagn. 2009;29:1193–203. https://doi.org/10.1002/pd.2379.

Weber R, Kantor P, Chitayat D, Friedberg MK, Golding F, Mertens L, Nield LE, Ryan G, Seed M, Yoo S-J, Manlhiot C, Jaeggi E. Spectrum and outcome of primary cardiomyopathies diagnosed during fetal life. JACC Heart Fail. 2014;2:403–11. https://doi.org/10.1016/j.jchf.2014.02.010.

Wieczorek A, Hernandez-Robles J, Ewing L, Leshko J, Luther S, Huhta J. Prediction of outcome of fetal congenital heart disease using a cardiovascular profile score. Ultrasound Obstet Gynecol. 2008;31:284–8. https://doi.org/10.1002/uog.5177.

6 First Trimester Fetal Echocardiography

Vita Zidere

Abstract

First trimester fetal echocardiography was introduced two decades ago. This service is usually available in specialist fetal medicine units but it is not included in routine prenatal screening programs. Early fetal heart assessment is important as it can provide early reassurance or diagnosis of a cardiac abnormality which may potentially instigate further investigation. First trimester fetal echocardiography also provides an insight into the early features and progression of certain forms of congenital heart disease (CHD). In this chapter, the technique of early fetal echocardiography, and first trimester sonographic markers for possible CHD are presented.

Keywords

Congenital heart disease · Fetal heart · First trimester · Evolution · First trimester markers of congenital heart disease

Electronic Supplementary Material The online version of this chapter (https://doi.org/10.1007/978-3-319-77461-9_6) contains supplementary material, which is available to authorized users.

V. Zidere
Evelina London Children's Hospital, Guy's and St Thomas' NHS Foundation Trust, London, UK

King's College Hospital NHS Foundation Trust, London, UK
e-mail: vita.zidere@gstt.nhs.uk

Introduction

With major improvements in ultrasound technology, detailed first trimester fetal echocardiography assessment is now possible. This can be performed transabdominally as early as 11 weeks gestation (Zidere et al. 2013).

An advantage of performing an early cardiac scan is the chance to provide some reassurance of normality to the patient or where there is an abnormality, to allow early counselling. Early cardiac examination is indicated particularly where there is a suspicion of a heart abnormality at the first trimester nuchal translucency scan or where there has been a previous pregnancy affected by major CHD, for example hypoplastic left heart syndrome. First trimester fetal cardiac assessment should be considered for fetuses with significantly increased nuchal translucency (above 99th centile or 3.5 mm) due to the high prevalence of cardiac abnormalities in this group (Hyett et al. 1997). The exact timing of early fetal echocardiography varies between units—at our centre this is typically offered at 13–14 weeks gestational age or earlier if CHD is suspected on an early scan for NT measurement.

The detection rate of cardiac abnormalities in the first trimester will depend on the local policy for timing of assessment of fetal cardiac anatomy and local expertise. At our own tertiary fetal medicine centre when nuchal translucency scans are performed, a four-chamber view, great

© Springer International Publishing AG, part of Springer Nature 2018

J. Simpson et al. (eds.), *Fetal Cardiology*, https://doi.org/10.1007/978-3-319-77461-9_6

arteries and three vessel trachea view is obtained both in grey scale and with colour Doppler imaging. No attempt is made to establish details of pulmonary or systemic venous drainage or other more subtle features. This approach permits early detection of major cardiac abnormities in the first trimester.

Limitations

If an 11–12 week fetal cardiac evaluation is not possible due to fetal size or an unfavourable fetal position, a repeat scan at 14 weeks maybe more conclusive as a result of growth.

With specialist early fetal echocardiography the main connections of the heart can usually be identified although such scanning is well-recognised to be technically challenging. Some types of cardiac abnormality may be overlooked in early pregnancy, even in experienced hands, for example abnormalities of the pulmonary veins or some types of ventricular septal defect. The identifiable structures of the fetal heart at 12–14 weeks are summarised in Table 6.1.

Conditions such as congenital complete heart block, cardiomyopathies and cardiac tumours do not usually become evident until later in pregnancy. Pulmonary valve and aortic valve stenosis are evolving conditions and therefore may become apparent or more severe as the pregnancy progresses (Zidere et al. 2013). Thus, sequential fetal echocardiography is indicated when these forms of CHD are diagnosed early in pregnancy.

A high degree of accuracy in the identification of CHD can be achieved by early fetal echocardiography specialist centres (Zidere et al. 2013). Early detection of CHD will clearly influence parental decision making, particularly for major fetal cardiac abnormalities. Furthermore, early recognition of associated anomalies may be prompted by diagnosis of CHD in the first trimester. For continuing pregnancies affected by CHD, later assessment in the second trimester remains vital to check for more subtle abnormalities, gauging of progression and ongoing discussion with the parents.

Table 6.1 Echocardiographic features which can be assessed at 12–14 weeks by specialist fetal cardiologist

2D-mode	Colour mapping	Comment
Position and size of the heart	Not applicable	Apex anterior and leftward
Four chamber view	Symmetrical filling of ventricles	Balanced size of ventricles
Atrioventricular valves	With or without regurgitation	Mild TR may be normal variant
Interventricular septum	Absence of colour flow crossing septum	Normal findings do not 100% exclude VSDs
Centre of the heart, "offsetting"	Not applicable	Offsetting of valves may be difficult to confirm
Left outflow tract, aorta and transverse arch	Antegrade or reverse flow	Aorta committed to left ventricle
Right outflow tract, pulmonary artery and arterial duct	Antegrade or reverse flow	Normal anteroposterior orientation of right ventricular outflow tract
Head and neck vessels	Antegrade flow	May be difficult to visualise, use of low velocity colour scales
Pulmonary veins	Flow towards left atrium	May be difficult to visualise, use of low velocity colour scales
Cardiac situs Position of abdominal vessels/stomach	Pulsatile flow in descending aorta Flow in inferior vena cava	

Technique

Advanced high-resolution ultrasound systems allow transabdominal assessment of the fetal heart rather than a transvaginal approach. This technique is extensively used by fetal medicine specialists and paediatric cardiologists, although some may prefer a transvaginal scan when the heart is examined at the time of the first trimester nuchal scan.

The main structures are assessed by means of conventional two-dimensional echocardiography using dedicated first trimester fetal heart ultrasound settings. These settings use a high frequency ultrasound, most commonly utilising harmonic imaging and with a narrow image sector which is zoomed to optimise both spatial and temporal resolution. The use of colour flow Doppler mapping enables easier visualisation of filling of the chambers and direction of flow in the great arteries in a small heart.

Although the fetal heart is small in the first trimester, the principles of echocardiography are the same as at second trimester. Accurate diagnosis of CHD depends on a systematic sequential assessment of all the heart connections in an analogous manner to the second trimester. With advances in ultrasound technology, image quality has move closer to that achievable in the second trimester but the resolution of ultrasound still means that some findings may not be clear until later in gestation. Some major themes or patterns are described below, but this does not substitute for sequential assessment as described in Chap. 2.

Cardiac Situs and Four Chamber View

The location of the apex of the heart and the stomach should be assessed. The normal position of the stomach and the heart is on the left side of the fetus and any variation in this should raise the suspicion of laterality disturbance (isomerism), particularly when the heart and stomach are on opposite sides This is described in Chap. 10. The standard four-chamber view is visualised to assess heart size, position, chamber sizes and the crux (Fig. 6.1, Video 6.1). In addition, patency of both atrioventricular valves and the relative size of both ventricles is assessed by means of colour flow Doppler (Fig. 6.2, Video 6.1). The position of the heart within the chest should be identified. The heart occupies 1/3 of the chest with its angle of around 50° (McBrien et al. 2013) at 11–14 weeks. Any deviation from normal should raise a suspicion of either CHD or an extracardiac anomaly such as diaphragmatic hernia. Some forms of CHD such as common arterial trunk, tetralogy of Fallot and its variations may exhibit leftward rotation of the heart (Smith et al. 1995).

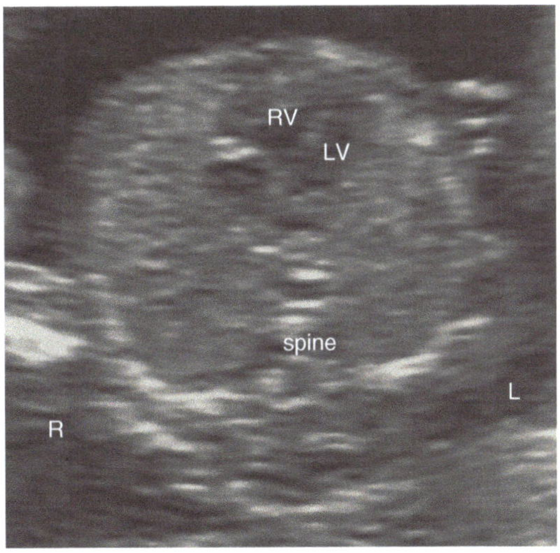

Fig. 6.1 The heart is seen in an apical four-chamber view. It occupies about one-third of the thorax. If the angle between the interventricular septum and the midline of the thorax is measured, the normal value at first trimester is about 50°. The two atriums and ventricles are seen in transverse cut. The atria and ventricles are equal cavity size. There is a subtle 'off-setting' of the atrioventricular valves as the septal leaflet of the tricuspid valve is inserted lower in the ventricular septum than the mitral valve. The ventricular septum appears intact from apex to crux. This is a normal four-chamber appearance in the first trimester

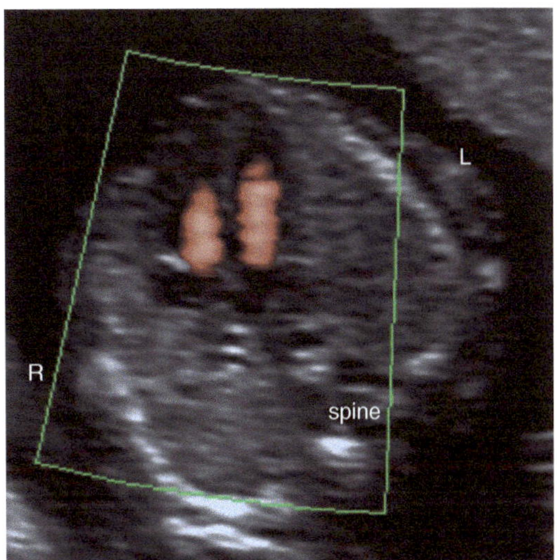

Fig. 6.2 In this transverse plane, the fetal heart is seen in an apical four-chamber view at 13 weeks gestation. Colour flow Doppler demonstrates equal ventricular filing of the left and right ventricles

Abnormalities of the Four-Chamber View

Loss of the normal crux of the heart is consistent with a diagnosis of an atrioventricular septal defect (Fig. 6.3, Video 6.2). It should be emphasised that some subtle varieties of this abnormality may be overlooked at this early stage of pregnancy. Absence of offsetting of the atrioventricular valves may be seen in some types of ventricular septal defects, but lack of offsetting may be very difficult to visualise at an early gestation.

The presence of asymmetry of the size of the ventricles should raise the suspicion of underlying CHD. In this assessment it is crucial to have good orientation to the four chamber plane because otherwise a false impression of asymmetry may be created. It is important to determine whether one ventricle is larger than normal or the other ventricle is smaller than normal to assist in differential diagnosis. Colour flow Doppler is also valuable to confirm patency of the atrioventricular valves and detect regurgitation of these valves. For example, tricuspid valve dysplasia or Ebstein's anomaly (Fig. 6.4a, Video 6.3), leads to enlargement of the right ventricle and right atrium due to regurgitation of the tricuspid valve. The left heart structures are "compressed" leading to an asymmetrical appearance. Assessment of the flow pattern across the mitral valve and presence of significant tricuspid regurgitation taking its origin from an apically displaced tricuspid valve (Fig. 6.4b, c) allows accurate diagnosis of this lesion.

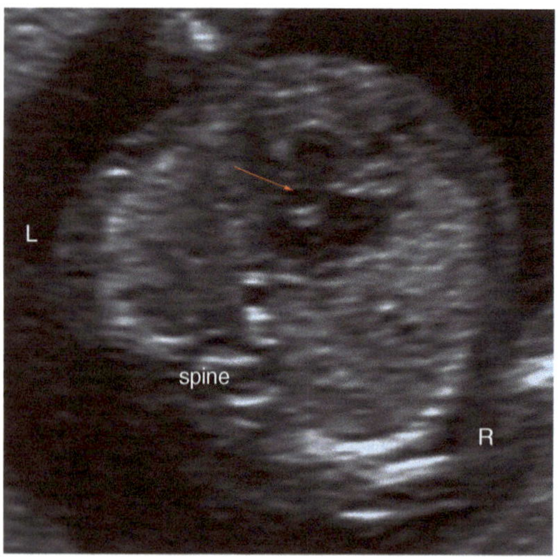

Fig. 6.3 This is an apical four-chamber view demonstrating a complete atrioventricular septal defect (red arrow) as there is loss of offsetting of the atrioventricular valves. The primum atrial septum is not extending to the atrioventricular junction

Asymmetry of the heart with a dominant right side and underdevelopment of the left ventricle can have a number of causes, this is described in Chap. 7. Flow into both the left and right ventricles should be assessed with colour flow Doppler.

If there is little or no flow into a hypoplastic left ventricle, this indicates mitral stenosis or atresia which is usually part of hypoplastic left heart syndrome (Fig. 6.5a–c). In other cases, there may be asymmetry of ventricular size (right dominant) but with no evidence of obstruction to left ventricular inflow. In such cases, there is typically asymmetry of great arterial size with hypoplasia of the aortic arch raising a suspicion of coarctation of the aorta. Such asymmetry is also observed in fetuses with underlying aneuploidy such as 45XO.

Cardiac asymmetry with dominance of the left ventricle and hypoplasia of the right ventricle is most commonly indicative of tricuspid atresia or pulmonary atresia with an intact ventricular septum. In this situation, the colour Doppler will prove that there is no flow/minimal flow across the tricuspid valve. Major four-chamber abnormalities commonly seen at first trimester are summarised in Table 6.2.

First Trimester Abnormalities of the Great Arteries

In some major congenital heart disease, for example tetralogy of Fallot and transposition of the great arteries, the four-chamber view is normal and the diagnosis is made only by examining the great arteries. This group of abnormalities can be diagnosed in the first trimester by careful examination of the outflow tracts.

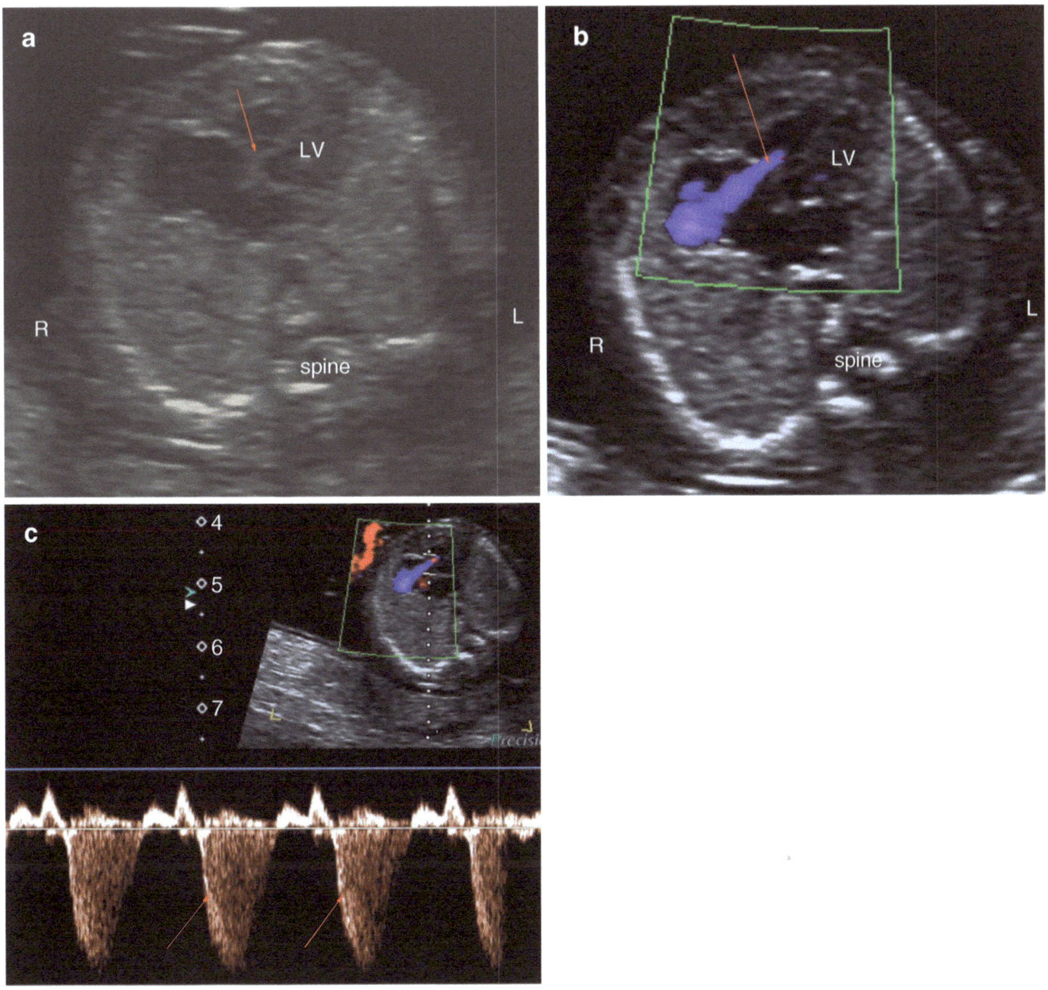

Fig. 6.4 (**a**) Transverse plane at the four-chamber view demonstrates asymmetry due to enlargement of the right atrium and right ventricle. In this view, there does appear to be normal offsetting of the tricuspid and mitral valves. (**b**) Colour Doppler demonstrates regurgitation of the tricuspid valve (red arrow). Note that the origin of the regurgitant jet is well into the right ventricle, consistent with displacement of the tricuspid valve. The displacement of the TV became increasingly evident later in gestation. (**c**) Pulsed Doppler shows holosystolic tricuspid regurgitation (red arrows) at a velocity of 138 cm/s obtained in apical four–chamber view at the level of tricuspid valve at 14 weeks gestation

The great arteries, aortic arch and arterial duct (Figs. 6.6, 6.7a, b and 6.8) can be examined by a gentle continuous sweep towards the fetal head from the four-chamber plane. As in the second trimester the great arteries are of equal size. It is essential to recognise normal relationships of the great arteries. The presence and position of the "V" sign (Fig. 6.9, Video 6.4) formed by the ductal and aortic arches must be recognised. Optimised colour flow Doppler may assist in identifying the arteries. Flow velocities in the great arteries are lower in the first trimester than second trimester. Therefore, colour scales need to be adjusted, typically to around 30–40 cm/s.

If only one great artery is seen, this usually indicates that the other great artery is smaller

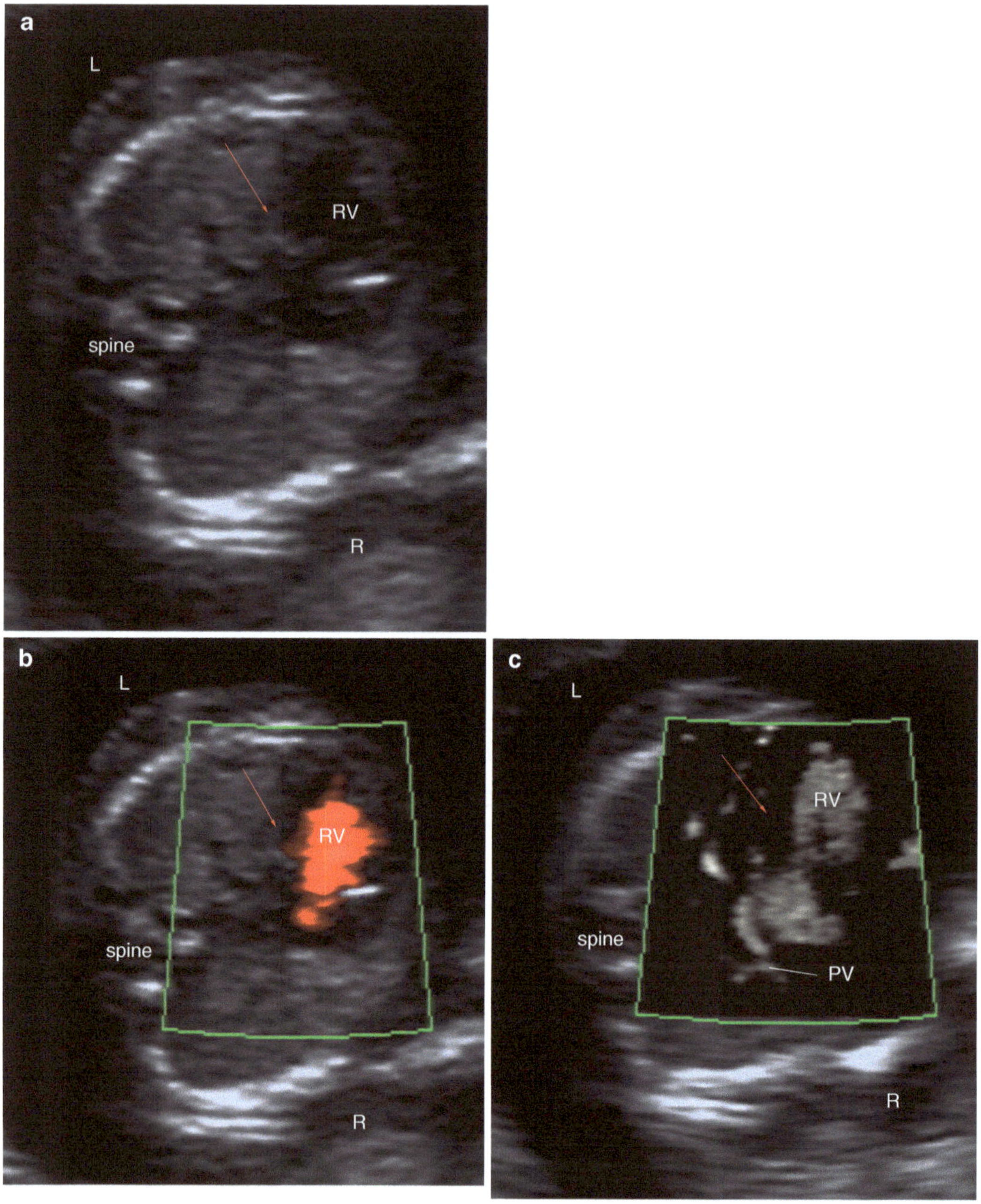

Fig. 6.5 (**a**) The heart is seen in an apical four-chamber view at 13 weeks gestation. There is only one atrioventricular valve and one ventricle seen on the right side on 2D-mode. There is no patent atrioventricular valve or ventricle seen on the left side (red arrow). (**b**) The colour Doppler demonstrates filling only in one, right ventricle. This is an example of mitral atresia (red arrow). (**c**) Superb microvascular imaging reinforces the findings demonstrating no filing in the left ventricle (red arrow) and only a single inflow to the right ventricle

Table 6.2 Differential diagnosis of potential major cardiac abnormalities seen in four-chamber view 2D-Mode and with Colour Doppler at first trimester scan

2D-mode	Colour mapping	Likely diagnosis
Equal size chambers and patent atrio-ventricular valves	Equal width and length of ventricular filling	Normal[a]
Asymmetry (left ventricle < right ventricle mitral valve < tricuspid valve aorta < pulmonary artery)	Asymmetrical filling (left ventricle < right ventricle)	Coarctation of the aorta
Symmetrical or asymmetrical ventricles but no offsetting and abnormal crux of the heart	Equal or asymmetrical filing; atrio-ventricular valve regurgitation	Atrioventricular septal defect
Only one atrio-ventricular opening on the right	No flow across the left atrio-ventricular valve	Mitral valve atresia (HLHS)
Only one atrio-ventricular opening on the left	No flow across the right atrio-ventricular valve	Tricuspid valve atresia or Pulmonary artery atresia with intact ventricular septum
Stomach and heart in discrepant positions or heart and stomach on the right	Absence of IVC draining into the right atrium and/or parallel vessel posterior to the descending aorta in sagittal view (in left isomerism only)	Likely laterality disturbance, isomerism (heterotaxy)
Persistently slow heart rate		Sinus bradycardia (possible long QT syndrome) or complete heart block as in left isomerism
Persistently fast heart rate		Sinus tachycardia or supraventricular tachycardia

[a]Note that normal four-chamber view will not exclude all VSDs

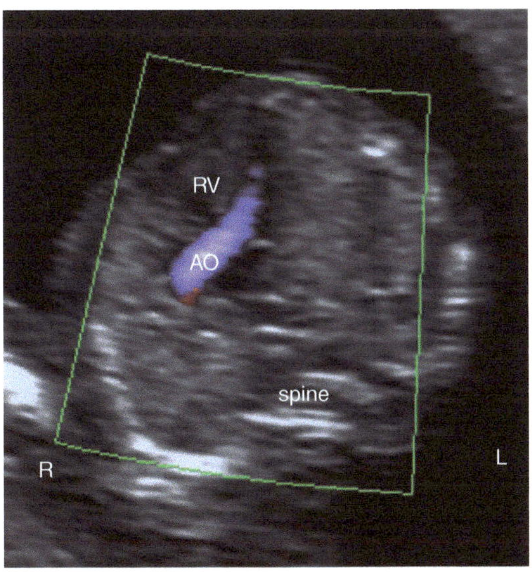

Fig. 6.6 Slight angulation cranially from the four–chamber view reveals the left ventricular outflow tract arising from the left ventricle on colour flow Doppler

than normal or even absent. The differential diagnosis includes common arterial trunk, aortic atresia or pulmonary atresia. These can be differentiated by the position, size and flow pattern of the great artery. A large and easily visible main pulmonary artery with no obvious aorta is typical of aortic atresia or a severe coarctation. Reversal of flow in the aortic arch on colour flow Doppler provides supportive evidence of severe left ventricular outflow tract obstruction. A large aorta with a small or no pulmonary artery identified is likely to represent severe pulmonary stenosis or atresia. Reversed flow in the arterial duct may be seen. In common arterial trunk, there is a single arterial outlet arising from the middle of the heart which typically overrides the ventricular septum. The pulmonary arteries arise from the trunk and demonstrate pulsatile antegrade flow. Stenosis and regurgitation of the

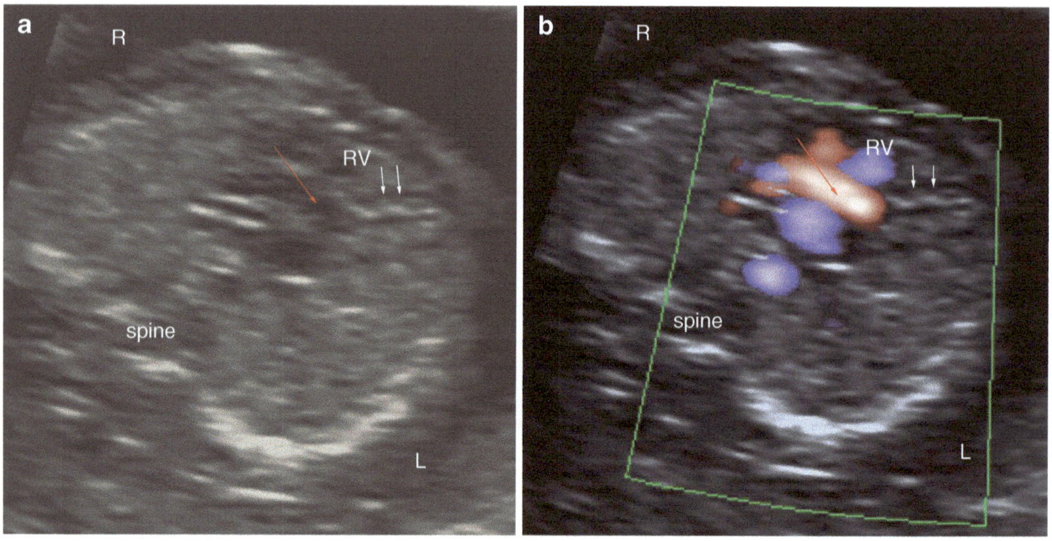

Fig. 6.7 (**a**) The transverse cut in 2D-mode demonstrates the left ventricular outflow tract (red arrow). The anterior wall of the aorta is in continuity with interventricular septum (white arrows) and the posterior wall is in continuity with the mitral valve. (**b**) Colour Doppler confirms antegrade (red arrow) flow in normal sized aorta

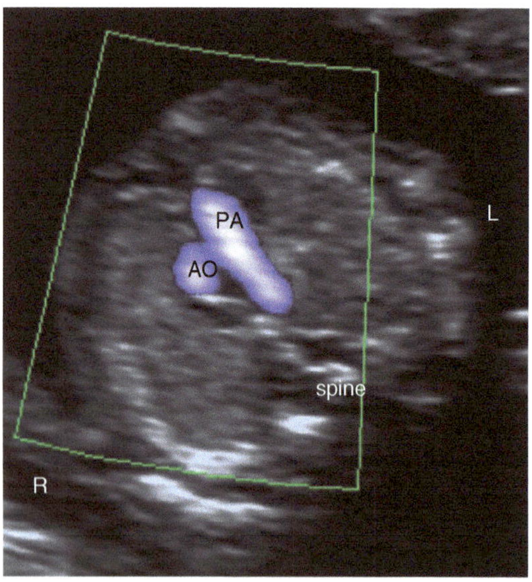

Fig. 6.8 This is a transverse plane using a colour flow Doppler at the level of the three-vessel view demonstrating the anteroposterior direction of the pulmonary artery in continuity with the arterial duct. The ascending aorta is shown in short axis. Both arteries have antegrade flow

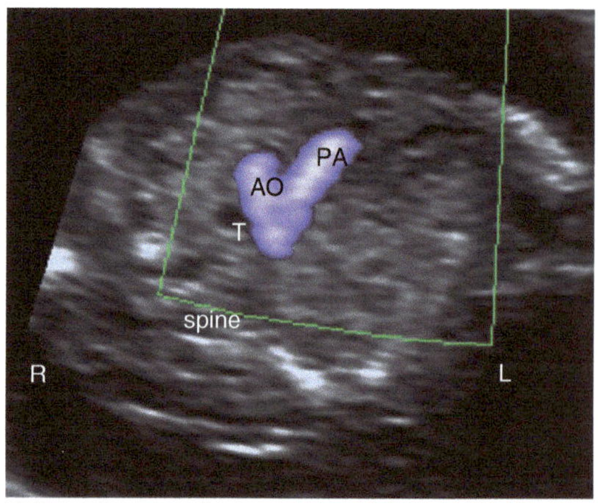

Fig. 6.9 First trimester three vessel—trachea view. In this transverse cut using colour flow Doppler, the transverse aortic arch and the pulmonary artery meet in a "V" shape anterior to the trachea. Both arteries have antegrade flow and appear equal in size

truncal valve frequently accompanies this diagnosis and can be confirmed by colour flow and pulsed wave Doppler.

If the great arteries have lost their normal "crossover" relationship and the normal "V" sign cannot be seen in the three-vessel trachea view, a diagnosis of the transposition of the great arteries should be suspected at this early stage of pregnancy. The great arteries have a more parallel arrangement than normal and tend to overlie each other so that only two vessels may be visible rather than the normal "three vessel" view (Fig. 6.10 and Video 6.5).

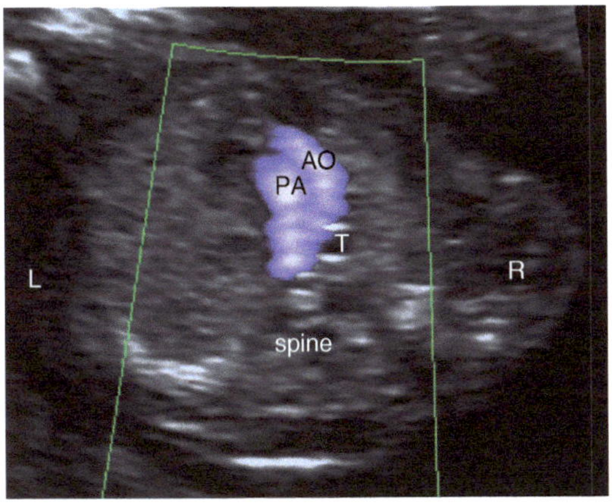

Fig. 6.10 This is a transverse plane at the level of the three-vessel-trachea view using colour flow Doppler. The normal "V" sign is not seen, and the vessels are seen in parallel. This fetus had transposition of the great arteries to account for the abnormal appearance

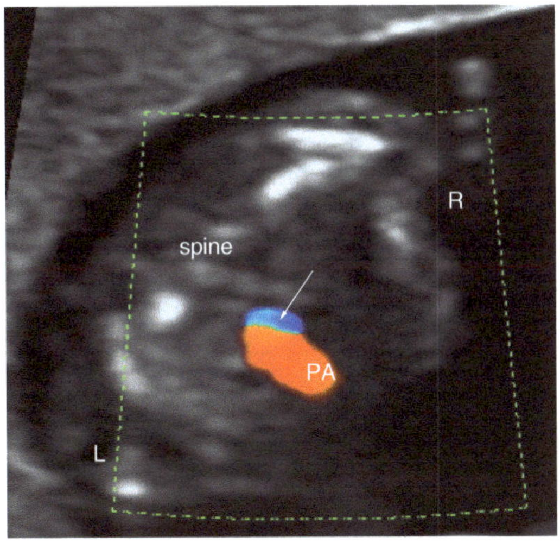

Fig. 6.11 The transverse plane at the level of transverse arch demonstrates diminutive transverse arch with reverse flow (white arrow) and forward flow in the arterial duct and pulmonary artery using colour Doppler at 13 weeks gestation. These appearances are consistent with aortic atresia in in the setting of hypoplastic left heart syndrome

Additional examination of the outflow tract may demonstrate the large outlet ventricular septal defect with aortic override typical of tetralogy of Fallot (Video 6.6). If a ventricular defect is not well seen and there is only mild asymmetry of the great arteries, the diagnosis of tetralogy of Fallot may become more obvious later in pregnancy. A ventricular septal defect in combination with aortic valve override and a normal size pulmonary artery can be indicative of aneuploidy, particularly trisomy 18.

Colour flow mapping is an additional tool to delineate great artery abnormalities which is particularly helpful in the first trimester. The presence of normally related great arteries with a normal antegrade laminar flow pattern should provide reassurance at early gestation.

Flow velocities in the first trimester are lower than later in pregnancy. Thus, the velocity range should be set at around 0.3 m/s. Abnormal flow patterns such as elevated velocity across the aortic or pulmonary valve or reversal of flow direction within the great arteries, aortic arch or ductal arch should raise the suspicion of an underlying abnormality.

Forward flow in a small aorta is usually observed in coarctation of the aorta. However, reverse flow in the aortic arch is an indicator of critical obstruction or atresia of the aortic valve (Fig. 6.11). Antegrade flow in a hypoplastic main pulmonary artery can be an indicator of pulmonary valve stenosis even in the absence of an increased flow velocity for example in the setting of tetralogy of Fallot. Increased Doppler flow velocity across the pulmonary valve may only become evident as the pulmonary vascular resistance falls after birth. Retrograde flow in the arterial duct is typical of critical pulmonary stenosis or pulmonary atresia. Bidirectional flow across the aortic or pulmonary valve is generally rarely observed. It can be seen either in one or both of the great arteries and is strongly associated with chromosomal anomalies at first trimester, particularly trisomy 18 (Zidere et al. 2007). Presence of bidirectional flow in the pulmonary artery may indicate absent pulmonary valve syndrome.

A summary of some of the more common types of congenital heart disease diagnosed in the first trimester are shown in Table 6.3.

There have been some recent developments in ultrasound technology which have particular advantages in the first trimester. Conventional ultrasound shows the blood pool as black and solid structures with a variable greyscale. In contrast, some modalities show blood flow

Table 6.3 Differential diagnosis of potential major cardiac abnormalities seen in Three-Vessel and Arch views in 2D-Mode and with Colour Doppler at first trimester scan

2D-mode	Colour mapping	Likely diagnosis
Crossover, equal size great arteries and patent arterial valves	Antegrade flow, equal width of great artery filling, forming "V" sign	Normal
Asymmetry (aorta < pulmonary artery; transverse aortic arch < arterial duct)	Antegrade flow but asymmetrical filling (aorta < pulmonary artery)	Coarctation of the aorta
Asymmetry (aorta ≤ pulmonary artery; transverse aortic arch ≤ arterial duct)	Aliased flow in aorta	Aortic stenosis
Asymmetry (aorta < pulmonary artery; transverse aortic arch < arterial duct)	Retrograde flow in aortic arch and asymmetrical filling (aorta < pulmonary artery; aortic arch < arterial duct)	Aortic atresia
Asymmetry (aorta > pulmonary artery; transverse aortic arch ≥ arterial duct)	Antegrade flow but asymmetrical filling (aorta > pulmonary artery)	Small pulmonary artery in case of tetralogy of Fallot
Asymmetry (aorta ≥ pulmonary artery; transverse aortic arch ≥ arterial duct)	Aliased flow in pulmonary artery	Pulmonary artery stenosis
Asymmetry (aorta ≥ pulmonary artery; transverse aortic arch ≥ arterial duct)	Retrograde flow in pulmonary arteria/arterial duct and asymmetrical filling (aorta > pulmonary artery; transverse arch > arterial duct)	Pulmonary artery atresia
No crossover, parallel equal size great arteries and patent arterial valves	Antegrade flow, equal width of great artery filling, no "V" sign formed	Transposition of the great arteries
Only one great artery seen	Antegrade flow (no second vessel seen with reversed flow)	Common arterial trunk

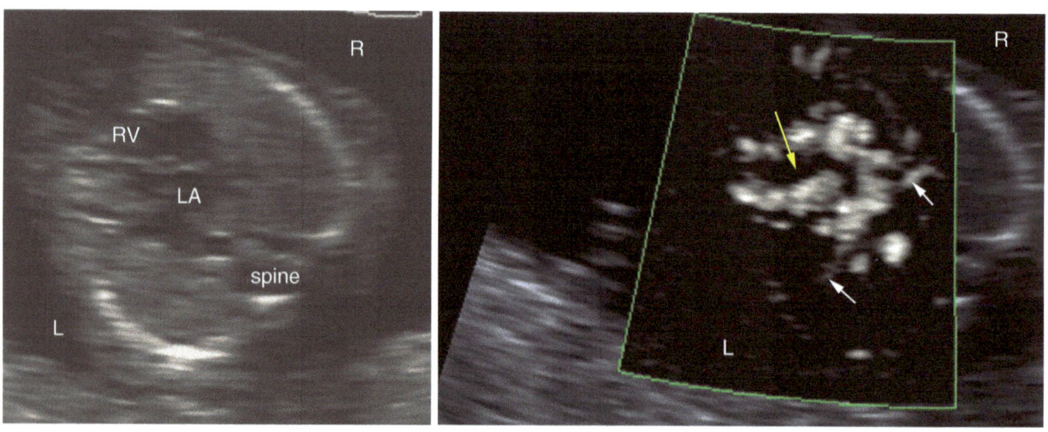

Fig. 6.12 On the left-side panel, transverse cut in 2D-mode demonstrates the heart in a lateral four-chamber view. This is a favourable orientation for examining the ventricular septum. On the right-side panel, the simultaneous image of the microvascular imaging emphasises the intact interventricular septum (yellow arrow) and two pulmonary veins (white arrows) draining into the left atrium in this fetus at 13 weeks gestation

within the cardiac chambers and vessels as "bright blood" and the solid structures, such as the myocardium, as dark. This facilitates delineation of very small structures such as interventricular septum, pulmonary veins, pulmonary arteries, and head and neck vessels during early fetal cardiac assessment (Figs. 6.12, 6.13, 6.14, 6.15 and 6.16).

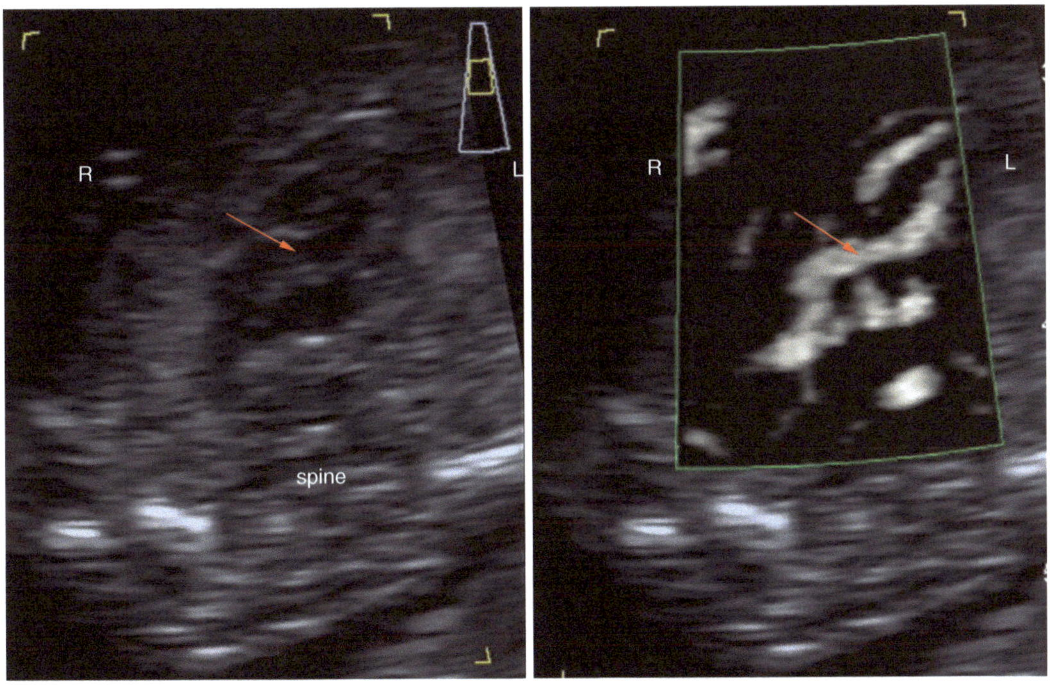

Fig. 6.13 On the left-side panel, this transverse cut in 2D-mode demonstrates the left ventricular outflow tract with arising great artery (red arrow). On the right-side panel, the simultaneous image of the microvascular imaging delineates the interventricular septum and shows that the vessel arising from the left ventricle has no early branching and therefore is aorta (red arrow) in this fetus at 13 weeks gestation

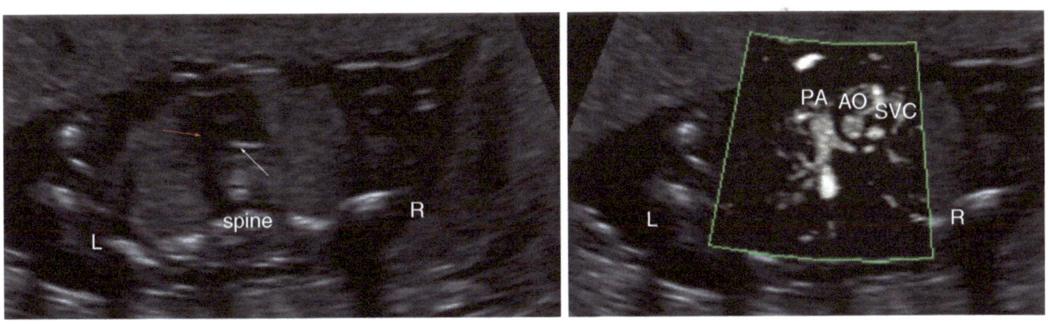

Fig. 6.14 On the left-side panel, the branch pulmonary artery (red arrow) in continuity with the arterial duct and the right pulmonary artery (white arrow) are seen in the transverse plane. This plane is obtained in slightly lower cut than in classic three-vessel view in this fetus at 13 weeks gestation. On the right-side panel, the simultaneous image using superb microvascular imaging clearly confirms the anatomy of the pulmonary artery showing both branch pulmonary arteries and the arterial duct. In addition, the aorta and superior vena cava are seen in transverse section

Fetal Heart Rhythm and Arrhythmias

The normal fetal heart rate at first trimester is higher than during the second and third trimesters. Figure 6.17 shows the range of heart rates observed related to gestational age based on our own departmental data. Pathological arrhythmias in first trimester fetus are rarely seen. Ectopic beats in the fetus are usually not observed during early scans.

A persistent bradycardia can indicate either a poor overall status of the fetus with an otherwise

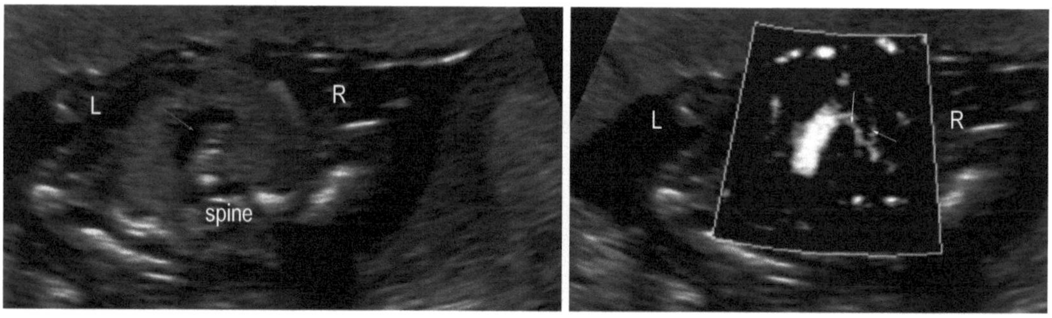

Fig. 6.15 On the left-side panel, a normal transverse aortic arch (red arrow) seen crossing the midline in front of trachea in the transverse plane in this fetus at 13 weeks gestation. On the right-side panel, a simultaneous image using superb microvascular imaging confirming normal origin of the right subclavian artery (yellow arrow) and the internal mammary artery arising from it (white arrow) at 13 weeks gestation is seen

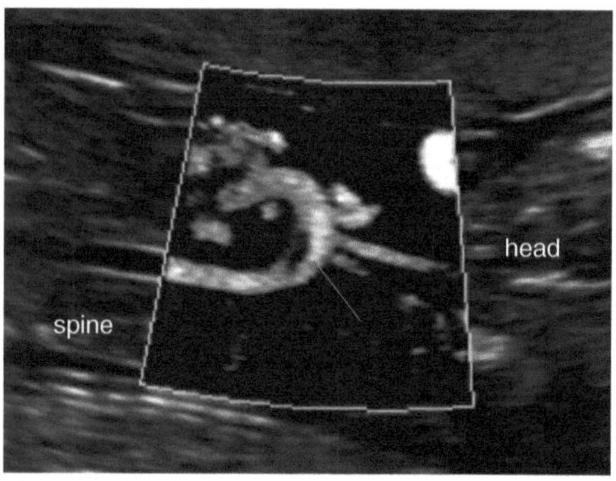

Fig. 6.16 The sagittal plane demonstrates a complete aortic arch (red arrow) with head and neck vessels using superb microvascular imaging at 13 weeks gestation

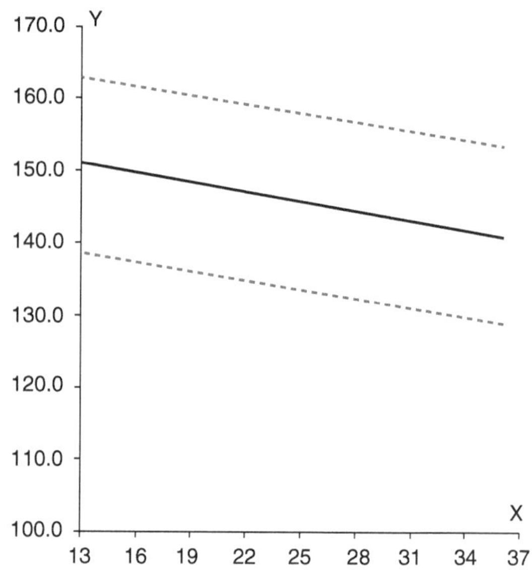

Fig. 6.17 This table demonstrates a graph of normal fetal heart rate and its physiological trend to decrease as pregnancy progresses (x-axis = weeks of gestation and y-axis = fetal heart rate in beats per minute, solid black line = mean, dashed red lines = 95% confidence intervals)

normal heart. Complete heart block may be result of CHD of which left atrial isomerism or discordant atrioventricular connections are the commonest lesions. Complete heart block in the fetus in the first trimester is not usually immune mediated as maternal anti-Ro(SS-A) and anti-LA (SS-B) antibodies cross the placenta after 16 weeks gestation.

Pathological fetal tachycardias normally have a ventricular rate in excess of 200 beats per minute, most commonly around 240–250 beats per minute. Supraventricular tachycardia is extremely rare in the first trimester but has been documented. Less pronounced tachycardia may indicate an underlying fetal chromosomal abnormality. The management of fetal arrhythmias is described in Chap. 11.

First Trimester Cardiac Markers

There is evidence from large screening studies that assessment of the tricuspid valve pulsed wave Doppler, origin of the right subclavian artery and ductus venosus Doppler profile can improve the detection of fetal aneuploidies and congenital heart disease (Faiola et al. 2005; Pereira et al. 2011; Borenstein et al. 2008; Prats et al. 2012).

Tricuspid Valve Assessment and Tricuspid Regurgitation

Tricuspid valve assessment requires a correct apical four-chamber plane, a pulsed Doppler sample gate between 2.0 and 3.0 mm is placed across the tricuspid valve with an insonation angle of less than 30°. Care should be taken not to erroneously interrogate with aortic valve flow as there is often a risk of an overlap at early gestation. Tricuspid regurgitation which occupies half the duration of systole and with a velocity of greater than 0.6 m/s should be considered abnormal (Fig. 6.18). As visualisation of the four-chamber is required for this assessment, major four-chamber abnormalities for example atrioventricular septal defect, hypoplastic left heart syndrome may be detected.

Data derived from our routine screening population (Pereira et al. 2011) demonstrates that the prevalence of tricuspid regurgitation in low risk population is 1.3%, which usually resolves by the second trimester. In fetuses with tricuspid regurgitation at first trimester, CHD will be present in 2.2% in the absence of increased nuchal translucency and abnormal ductus venous flow pattern. Thus, the fetal heart structure should be carefully assessed when tricuspid valve regurgitation is observed in the first trimester.

The anatomy of the aberrant right subclavian artery is covered in Chap. 9. This vessel arises from the descending aorta and passes behind the trachea below the transverse aortic arch at the level of the arterial duct. This is shown in Fig. 6.19 and Video 6.7 and discussed further in Chap. 9. This finding has implications for the risk of chromosomal abnormality or associated CHD, and may occasionally give rise to respiratory or gastro-intestinal symptoms postnatally by compression of the trachea or oesophagus respectively.

Abnormal **ductus venosus** flow is measured by Pulsed Doppler during the first trimester nuchal scan as part of the assessment of fetal well-being but is not specific to any particular structural heart abnormality in the fetus. A persistently abnormal ductus venosus flow (Fig. 6.20) may indicate underlying chromosome anomaly or imminent fetal demise. The limitation in using this particular marker is that it can be inconsistent during the same scan making difficult to interpret.

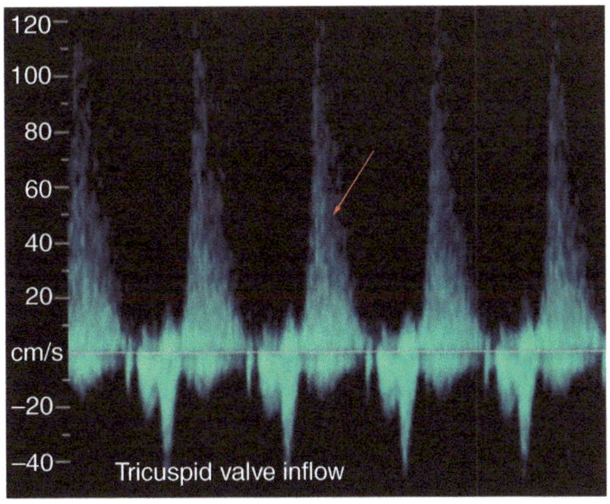

Fig. 6.18 Pulsed Doppler shows holosystolic tricuspid regurgitation (red arrow) at a velocity of 100 cm/s obtained in apical four–chamber view at the level of tricuspid valve

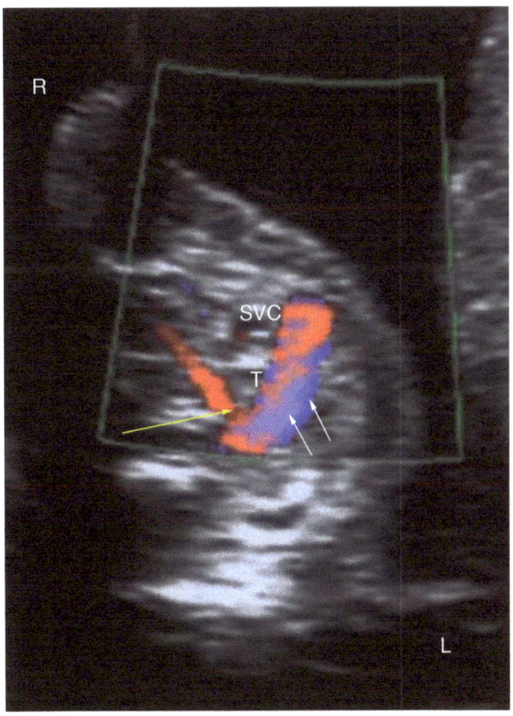

Fig. 6.19 This first trimester image demonstrates left aortic arch (white arrows) and an aberrant right subclavian artery (yellow arrow) arising from the descending aorta behind the trachea and below the transverse aortic arch and heading towards the right shoulder

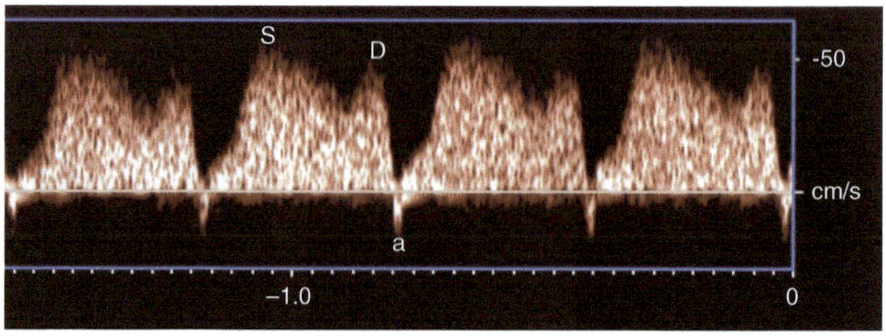

Fig. 6.20 This figure shows flow in the ductus venosus which flows towards the heart during ventricular systole (S) and early diastole (D) with reversal of flow direction with atrial contraction (a)

References

Borenstein M, Cavoretto P, Allan L, Huggon I, Nicolaides KH. Aberrant right subclavian artery at 11 + 0 to 13 + 6 weeks of gestation in chromosomally normal and abnormal fetuses. Ultrasound Obstet Gynecol. 2008;31:20–4. https://doi.org/10.1002/uog.5226.

Faiola S, Tsoi E, Huggon IC, et al. Likelihood ratio for trisomy 21 in fetuses with tricuspid regurgitation at the 11 to 13 + 6-week scan. Ultrasound Obstet Gynecol. 2005;26:22–7. https://doi.org/10.1002/uog.1922.

Hyett JA, Perdu M, Sharland GK, et al. Increased nuchal translucency at 10–14 weeks of gestation as a marker for major cardiac defects. Ultrasound Obstet Gynecol. 1997;10:242–6. https://doi.org/10.1046/j.1469-0705.

McBrien A, Howley L, Yamamoto Y, et al. Changes in fetal cardiac axis between 8 and 15 weeks' gestation. Ultrasound Obstet Gynecol. 2013;42:653–8. https://doi.org/10.1002/uog.12478.

Pereira S, Ganapathy R, Syngelaki A, et al. Contribution of fetal tricuspid regurgitation in first-trimester screening for major cardiac defects. Obstet Gynecol. 2011;117:1384–91. https://doi.org/10.1097/AOG.0b013e31821aa720.

Prats P, Ferrer Q, Comas C, Rodríguez I. Is the addition of the ductus venosus useful when screening for aneuploidy and congenital heart disease in fetuses with normal nuchal translucency? Fetal Diagn Ther. 2012;32:138–43. https://doi.org/10.1159/000335489.

Smith RS, Comstock CH, Kirk JS, Lee W. Ultrasonographic left cardiac axis deviation: a marker for fetal anomalies. Obstet Gynecol. 1995;85:187–91. https://doi.org/10.1016/0029-7844(94)00350-M.

Zidere V, Allan LD, Huggon IC. Implications of bidirectional flow in the great arteries at the 11-14-week scan. Ultrasound Obstet Gynecol. 2007;30:807–12. https://doi.org/10.1002/uog.5162.

Zidere V, Bellsham-Revell H, Persico N, Allan LD. Comparison of echocardiographic findings in fetuses at less than 15 weeks' gestation with later cardiac evaluation. Ultrasound Obstet Gynecol. 2013;42(6):679–86.

Abnormalities of the Four Chamber View

7

Owen I. Miller, John Simpson, and Vita Zidere

Abstract

The four-chamber view (4ChV) is fundamental to fetal echocardiography, as it will show some, but not all the evidence for most fetal cardiac abnormalities. The 4ChV provides the base view from which further views can be developed and is fundamental in the assessment of ventricular proportions and imbalance, ventricular inlets, evaluation of the crux and for septal defects. Additionally, the 4ChV is the ideal view for initial evaluation of heart rhythm and extracardiac abnormalities such as a pericardial effusion, mass lesions and abnormalities of heart position. This chapter will explore abnormalities seen in the 4ChV and discuss common associations and outcomes for each lesion to guide counselling.

Electronic Supplementary Material The online version of this chapter (https://doi.org/10.1007/978-3-319-77461-9_7) contains supplementary material, which is available to authorized users.

O. I. Miller (✉) · J. Simpson
Evelina London Children's Hospital, Guy's and St Thomas' NHS Foundation Trust, London, UK
e-mail: Owen.Miller@gstt.nhs.uk; john.simpson@gstt.nhs.uk

V. Zidere
Evelina London Children's Hospital, Guy's and St Thomas' NHS Foundation Trust, London, UK

King's College Hospital NHS Foundation Trust, London, UK
e-mail: vita.zidere@gstt.nhs.uk

Keywords

Congenital heart disease · Septal defects · Coarctation of the aorta · Hypoplastic left heart · Aortic stenosis · Pulmonary atresia · Tricuspid atresia · Double inlet left ventricle · Ebstein's anomaly of the tricuspid valve · Primary cardiac tumours

Introduction

The four-chamber view is the most crucial view of the fetal cardiac examination, as it will be abnormal in the majority of pathological lesions seen in the fetal heart. However, some abnormalities will only be suspected with views of the outflow tracts (Chap. 8). Comment should be made on several key features, including heart position, size, structure and function. For a detailed description of the normal appearances the reader is referred to Chap. 2. The 4ChV should function as the plane of reference before embarking on a sequential evaluation of other heart structures, and is the standard view to demonstrate several major congenital heart lesions which will be addressed in more detail in this chapter. Abnormalities of the heart position and/or size will also be discussed. In some fetuses, the right and left sides of the heart may show asymmetry, but this is not a unifying diagnosis and the potential underlying causes of such an asymmetric appearance will be outlined.

© Springer International Publishing AG, part of Springer Nature 2018

J. Simpson et al. (eds.), *Fetal Cardiology*, https://doi.org/10.1007/978-3-319-77461-9_7

Abnormal Cardiac Position

The normal fetal heart occupies around 1/3 of the fetal thorax and the apex is orientated around 40–45° anterior and to the left. A summary of potential causes of abnormal cardiac position are shown in Fig. 7.1. In fetuses with CHD, the heart position may be abnormal due to the underlying lesion itself. In many fetuses with abnormalities of the outflow tracts, notably tetralogy of Fallot and its variants (Fig. 7.2), the heart is rotated to the left. The reader is referred to Chap. 14 for more information on extracardiac abnormalities.

When assessing the fetus with abnormal cardiac position, our preference is to describe the cardiac situs and the position of the apex (Fig. 7.3) rather than using less clear terms, such as dextrocardia, dextroposition or dextroversion. The cardiac connections should be described in the usual sequential segmental fashion.

Abnormal Cardiac Size

There are both cardiac and extracardiac causes for an abnormal cardio-thoracic ratio (CTR),

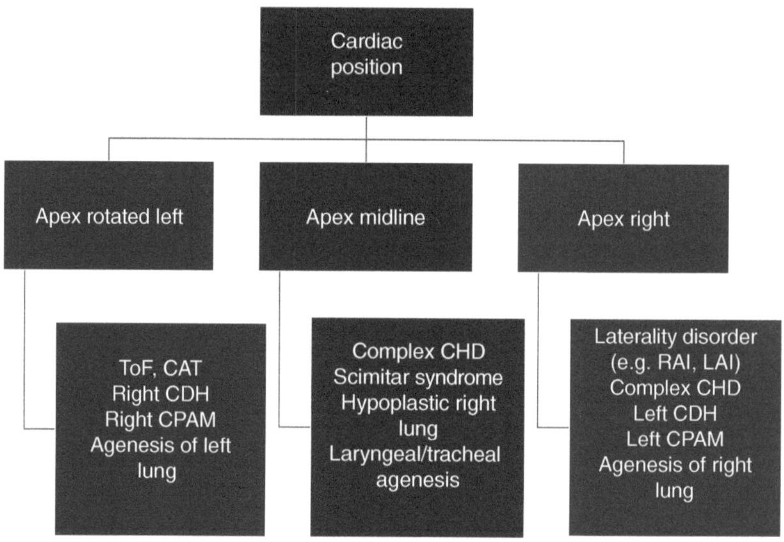

Fig. 7.1 This flowchart demonstrates abnormalities of fetal cardiac position. *ToF* tetralogy of Fallot, *CAT* common arterial trunk, *CDH* congenital diaphragmatic hernia, *CPAM* congenital pulmonary airway malformation, *CHD* congenital heart disease, *RAI* right atrial isomerism, *LAI* left atrial isomerism

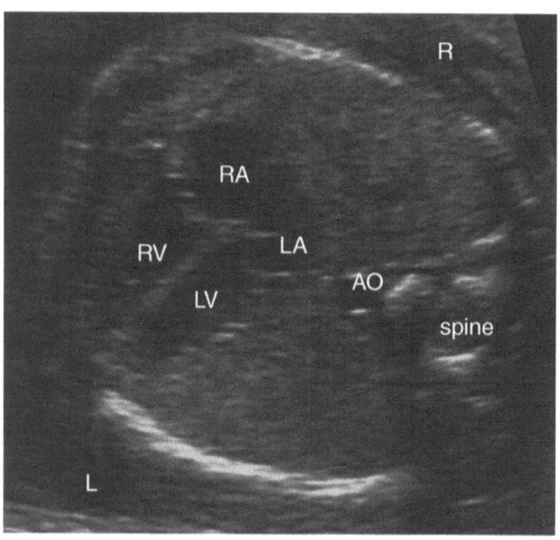

Fig. 7.2 The four-chamber view demonstrates cardiac apex rotated to the left. This appearance is often seen in tetralogy of Fallot or in common arterial trunk

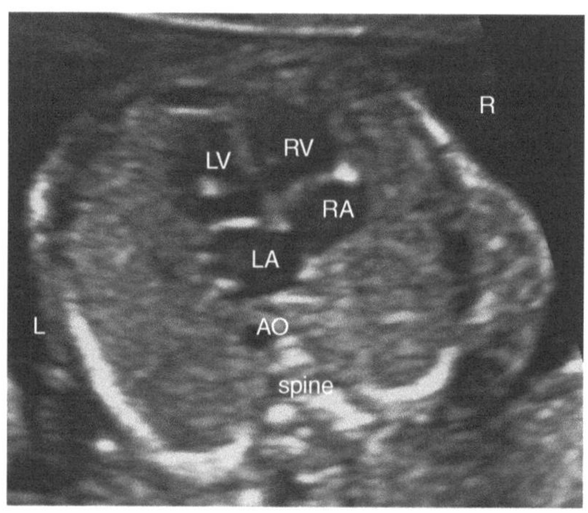

Fig. 7.3 The midline cardiac apex is seen in this example. The anatomy of the four-chambers appears within normal limits but the fetus was proven to have an unbalanced translocation

which can be increased or rarely decreased. An elevated CTR is usually due to increased size of the heart. However, in cases where there is intrauterine growth restriction, oligohydramnios caused by renal abnormality or thoracic/skeletal dysplasia the actual thorax is small but the heart is normal in size. In such cases, the smaller thorax accounts for the increased CTR.

Cardiomegaly may be due to reduced function (reduced contractility), or abnormal cardiac loading conditions due to either a cardiac abnormality or extracardiac shunt (Fig. 7.4a, b). Causes of reduced cardiac function include viral myocarditis (e.g. Coxsackie or Parvovirus), inborn errors of metabolism or structurally abnormal myocardium (e.g. non-compaction of the myocardium). This is discussed further in Chap. 5. Abnormal loading conditions causing increased stroke volume result in vigorous rather than decreased contractility. In case of severe, untreated arrhythmia such as supraventricular tachycardia, atrial flutter or complete heart block (see Chap. 11) the fetus can present with cardiomegaly with or without fetal hydrops. Cardiomegaly can be also caused by severe valve regurgitation in the context of congenital heart disease. For example, severe mitral valve regurgitation in critical aortic stenosis (Fig. 7.5, Video 7.1), pulmonary regurgitation in absent pulmonary valve syndrome and tricuspid valve regurgitation in Ebstein's anomaly or tricuspid valve dysplasia (Fig. 7.6). Rarely, an enlarged and poorly contracting right ventricle can occur in isolation. Such appearance should prompt evaluation of the arterial duct to exclude premature constriction which may present with right ventricular enlargement and failure.

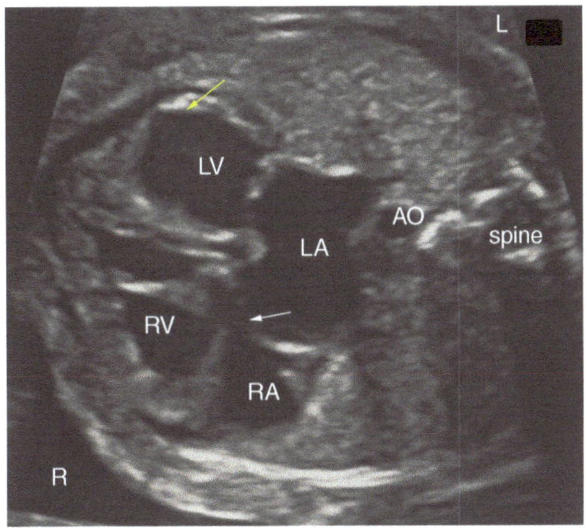

Fig. 7.5 The four-chamber view demonstrates cardiomegaly in example of critical aortic stenosis. A dilated, echogenic (yellow arrow) and non-apex forming left ventricle is seen. The left atrium appears dilated due to mitral regurgitation (seen on Video 7.1) and restrictive atrial septum (white arrow)

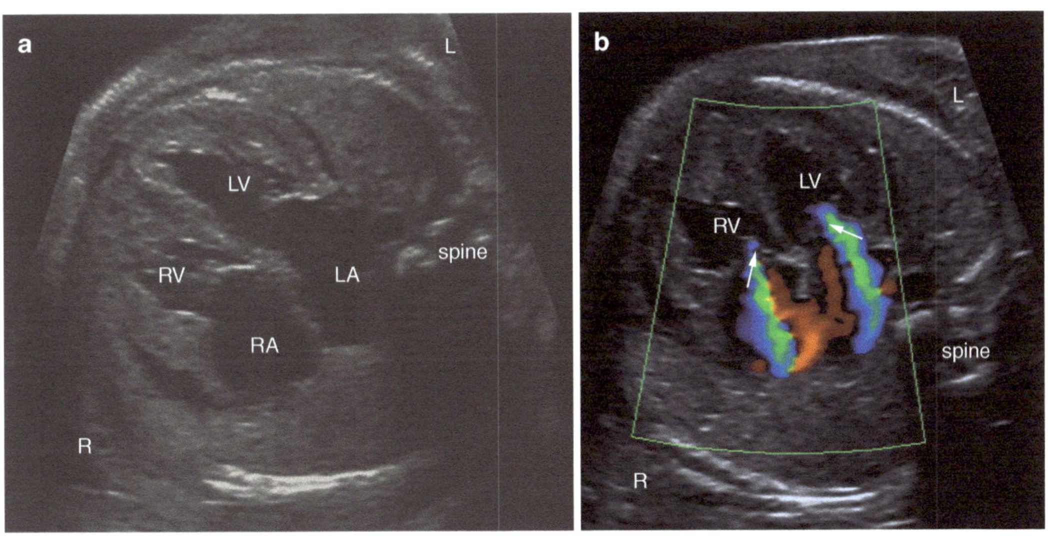

Fig. 7.4 (**a**) There is marked cardiomegaly and biventricular hypertrophy in this recipient twin in the setting of Twin to Twin transfusion syndrome. (**b**) Colour Doppler on the four-chamber view in the recipient twin demonstrates (arrows)

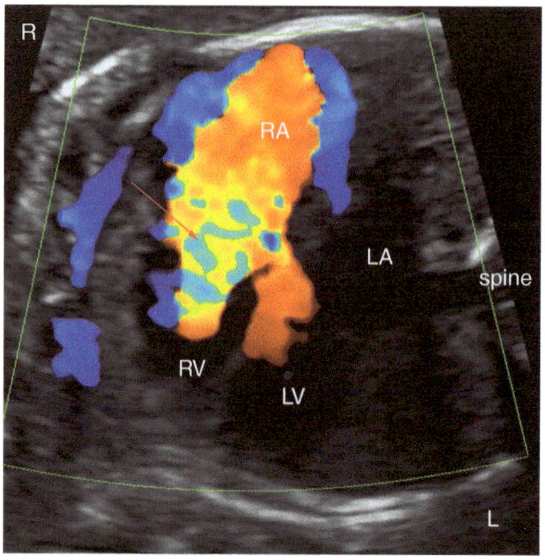

Fig. 7.6 Colour Doppler at the four-chamber view demonstrates severe tricuspid valve regurgitation (red arrow) in this case of tricuspid valve dysplasia. Note the significant enlargement of the right atrium

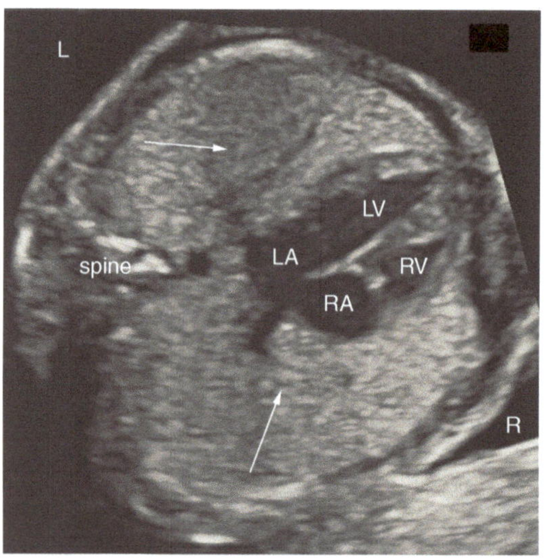

Fig. 7.7 The fetal heart appears small with midline apex. This is due to enlarged, echogenic (congested) lungs caused by tracheal atresia

The cardio-thoracic ratio may be decreased due to the heart being compressed by extracardiac lesions within the chest such as congenital diaphragmatic hernia (Video 7.2) or large pleural effusions. In cases of tracheal atresia, fluid retention in the lungs causes distension and mass effect (Fig. 7.7).

Common causes of either an increased or decreased CTR are summarised in Fig. 7.8. Treatment of the underlying cause is key in affected cases.

Pericardial Effusion

Pericardial effusion is best evaluated in the four-chamber view. A thin black rim of relatively uniform thickness around the ventricles represents a normal finding (see Chap. 2). As there many potential causes of a pericardial effusion, the finding is non-specific, it is therefore essential to confirm that the cardiac structure and function are normal. Cardiomyopathy, arrhythmia or structural abnormalities may all lead to development of a pericardial effusion as a marker of incipient cardiac failure. Rare, but important causes of a pericardial effusion include cardiac tumours (Fig. 7.9) or an outpouching of the left or right ventricle (Fig. 7.10). However, comprehensive fetal medicine review is essential to exclude intra-uterine infection, anaemia and any possible associated genetic abnormalities.

Septal Defects

Ventricular Septal Defects

Isolated ventricular septal defect (VSD) is the commonest congenital heart lesion (about 30% of all CHD) detected postnatally, with incidence of 2/1000 live birth (Ferencz et al. 1985). Ventricular septal defects are seen in association with many more complex forms of congenital heart disease, for example, tetralogy of Fallot. These specific lesions are described in detail in respective chapters. This chapter focuses on isolated VSDs or where the VSD is the dominant cardiac lesion.

Ventricular septal defects are normally categorised according to their position when visualised from the right ventricular aspect (Fig. 7.11), the categories being:

- **Perimembranous**, which are located in the thin membranous portion of the ventricular

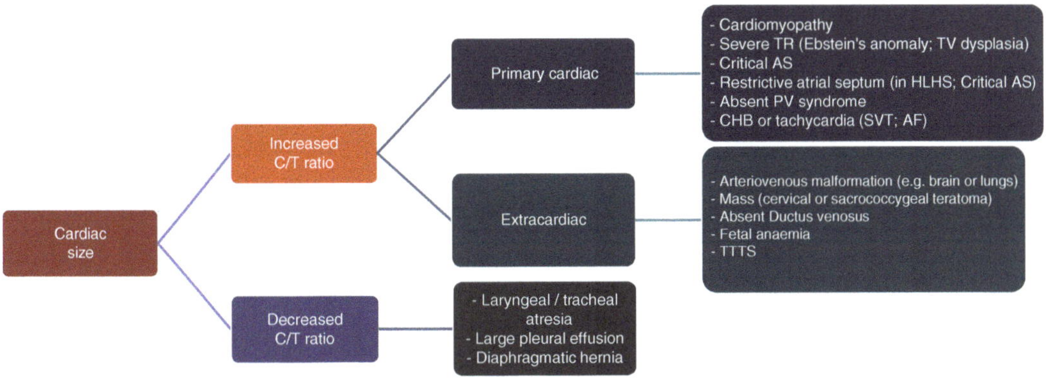

Fig. 7.8 Cardiac and extracardiac reasons for increased or decreased cardiothoracic ratio are demonstrated in this flowchart. *TR* tricuspid regurgitation, *AS* aortic stenosis, *HLHS* hypoplastic left heart syndrome, *PV* pulmonary valve, *SVT* supraventricular tachycardia, *AF* atrial flutter, *TTTS* Twin to Twin transfusion syndrome

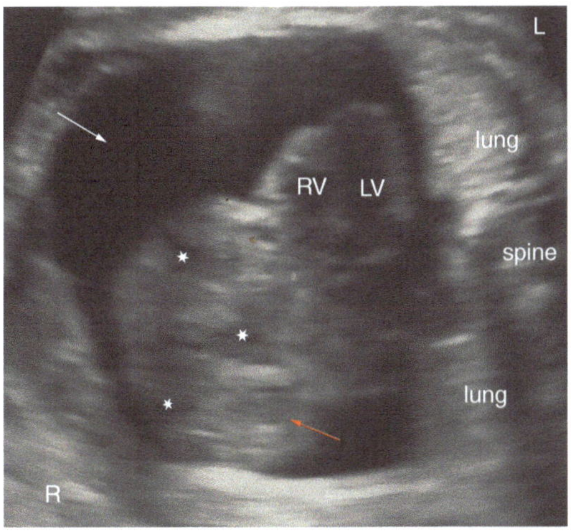

Fig. 7.9 This demonstrates a large, solitary (red arrow) multi-cystic (*) mass on the surface of the heart in association with a widespread pericaridial effusion (white arrow) which is typical of a cardiac teratoma

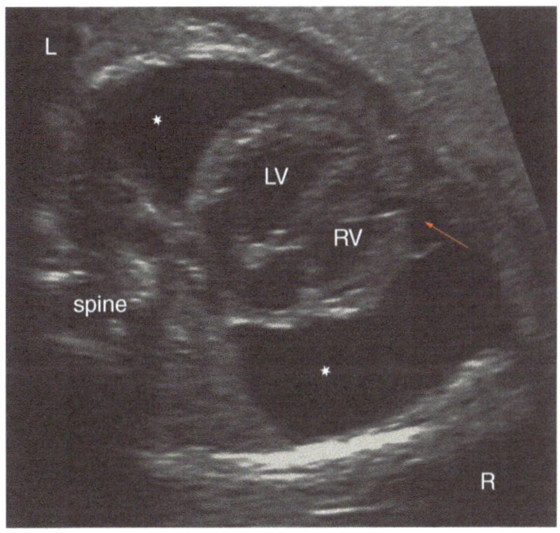

Fig. 7.10 A large pericardial effusion (*) is seen in the four-chamber view. Both lungs are pushed towards the fetal spine. This is likely due to the irritative process caused by the right ventricular outpouching (red arrow)

septum, adjacent to the tricuspid valve, but may have extension into the ventricular inlet or outlet.

- **Doubly committed subarterial**, located in a superior position with fibrous continuity between the aortic and pulmonary valves.
- **Muscular defects**, which have entirely muscular boundaries and can be located anywhere in the muscular ventricular septum.

Although isolated VSDs can be diagnosed prenatally, the diagnosis of VSD during fetal life presents a number of challenges. The right and left ventricular pressures are equal so there is no major left to right shunt, hence the flow pattern across defects is typically low velocity and bidirectional. The membranous portion of the ventricular septum is thin and prone to ultrasound image 'drop out', with potential for both false-positive and false-negative diagnoses. It is important that suspected VSDs are visualised in multiple sonographic projections to differentiate between true VSD and "drop out". The ability to diagnose an isolated VSD is influenced by sonographer's expertise in cardiac evaluation, the quality of the image obtained, the angle of

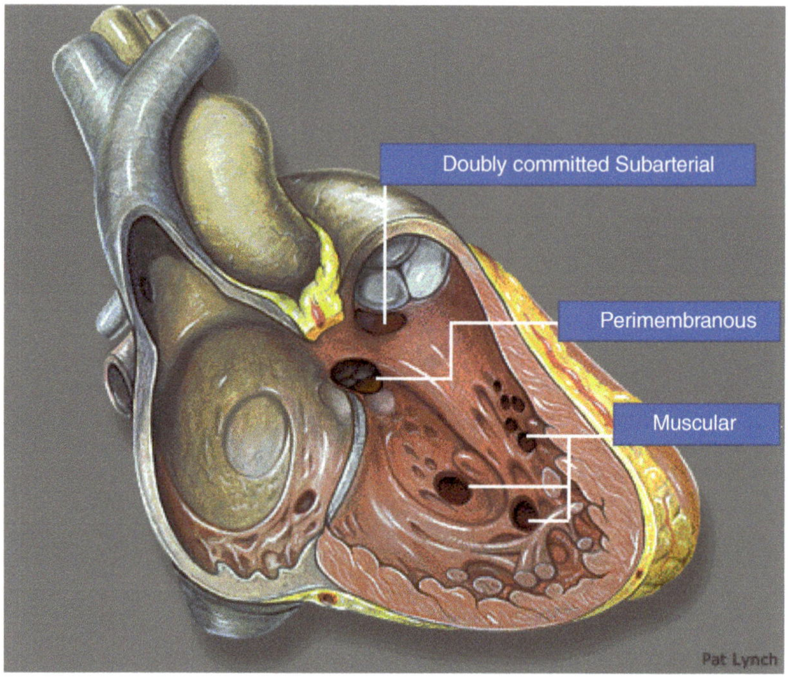

Fig. 7.11 This drawing demonstrates types of ventricular septal defect as seen from the right ventricle aspect

insonation, the size of the defect, use of colour flow Doppler and the gestational age at the time of the scan.

Furthermore, a confident diagnosis for some VSD types is quite difficult during fetal life. For example, in cases doubly committed subarterial defect the required sonographic views may not be readily obtainable in the fetus. Small VSDs, particularly muscular lesions, are not readily seen on grey-scale cross-sectional images alone and may be diagnosed only using colour flow Doppler. Hence, it is not unusual to overlook small VSDs during a second trimester scan. These may become easier to identify in the third trimester but many are only identified after birth.

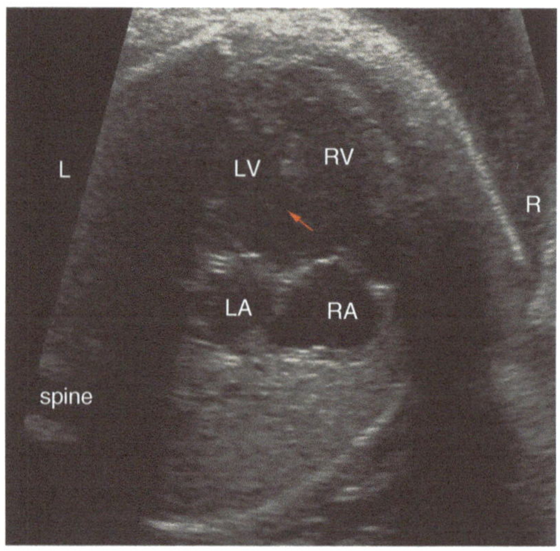

Fig. 7.12 A large perimembranous to inlet ventricular septal defect (red arrow) is seen in an apical four-chamber view in this fetus. There is the loss of off-setting of the atrioventricular valves. However, this is not an atrioventricular septal defect as there are two separate atrioventricular valves and the primum atrial septum is present

Echocardiographic Features

Perimembranous defects are seen at the crux of the heart, in the thin portion of the ventricular septum. This is the most difficult group to distinguish between a true defect and "drop out" in the ventricular septum. In some perimembranous defects there is loss of differential insertion of the atrioventricular valves (Fig. 7.12, Video 7.3). However, in contrast to an atrioventricular septal defect, the primum atrial septum is present and the atrioventricular valves have normal morphology. Perimembranous defects may extend inferiorly into the inlet septum, thus continue to be seen on caudal angulation of the transducer. They may also extend towards the outlets of the heart and so remain visible when the transducer is angulated cranially towards the outflow tracts (Fig. 7.13).

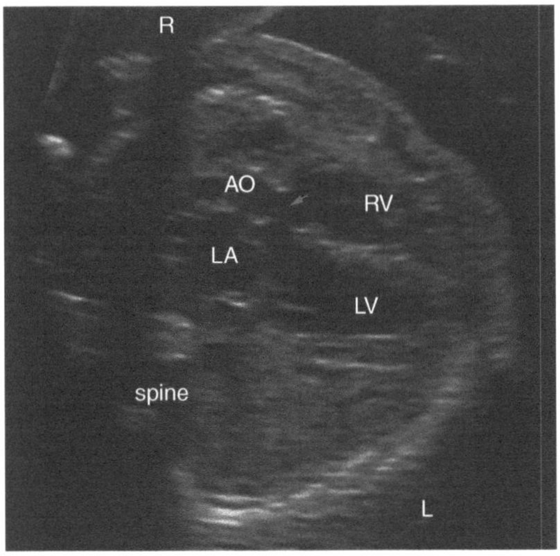

Fig. 7.13 A large perimembranous ventricular septal defect (red arrow) with outlet extension is seen in this example. The image is obtained by angulating cranially towards the left outlet from a four-chamber view

Muscular VSDs have purely muscular boundaries and may be seen in any portion of the ventricular septum (Fig. 7.14, Videos 7.4a and 7.4b). These are most commonly seen in the mid trabecular and apical trabecular portions of the ventricular septum.

Associations

Ventricular septal defects should not be considered together as a single group when considering the potential associations.

Perimembranous VSDs

Perimembranous VSDs may be associated with chromosomal abnormalities (including major aneuploidies) and extracardiac abnormalities (Mosimann et al. 2014). Detailed anomaly scanning and reference to screening results is important in all cases. Data from our group has shown that the incidence of an underlying karyotypic abnormality is higher if there are abnormal screening results or other abnormal sonographic findings. Fetal karyotyping should be discussed in all cases of a confirmed perimembranous VSD. If there is associated overriding of the aorta, with a normal sized pulmonary artery, this is suggestive of underlying trisomy 18.

Muscular VSDs

Muscular VSDs may be associated with extracardiac anomalies and karyotypic abnormalities but with a less strong association than the perimembranous group. Our experience has been that the incidence of an underlying genetic cause is very low in the absence or other sonographic abnormalities and normal background screening investigations.

Management and Outcome

Isolated VSDs do not require delivery at a specialist cardiac centre as early neonatal compromise is highly unlikely. Affected babies are assessed routinely 2–6 weeks after birth to coincide with the natural fall in pulmonary vascular resistance, to gauge the extent left to right shunting of blood. Left to right shunting across the VSD results in high pulmonary blood flow leading to increased respiratory rate, poor weight gain and signs of congestive cardiac failure. Surgery for such defects is typically undertaken in the first 3–4 months of life, with overall good results from surgery. Some perimembranous and muscular defects are small enough to manage conservatively as there is a natural tendency for spontaneous closure, particularly for smaller muscular defects (Mosimann et al. 2014). In such cases, surgery is not required but ongoing cardiac review is indicated until the defect has closed.

Atrioventricular Septal Defect (AVSD)

An atrioventricular septal defect is one of the commonest four chamber abnormalities with an incidence of 3 per 10,000 live births. A schematic diagram of an AVSD is shown in Figs. 7.15 and 7.16. This lesion is an abnormality of the junction between the atriums and the ventricles, characterised by a common atrioventricular junction in contrast to the normal separate mitral and tricuspid valves.

Echocardiographic Features

Determination of cardiac situs is essential in the echocardiographic assessment of this group of lesions. Interruption of the inferior vena cava (left atrial isomerism) or the aorta and IVC lying

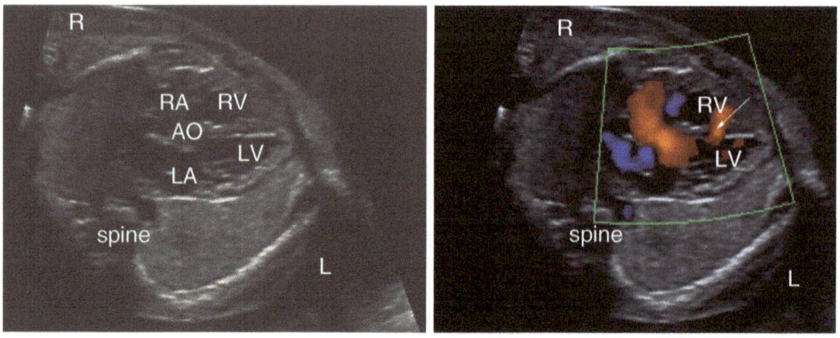

Fig. 7.14 A small mid-muscular ventricular septal defect seen on colour flow Doppler (white arrow) in the four-chamber view on the right panel. Note that there is no obvious defect seen on 2D grey scale, left sided panel. A bidirectional flow pattern can be confirmed through the cardiac cycle on moving image using colour flow Doppler and/or Pulsed wave Doppler

Fig. 7.15 A schematic diagram of an atrioventricular septal defect is demonstrated in this drawing

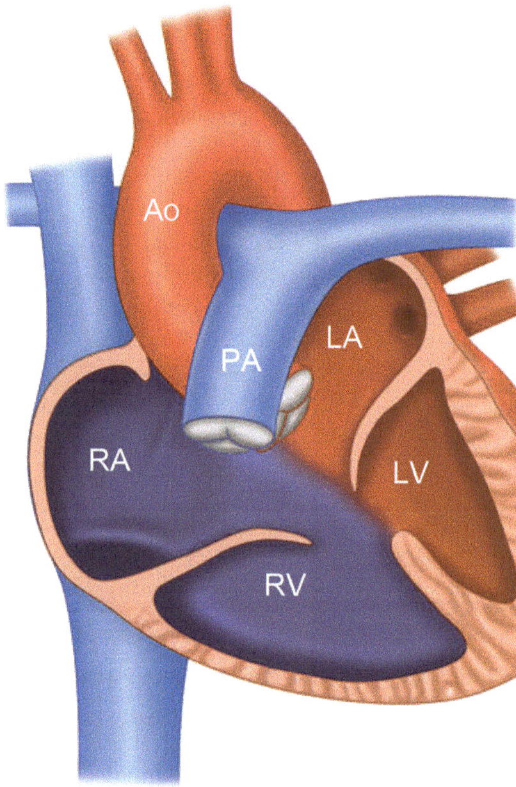

to the same side of the spine should raise the suspicion of a laterality disturbance. This is critical because the associations of AVSD with abnormal situs (laterality) are completely different from AVSD with normal situs. The four-chamber view of an AVSD is shown in Fig. 7.17a–c and in Videos 7.5a, 7.5b, 7.5c and 7.5d. There is loss of differential insertion of the atrioventricular valves. There is a communication between the atriums just above the atrioventricular valves with loss of the normal primum septum in this region (the "primum" defect). There is usually a defect between the ventricles which is of variable size. The term "partial" atrioventricular septal defect is often applied to the AVSD where there is no ventricular component to the defect and there is only a communication between the atriums. In most cases, the size of the left and

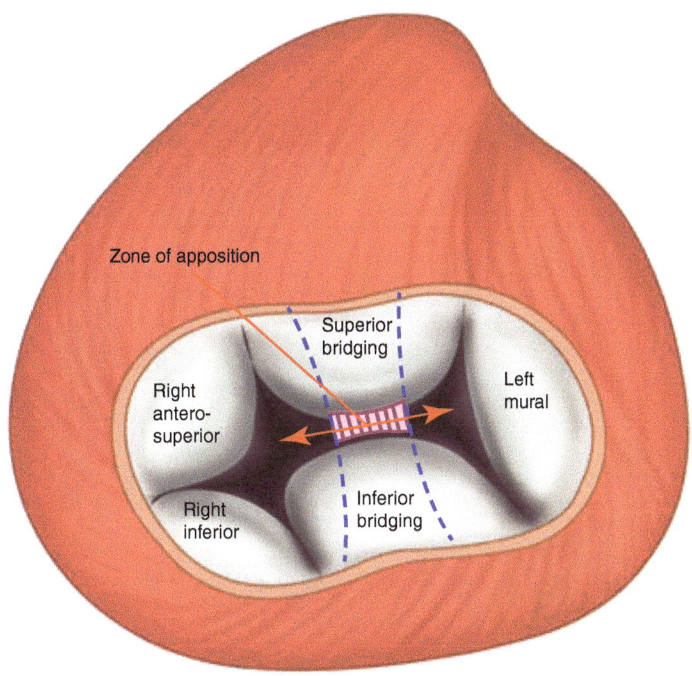

Fig. 7.16 A common atrioventricular junction, seen en face from below. In contrast to the normal separate mitral and tricuspid valves, there are valve leaflets which span across the ventricular septum known as the superior and inferior "bridging" leaflets and more lateral mural leaflets

right ventricles is similar and the AVSD is described as "balanced". However, in a minority of cases there is a discrepancy between the sizes of the right and left ventricles, in which case the defect is described as "unbalanced". Imbalance in the ventricular size is normally matched by an imbalance in the size of the corresponding great artery. Although the four-chamber view of the fetal heart permits diagnosis of the lesion, understanding the anatomy of the atrioventricular junction depends on additional short-axis views of the atrioventricular junction.

For the advanced sonographer, details of the AV valves may be appreciated on fetal echocardiography. In the normal fetal heart, the mitral and tricuspid valves are separate and the aorta is wedged between the two atrioventricular valves. In contrast, the atrioventricular septal defect is characterized by a common atrioventricular junction (Video 7.6). Two of the valve leaflets span across the ventricular septum and are known as the superior and inferior "bridging" leaflets. Appreciation of the valvar anatomy in this way depends on a favourable fetal lie and high-resolution imaging.

Once the diagnosis of AVSD is established by the absence of AV valve offsetting using 2D echo, colour flow Doppler adds value by looking for balance in size of the inflow signals during diastole and looking for jets of AV valve regurgitation during systole. AV valvar regurgitation is common, usually to a minor degree in most cases of AVSD (Video 7.7). More extensive AV valve regurgitation is associated with a higher risk (Delisle et al. 1999) and will thus influence antenatal counselling.

Abnormalities of the outflow tracts may coexist with the AVSD. In most cases, the great arteries are normally related but overriding of the aorta with pulmonary stenosis (AVSD with tetralogy of Fallot) may occur. Evaluation of the outflow tract is not part of the 4ChV but is an essential component of AVSD evaluation, as this lesion may be associated with left ventricular outflow tract obstruction or other serious outlet malformations such as double outlet right ventricle where both great arteries arise from the right ventricle (see Chap. 8). More complex abnormalities of the great arterial arrangement occur particularly in the context of abnormal cardiac situs.

Associations

Atrioventricular septal defect may be associated with laterality disturbance (left atrial or right atrial isomerism) (Chap. 10). Fetal karyotype abnormalities are very rare in the context of a laterality disturbance. In the context of normal cardiac situs, this lesion is strongly associated with

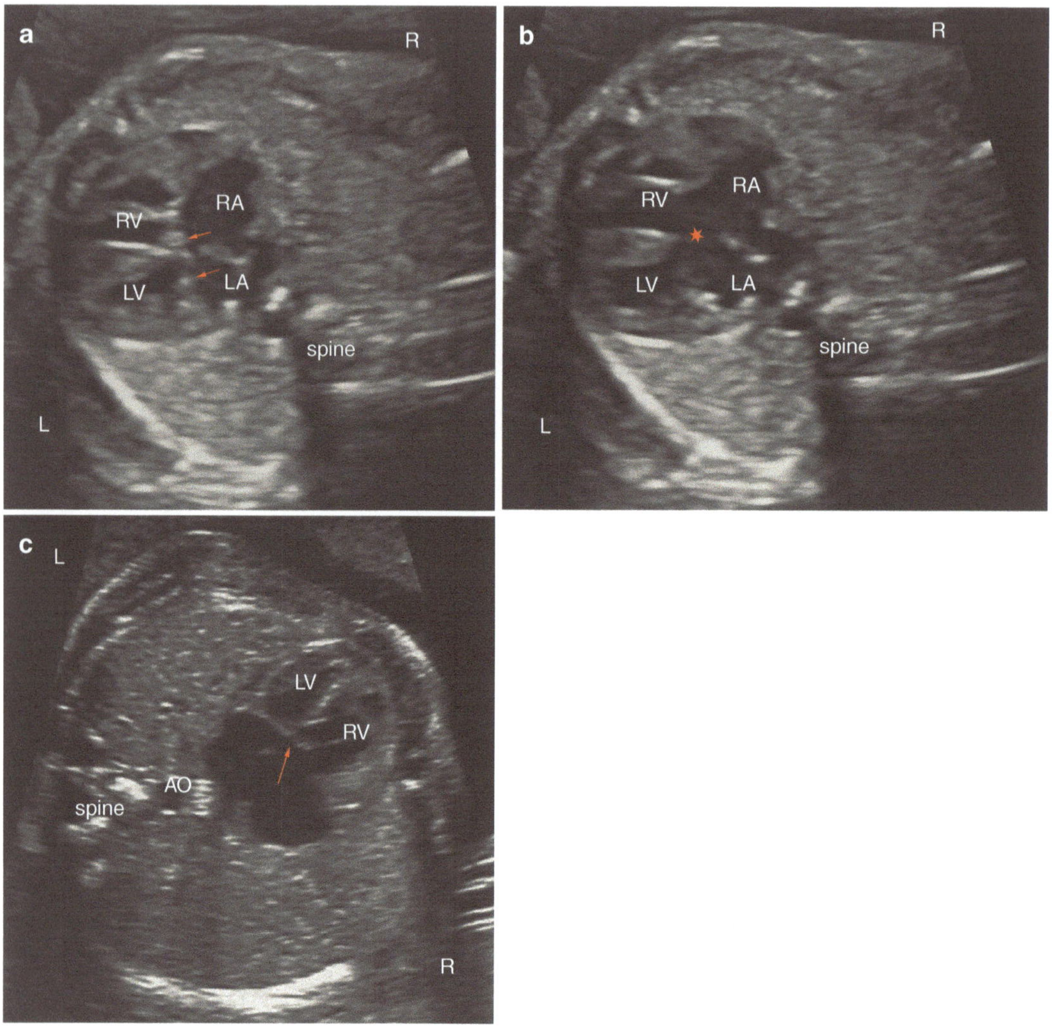

Fig. 7.17 (**a**) This apical four-chamber view demonstrates a loss of off-setting due to a common atrioventricular valve. This appears as a straight line in ventricular systole (red arrows). (**b**) A large atrioventricular septal defect (*) is seen in this apical four-chamber view during ventricular diastole. (**c**) This is another example of a complete atrioventricular septal defect but without an obvious ventricular component. The fetal heart is seen in a four-chamber view. There is loss of off-setting with the atrioventricular valves forming a straight line (red arrow) in ventricular systole

chromosomal abnormalities (Mogra et al. 2011), particularly trisomy 21. In fetal series, the incidence of trisomy 21 is 50–90%.

Postnatal Management

The fetus with a balanced AVSD without left or right heart obstruction does not require delivery at a high level cardiac centre. Once the pulmonary vascular resistance falls, there will be an increased left to right shunt, analogous to VSD. Surgical repair is normally undertaken in the first 3–6 months and consists of closure of the atrial and ventricular components of the defect coupled with repair of the left atrioventricular valve. The surgical mortality is less than 2% but the overall prognosis is heavily influenced by associated anomalies. If there is significant atrioventricular valve regurgitation, surgery may have to be undertaken earlier with a higher operative risk. More complex or unbalanced AVSD is managed on an individualised basis according to the individual anatomy.

Hypoplastic Left Heart

Hypoplastic left heart (HLH) refers to a group of conditions characterised by underdevelopment of the mitral valve, left ventricle and aorta so that the left heart is incapable of supporting the systemic arterial circulation after birth. "Classical" HLH is defined as atresia of the aortic valve coupled with atresia or stenosis of the mitral valve, in an otherwise normally connected heart. HLH "variants" should not be confused with the classical form of the lesion because the management and associations may be significantly different. HLH "variants" include critical aortic stenosis with hypoplasia of the mitral valve and left ventricle, severe coarctation of the aorta (both mitral and aortic valves are patent) and an unbalanced atrioventricular septal defect where the left ventricle and aorta are small.

"Classical" Hypoplastic Left Heart

"Classical" HLH has an incidence of 2–3 per 10,000 live births and constitutes around 3% of all congenital heart lesions, although a higher proportion are seen during fetal life due to ascertainment bias on four chamber screening. A schematic diagram of classical HLH is shown below (Fig. 7.18). All blood returning to the left atrium must pass across the atrial septum into the right atrium. From there, blood flows into the right ventricle and pulmonary artery. Systemic perfusion is maintained by blood flow from the arterial duct into the descending aorta. Brain perfusion is maintained by retrograde flow from the arterial duct into the aortic arch. Systemic perfusion can only be maintained for as long as the arterial duct remains patent.

Echocardiographic Features

There are two major subgroups of classical HLH; mitral atresia/aortic atresia (MA/AA) and mitral stenosis/aortic atresia (MS/AA) with slightly different echocardiographic features. In the MA/AA group the left ventricle is slit-like with no discernible cavity and the mitral valve is either imperforate or absent (Fig. 7.19a, b, Videos 7.8 and 7.9). The MS/AA subtype, in contrast, typically has a globular left ventricle with increased echogenicity. A small jet of antegrade flow may be visible on colour flow Doppler with a variable degree of mitral valve regurgitation. Blood flow at atrial level is from left to right, in contract to the normal

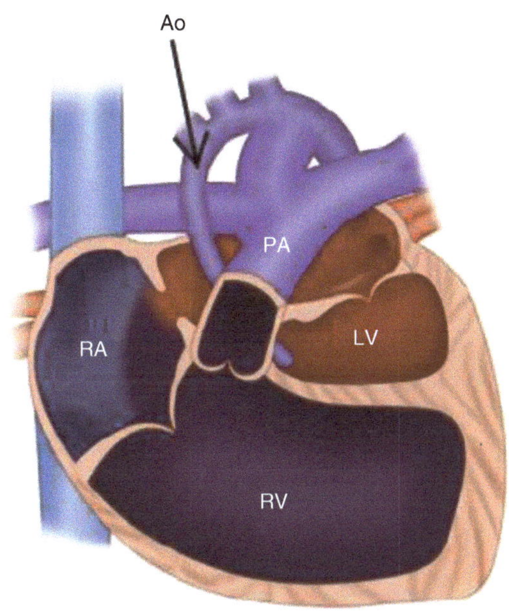

Fig. 7.18 Classical hypoplastic left heart showing severe underdevelopment of left heart structures is seen in this drawing

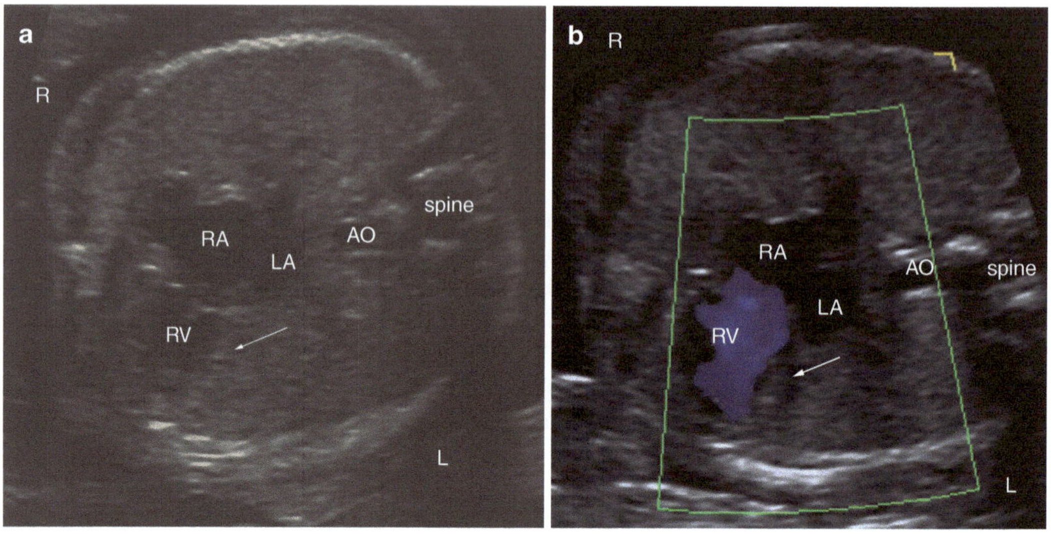

Fig. 7.19 (**a**) This apical four-chamber view shows a diminutive, slit-like left ventricle which is not forming the apex of the heart (white arrow). This appearance is indicative of mitral valve atresia in the setting of hypoplastic left heart syndrome. (**b**) There is no flow across the mitral valve or within the left ventricle (white arrow) on colour flow Doppler

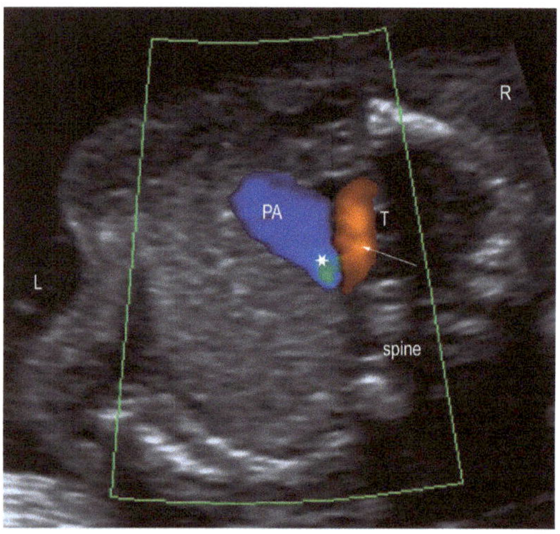

Fig. 7.20 This image demonstrates an example of hypoplasia of the aortic arch. There is forward flow in the pulmonary artery and arterial duct (asterisk) but reversed flow (white arrow) in the left aortic arch indicating aortic atresia

pattern. Colour flow Doppler confirms that all blood enters the heart across the tricuspid valve. From the right ventricle, antegrade flow is seen across the pulmonary valve and arterial duct. In the 3VT view, the aortic arch is usually hypoplastic with reversal of flow (Fig. 7.20, Video 7.10).

Some echocardiographic features merit particular attention because of their impact on prognosis. In most cases, right ventricular function is good and there is little or no tricuspid valve regurgitation, but in a minority of cases there is significant right ventricle dysfunction and/or tricuspid valve regurgitation. Both of these features have an adverse effect on postnatal prognosis because the right ventricle has to support the high pressure systemic arterial circulation after birth (Chap. 18). A further specific consideration in HLH is whether there is any obstruction to blood flow leaving the left atrium across the atrial septum. If there is significant obstruction due to the atrial septum being "restrictive", this leads to high pressure in the left atrium (Fig. 7.5) which is transmitted back to the pulmonary vasculature leading to pulmonary vascular disease or abnormal lymphatic development (pulmonary lymphangiectasia). This can lead to high resistance in the pulmonary circulation after birth which can mean that single ventricle palliation is either very high risk or not feasible at all (Chap. 18). Interrogation of pulmonary venous flow is widely used to predict septal restriction (Fig. 7.21a–c). In recent years, fetal cardiac MRI has been use with the aim of identifying pulmonary lymphangiectasia before birth. The term "nutmeg" lung has been used to describe the appearances of the lung in this context as the appearance is thought to resemble a cut nutmeg. Fetal intervention to perforate the

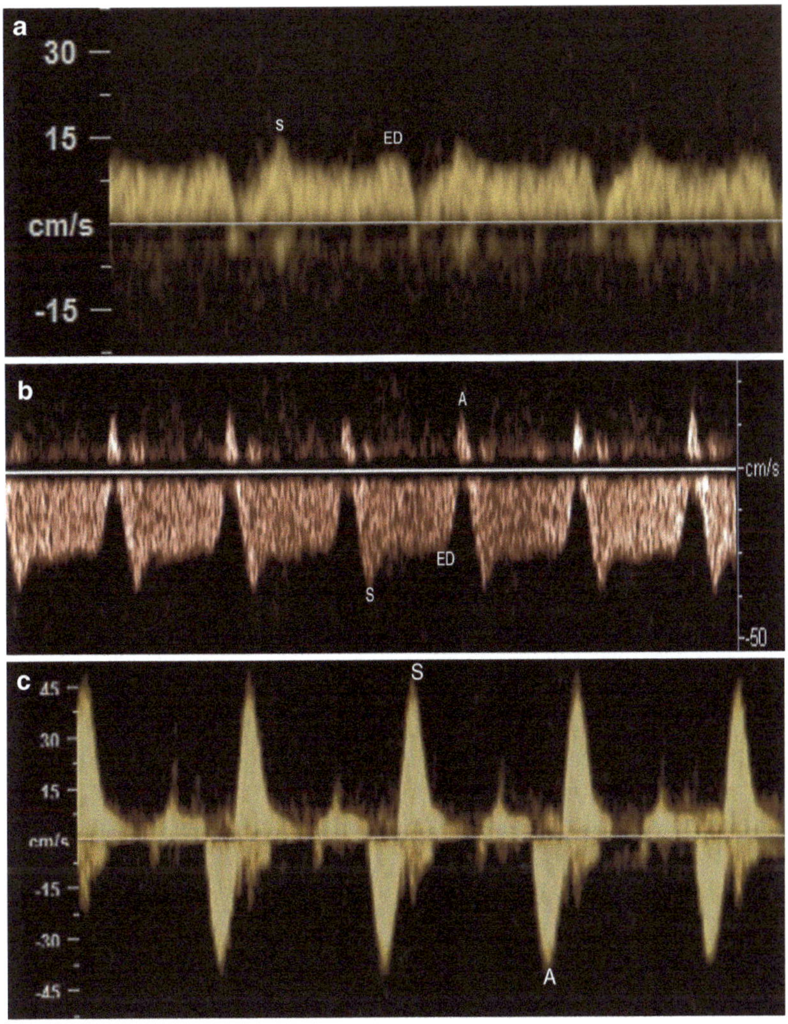

Fig. 7.21 (**a**) Normal pulmonary vein profile demonstrated using a Pulsed Wave Doppler with almost equal peaks in systole (S) and early diastole (ED). (**b**) This is an example of potentially mild restriction at the foramen ovale as this shows a lower wave then normal in early diastole (ED) and a reverse flow in atrial systole (A). (**c**) A severe case of restriction at foramen ovale is demonstrated in this Pulsed Wave Doppler example. There is an absent flow in early diastole and high velocity reversal flow (A)

atrial septum has been undertaken in selected cases in an attempt to prevent or reverse pulmonary vascular changes and lymphangiectasia and to improve postnatal oxygenation in affected fetuses. Even in technically successful cases, the atrial septum may become restrictive so that in some cases stent implantation across the atrial septum has been employed to maintain patency of the atrial septum.

Associations

There is considerable variation in the incidence of associated structural and chromosomal abnormalities in the published literature ranging from around 5 to 30%. This depends to a large extent on the definition of HLH which is used. In our own series, the incidence is 5% where a strict definition of classical HLH is used. All affected cases are offered detailed anomaly scanning as a minimum and the option of fetal karyotyping is discussed.

Hypoplastic Left Heart "Variants"

Critical Aortic Stenosis with Hypoplastic Left Heart Structures

Critical aortic valve stenosis may progress with advancing gestational age (see Chap. 8). Left ventricle growth tends to be suboptimal in fetuses with aortic valve stenosis so that by term the left ventricle is hypoplastic and unable to support the systemic circulation (Fig. 7.22, Video 7.11). In this setting, management is that of classical

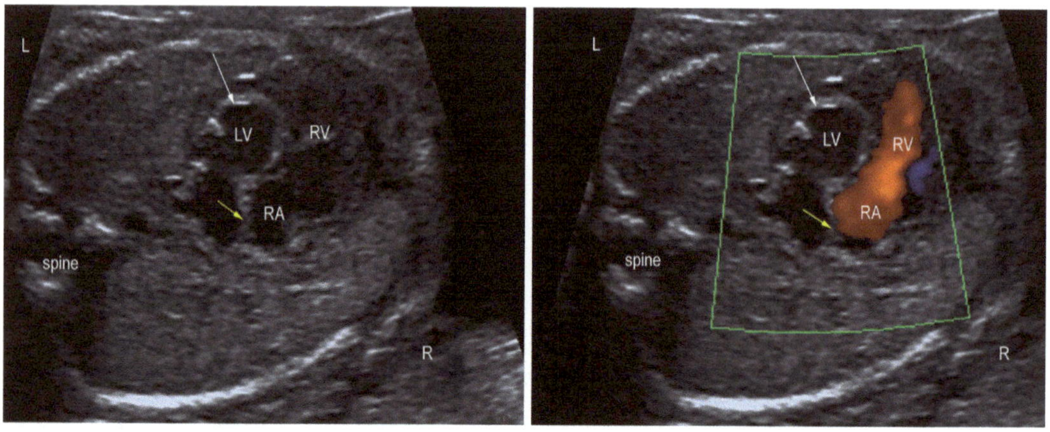

Fig. 7.22 The four-chamber view demonstrates a dilated, echogenic (white arrow) and non-apex forming left ventricle. This is a typical example of critical aortic stenosis. In addition, a restrictive atrial septum is seen (yellow arrow). The right-hand panel demonstrates flow across the right atrioventricular valve and within the right ventricle only. The video image 7.11 showed poor left ventricular contractility

HLH. In selected cases, fetal cardiac intervention has been undertaken to dilate the aortic valve in utero with the aim of promoting growth and function of the left heart (see Chap. 8). Chromosomal and extracardiac abnormalities are not common in this group.

Severe Coarctation of the Aorta

Coarctation of the aorta is described fully in Chap. 9. This lesion can present with a severe degree of asymmetry between the size of the right and left ventricle (Videos 7.12a and 7.12b) and a similar discrepancy between the size of the ductal and aortic arches (Video 7.12c). Thus, the term "HLH" has been loosely applied to this group. However, in contrast to classical HLH both the mitral and aortic valves are patent. Reversal of flow in the aortic arch is universal in classical HLH but variable in suspected coarctation of the aorta. A minority of cases of fetal coarctation of the aorta undergo single ventricle palliation after birth but in most cases a biventricular repair is achieved. The reader is referred to Chaps. 9 and 18 for more information on fetal coarctation and postnatal management respectively.

Unbalanced Atrioventricular Septal Defect

Some atrioventricular septal defects are severely unbalanced with a hypoplastic left ventricle and dominant right ventricle (Video 7.13). In the worst affected cases, the imbalance of ventricular size is such that a biventricular repair is not feasible. Atrioventricular valve regurgitation is frequent in such cases which represents an adverse prognostic sign. Due to the nature of the atrial communication ("primum" defect) restriction of left to right blood flow at the level of the atrial septum does not occur. Chromosomal abnormalities, including major trisomy, may co-exist with this group of lesions as well as defects of laterality (left or right atrial isomerism). The prognosis for unbalanced AVSD is very guarded if a single ventricle repair is undertaken because of progressively severe atrioventricular valve regurgitation.

Postnatal Management

Hypoplastic left heart will be duct dependent and therefore should be delivered in a centre with immediate access to congenital cardiac support and newborn intensive care. In most cases a normal delivery is planned but in fetuses with severely restrictive or intact atrial septum then Caesarian delivery may be necessary so that immediate intervention may be feasible after birth.

For any form of classical or variant HLH, if the left heart is unable to support the systemic arterial circulation after birth, a "single ventricle" form of surgical approach is adopted. Initially, a prostaglandin E infusion is commenced after birth to maintain ductal patency. There are a number of alternatives for initial surgery including the Norwood operation (aortic arch reconstruction, removal of atrial septum, insertion of systemic to pulmonary artery shunt), the Sano operation (utilizes a shunt from right ventricle to pulmonary arteries) or the Hybrid operation (stenting of the arterial duct coupled with banding of the branch pulmonary arteries). In all cases, the eventual management is towards a total cavopulmonary connection where the systemic veins are connected to the pulmonary arteries and the right ventricle pumps the systemic arterial circulation. The indications and specific techniques for both Norwood-type surgery and Hybrid-type catheter intervention are continually evolving and will be described in more detail in Chap. 18. Adverse prognostic factors include poor right ventricle function, significant tricuspid valve regurgitation, prematurity/low birth weight, genetic comorbidities and significant airway or lung pathology.

Hypoplasia of the Right Heart

Hypoplasia of the right heart may be due to anatomic obstruction of inflow to the right ventricle (e.g. tricuspid atresia) or obstruction to pulmonary blood flow (e.g. critical pulmonary stenosis or pulmonary atresia with intact ventricular septum). These lesions will be described in detail.

Tricuspid Atresia

Tricuspid valve atresia is very rare cardiac condition with a prevalence of 0.3 per 10,000 live births (Ferencz et al. 1985). There are two major forms of this lesion. The first, most common type, is absence of the right atrioventricular connection where there is an infolding of tissue between the right atrium and right ventricle so that there is no potential communication between the right atrium and right ventricle. In the second form, the tricuspid valve is present but is imperforate so that no flow can occur from the right atrium to the right ventricle. In physiological terms, the two varieties cause the same haemodynamic disturbance. In virtually all cases there is a ventricular septal defect. Most commonly, the great arteries are normally related: the pulmonary valve may be normally formed, stenotic or atretic and is typically smaller than the aortic valve. A diagram of tricuspid atresia with normal related great arteries is shown in Fig. 7.23.

In a minority if cases, the great arteries are transposed. In this context, the pulmonary artery arises from the left ventricle and is enlarged and the aorta arises from the smaller right ventricle and is hypoplastic.

Echocardiographic Features

In the 4ChV there will be a normally formed mitral valve and left ventricle. The right sided atrioventricular connection will not be patent and bright tissue will be visualised between the right atrium and a very small (hypoplastic) right ventricle (Fig. 7.24, Video 7.14). There will be no demonstrable flow from the right atrium to the right ventricle when using colour flow Doppler (Video 7.15). A single band of colour flow will be seen from the left atrium to the left ventricle. The right

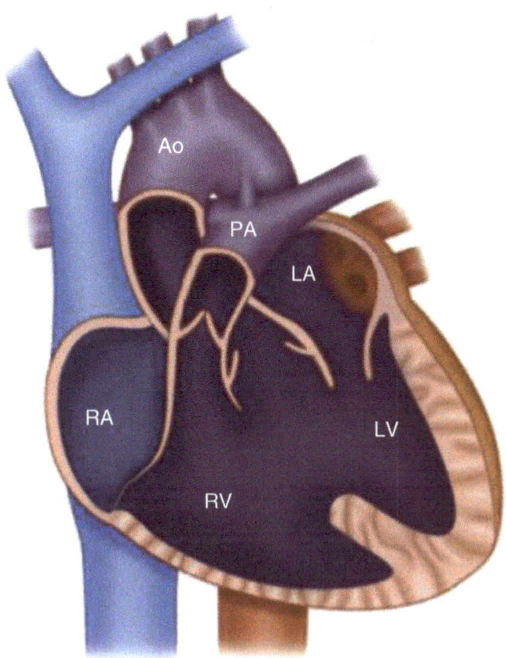

Fig. 7.23 A diagram of tricuspid atresia with normal related great arteries, associated hypoplasia of right ventricle and main pulmonary artery is shown in this drawing

ventricle varies in size and flow through the pulmonary artery is dependent on left to right flow of blood from the left ventricle into the right ventricle through the VSD. Views of the outflow tracts are essential to determine the relationship of the great arteries. If these are normally related (Video 7.16), then evaluation is to evaluate associated pulmonary stenosis or atresia. If the great arteries are transposed (discordant ventriculoarterial connections) which occurs in up to 40% of cases (Berg et al. 2010) (Fig. 7.25, Videos 7.17a and 7.17b) the aorta is committed to the right ventricle. The blood flow to the aorta and its size would largely depend on blood flow through the VSD. Coarctation of the aorta is frequently associated with a transposed arrangement of the great arteries.

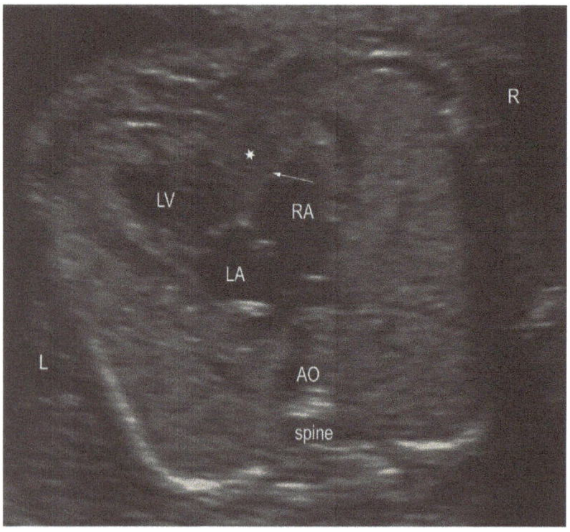

Fig. 7.24 This apical four-chamber view shows tricuspid atresia. The tricuspid valve is not present (white arrow) and there is no connection between the right atrium and the right ventricle. This results in a small right ventricle (asterisk)

Tricuspid atresia may be difficult to distinguish from severe pulmonary stenosis/atresia with an intact interventricular septum. The appearance of the four-chamber view can be quite similar in both malformations. In pulmonary atresia with intact ventricular septum the right ventricle may appear globular, echogenic and poorly contracting but the tricuspid valve is patent, although very small with limited excursion. A trace of flow across the tricuspid valve can be demonstrated with colour flow Doppler in pulmonary stenosis but not in tricuspid atresia as brightly echogenic tissue will be visible in the position of the tricuspid valve. Furthermore, in tricuspid valve atresia there is an associated VSD in contrast to pulmonary atresia with intact ventricular septum.

Associations

Tricuspid atresia is usually an isolated condition but can be associated with chromosomal anomalies such as trisomy 18. Extracardiac anomalies including VACTERL and renal tract abnormalities have been described (Berg et al. 2010).

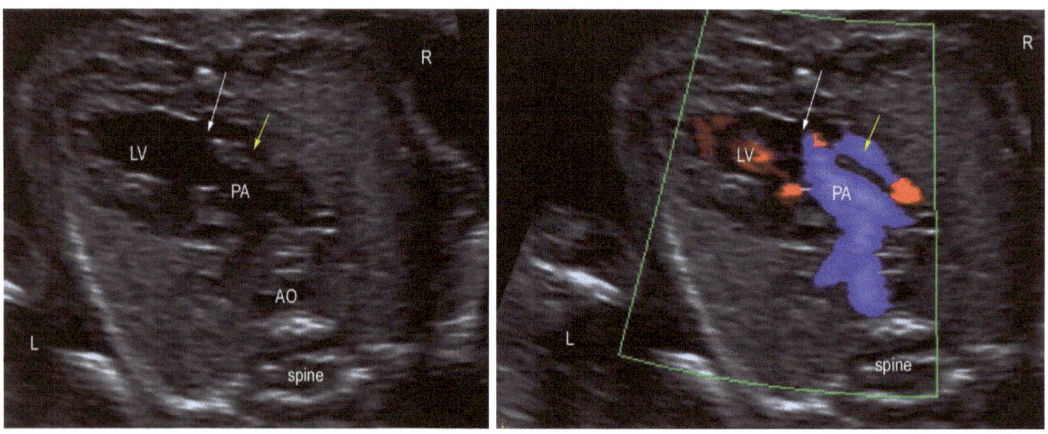

Fig. 7.25 Looking towards the outflow tracts there is an abnormal appearance of the ventricles and the great arteries. The left ventricle is dominant and the right ventricle is hypoplastic and an outlet ventricular septal defect (white arrow) is seen. The great arteries are parallel indicating ventriculoarterial discordance (transposed great arteries). The aorta (yellow arrow) is much smaller that the pulmonary artery suggestive of coarctation of the aorta

Management

Tricuspid atresia with associated pulmonary atresia will be duct-dependent and therefore should be delivered in a centre with immediate access to congenital cardiac support and newborn intensive care. However, mode of delivery will follow routine obstetric principles.

Tricuspid atresia but with adequate pulmonary blood flow will not be duct dependent and site of delivery is more negotiable. Our own practice is to deliver all “single ventricle” fetuses in our perinatal cardiac centre for immediate postnatal cardiac evaluation and access to newborn intensive care.

Given the obligate right to left atrial shunt, the newborn will be desaturated but to a variable degree depending on the amount of pulmonary blood flow either from the arterial duct or antegrade across the pulmonary valve.

For duct-dependent newborns with tricuspid atresia, a more sustainable source of pulmonary blood flow will be required before hospital discharge and this is most commonly achieved by the creation of a surgical systemic to pulmonary artery shunt (e.g. Blalock-Taussig shunt). However, catheter intervention with endovascular stenting of the arterial duct may be employed in selected case according to clinical status or centre preference. The eventual management of all cases of tricuspid atresia is towards a single ventricle (Fontan) circulation (Fontan and Baudet 1971) which is described in greater detail in Chap. 18. This approach is not curative and carries a guarded long-term prognosis.

Pulmonary Atresia with Intact Ventricular Septum (PAIVS)

Pulmonary atresia with intact ventricular septum is associated with an abnormal 4ChV of the heart. The right ventricular size is variable but this typically appears hypoplastic, globular and poorly contracting. The tricuspid valve appears patent but small with limited excursion of the valve leaflets (Fig. 7.26). A degree of tricuspid valve regurgitation is usually evident on colour flow Doppler but varies in its severity. In some cases, colour flow Doppler may show abnormal flow patterns over the right ventricle due to abnormal coronary development, including right ventricular to coronary communications (Video 7.18). Some infants will prove to have coronary stenosis or interruption but this cannot be reliably diagnosed by fetal echocardiography.

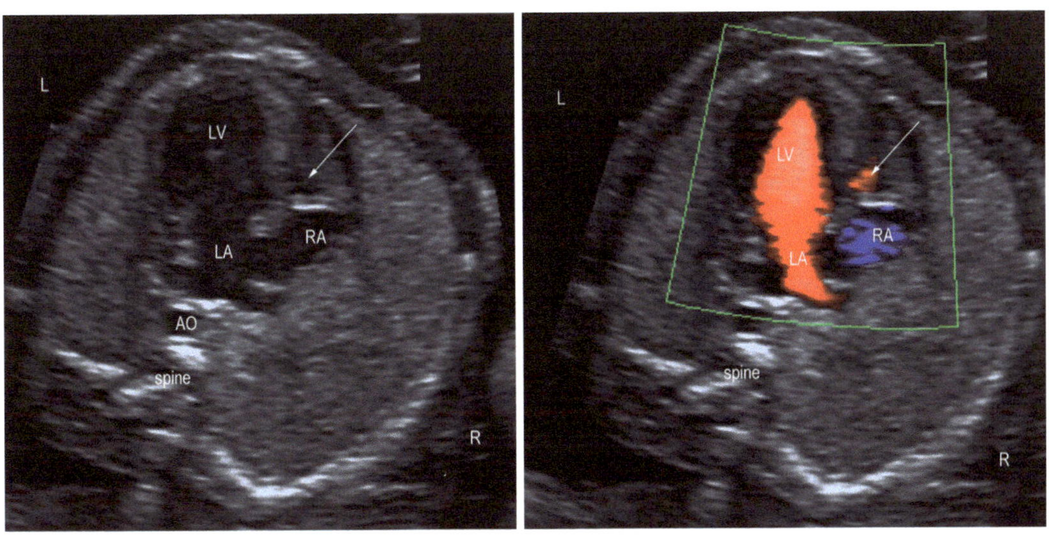

Fig. 7.26 This is an example of abnormal four-chamber view in case of a pulmonary atresia with intact ventricular septum. The right ventricle is hypertrophied and hypoplastic (white arrow). On the right sided panel, colour flow Doppler demonstrates flow within both ventricles including the hypoplastic right ventricle (white arrow). There was a small but patent tricuspid valve

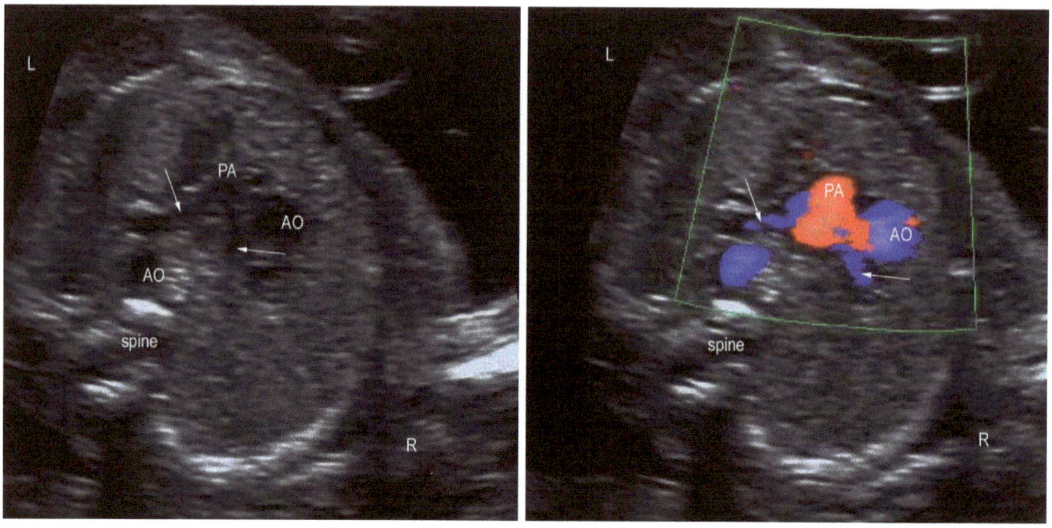

Fig. 7.27 The three-vessel view in this same fetus shows the pulmonary artery is slightly smaller than the aorta. The pulmonary artery branches (white arrows) are slender but confluent. On the right-hand panel, retrograde flow in the main pulmonary artery is seen with colour flow Doppler

Views of the outflow tracts will show underdevelopment of main pulmonary artery (Video 7.19). Blood flow to the pulmonary circulation is maintained by retrograde flow from the arterial duct which can be observed using colour flow Doppler (Fig. 7.27). In some cases, the right ventricular outflow tract is patent up to the level of the pulmonary valve (membranous atresia) but in others muscle separates the right ventricle from the pulmonary arteries. This distinction is important for management, as described later.

Associations

Pulmonary atresia with intact ventricular septum is usually an isolated lesion but may be associated with chromosomal abnormalities in around 5% of cases. In all cases detailed fetal anomaly scanning should be undertaken and fetal karyotyping is discussed in the light of screening investigations and associated anomalies.

Postnatal Management

Prostaglandin E is commenced in all cases after birth to maintain pulmonary blood flow. The fundamental decision after birth is whether the right ventricle is sufficiently developed to support pulmonary blood flow. If the right heart is judged inadequate then management is towards a single ventricle (Fontan) circulation (Chap. 18). Severe hypoplasia of the tricuspid valve, right ventricle and the presence of coronary abnormalities all influence management towards a single ventricle circulation. If the right ventricle is judged adequate then reestablishment of flow from the right ventricle to the pulmonary circulation is achieve either by interventional cardiac catheterisation or surgery. Insertion of a systemic to pulmonary artery shunt or stenting of the arterial duct is frequently also required to maintain pulmonary blood flow.

Other Abnormalities of the Crux

The normal 4ChV will display a clear centre of the heart, the so called "crux". The differential insertion (tricuspid valve slightly closer to the apex than the mitral) is also termed "atrioventricular valve offsetting" (see Chap. 2). Cardiac lesions where atrioventricular valve offsetting is abnormal can signify a major structural abnormality. Atrioventricular septal defect and inlet ventricular septal defect both have minimal or loss of atrioventricular valve offsetting and have been described above. There are a number of additional miscellaneous abnormalities, which are also recognisable from the 4ChV and have abnormal atrioventricular valve offsetting.

Double Inlet Left Ventricle

Double Inlet Left Ventricle (DILV) is a rare condition with incidence of 1 per 10,000 live birth (Allen et al. 2000). It is defined as both atrioventricular valves opening into a single dominant ventricular chamber which is usually the left ventricle. Typically, the right ventricle is severely hypoplastic and usually superior to the left ventricle. The great arteries are transposed in the majority of cases so that a large pulmonary artery arises from the left ventricle and a small aorta arises from the right ventricle. There is a ventricular septal defect, which is often not in a standard plane and may be difficult to visualise.

Echocardiographic Features

In the 4ChV, atrioventricular valve offsetting is minimal or absent and there is no visible interventricular septum reaching the crux of the heart and dividing ventricles equally. The ventricular septum is seen above the 4ChV when it divides the main inlet ventricle from the anterior outlet which is usually the right ventricle. The right ventricle can be very small or rudimentary and is connected to the left ventricle via a VSD, which varies in size (Figs. 7.28 and 7.29).

Outflow tract assessment is required, as in this condition the great arteries are usually transposed. The pulmonary artery often arises from the inlet ventricle, is wedged between the two atrioventricular valves and appears to be of good size. In contrast, the aorta will arise above the pulmonary artery from the small outlet (right) ventricle. The size of the aorta in this arrangement varies, but is commonly small as there is a frequent association with coarctation of the aorta (Video 7.20).

Associations

Double inlet left ventricle is not usually associated with major genetic syndromes or extracardiac abnormalities.

Management

Double inlet left ventricle can be a difficult fetal diagnosis, and requires detailed postnatal cardiac evaluation. The newborn will also have a func-

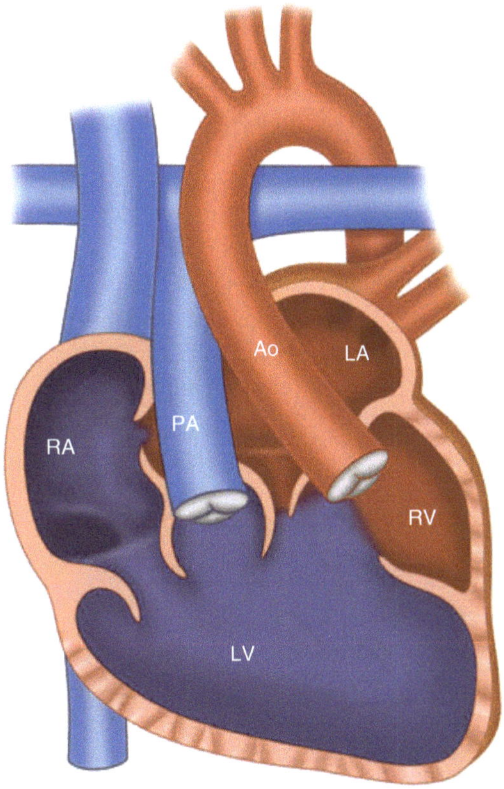

Fig. 7.28 This drawing demonstrates anatomy of the double inlet left ventricle

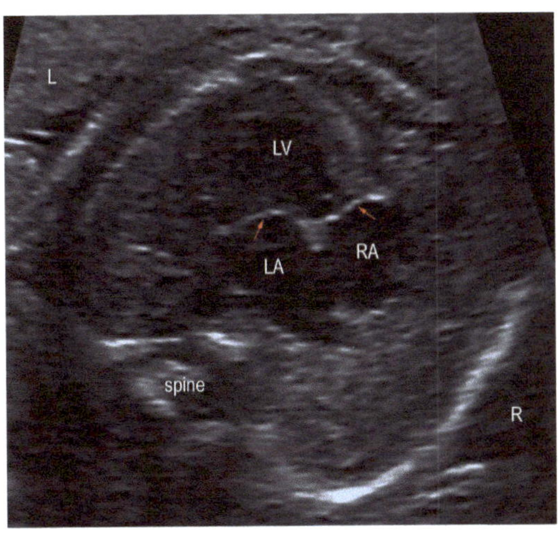

Fig. 7.29 The apical four-chamber view demonstrates an example of double inlet ventricle at 20 weeks gestation. In this view, there are two atria and two atrioventricular valves (red arrows) opening into a single (usually anatomically left) ventricle. Typically, there is loss of offsetting of the atrioventricular valves and no ventricular septum is seen dividing the ventricular mass

tionally single ventricle circulation which may be unstable. For this reason, our practice is to plan delivery in a centre with access to congenital cardiac support to allow timely postnatal review and cardiac management planning. Mode of delivery usually will follow routine obstetric principles.

Outcome

Double inlet left ventricle is not compatible with a biventricular circulation and therefore infants born with this lesion will need to follow a single ventricle palliative surgical pathway (see Chap. 18) with a guarded prognosis.

Ebstein's Anomaly of the Tricuspid Valve

Ebstein's anomaly of the tricuspid valve is a rare congenital heart disease, with a birth prevalence of 1 per 20,000 live birth (Ferencz et al. 1985), accounting for about 0.5% of all congenital heart disease diagnosed in the first year of life.

The cardinal feature of Ebstein's anomaly is apical displacement of the tricuspid valve into the right ventricle (Fig. 7.30). The tricuspid valve has three leaflets, the antero-superior, septal and inferior (posterior) which normally insert near the crux of the heart. Two of these leaflets (the septal and inferior) are displaced into the right ventricle in Ebstein's anomaly. This anatomy is associated with a variable degree of tricuspid valve regurgitation.

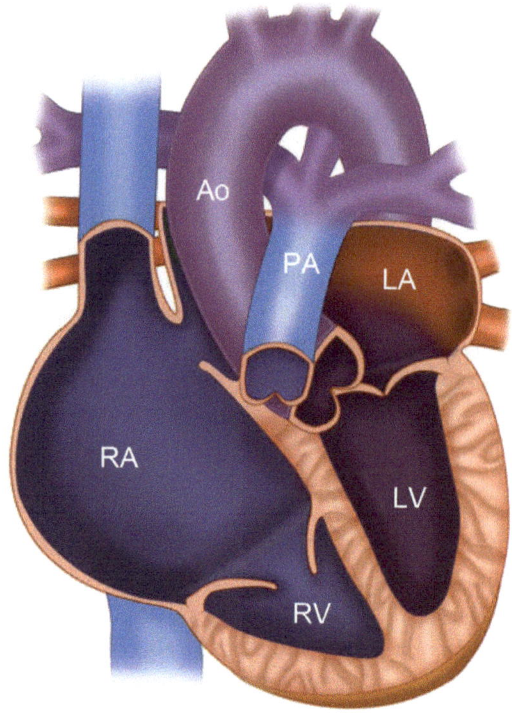

Fig. 7.30 This drawing demonstrates the anatomy of the tricuspid valve in Ebstein's anomaly of the tricuspid valve. The typical apical displacement of the tricuspid valve into the right ventricle is seen in this drawing

Echocardiographic Features

The 4ChV in Ebstein's anomaly will show exaggerated atrioventricular valve offsetting with the hinge point of the tricuspid valve more apically displaced than normal. The right atrium appears bigger than usual as a result of the "atrialisation" of the right ventricular, due to displacement of the tricuspid valve (Fig. 7.31a).

A fetal diagnosis of Ebstein's anomaly may be challenging as an echogenic tricuspid annulus appearing in the correct position can be misleading. A close inspection of the tricuspid valve leaflets will demonstrate their apical displacement (Fig. 7.31b).

Depending on the severity of the displacement the functional volume of the right ventricle may be reduced. A variable amount of tricuspid regurgitation may be seen with colour flow Doppler (Video 7.21). Presence of severe tricuspid regurgitation (Fig. 7.32) would cause right ventricle volume load and left ventricular compression, dilatation of the right atrium and subsequently increased central venous pressure, which may trigger fetal hydrops. The cardiomegaly caused by right heart dilatation may increase the risk of secondary lung compression and hypoplasia adding to a probability of a poor outcome.

In cases with severe tricuspid regurgitation, there may be little or no forward flow into the main pulmonary artery. It may be difficult to distinguish between anatomic and functional pulmonary atresia, although trace pulmonary regurgitation on colour Doppler may be a clue to support functional rather than anatomic pulmo-

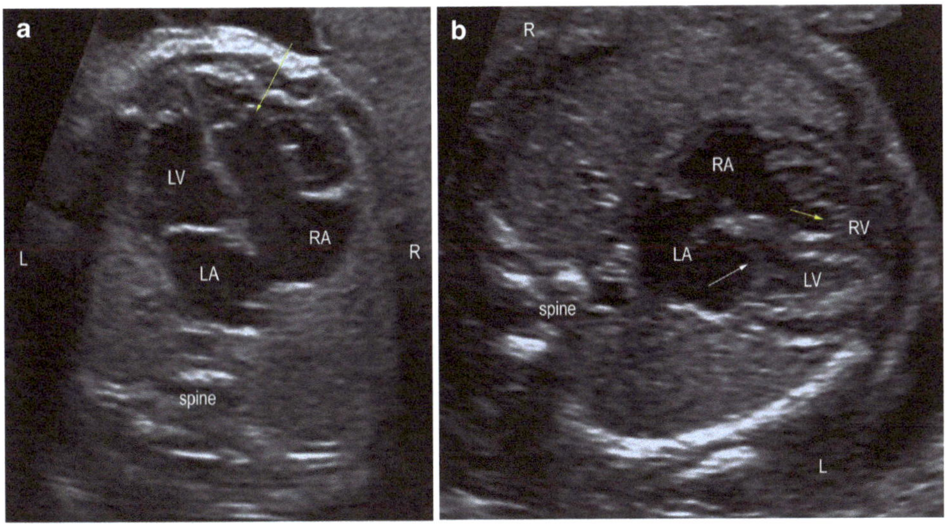

Fig. 7.31 (**a**) This four-chamber view demonstrates Ebstein's malformation of the tricuspid valve. The attachment of the septal leaflet of the tricuspid valve (yellow arrow) is significantly displaced towards the apex of the right ventricle compared to the mitral valve in the expected normal position. The right atrium is enlarged (atrialised right ventricle) due to a displacement of the tricuspid valve. (**b**) This is another example of Ebstein's malformation of the tricuspid valve. The displacement of the tricuspid valve (yellow arrow) is less obvious and the right atrium is mildly enlarged. The white arrow points to normal position of the mitral valve

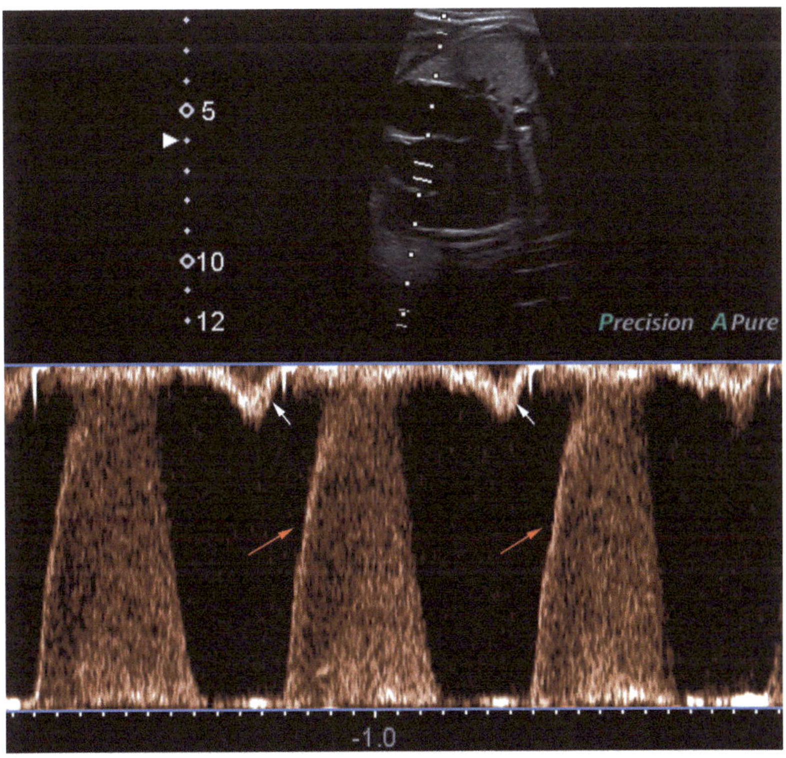

Fig. 7.32 Pulsed wave Doppler demonstrates holosystolic (red arrows) in a case of Ebstein's anomaly of the tricuspid valve

nary atresia. The flow assessment across the pulmonary artery and arterial duct are essential criteria as this information helps prognostication of postnatal outcome (Video 7.22). Reversal of flow in the arterial duct occurs in severely affected cases.

A fetal scoring system has been developed to assist in predicting outcome and key factors associated with increased mortality included increased cardiothoracic ratio, enlarged atrialised right atrium/right ventricle ratio and right-left ventricular ratio; reduced/absent pulmonary valve flow, and retrograde duct flow (Andrews et al. 2008).

Ebstein's anomaly can be suspected as early as the first trimester when some degree of exaggerated atrioventricular valve offsetting is seen with or without tricuspid regurgitation. This condition can progress during pregnancy, so that sequential review is essential. In our experience, early presentation with what may appear to be a subtle form of this condition having minimal tricuspid valve displacement, trace tricuspid regurgitation and forward flow in good size pulmonary artery may not necessarily predict a good outcome. Later scans may demonstrate distinct tricuspid valve displacement with significant regurgitation and associated functional pulmonary atresia leading to a less optimistic postnatal prognosis. In worse case scenarios, severe tricuspid valve regurgitation can result in severe cardiomegaly leading to lung compression, development of hydrops and subsequent fetal demise.

Fetuses with Ebstein's anomaly are at risk of arrhythmias, most commonly atrial flutter (due to atrial stretch) or supraventricular tachycardia (due to coexistent accessory conduction pathways).

Associations

Ebstein's anomaly of the tricuspid valve may be associated with extracardiac and genetic conditions including trisomy 21, trisomy 18, microdeletion of 1p36 and 8p23. CHARGE and VACTERL associations have been reported in association with this lesion (Digilio et al. 2011).

Management and Outcome

Management and prognosis will depend on anatomical severity of the condition. Cases diagnosed during fetal life are detected on the basis of abnormal four chamber views, cardiac enlargement or hydrops and so there is an ascertainment bias towards more severely affected cases. However, a broad spectrum of severity of this lesion is seen during fetal life.

The management is dictated by the underlying physiology. In less severe cases, the fall in pulmonary vascular resistance postnatally means that tricuspid valve regurgitation improves and antegrade flow of blood into the pulmonary circulation becomes adequate, so no intervention is required. At the other end of the spectrum, chronic cardiomegaly may lead to pulmonary hypoplasia and poor ventilatory status. If tricuspid valve regurgitation is severe, there may be poor antegrade pulmonary artery flow despite treatments such as inhaled nitric oxide and oxygen to further reduce pulmonary vascular resistance. Ideally, administration of Prostaglandin E is withheld to allow the arterial duct to close and promote antegrade flow into the pulmonary circulation from the right ventricle. Management of these cases needs to be undertaken in a high level neonatal facility with close cardiology input. There is relatively high rate of fetal and neonatal loss particularly in those with adverse prognostic features (Andrews et al. 2008). Postnatal scoring systems are used to grade Ebstein's anomaly after birth (Celermajer et al. 1992). Later in childhood or adolescence some cases may be considered for reconstructive tricuspid valve surgery.

Tricuspid Valve Dysplasia

The tricuspid valve may be abnormal with thickened or deformed leaflets (Fig. 7.33), but not apically displaced with normal atrioventricular valve offsetting and can occur as isolated lesion (Lang et al. 1991). Such tricuspid valve dysplasia demonstrates a variable degree of tricuspid regurgitation. Significant regurgitation can lead to enlargement of the right atrium and subsequently to cardiomegaly seen in the 4ChV (Fig. 7.6, Video 7.23). Severe regurgitation can further lead to reduce outflow and therefore functional or anatomical pulmonary stenosis or atresia. This is an evolving lesion and serial fetal cardiac scans are essential.

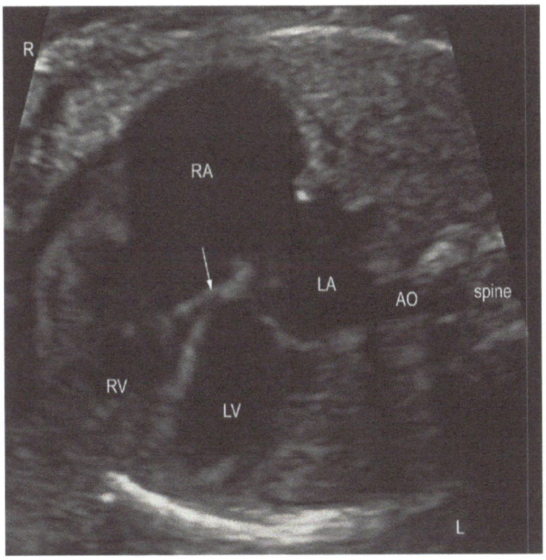

Fig. 7.33 There is marked cardiomegaly due to an enlarged right atrium caused by severe tricuspid valve regurgitation. The tricuspid valve is not displaced (white arrow) but appears thickened. This is a case of tricuspid valve dysplasia seen in the third trimester

Associations

Association with trisomy 18 is possible, particularly if other valves appear dysplastic.

Management and Outcome

Although there are morphological differences in the anatomy of the tricuspid valve between tricuspid dysplasia and Ebstein's anomaly; the hemodynamic consequences are similar as are the management and outcome. Recent multicentre experience continues to show a high rate of fetal and neonatal mortality (Freud et al. 2015) explaining why this cardiac lesion is seen more commonly in fetal life than postnatally.

Discordant Atrioventricular and Ventriculoarterial Connections

Atrioventricular and ventriculoarterial discordance, also called "congenitally corrected transposition", is a rare cardiac condition with a prevalence of 0.45 per 10,000 live birth (Ferencz et al. 1985) accounting for 0.05% of congenital heart disease.

In the majority of cases with this condition, the heart lies midline or in the left chest but can also lie in the right chest. In atrioventricular discordance, the morphological left atrium leads to a morphological right ventricle and the morphological right atrium connects to a morphological left ventricle. The arterial connections are also discordant meaning that the pulmonary artery is connected to the morphologically left ventricle and the aorta to the morphologically right ventricle. Thus, the oxygenated blood would still be delivered to the body where the venous blood flow would return to the lungs not causing imminent hemodynamic issues after birth (Fig. 7.34).

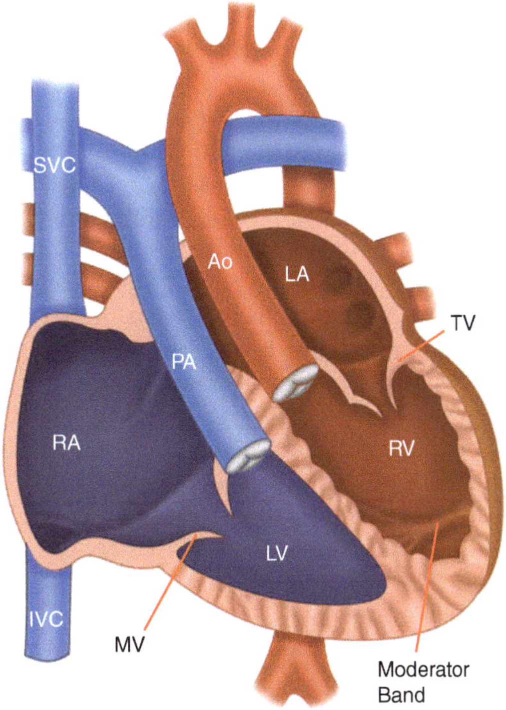

Fig. 7.34 This drawing demonstrates atrioventricular and ventriculoarterial discordance

Echocardiographic Features

In the 4ChV, atrioventricular valve off-setting will appear reversed, as the valve between the left atrium and the left-sided ventricle will be the tricuspid, its septal hinge point will be more apically placed. The atrioventricular valves follow their morphological ventricles. Thus, this ventricle will have a coarse trabeculation and the moderator band at the apex as in morphological right ventricle. In contrast, the valve between the right atrium and the smooth walled left ventricle will be the mitral valve (Fig. 7.35, Video 7.24). A careful assessment of the tricuspid valve is advisable as it may be dysplastic or significantly displaced into the right ventricle as in Ebstein's anomaly. The interventricular septum should be evaluated in view of possible ventricular septal defects in this cardiac lesion. Further outflow tract assessment will reveal that the pulmonary artery arises from the morphologically left ventricle and will be seen first on sweeping cranially with the aorta arising anterior and to the left from the morphologic right ventricle (Video 7.25). Assessment of the great artery size on 2D grey-scale as well as Doppler flow pattern analysis is essential to exclude additional artery stenosis, in particular the pulmonary artery.

Associations

Atrioventricular and ventriculoarterial discordance is rarely associated with chromosomal and extracardiac anomalies. Conduction disorders, predominantly complete heart block may be seen in the fetus (Hunter and Simpson 2015) but more commonly develops during childhood or later in adulthood.

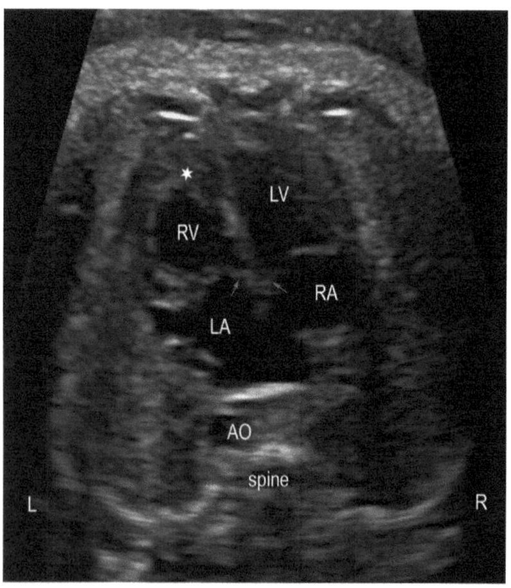

Fig. 7.35 This apical four-chamber view demonstrates atrioventricular discordance. The pulmonary venous chamber (left atrium) is anterior to the spine. This connects to a ventricle with a moderator band at the apex (asterisk). On closer inspection of the atrioventricular valves there is reversed off-setting (red arrows). The left-sided atrioventricular valve arises closer to the apex indicating that this is the tricuspid valve. These features are consistent with atrioventricular discordance, the morphological right ventricle is on the left side

Management and Outcome

The perinatal management can follow usual obstetric pathways unless there is fetal complete heart block, which may impair fetal monitoring during labour. Thus, Caesarean section may be considered. Most newborns, even those with complete heart block will have a stable circulation, which does not require immediate intervention.

The management of the patient with atrioventricular and ventriculoarterial discordance is dictated by the underlying anatomy and associated lesions.

Patients with unoperated isolated atrioventricular and ventriculoarterial discordance will have a morphological right ventricle pumping at high pressure and high afterload via the aorta to the systemic circulation. This will inevitably lead to the right ventricular dysfunction and often frank failure. The time course for the onset of symptomatic right ventricular dysfunction is however highly variable with some unoperated adults still asymptomatic. However, the lifetime risk of right ventricular failure has led to various surgical strategies including radical corrective surgery where the atrial venous return is redirected to the opposite ventricle (atrial switch) and the ventricular outlets are reconnected surgically to the opposite artery (arterial switch), thus allowing the left ventricle to function as the systemic ventricle. This surgery is termed the "double switch" operation, and due to its complexity, high surgical risk and uncertain long-term benefit is performed in only selected cases. For these reasons, the ultimate prognosis for the fetus with an atrioventricular and ventriculoarterial discordance remains variable.

More complex forms of this group of lesions are managed on an individualised basis with options ranging from conservative management through to single ventricle repair. Established complete heart block will usually require the postnatal insertion of an artificial pacemaker, which can be achieved at low surgical risk, but will require regular ongoing surveillance and periodic replacement during the patient's lifetime.

Asymmetry of the 4ChV

Cardiac "asymmetry" is a descriptive term usually applied to a situation where left heart structures appear smaller than those on the right but with blood flow into the heart across both the mitral and tricuspid valves and blood flow out of the heart through the aorta and pulmonary artery. This contrasts with structural lesions with either severe stenosis or atresia of the atrioventricular valves or great arteries. There are a number of causes of such asymmetry including primary cardiac or extracardiac aetiology.

The asymmetrical heart usually presents with both left atrium and left ventricle appearing smaller than the right but with patent mitral and tricuspid valves. It is important to remember that the appearance of asymmetry may be physiological in the last 10 weeks of pregnancy (Fig. 7.36), however fetal cardiac structures should be carefully assessed before such a conclusion is drawn.

The 4ChV is the primary view for judging ventricular and atrial size. Although asymmetry may be evident between the ventricles, the imbalance is rarely just ventricular but rather represents a more extensive problem. The initial decision for the fetal echocardiographer is to determine whether any asymmetry is due to one side of the heart being smaller than expected or the other being larger than expected. In the normal 4ChV the ventricles both reach the apex and failure of either ventricle to form the cardiac apex should be viewed as abnormal. Such a judgment is usually made subjectively. However, measurement of the inlet (mitral and tricuspid) valves and expressing these annulus measurements as Z-scores can be used to inform that decision.

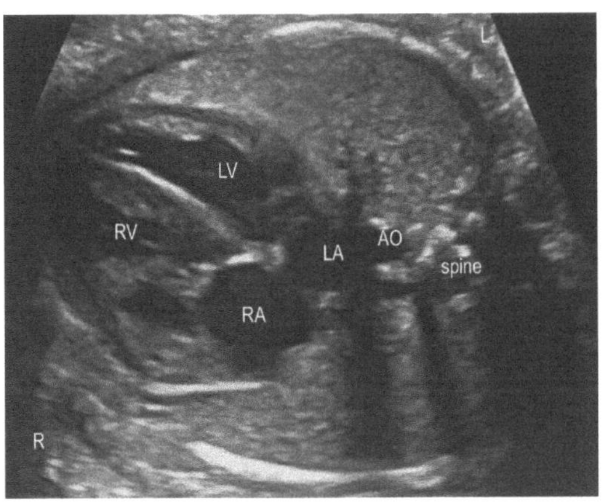

Fig. 7.36 The fetal heart is seen in an apical four-chamber view at 33 weeks gestation. There is a degree of asymmetry with right ventricular dominance which is common in the third trimester. The left ventricle reaches the apex

Primary Cardiac Causes of 4ChV Asymmetry

Coarctation of the Aorta

Coarctation of the aorta is the most common cause of asymmetry. Suspicion is first raised during four-chamber assessment but examination of the great arteries and aortic arch confirms this diagnosis. The left ventricle is smaller than the right ventricle and the mitral valve annulus may be small for gestation (Fig. 7.37). The asymmetry of the ventricles varies, as it is dependent on the severity of coarctation. Even more important is the associated disparity of size of the great arteries with hypoplasia of the aortic arch being a particularly strong marker of coarctation of the aorta. This lesion is addressed more fully in Chap. 9.

Anomalous Pulmonary Venous Connection (TAPVC)

Total anomalous pulmonary venous connection (TAPVC) results in absence of pulmonary venous return to the left atrium. In TAPVC, the pulmonary venous drainage, by definition, drains instead to the right heart. Flow to the left heart is only achieved by right to left shunting of blood at atrial level. Thus, the left atrium and the left ventricle appear smaller than normal. It is essential that in any case of cardiac asymmetry that the pulmonary venous drainage is thoroughly assessed. In addition to asymmetry seen on 2D grey-scale, colour flow Doppler will confirm an absence of blood from the pulmonary veins to the posterior left atrium. The sonographer should also look for an additional venous channel draining either above the heart (usually into the innominate vein) or inferiorly (usually into the liver) in cases of suspected TAPVC. This lesion is discussed in greater detail in Chap. 10.

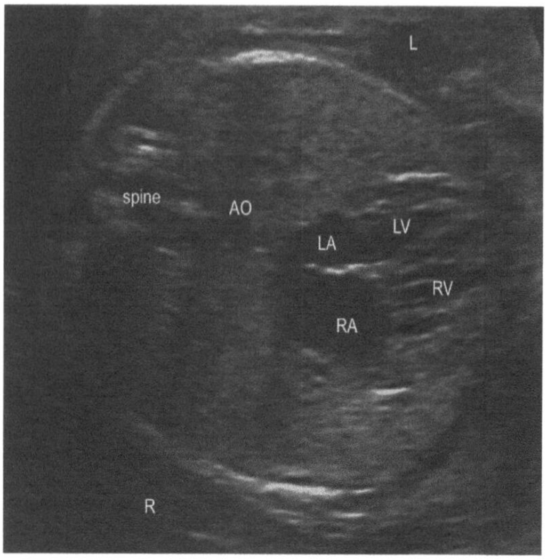

Fig. 7.37 An apical four-chamber view at 20 weeks gestation demonstrating moderate ventricular disproportion. Ventricular disproportion in the first or second trimester is not normal and therefore the aetiology should be sought. This fetus had coarctation of the aorta

Persistent Left Superior Vena Cava (PLSVC)

Presence of the persistent left superior vena cava in the fetus may be associated with asymmetry in 4ChV. The coronary sinus is dilated as it typically receives the PLSVC. There is a recognised association between PLSVC and coarctation of the aorta so that careful assessment and measurement of the aortic arch is essential to ensure that coarctation of the aorta is not overlooked. Further discussion of PLSVC can be found in Chap. 10.

Extracardiac Causes for 4ChV Asymmetry

There are several groups of extracardiac abnormalities which can lead to cardiac asymmetry which are summarised in Fig. 7.38. Extracardiac abnormalities (Fig. 7.39) are discussed in Chap. 14 and agenesis of the ductus venosus in Chap. 10.

Fetal growth restriction (FGR) merits particular consideration because it can present with asymmetry of ventricular size as well as hypoplasia of the aortic arch, which frequently raises a suspicion of coarctation of the aorta. In FGR, flow in the distal aortic arch may be bidirectional (with flow reversal in diastole) or reversed (Video 7.26). In FGR changes in peripheral vascular resistance (cerebral vasodilation and systemic and pulmonary vasoconstriction) are thought to preferentially divert blood supply to the vital organs (brain, myocardium and the adrenal glands), thus the reverse flow in the aortic arch during diastole is seen. This so called 'the brain sparing effect' is discussed in Chap. 14. These circulatory changes may be reflected at the level of the fetal heart by reduced left ventricular afterload (due to cerebral vasodilation) and increased right ventricular afterload (due to systemic and pulmonary vasoconstriction). Differentiation from true coarctation of the aorta during fetal life can be difficult.

Primary Cardiac Tumours

The most common primary fetal cardiac tumours are described in this chapter. Primary cardiac tumours are rare in fetuses, neonates and children found in only 0.08% of children referred for a cardiac examination (Isaacs Jr. 2004).

Rhabdomyoma

Rhabdomyoma is the commonest (60%) cardiac tumour seen during fetal life. Teratoma and fibroma are the next commonest type of primary fetal cardiac tumour (Isaacs Jr. 2004). Myxoma, lipoma and cardiac vascular tumours are also rarely described.

Primary fetal cardiac tumours tend to appear after 20 weeks of gestation and they are usually seen in the four-chamber view. Mediastinal tumours can occupy space but may also affect cardiac function. Depending on location (mediastinum/thorax or intracardiac) and size of the mass, it may result in an increased cardio-thoracic ratio.

Prognosis will be determined by diagnosis, haemodynamic effect of the tumour and response to treatment or spontaneous regression. Tumour size per se is not the primary determinant of outcome, but rather position of the tumour in the heart or mediastinum and whether there is a

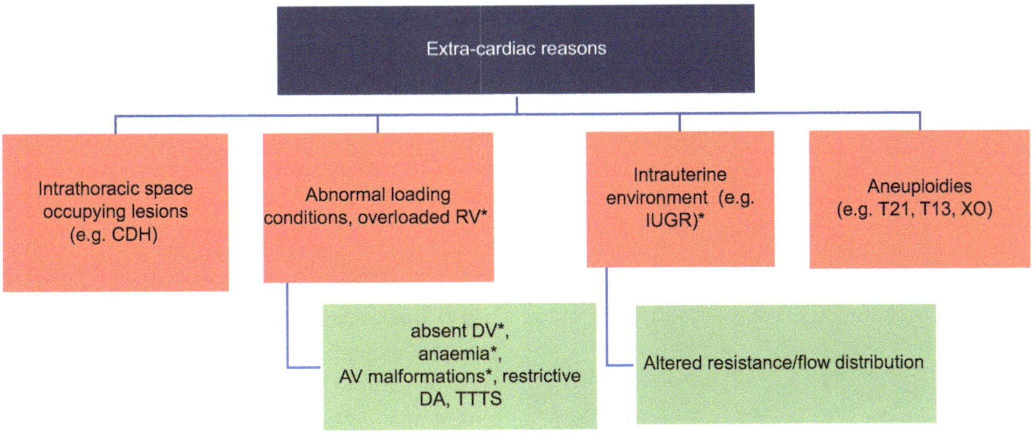

Fig. 7.38 This flowchart demontrates potential reasons for caridac asymetry in extracardiac fetal anomalies. Asymetrical four-chamber appearance in extracardiac fetal anomalies. *Typically together with cardiomegally. *DA* ductus arteriosus, *DV* ductus venosus, *CDH* congenital diaphragmatic hernia, *RV* right ventricle, *IUGR* intrauterine growth restriction, *T21* trisomy 21, *T13* trisomy 13, *XO* Turner syndrome, *TTTS* twin-to-twin transfusion syndrome

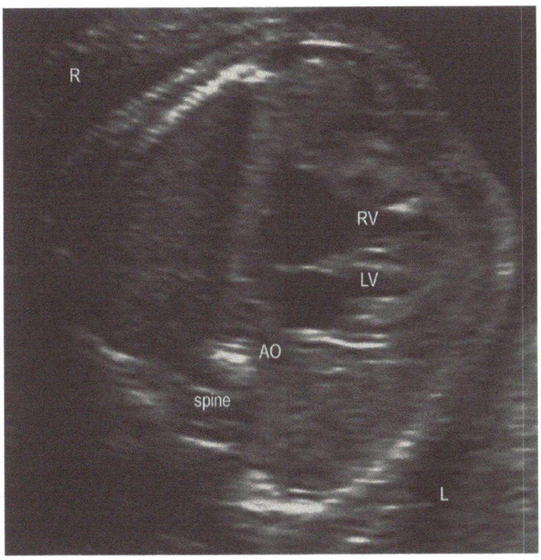

Fig. 7.39 The heart is seen in an apical four-chamber view at 19 weeks gestation with confirmed trisomy 13. There is moderate ventricular disproportion but the transverse aortic arch appeared normal on further assessment

physiological effect such as obstruction to blood flow (Lacey and Donofrio 2007).

Rhabdomyomas can lie anywhere within the atrial or ventricular wall. They vary in size appearing as a homogeneous mass, slightly more echogenic than myocardium but less than echogenic foci (Fig. 7.40). Although a solitary rhabdomyoma may be observed, multiple tumours are more often found. If a single tumour is seen at 20 weeks there is a high chance of additional tumours becoming evident with advancing gestational age. The occurrence of multiple tumours strongly supports the diagnosis of a rhabdomyoma in contrast to other tumours which are usually solitary. Protrusion into the cardiac cavity rarely causes intracardiac flow obstruction. Fetal arrhythmias also occur in a minority of cases.

Associations

Cardiac rhabdomyomas are strongly associated with Tuberous Sclerosis in the fetus. Investigation by fetal brain MRI is often undertaken to investigate for additional supportive features such as tubers in the brain. This is further discussed in Chap. 15.

Management and Outcome

Rhabdomyomas may cause arrhythmia in a minority of cases and rarely hydrops due to intracardiac blood flow obstruction. Rhabdomyomas have a natural tendency to regress after birth, usually resolving over the first few years. If no clinically significant obstruction is evident postnatally then surgical treatment is unnecessary.

Postnatal follow-up with cardiologist is required until the cardiac masses have resolved spontaneously. Genetics review is recommended in all cases, with and without obvious signs of tuberous sclerosis.

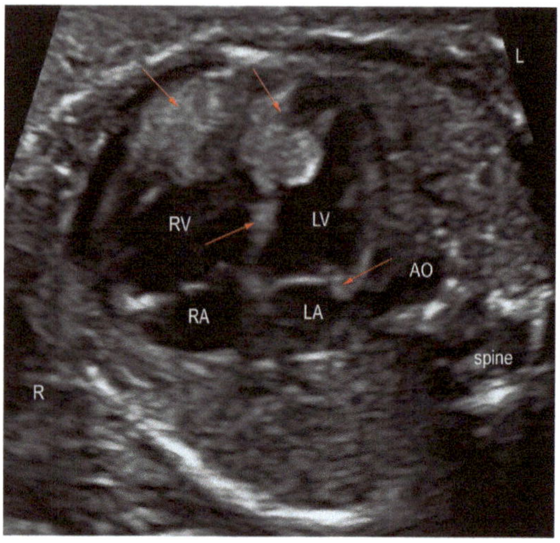

Fig. 7.40 This four-chamber view demonstrates multiple homogenous masses of varying size within the myocardium (red arrows). The texture is homogenous and slightly brighter than myocardium and is typical of rhabdomyomas

Teratoma

Teratoma is a solitary tumour lying on the surface of the heart usually attached to the great vessels, protruding into the pericardial sac. Its distinctive features are multiple cysts of varying sizes and an associated large pericardial effusion (Fig. 7.9). Both the tumour and/or pericardial effusion can obstruct venous return, causing fetal hydrops and subsequent demise.

Associations

Underlying or extracardiac lesions have not been observed in teratoma.

Management and Outcome

In severe cases, prenatal pericardial fluid drainage and thoraco-amniotic shunt insertion may be considered in order to prevent further lung compression increasing the chance of survival. Spontaneous regression is not observed in this type of cardiac mass. In surviving cases, surgical treatment, performed soon after birth, may be successful if the whole tumour can be completely excised. No recurrence of this type of cardiac tumour has been reported.

Fibroma

Fibroma occurs most frequently within the left ventricular free wall or interventricular septum but occasionally is seen in the right ventricle. It is a single, usually large, homogeneous soft-tissue mass that may be either sharply marginated or infiltrative with commonly associated calcifications. Associated arrhythmias or intracardiac blood flow obstruction may lead to heart failure or sudden death. Spontaneous regression of this type of cardiac mass has not been observed. In symptomatic cases, surgical intervention postnatally may be considered. The success of surgical intervention and long term functional result would depend on the location and resectability of the mass (Zidere et al. 2002).

References

Allen LD, Hornberger LK, Sharland GK. Double inlet left ventricle in the fetus. In: Fetal cardiology. London: Greenwich Medical Media; 2000. p. 174–82.

Andrews RE, Tibby SM, Sharland GK, Simpson JM. Prediction of outcome of tricuspid valve malformations diagnosed during fetal life. Am J Cardiol. 2008;101(7):1046–50.

Berg C, Lachmann R, Kaiser C, Kozlowski P, Stressig R, Schneider M, Asfour B, Herberg U, Breuer J, Gembruch U, Geipel A. Prenatal diagnosis of tricuspid atresia: intrauterine course and outcome. Ultrasound Obstet Gynecol. 2010;35:183–90.

Celermajer DS, Cullen S, Sullivan ID, Spiegelhalter DJ, Wyse RKH, Deanfield JE. Outcome in neonates with Ebstein's anomaly. J Am Coll Cardiol. 1992;19(5):1041–6.

Delisle MF, Sandor GG, Tessier F, Farquharson DF. Outcome of fetuses diagnosed with atrioventricular septal defect. Obstet Gynecol. 1999;94:763–7.

Digilio MC, Bernardini L, Lepri F, Giuffrida MG, Guida V, Baban A, Versacci P, Capolino R, Torres B, De Luca A, Novelli A, Marino B, Dallapiccola B. Ebstein anomaly: genetic heterogeneity and association with microdeletions 1p36 and 8p23.1. Am J Med Genet. 2011;155A:2196–202.

Ferencz C, Rubin JD, McCarter RJ, Brenner JI, Neill CA, Perry LW, Hepner SI, Downing JW. Congenital heart disease: prevalence at livebirth. The Baltimore-Washington Infant Study. Am J Epidemiol. 1985;121(1):31–6.

Fontan F, Baudet E. Surgical repair of tricuspid atresia. Thorax. 1971;26(3):240–8.

Freud LR, Escobar-Diaz MC, Kalish BT, Komarlu R, Puchalski MD, Jaeggi ET, Szwast AL, Freire G, Levasseur SM, Kavanaugh-McHugh A, Michelfelder EC, Moon-Grady AJ, Donofrio MT, Howley LW, Tierney ES, Cuneo BF, Morris SA, Pruetz JD, van der Velde ME, Kovalchin JP, Ikemba CM, Vernon MM, Samai C, Satou GM, Gotteiner NL, Phoon CK, Silverman NH, McElhinney DB, Tworetzky W. Outcomes and predictors of perinatal mortality in fetuses with Ebstein anomaly or tricuspid valve dysplasia in the current era: a multi-center study. Circulation. 2015;132:481–9.

Hunter LE, Simpson JM. Atrioventricular block in fetal life. J Saudi Heart Assoc. 2015;27:164–78.

Isaacs H Jr. Fetal and neonatal cardiac tumors. Pediatr Cardiol. 2004;25(3):252–73. Review. PubMed PMID: 15360117.

Lacey SR, Donofrio MT. Fetal cardiac tumors: prenatal diagnosis and outcome. Pediatr Cardiol. 2007;28:61–7.

Lang D, Oberhoffer R, Cook A, Sharland G, Allan L, Fagg N, Anderson RH. Pathological spectrum of malformations of the tricuspid valve in prenatal and neonatal life. J Am Coll Cardiol. 1991;17:1161–7.

Mogra R, Zidere V, Allan LD. Prenatally detectable congenital heart defects in fetuses with Down syndrome. Ultrasound Obstet Gynecol. 2011;38(3):320–4.

Mosimann B, Zidere V, Simpson JM, Allan LD. Outcome and requirement for surgical repair following prenatal diagnosis of ventricular septal defect. Ultrasound Obstet Gynecol. 2014;44(1):76–81.

Zidere V, Lubaua I, Lacis A. Giant fibroma of the right ventricle. Cardiol Young. 2002;12(6):584–6.

8 Abnormalities of the Great Arteries

John Simpson

Abstract

This chapter describes the sonographic features of major abnormalities of the outflow tracts including transposition of the great arteries, common arterial trunk, tetralogy of Fallot and double outlet right ventricle as well as aortic and pulmonary valve stenosis. The sonographic features of each lesion are illustrated and contrasted with the normal anatomy of the fetal cardiac outflow tracts. The associations of the different abnormalities and the approach to postnatal management are also discussed.

Keywords

Fetal heart · Outflow tracts · Great arteries · Congenital heart disease

Introduction

Diagnosis of abnormalities of the great arteries during fetal life poses a significant challenge in terms of their recognition during routine obstetric screening. In many fetuses, the four chamber view of the heart may appear normal and an abnormality only recognised if the echocardiographer has a clear understanding of the normal anatomy of the great arteries (Chap. 2). Results of screening for congenital heart disease show that the detection of abnormalities of the outflow tracts is much lower than abnormalities where the four chamber view is abnormal. For the specialist, differential diagnosis of different abnormalities may sometimes be difficult and even when a firm diagnosis has been reached, prognostication may depend on details of the individual anatomy. This chapter focuses on the sonographic features of the commoner groups of abnormalities of the great arteries. The sonographic features are compared to normal and important details are highlighted. The emphasis is on a systematic approach to assessment. A brief overview of the approach to postnatal management is also provided.

Transposition of the Great Arteries

Transposition of the great arteries (TGA) is a form of CHD where the pulmonary artery arises exclusively or predominantly from the morphologic left ventricle and the aorta arises exclusively or predominantly from the morphologic right ventricle. The term "simple" TGA is used to describe this anatomy where there are no other associated cardiac lesions (Table 8.1). However, transposition of the great arteries can

Electronic Supplementary Material The online version of this chapter (https://doi.org/10.1007/978-3-319-77461-9_8) contains supplementary material, which is available to authorized users.

J. Simpson
Evelina London Children's Hospital, Guy's and St Thomas' NHS Foundation Trust, London, UK
e-mail: john.simpson@gstt.nhs.uk

© Springer International Publishing AG, part of Springer Nature 2018

J. Simpson et al. (eds.), *Fetal Cardiology*, https://doi.org/10.1007/978-3-319-77461-9_8

Table 8.1 Summary of groups of CHD where transposition of the great arteries has been described. TGA may be observed in conjunction with a diverse group of cardiac lesions

Feature	Diagnostic group	Four chamber view
Abnormal cardiac situs	Right atrial isomerism	Abnormal Usually AVSD
Abnormal atrioventricular connections	Tricuspid atresia Double inlet left ventricle	Abnormal
NORMAL atrioventricular connections	Simple TGA TGA with VSD TGA with VSD and PS TGA with VSD and Coarctation	Normal Normal or VSD seen only towards the ventricular outlets.
Size of great arteries	Simple TGA TGA with VSD TGA with VSD and PS TGA with VSD and Coarctation	Ao = PA Ao = PA Ao > PA PA > Ao
Three vessel trachea view	Aortic arch and ductal arch meet in a "V" shape	Aorta frequently courses directly above ductal arch so Aortic arch and SVC in "two vessel" view

occur in the setting of abnormalities of the atrioventricular connections, notably tricuspid valve atresia, double inlet left ventricle and right atrial isomerism. In that situation, management is usually towards a functionally single ventricle circulation which is covered in Chap. 18. Those cases are usually initially detected because of an abnormal four chamber view in addition to abnormal views of the outflow tracts and their diagnosis and management is not discussed further here.

The focus of this chapter relates to the sonographic features, associations and management of fetuses where there are normal atrioventricular connections and the dominant abnormality is TGA (Pascal et al. 2007). In this context, however, TGA may co-exist with other abnormalities including a ventricular septal defect, coartctation of the aorta, pulmonary valve stenosis, subpulmonary stenosis and abnormalities of the mitral valve. Simple TGA has an incidence of 3.5 per 10,000 live births and accounts for 5% of CHD. A schematic illustration of this lesion is shown in Fig. 8.1.

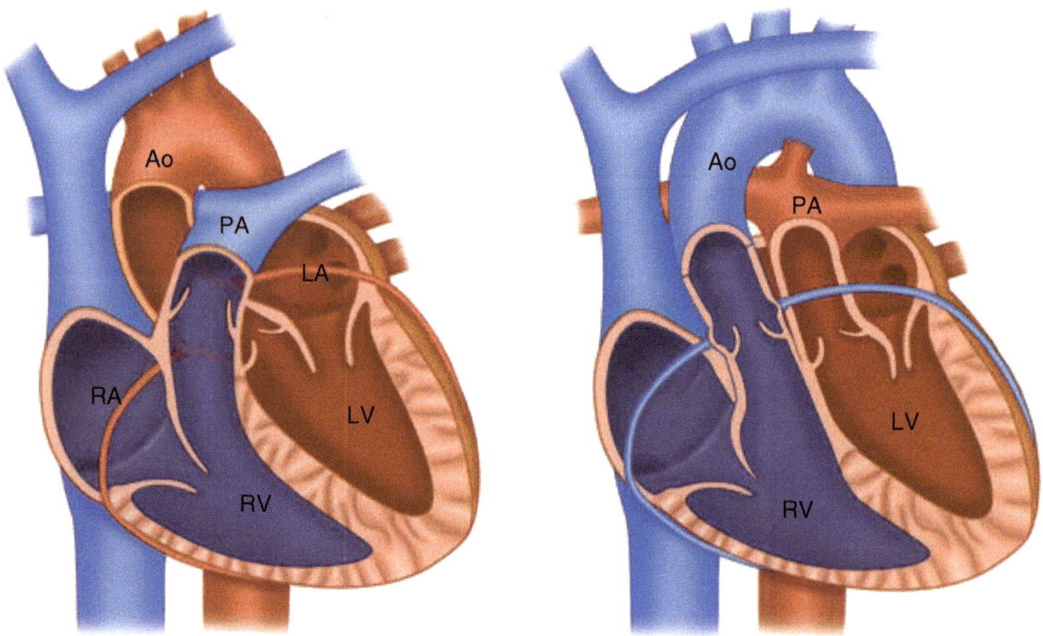

Fig. 8.1 This diagram compares the anatomy of the normal heart versus simple transposition of the great arteries (TGA). In TGA, the pulmonary artery arises from the left ventricle and the aorta from the right ventricle. The orientation is more parallel than normal so that the normal spiral or "crossing" orientation of the great arteries is lost

Echocardiographic Features

In simple transposition of the great arteries the four-chamber view of the fetal heart is typically normal (Video 8.1). Detection of the lesion depends on visualisation of the outflow tracts. The detection rate for simple TGA was previously very low but has improved as views of the outflow tracts have been incorporated into screening programmes.

On sweeping the transducer cranially from the four-chamber view in the normal heart, the first vessel to be observed is the aorta arising from the left ventricle which is directed towards the right shoulder of the fetus. In contrast, in simple TGA the first vessel is the main pulmonary artery which hooks posteriorly towards the spine and may be observed to bifurcate (Fig. 8.2a, Video 8.2). On angulating further cranially, in simple TGA the aorta arises from the RV anterior to the pulmonary artery and continues into the aortic arch which typically passes directly superior to the ductal arch (Fig. 8.2b, Video 8.2). The effect of this is that the normal "V" shape of the arterial duct and aortic arch in the "three vessel" and trachea (3VT) view is lost. Thus, there may only be two vessels visible in the 3VT view (Fig. 8.2c, Videos 8.3 and 8.4). Views of the upper mediastinum also demonstrate the abnormal relative position of the great arteries with the aorta usually anterior and to the right of the pulmonary artery (Fig. 8.2d). If the transducer is rotated slightly, the aorta and pulmonary artery may be observed to arise in parallel (Fig. 8.2e, Videos 8.5 and 8.6)

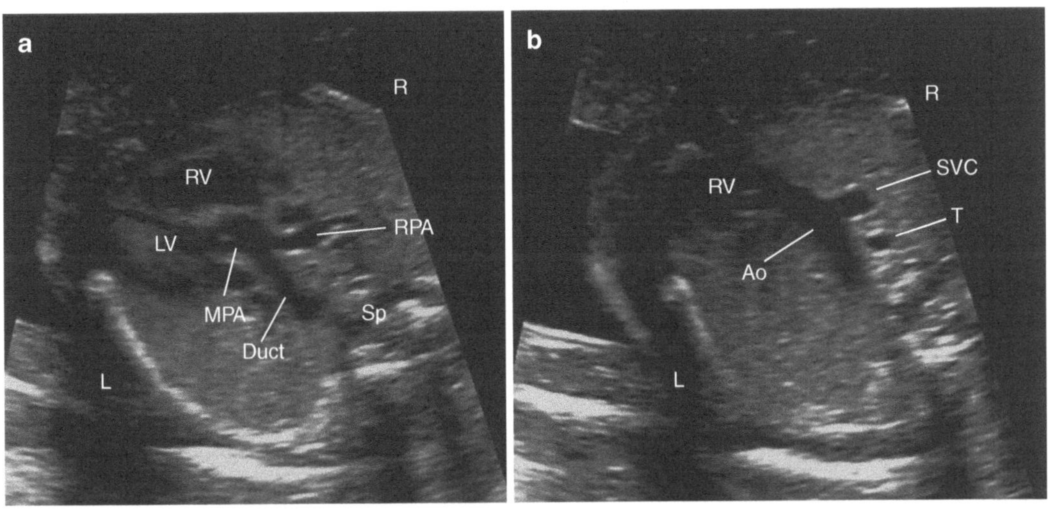

Fig. 8.2 Simple transposition of the great arteries. (**a**) Pulmonary artery arising from the left ventricle. On sweeping cranially from the four chamber view, the first vessel is the pulmonary artery which turns posteriorly towards the spine rather than being directed towards the right shoulder. The main pulmonary artery bifurcates, with the arterial duct and right pulmonary artery visible in this example. (**b**) Aorta arising from the right ventricle. As the transducer is angle even further cranially, the aorta can be seen arising from the right ventricle. The orientation is similar to that of the pulmonary artery. In this example, the aorta passes to the left of the trachea. (**c**) This is the equivalent of the normal three vessel and trachea view (3VT) view in the normal heart. Note that only the aorta alone is visible, thus there are only two vessels visible—the aorta and the superior vena cava. In this example, the aortic arch is left sided and the SVC is seen to the right. (**d**) This projection is obtained on cranial angulation of the transducer from the four-chamber view. This shows the abnormal relationship of the great with the aorta anterior and to the right of the pulmonary artery. (**e**) Parallel orientation of the great arteries. If the transducer is rotated obliquely then the parallel orientation of the great arteries in TGA can be appreciated. The aorta is superior to the pulmonary artery and duct. Note that the great arteries are seen in long axis in the same sonographic cut which is not possible in the normal fetal heart. (**f**) Foramen ovale size in transposition of the great arteries The foramen ovale is well seen in the four chamber view. In TGA the appearances of the PFO vary. In some cases this is large as shown whereas in others the PFO is small. This impacts mixing of oxygenated and deoxygenated blood postnatally

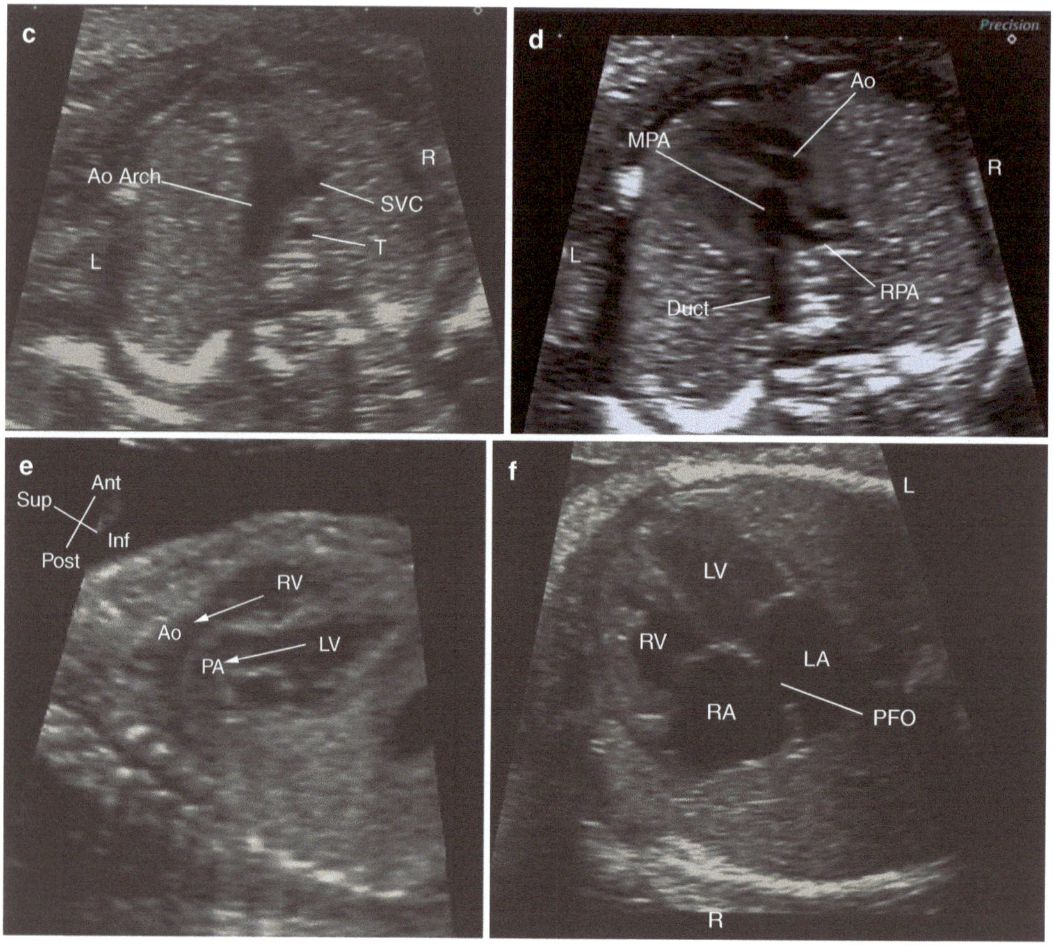

Fig. 8.2 (continued)

Table 8.2 Summary of echocardiographic features of simple TGA

Feature	Normal heart	Simple TGA
4 chamber view	Normal	Normal
LVOT	Aorta directed towards right shoulder	Pulmonary artery "hooks" towards spine
Relationship of GA	Aorta and PA cross each other with PA anterior	Aorta and PA in parallel orientation
Size of great arteries	Aorta similar to PA	Aorta similar to PA
Three vessel trachea view	Aortic arch and ductal arch meet in a "V" shape	Aorta frequently courses directly above ductal arch so Aortic arch and SVC in "two vessel" view

in contrast to the normal spiralling pattern. The size and other features of the foramen ovale are also seen in the four chamber view (Fig. 8.2f). The echocardiographic features of simple TGA are summarised in Table 8.2 and contrasted with the normal heart.

Associated lesions include ventricular septal defects (Fig. 8.3, Video 8.7) which can occur in any portion of the ventricular septum. Some of these VSDs are visualised above the level of the four-chamber view in a subpulmonary location. The size of defects is highly variable and they are

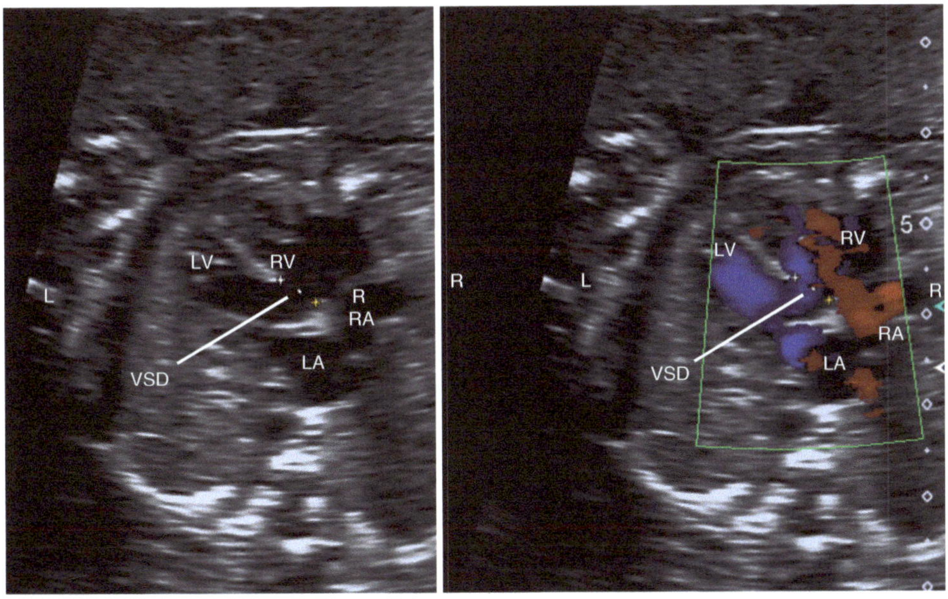

Fig. 8.3 Transposition of the great arteries with ventricular septal defect. In the left pane the VSD is evident in the four chamber view and is being measured by calipers. In the right pane colour flow Doppler confirms the presence of the defect. The location of the VSD is variable, some are evident only on views of the outflow tracts

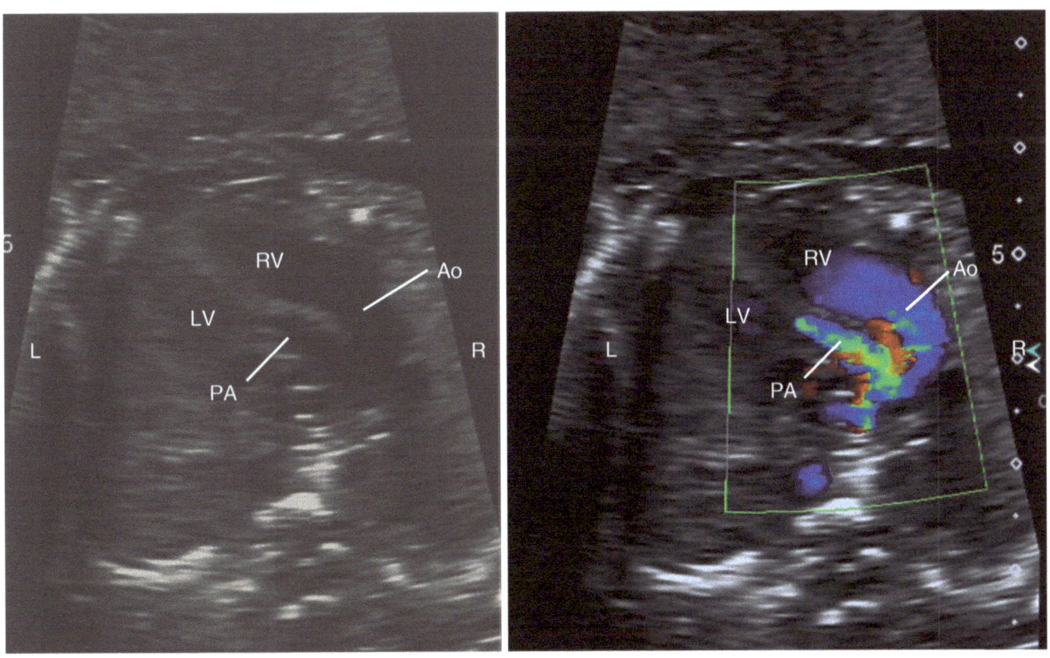

Fig. 8.4 Transposition of the great arteries with pulmonary stenosis. The left pane shows that the aorta is significantly larger than the pulmonary artery. Use of colour flow (*right pane*) confirms aliasing of colour flow due to obstruction of pulmonary blood flow

often an irregular shape or slit-like in their morphology. Subpulmonary or pulmonary valve stenosis should be suspected if the pulmonary artery is smaller than the aorta (Figs. 8.4 and 8.5, Video 8.8). In most cases, there is an associated ventricular septal defect. Views of the left ventricular outflow tract are essential to define the level of obstruction. Doppler interrogation has a limited role in estimating the severity of pulmonary valve stenosis because of high pulmonary vascular resistance and patency of the arterial duct during fetal life. Hypoplasia of the pulmonary artery and reversal of flow in the arterial duct during systole are good markers of severity (Figs. 8.4 and 8.5, Video 8.8). The assessment of the degree of obstruction to pulmonary blood flow has critical importance with respect to the postnatal operative options. Coarctation of the aorta in association with TGA is suspected when a discrepancy between the size of the great arteries (Aorta <PA) is observed as well as hypoplasia of the transverse aortic arch (Fig. 8.6a, b). Signs of both PS and coarctation of the aorta may evolve or progress with advancing gestational age. In the majority of fetuses with TGA and signs of coarctation of the aorta there will be an associated VSD. The mitral valve should be carefully visualised in all cases of TGA. The normal MV only has attachments to the free wall of the LV and none to the ventricular septum. The most common MV abnormality in TGA is a true cleft in the anterior leaflet. This can be confirmed on short axis views of the valve which shows a "trileaflet" appearance and septal attachments of the MV frequently occur.

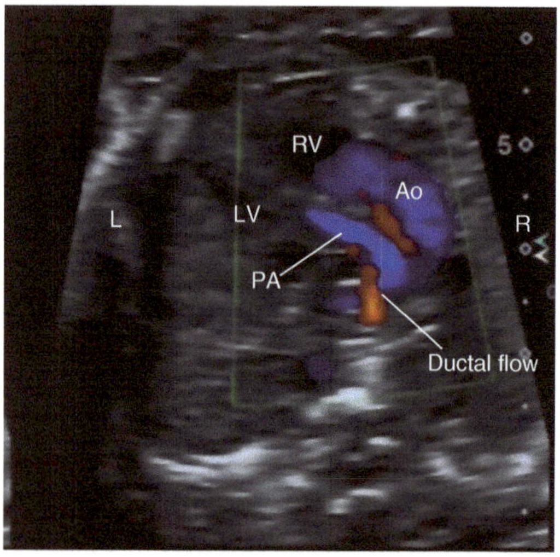

Fig. 8.5 TGA with pulmonary stenosis. The aorta is larger than the pulmonary artery. Retrograde flow is seen in the arterial duct confirming significant obstruction to pulmonary blood flow

During the transition to postnatal life, adequate mixing of oxygenated and deoxygenated blood is important to maintain systemic arterial oxygen saturations. Prediction of whether the atrial septum will become restrictive or not has been investigated

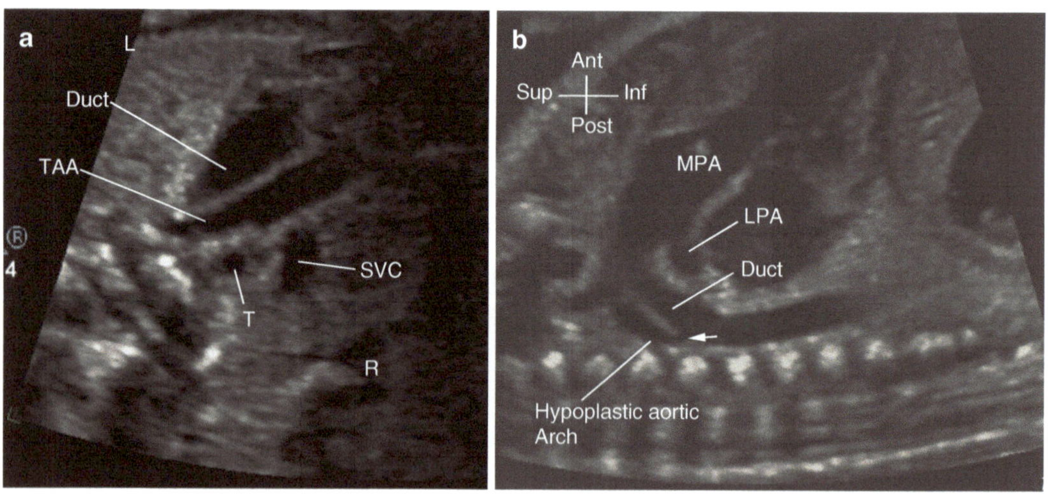

Fig. 8.6 Transposition of the great arteries with coarctation of the aorta. (**a**) In this fetus with transposition of the great arteries, the arteries were in a side by side orientation so that the transverse aortic arch (TAA) and arterial duct could be compared. The aortic arch was much smaller than the pulmonary artery and arterial duct, raising the suspicion of coarctation of the aorta. (**b**) The sagittal view confirmed severe hypoplasia of the aortic arch which is much smaller than the arterial duct. Severe narrowing at the point of the aortic arch joining the arterial duct is evident (*arrowed*) indicative of coarctation of the aorta which was confirmed after birth

in several studies. Data from our own unit has suggested that a small size of the foramen ovale in relation to total septal length is most predictive (Vigneswaran et al. 2017) but other groups have reported a hypermobile atrial septum or "fixed" appearance as being most predictive. In current practice, prediction of atrial septal restriction remains imperfect. The potential requirement for emergency balloon atrial septostomy is an important consideration with respect to site of delivery.

Associations

In simple TGA it is rare for there to be major abnormalities of the fetal karyotype. Non-cardiac malformations are not common but all such cases should have detailed assessment for non-cardiac malformations, with the offer of fetal karyotyping particularly if there are any associated abnormalities or abnormal first trimester screening results.

Management

In our own practice, delivery of cases of TGA is at the tertiary cardiac centre, ideally at term, but there is typically no cardiac indication for a Caesarian section (see Chap. 18). After delivery, a prostaglandin E (PGE) infusion is commenced to maintain ductal patency and improve mixing of oxygenated and deoxygenated blood. Monitoring of pre- and post-ductal oxygen saturations is mandatory. In some cases, there are very low oxygen saturations despite administration of PGE due to restriction of left to right blood flow across the atrial septum. In this situation a balloon atrial septostomy is undertaken. This procedure involves passing a balloon tipped catheter across the atrial septum and rapidly pulling the inflated balloon back from the left atrium to the right atrium to tear the atrial septum and increase left to right shunting of oxygenated blood to improve delivery of oxygenated blood to the systemic arterial circulation.

The definitive surgical treatment of simple TGA is to switch the position of the great arteries (arterial switch operation) which is illustrated in Fig. 8.7. This procedure uses cardiopulmonary bypass and involves "switching" the position of the great arteries. As part of the procedure the coronary arteries are transferred to the new aorta, which carries the risk of kinking the coronaries resulting in myocardial ischaemia. There is variability of the anatomy of the coronary arteries which cannot be diagnosed confidently until after birth. If there is an associated VSD and / or coarctation of the aorta these are normally repaired during the initial surgery.

In cases with associated pulmonary valve stenosis or subpulmonary stenosis, the option of an arterial switch operation may be precluded because the pulmonary valve becomes the aortic valve which needs to be free of significant obstruction and leakage. If an arterial switch operation is not possible due to the severity of pulmonary valve stenosis then alternative strategies such as baffling the left ventricle to the aorta through the VSD and inserting a conduit between the RV and pulmonary arteries (Rastelli operation) or relocation of the aortic root to the pulmonary position (Nikaidoh operation) may need to be considered. In selected cases, redirection of the pulmonary and systemic venous return (Senning operation) or even single ventricle palliation may have to be considered.

All children who have undergone surgical repair of TGA and its variants will need to be followed up lifelong. Following an arterial switch, features which require review include aortic and pulmonary valve function, branch pulmonary artery stenosis, aortic root dilation and coronary perfusion.

Common Arterial Trunk

Common arterial trunk (or truncus arteriosus) is a type of CHD in which a single great artery leaves the heart and divides to supply the aortic arch and the pulmonary circulation. The incidence is approximately 10 per 100,000 livebirths, constituting less 1% of CHD diagnosed before birth. The trunk usually arises astride a ventricular septal defect and may be more committed to the right ventricle than the left. The truncal valve can be stenotic (narrowed) and / or regurgitant. In most cases the arterial duct is absent and the

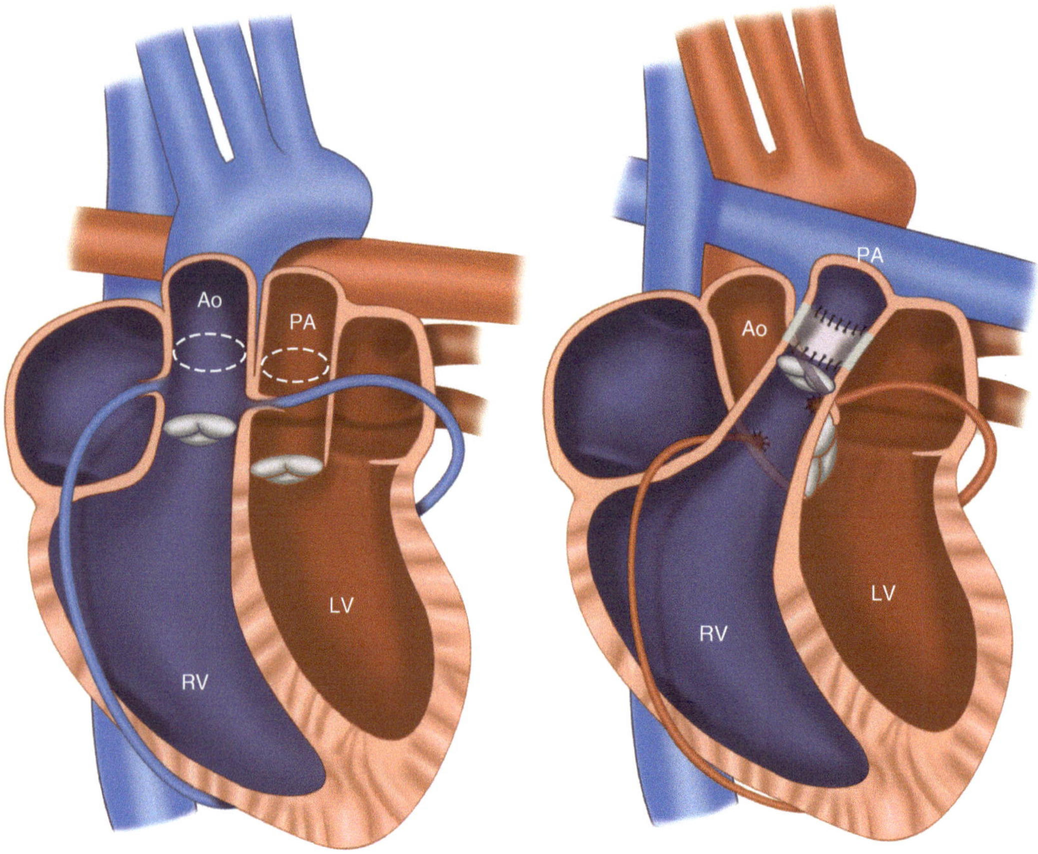

Fig. 8.7 —Arterial switch operation. The arterial switch operation. The aorta and pulmonary artery are transected above the level of the valve and the arteries are "switched". The coronary arteries have to be removed from the aorta on "buttons" of tissue and then attached to the neo-aorta. Following surgery the blood flow is physiologically corrected. The pulmonary artery is anterior to the aorta and both branch pulmonary arteries pass anterior to the aorta

aortic arch may either be left sided or right sided. In a small minority of cases the aortic arch is interrupted and the arterial duct supplies the descending aorta. Fig. 8.8 shows a diagrammatic representation of the lesion.

Echocardiographic Features

A summary of key features of common arterial trunk compared to the normal fetal heart is shown in Table 8.3. The four-chamber view of the fetal heart is usually normal although the apex may be rotated more to the left than normal (Vigneswaran et al. 2015). The ventricular septal defect in CAT is not usually seen in the four-chamber view but only when the transducer is angulated cranially towards the outflow tracts (Video 8.9). A single large artery exits the heart which continues into the aortic arch (Fig. 8.9a). The origin of the pulmonary arteries from the arterial trunk may be difficult to image clearly. There is variability of the pulmonary artery anatomy: in some cases the main PA arises from the trunk and then bifurcates (Type 1), in others the PAs arise at the same level but separately (Type 2) and in a minority the left and right pulmonary arteries arise separately and remote from each other (Type 3). Assessment of the PA anatomy is best done using a combination of grey scale and colour flow Doppler imaging (Fig. 8.9b–d, Videos 8.10, 8.11, and 8.12). The appearances of the truncal valve should be assessed, by colour flow and pulsed Doppler because truncal valve stenosis and regurgitation is a frequent co-existing finding (Video 8.13). If truncal valve stenosis is severe, then significant

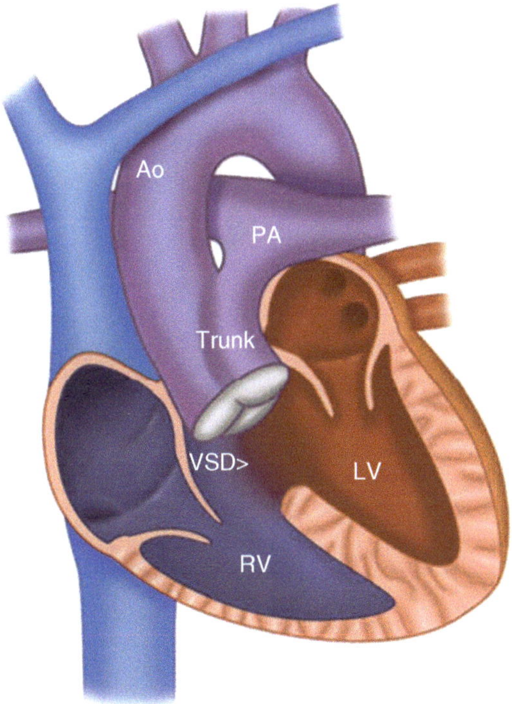

Fig. 8.8 Common arterial trunk. The common trunk arises above a ventricular septal defect and divides into the aorta and the pulmonary artery. The duct is usually absent and the aortic arch can be right sided, left sided or interrupted. The anatomy of the pulmonary artery origin is variable. The truncal valve is frequently stenotic and/or regurgitant which complicates management. The oxygen content of the blood in this diagram reflects the postnatal rather than prenatal circulation

Table 8.3 Summary of echocardiographic features of common arterial trunk

Feature	Normal heart	Common arterial trunk
4 chamber view	Normal	Normal/near normal
LVOT	Aorta directed towards right shoulder	Single great artery arises above a VSD
Relationship of GA	Aorta and PA cross each other with PA anterior	Single great artery giving rise to aortic and pulmonary circulation
Size of great arteries	Aorta similar to PA	Trunk larger than normal aorta
Three vessel trachea view	Aortic arch and ductal arch meet in a "V" shape	Single great artery and SVC. Aortic arch left or right sided Duct usually absent, unless interrupted aortic arch

ventricular hypertrophy and dysfunction may occur which can result in fetal hydrops in a small minority of cases. If sonographic windows are adequate the morphology of the truncal valve can be visualised which can range from bicuspid through to quadricuspid valves. In most cases, delineation of the truncal valve morphology can only be achieved after birth. It is important that sequential echocardiography is undertaken because truncal valve stenosis and regurgitation can become progressively more severe as the gestational age advances with an adverse impact on prognosis (Duke et al. 2001). The aortic arch may be either left or right sided with only two vessels visible in the equivalent of the normal 3VT view (Fig. 8.9e). In most cases, the arterial duct is absent, but in some cases, notably those with associated interruption of the aortic arch then the duct is present.

Associations

CAT is frequently associated with karyotypic abnormalities. The most frequent abnormality is 22q11 microdeletion which can occur in up to 30% of cases. Extracardiac abnormalities are also frequent in up to 40%, emphasising the importance of comprehensive assessment, including the offer of fetal karyotyping.

Management

The usual aim for cases of CAT is to deliver at term either at the cardiac centre or at a high level neonatal unit (Swanson et al. 2009). If there is evidence of significant truncal valve stenosis and/or regurgitation, careful cardiological oversight is essential because abrupt haemodynamic deterioration is well described.

Prostaglandin E infusion is not indicated in most cases and is administered only if there is interruption of the aortic arch and a duct dependent systemic circulation. Oxygen saturations are usually adequate (>85%) and tend to increase as the pulmonary vascular resistance falls after birth and pulmonary blood flow increases. Because there is only one outlet from the heart, high

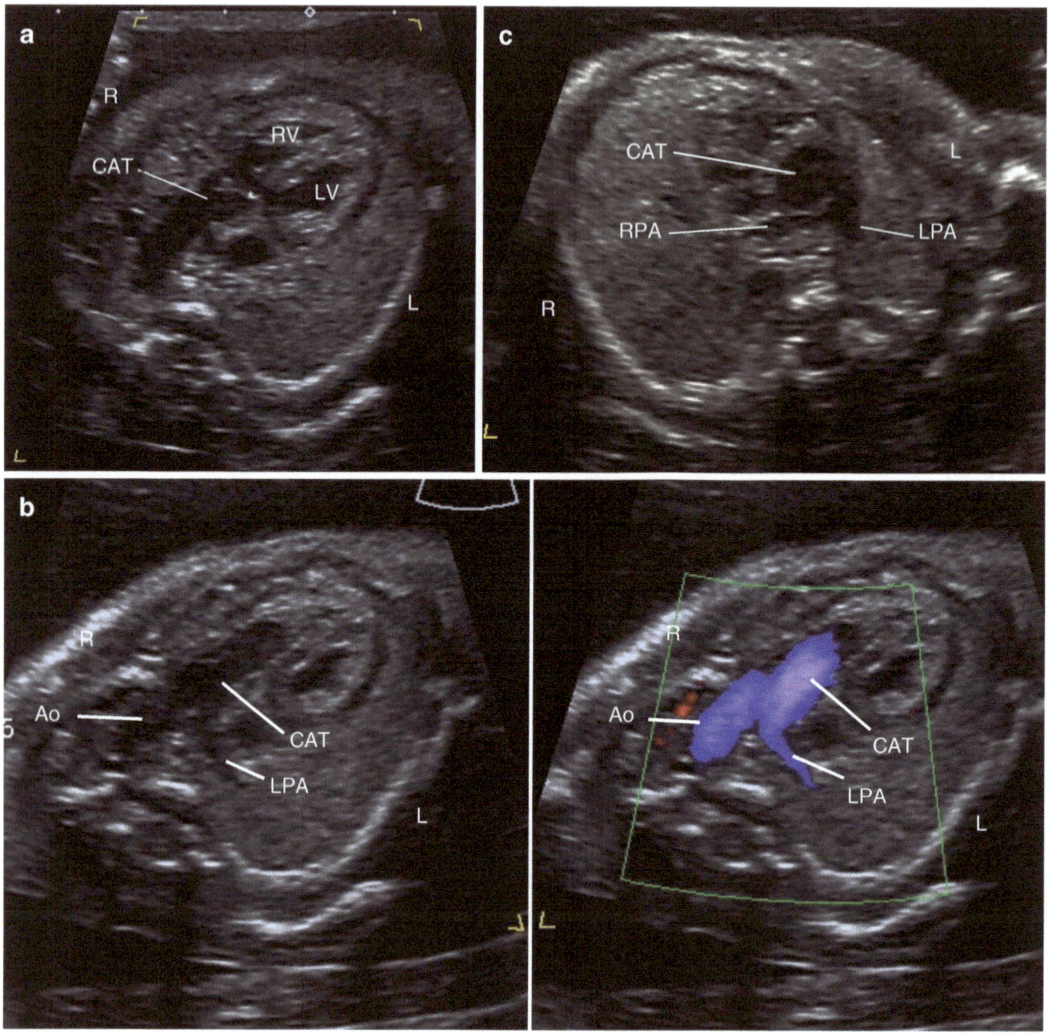

Fig. 8.9 (**a**) The common arterial trunk (CAT) arises astride a ventricular septal defect (*). The CAT is larger than the normal aorta or pulmonary artery. (**b**) The CAT gives rise to both the aorta and the pulmonary arteries. In this example the left pulmonary artery (LPA) can be seen arising from the CAT with antegrade flow into the LPA. (**c**) This short axis view shows the left and right pulmonary arteries arising from the CAT with a common origin. The usual point of origin is on the posterior and left side of the CAT but this is variable. (**d**) The left pane shows the origin of the pulmonary arteries from the CAT and the right pane confirms this with colour flow Doppler. Note that there is antegrade flow into the branch pulmonary arteries from the CAT. (**e**) The aortic arch is right sided in this case—the transverse aortic arch (TAA) passes to the right of the trachea (T). Only two vessels (TAA and SVC) are visible in contrast to the normal 3VT view

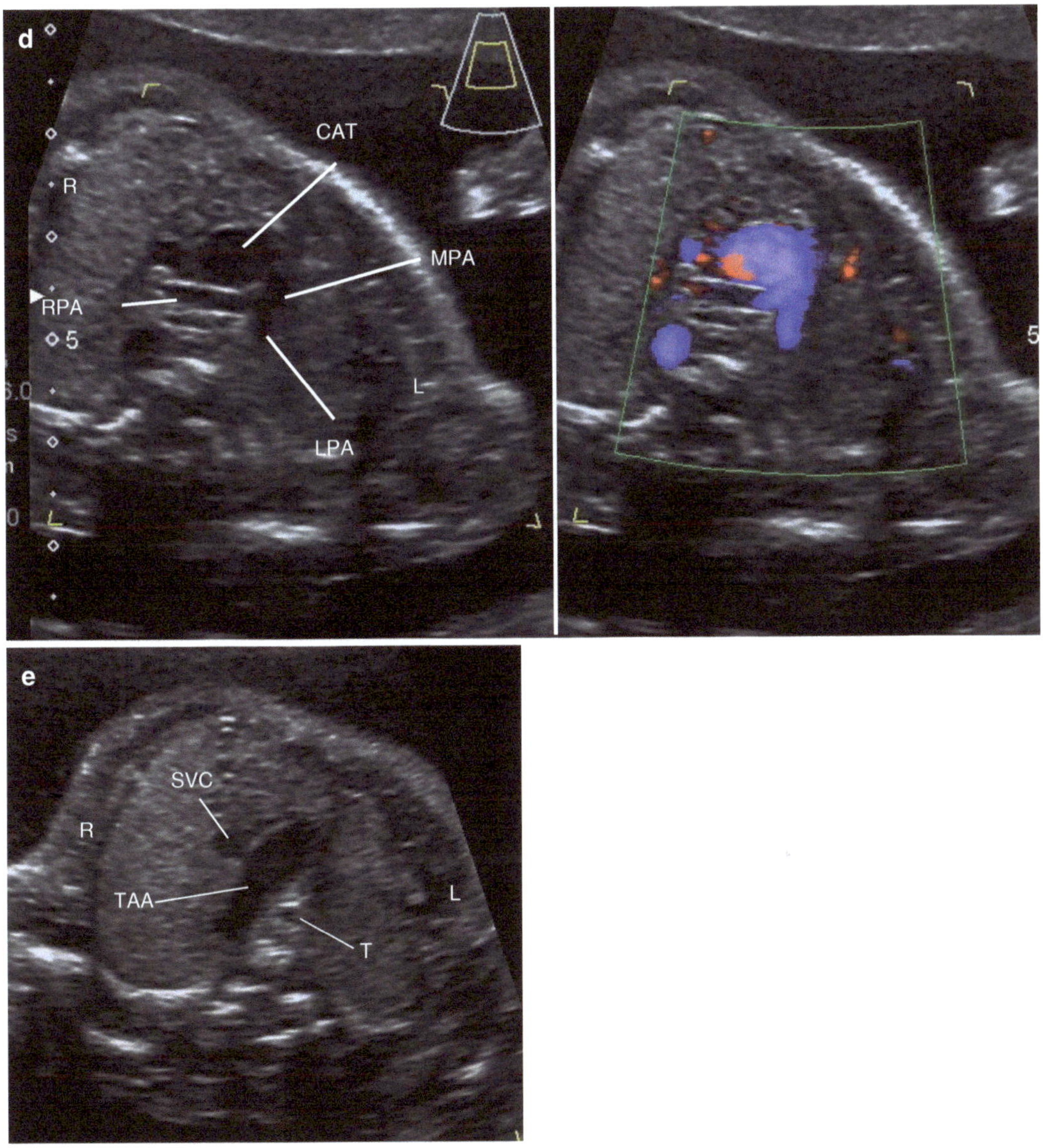

Fig. 8.9 (continued)

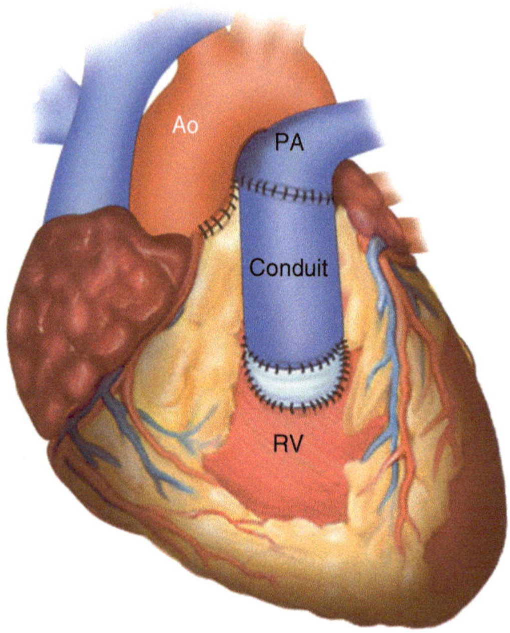

Fig. 8.10 Repair of common arterial trunk. The CAT is repaired by closing the VSD and connecting the right ventricle to the pulmonary arteries using a conduit

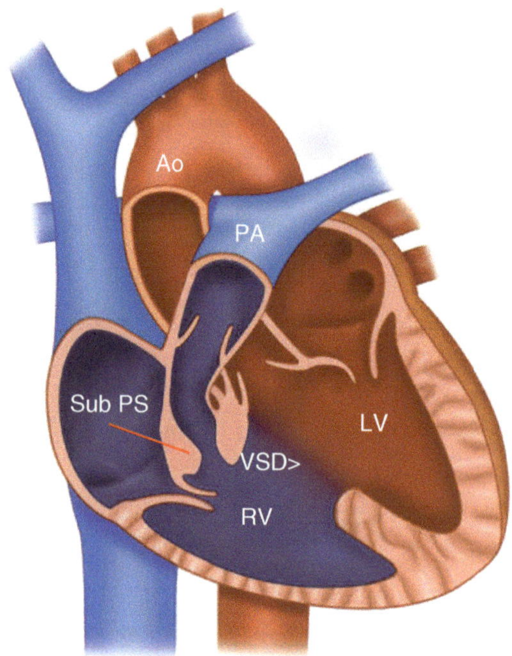

Fig. 8.11 Tetralogy of Fallot. Schematic diagram of tetralogy of Fallot. The aorta arises above a ventricular septal defect and there is obstruction to pulmonary blood flow which is typically muscular narrowing below the pulmonary valve and at the level of the pulmonary valve itself

pulmonary blood flow effectively "steals" from the systemic arterial circulation which can contribute to haemodynamic instability.

Surgical repair consists of patch closure of the VSD combined with connection of the right ventricle to the pulmonary circulation (Fig. 8.10). If the truncal valve is stenotic and / or regurgitant then this may be addressed at the time of initial surgery or else deferred until the child is bigger and older. All patients who have undergone repair of CAT will require lifelong cardiac review. The truncal valve becomes the aortic valve which will need to be monitored for stenosis, regurgitation and for associated dilation of the aortic root and ascending aorta. An integral part of the repair is insertion of a conduit between the right ventricle and pulmonary arteries. Monitoring for conduit stenosis, pulmonary regurgitation and branch pulmonary stenosis are important long-term considerations. Replacement of the right ventricle – pulmonary artery conduit is inevitable at some point during childhood.

Tetralogy of Fallot

Tetralogy of Fallot, as the name suggests, is characterised by four major features which include a ventricular septal defect, overriding of the aorta, obstruction to pulmonary blood flow and right ventricular hypertrophy (Fig. 8.11). During fetal life, right ventricular hypertrophy is not evident because the left and right ventricular pressures are equal in the same way as in the normal fetal heart. The incidence of tetralogy of Fallot is 3–5 per 10,000 live births and it makes up around 8% of congenital heart defects in liveborn infants.

In "classical" tetralogy of Fallot the ventricular septal defect is in the membranous portion of the ventricular septum and there is anterior deviation of the outlet septum which leads to a variable degree of obstruction of the right ventricular outflow tract. The aortic arch is right sided in around

30% of cases. During fetal life, if the obstruction to pulmonary blood flow is significant then flow in the arterial duct is from the aorta to the pulmonary circulation i.e. reversed. This is a useful marker of the severity of obstruction to pulmonary blood flow. The main and branch pulmonary arteries tend to be particularly small in fetuses with a severe degree of obstruction of the right ventricular outflow tract. If the pulmonary valve is atretic, some use the term pulmonary atresia with ventricular septal defect and others tetralogy of Fallot with pulmonary atresia – this is covered separately later in this chapter.

Echocardiographic Features

The echocardiographic features of tetralogy of Fallot are summarised in Table 8.4. The four-chamber view of the heart is usually normal. In some cases the cardiac axis is rotated to the left (Fig. 8.12, Video 8.14) which has been described more frequently in cases with 22q11 microdeletion. The VSD, although usually large, is not typically visible in the four-chamber view but becomes evident as the transducer is angulated cranially towards the aorta. The aorta arises astride the VSD (Fig. 8.13a, Video 8.15)—the degree of aortic override is variable so that in some cases the aorta is more committed to the right ventricle than the left ventricle. In this situation the term tetralogy of Fallot with double outlet right ventricle is sometimes used. The normal continuity of the ventricular septum with the anterior wall of the aorta is lost which is an important clue to the diagnosis (Fig. 8.13a). The pulmonary artery arises normally from the right ventricle and has a normal antero-posterior course (Fig. 8.13b, c, Video 8.16), but in the vast majority of cases the pulmonary artery is smaller than the aorta, in contrast to the normal heart (Video 8.17). The Doppler velocity across the pulmonary valve may be slightly increased (Fig. 8.13d) but is seldom markedly elevated. The aortic arch is left sided in 70% of cases (Fig. 8.13e), in which case the arterial duct is almost always left

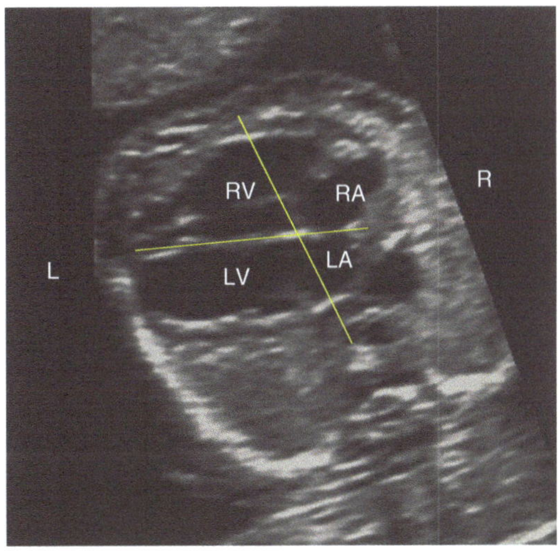

Fig. 8.12 Rotation of the heart to the left. In this 17 week gestation fetus there is clear rotation of the heart to the left so that the ventricular septum lies approximately transverse across the chest. Such rotation is often seen in fetuses with tetralogy of Fallot and its variants

Table 8.4 Summary of echocardiographic features of classical tetralogy of Fallot

Feature	Normal heart	Tetralogy of fallot
4 chamber view	Normal	Normal/near normal Apex may be rotated to left
LVOT	Aorta directed towards right shoulder Continuity between anterior wall of the aorta and ventricular septum	Aorta overrides a VSD Degree of override variable Loss of continuity between anterior wall of the aorta and ventricular septum
Relationship of GA	Aorta and PA cross each other with PA anterior	Normally related great arteries
Size of great arteries	Aorta similar to PA	Aorta larger than pulmonary artery
Three vessel trachea view	Aortic arch and ductal arch meet in a "V" shape	Aortic arch left or right sided Pulmonary artery and duct usually smaller than aorta Reversal of flow in arterial duct if pulmonary obstruction severe.

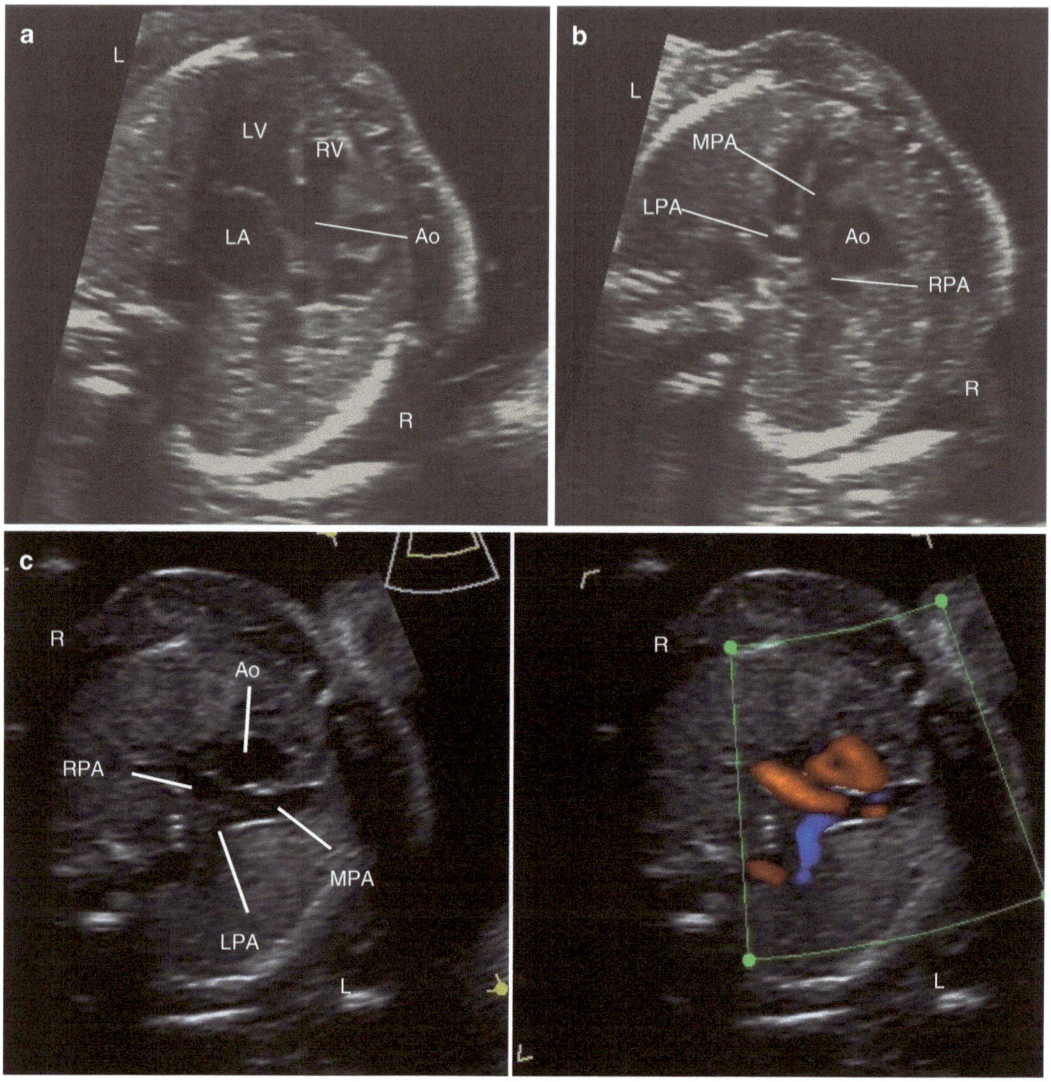

Fig. 8.13 Tetralogy of Fallot. (**a**) The aorta arises astride the ventricular septum so that both the RV and LV are in communication with the aorta. There is loss of continuity between the ventricular septum and the anterior wall of the aorta. (**b**) If the transducer is angled more cranially than the view in **a**, the pulmonary artery is visualised along with its bifurcation. The pulmonary artery is typically smaller than the aorta, reflecting obstruction to pulmonary blood flow. (**c**) The left pane shows the MPA branching into the LPA and RPA. This is confirmed by the use of colour flow Doppler which assists in the confirmation of antegrade blood flow across the pulmonary valve into the branch pulmonary arteries. (**d**) Pulsed Doppler interrogation of pulmonary blood flow typically shows a slightly elevated Doppler velocity across the pulmonary valve (110 cm/s in this case). This confirms antegrade flow but is not helpful in accurately determining the severity of obstruction to pulmonary blood flow. (**e**) In around 30% if cases of tetralogy of Fallot, the aortic arch is right sided. In this example there is a right aortic arch (RAA) passing to the right of the trachea (T). The discrepancy in size between the right ventricular outflow tract (RVOT) and the aortic arch is also evident. (**f**) In this short axis view, the anterior deviation of the muscular outlet septum can be seen as well as the typical "membranous" VSD (*) confirmed by the continuity of the tricuspid valve and the aorta

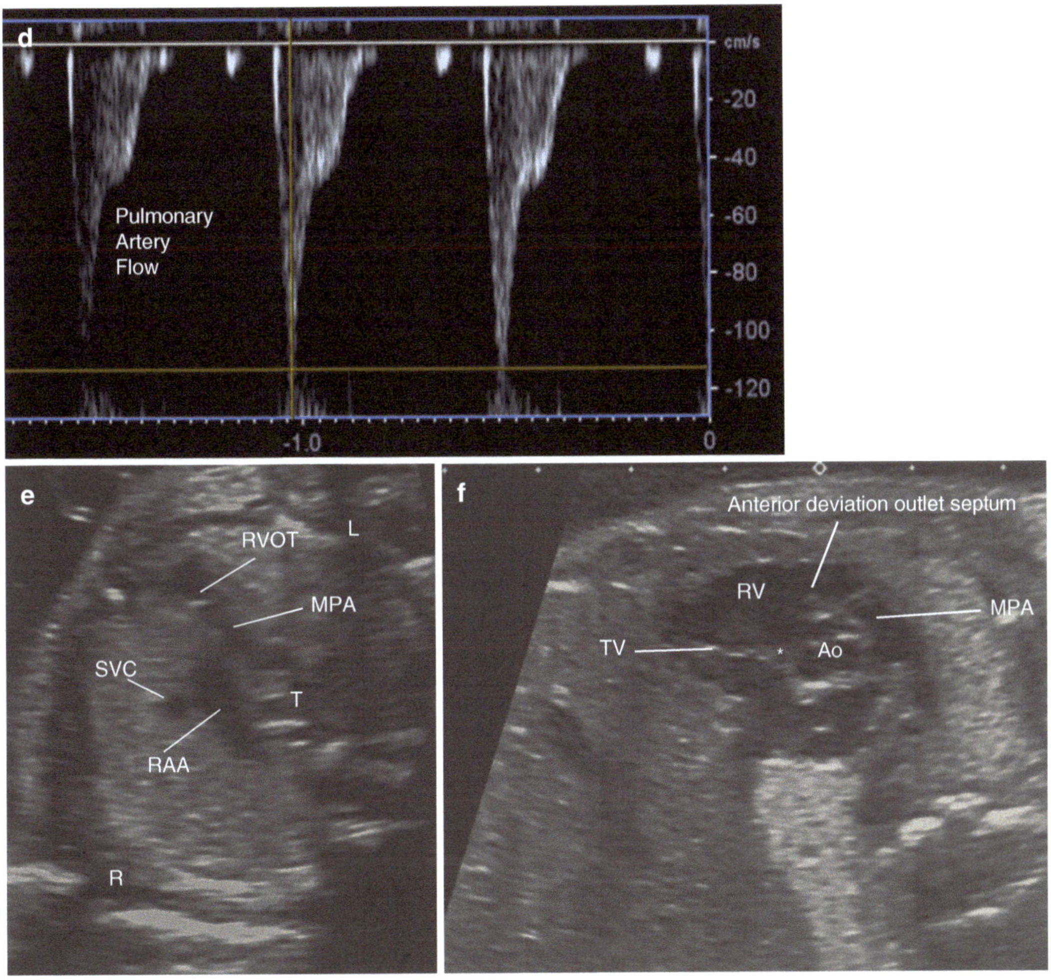

Fig. 8.13 (continued)

sided. The aortic arch is right sided in around 30% of cases with either a left or right sided arterial duct (Video 8.18). If the sonographic views are favourable, the anterior deviation of the outlet septum into the right ventricular outflow tract can be visualised (Fig. 8.13f, Video 8.19).

Associations

Tetralogy of Fallot may be associated with genetic abnormalities, most commonly trisomy 21 or chromosome 22q11 deletion, but a diverse range of genetic abnormalities have been described with Tetralogy of Fallot in up to 30% of cases (Zidere et al. 2006). Syndromes such as CHARGE and VACTERL association may be associated as are structural anomalies including exomphalos. In practice, detailed anomaly scanning and the offer of fetal karyotyping is important whenever this lesion is diagnosed prenatally because of the high frequency and diverse nature of associated anomalies.

Management of Tetralogy of Fallot

In tetralogy of Fallot there is rarely a cardiac indication to advise Caesarian delivery and usually the aim is for delivery at term. There will be institutional variation with respect to the site of delivery. In our practice, delivery is planned at the cardiac centre if the degree of pulmonary obstruction is felt to be severe i.e. with small pulmonary arteries and reversal of flow in the arterial duct (Pepas et al. 2003; Quartermain et al. 2013). In all cases, delivery should take place with appropriate neonatal support to monitor oxygen saturations and administer prostaglandin E to maintain ductal patency if saturations are suboptimal. If saturations are deemed adequate (>80–85% in air) then the arterial duct is allowed to close, with monitoring of oxygen saturations and echocardiographic assessment. If the oxygen saturations are inadequate then early surgery to augment pulmonary blood flow is undertaken. This usually consists of a systemic to pulmonary artery shunt. Some institutions will prefer to balloon dilate or stent the right ventricular outflow tract rather than insert a shunt.

The definitive repair of tetralogy of Fallot is surgical with closure of the ventricular septal defect and relief of obstruction to pulmonary blood flow (Fig. 8.14). Postoperatively, all patients with repaired tetralogy of Fallot will require long term follow-up. This is to monitor for obstruction to pulmonary blood flow and regurgitation of the pulmonary valve. The surgical repair results in pulmonary regurgitation in almost all cases and many patients will require surgical or interventional replacement of the pulmonary valve in the longer term. Other long-term complications include dilation of the aorta, branch pulmonary artery stenosis and arrhythmias.

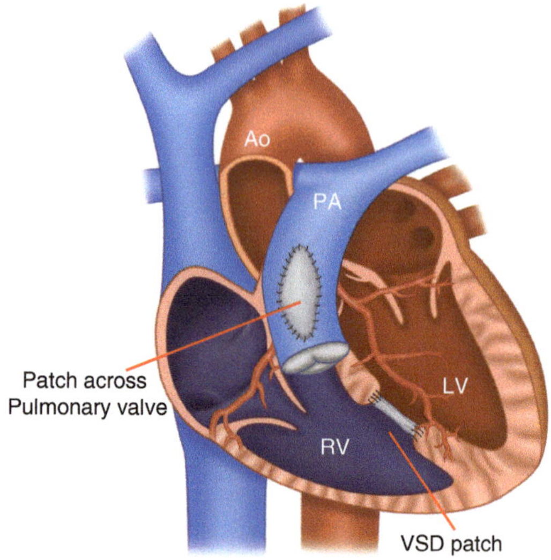

Fig. 8.14 Surgical repair of tetralogy of Fallot. This diagram shows the approach to surgical repair where the VSD is closed and obstruction to pulmonary blood flow is relieved by resection of subpulmonary muscle, dilation of the pulmonary valve and in many cases the size of the RV outflow tract is augmented by use of a patch

Tetralogy of Fallot with Pulmonary Atresia

Tetralogy of Fallot with pulmonary atresia refers to the group of patients who have a ventricular septal defect with aortic override but no antegrade flow across the pulmonary valve i.e. the valve is atretic. This lesion has an incidence of 7 per 100,000 livebirths and accounts for less than 1.5% of cardiac lesions identified before birth. Some authorities object to calling this variation "tetralogy of Fallot" at all and prefer the term "pulmonary atresia with ventricular septal defect", but the terms refer to the same group of lesions. The size and distribution of the branch pulmonary arteries is highly variable. In the "simplest" scenario, there are confluent central pulmonary arteries which are supplied retrograde via the arterial duct. However, in many cases the pulmonary arteries are very small or absent and the blood supply to the lungs is from multiple collateral arteries arising from the aorta or head and neck vessels. Major aortopulmonary collateral arteries (MAPCAS) have a highly variable course and distribution and the postnatal management is far more complex than classical tetralogy of Fallot. A diagrammatic representation of this lesion is shown in Fig. 8.15.

Echocardiographic Features

The echocardiographic features of tetralogy of Fallot with pulmonary atresia are summarised in Table 8.5. The four chamber appearances and overriding of the aorta are similar to classical tetralogy of Fallot (Video 8.20). The aortic arch is frequently right sided. On sweeping cranially from the four-chamber view to the three-vessel view, it may be impossible to view central pulmonary arteries due to the small size of these vessels and in some cases there are no central pulmonary arteries at all (Fig. 8.16a, Videos 8.21 and 8.22). Colour flow Doppler may assist in the visualisation of such small vessels. Retrograde

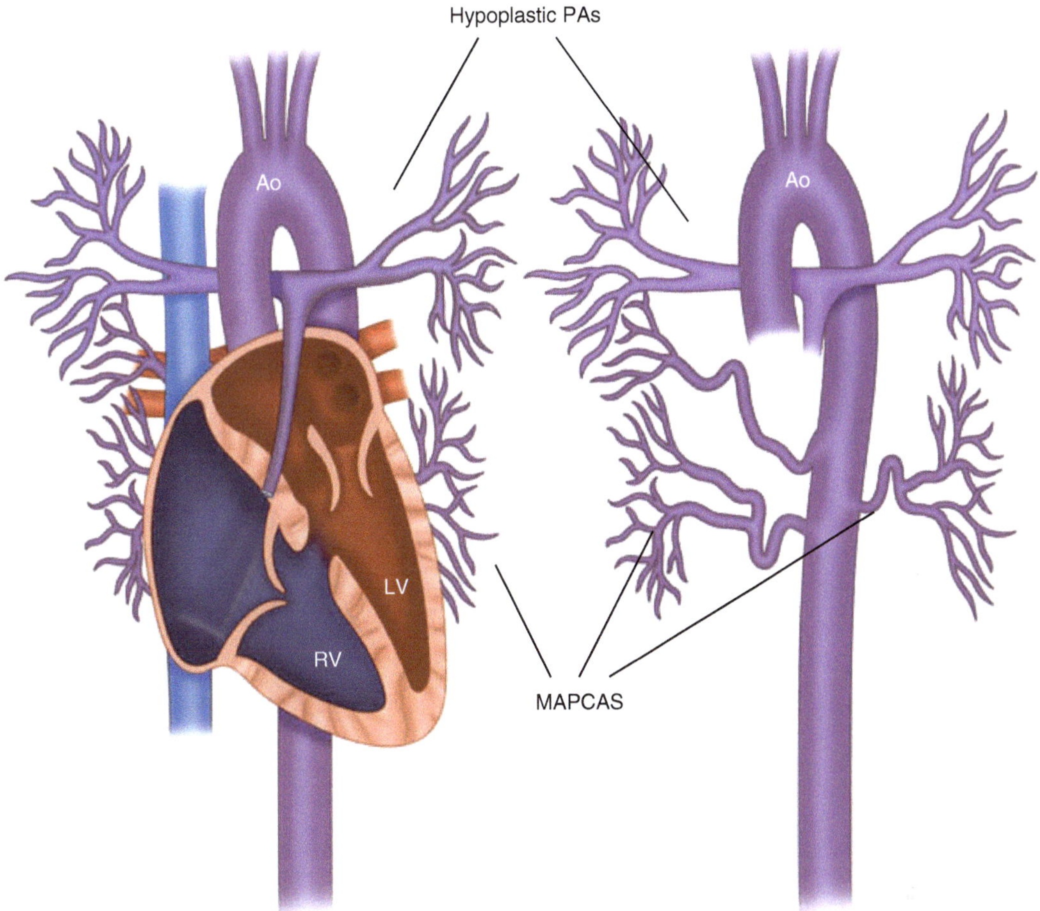

Fig. 8.15 Tetralogy of Fallot with pulmonary atresia. The anatomy of this lesion is complex and variable. There is a ventricular septal defect in all cases. The pulmonary arteries are not connected to the right ventricle and in this example are supplied via multiple aortopulmonary collateral arteries (MAPCAS). The size of the pulmonary arteries and the anatomy of the collateral supply is variable and difficult to determine during fetal life

Table 8.5 Echocardiographic features of Tetralogy of Fallot with pulmonary atresia

Feature	Normal heart	TOF with pulmonary atresia
4 chamber view	Normal	Apex normal or rotated to left
LVOT	Aorta directed towards right shoulder	Aorta overrides a VSD Degree of override variable
Relationship of GA	Aorta and PA cross each other with PA anterior	Main pulmonary artery absent or hypoplastic
Size of great arteries	Aorta similar to PA	Hypoplasia of main and central pulmonary arteries. Pulmonary arteries may be difficult to visualise or absent
Three vessel trachea view	Aortic arch and ductal arch meet in a "V" shape	Aortic arch left or right sided Retrograde flow in arterial duct MAPCAs visible in this view and sagittal views of Ao arch

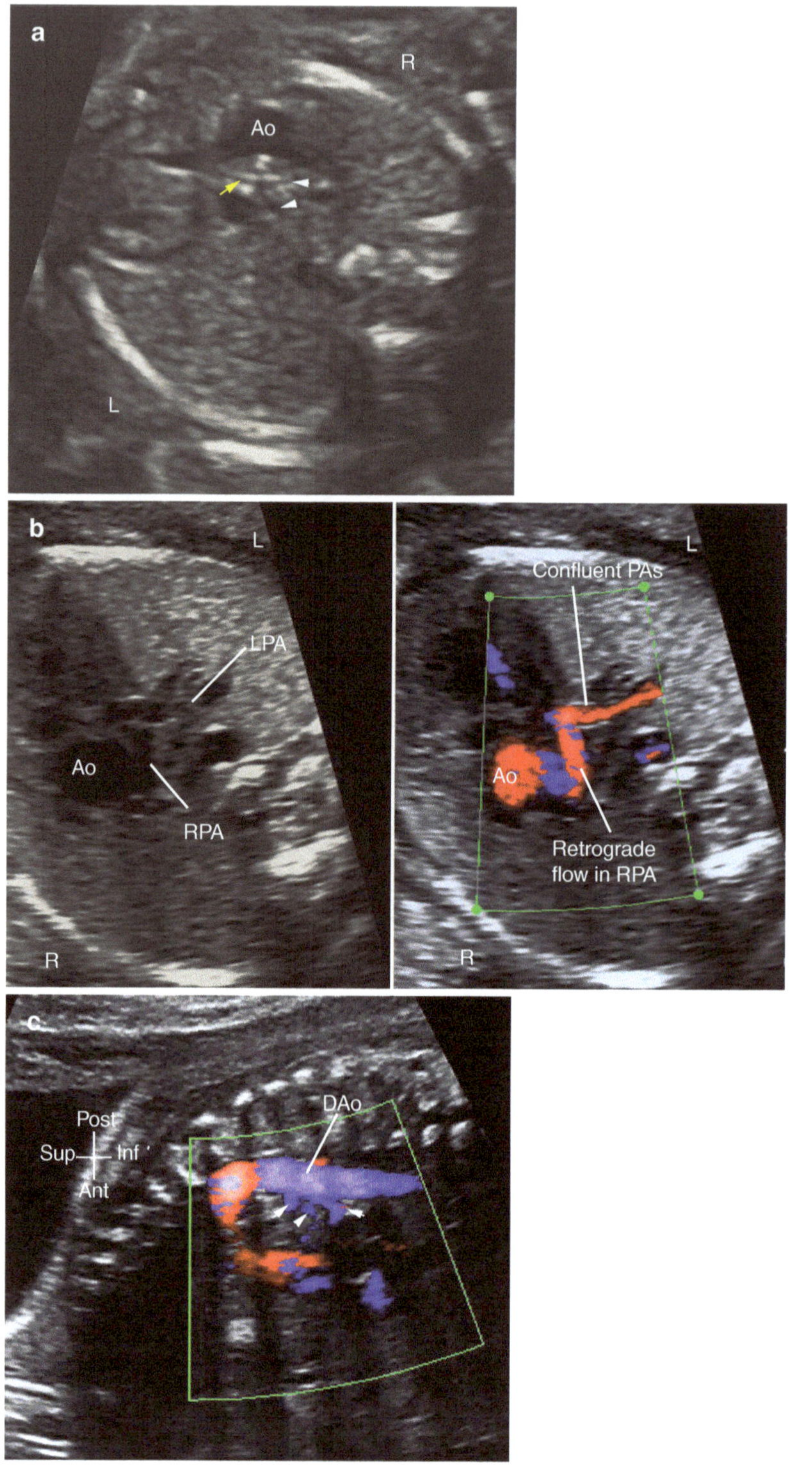

Fig. 8.16 (**a**) Hypoplastic central pulmonary arteries. The pulmonary arteries may be tiny and difficult to visualise. The main pulmonary artery is threadlike (yellow arrow) but it can be seen to bifurcate into branch pulmonary arteries (white arrowheads). (**b**) The left pane shows the aorta and the pulmonary arteries which are difficult to visualise. The use of colour flow Doppler shows flow from the aorta to the pulmonary arteries. Flow in the right pulmonary artery is retrograde. (**c**) This is a sagittal view showing three aortopulmonary arteries (arrow heads) arising from the descending aorta. The point of origin of the MAPCAS from the aorta can be seen but the precise course in the lungs cannot be determined reliably until after birth

flow in the arterial duct may be evident (Fig. 8.16b, Video 8.23). The duct in such cases normally arises from the underside of the aortic arch to supply the pulmonary arteries. In other cases, there may not be an arterial duct and blood supply the lungs is from MAPCAS (Fig. 8.16c). These vessels may be visualised using a combination of transverse and sagittal projection of the aortic arch and lung fields. These vessels are tortuous and it is rarely possible to define their course and distribution in a single sonographic cut. This adds to prognostic uncertainty with respect to postnatal management. In some cases the differential diagnosis between PATVSD and common arterial trunk can be difficult if the origin of the pulmonary arteries cannot be established i.e whether these arise from a common trunk or whether there is a pulmonary artery lying directly adjacent to the aorta (Vesel et al. 2006; Gomez et al. 2015).

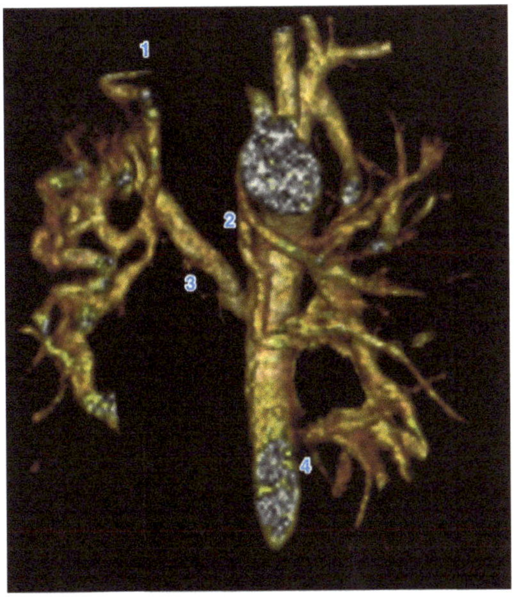

Fig. 8.17 This is a gadolinium enhanced postnatal cardiac MRI scan of MAPCAS arising from the descending aorta. The tortuous nature of the vessels can be appreciated as well as their size and distribution within the lungs

Associations

TOF with pulmonary atresia may be associated with genetic abnormalities and major extracardiac anomalies. In our own series, genetic abnormalities were detected in 10/27 cases, of which the commonest was 22q11 deletion followed by trisomy 13. Extracardiac abnormalities were identified in 20% of cases (Vesel et al. 2006). Detailed assessment of the fetal anatomy as well as the offer of fetal karyotyping is indicated in affected cases.

Postnatal Management

This lesion is highly variable and the postnatal surgical approach is dictated by the anatomy. Delineation of the detailed anatomy of the pulmonary circulation in this lesion via MAPCAS is not feasible currently until after the baby is born when a combination of CT / MRI and cardiac catheterisation is used (Fig. 8.17). The initial priority is to provide adequate pulmonary blood flow which involves either a systemic to pulmonary artery shunt or surgery on the right ventricular outflow tract to restore continuity between the right ventricle and the pulmonary arteries. In some cases, the MAPCAS provide sufficient pulmonary blood flow so that no such initial surgery is required. In the longer term the aim is to reconstruct the pulmonary arteries to provide a good vascular bed so that the right ventricle can be connected to the pulmonary arteries and the VSD closed surgically (Fig. 8.18). In all cases, long term follow-up is required and in some cases the "ideal" repair outlined above cannot be achieved. The management of such cases requires highly specialised imaging, catheter intervention and surgery. The prognosis is highly dependent on the anatomy of the pulmonary circulation and reintervention on the branch pulmonary arteries may be required either by surgery or interventional cardiac catheterisation. The conduit between the right

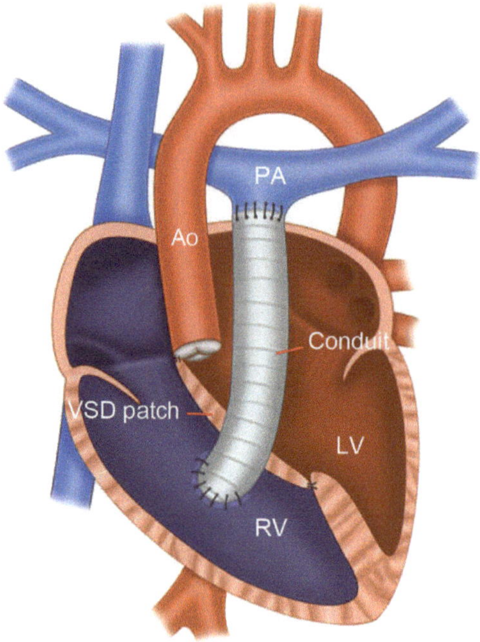

Fig. 8.18 The surgical repair of tetralogy of Fallot with pulmonary atresia consists of closure of the ventricular septal defect coupled with insertion of a conduit between the right ventricles and pulmonary arteries. The feasibility of achieving this repair is dependent on well-developed pulmonary arteries with low resistance to blood flow

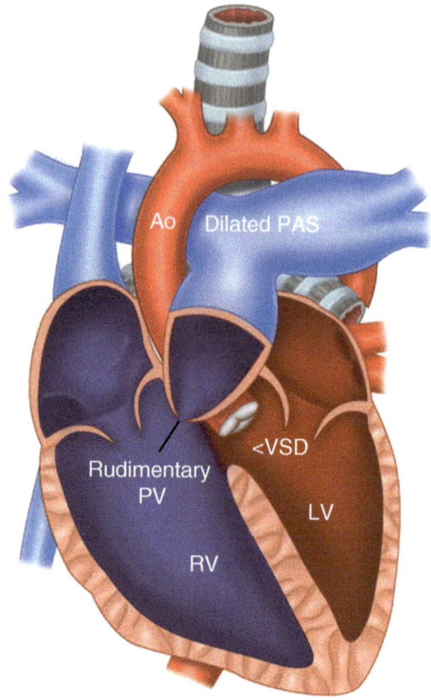

Fig. 8.19 Schematic diagram of tetralogy of Fallot with absent pulmonary valve. There is a stenotic, rudimentary valve ring (1) and dilated main and branch pulmonary arteries (2). There is typically a ventricular septal defect with aortic override (3). The arterial duct is absent

ventricle and pulmonary arteries will require replacement in all cases after the initial surgical repair.

Tetralogy of Fallot with Absent Pulmonary Valve/Absent Pulmonary Valve Syndrome

Tetralogy of Fallot with absent pulmonary valve is characterised by a ventricular septal defect and overriding of the aorta, consistent with classical tetralogy of Fallot. In this variant, however, there is a rudimentary valve ring rather than a true pulmonary valve. There is obstruction to pulmonary blood flow at the level of this ring accompanied by pulmonary regurgitation due to the lack of a functioning pulmonary valve. The branch pulmonary arteries are dilated, sometimes severely, and the arterial duct is absent in the vast majority of cases. Some prefer the term "Absent pulmonary valve syndrome" which would also encompass rare cases without a ventricular septal defect or aortic override but with the same abnormality of the branch pulmonary arteries. Around 3% of cases of tetralogy of Fallot have associated absent pulmonary valve, which accounts for around 1% of CHD diagnosed before birth. A schematic diagram of this lesion is shown in Fig. 8.19.

Echocardiographic Features

The echocardiographic features of tetralogy of Fallot with absent pulmonary valve are summarised in Table 8.6. The initial abnormalities which prompt referral are normally cardiomegaly, visualisation of hugely dilated branch

Table 8.6 Summary of echocardiographic features of tetralogy of Fallot with absent pulmonary valve

Feature	Normal heart	TOF with absent pulmonary valve
4 chamber view	Normal	Normal/ Cardiomegaly Apex normal or rotated to left
LVOT	Aorta directed towards right shoulder	Aorta overrides a VSD Degree of override variable
Relationship of GA	Aorta and PA cross each other with PA anterior	Normally related great arteries
Size of great arteries	Aorta similar to PA	Dilated main and branch pulmonary arteries Pulmonary stenosis/ regurgitation
Three vessel trachea view	Aortic arch and ductal arch meet in a "V" shape	Aortic arch left or right sided Branch pulmonary arteries dilated Duct usually absent

pulmonary arteries or rotation of the heart to the left (Fig. 8.20a, b, Videos 8.25, 8.26, 8.27, and 8.28) (Razavi et al. 2003; Wertaschnigg et al. 2013). The aorta arises astride a ventricular septal defect and the pulmonary artery is in its usual anteroposterior orientation. Use of colour flow Doppler confirms turbulent antegrade flow into the branch pulmonary arteries and regurgitant flow from the pulmonary arteries into the right ventricle (Figs. 8.20c–e, Videos 8.29 and 8.30). In most cases the arterial duct is absent but this is not invariable. In some cases, there is no ventricular septal defect but the dilation of the branch pulmonary arteries and appearance of the rudimentary pulmonary valve ring is similar. In severe cases, there is severe RV dysfunction due to volume and pressure overload and in a minority of cases fetal hydrops may develop. In common with classical tetralogy of Fallot, the heart may be rotated to the left providing a further clue to an underlying cardiac abnormality.

Associations

Tetralogy of Fallot with absent pulmonary valve is strongly associated with chromosome 22q11 deletions which is by far the commonest genetic association, occurring in up to 40% of cases. If there is severe regurgitation, RV volume loading and dysfunction may lead to fetal hydrops. Extracardiac malformations may occur and detailed anomaly scanning with the offer of fetal karyotyping is mandatory.

Management

The prognosis of this form of congenital heart disease is not simply related to the cardiac lesion. The severe enlargement of branch pulmonary arteries compresses surrounding the surrounding lung tissue and bronchial tree. Some infants have intrinsically abnormal, floppy airways due to abnormal development of cartilage (tracheobronchomalacia). Postnatally, some infants are relatively asymptomatic with acceptable oxygen saturations and little or no evidence of respiratory distress. In this setting, management is initially conservative. Elective repair is undertaken later in infancy, consisting of closure of the VSD, relief of stenosis at the level of the pulmonary valve ring and plication of the branch pulmonary arteries to reduce their size (Fig. 8.21). Long term review is required and replacement of the pulmonary valve to reduce pulmonary regurgitation is necessary later in life. In contrast to the scenario outlined above, some infants with this lesion develop severe respiratory distress after birth such that ventilation is required early. Air-trapping in the lungs results from the associated bronchomalacia. This scenario has a much worse prognosis because early surgery is indicated to repair the cardiac lesion and plicate the pulmonary arteries to relieve airways compression. Even when this is technically successful, ongoing respiratory complications may occur with an adverse effect on outcome. Some infants may require longer term ventilation and stenting of airways to improve respiratory status.

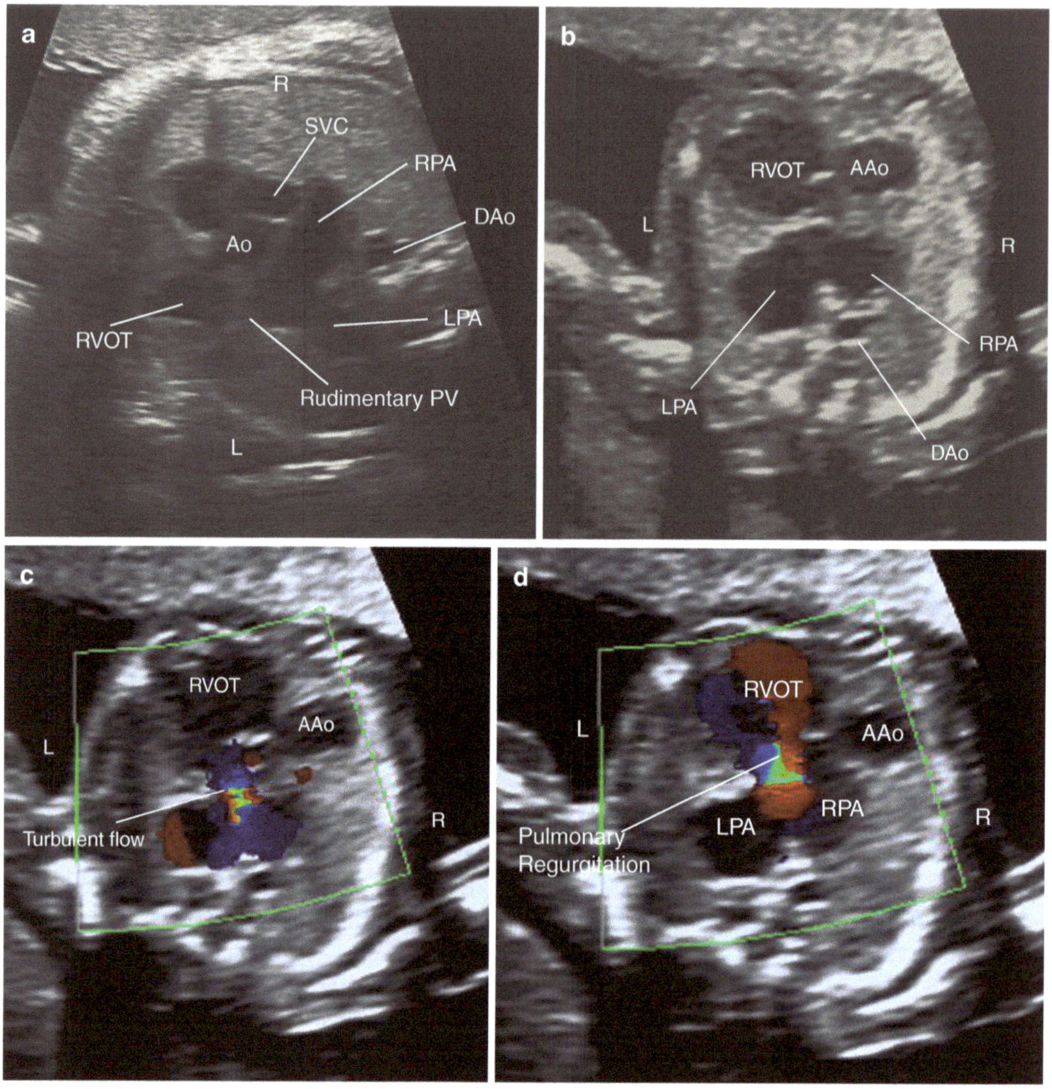

Fig. 8.20 Absent pulmonary valve syndrome. (**a**) This is a classical view of absent pulmonary valve syndrome. There is only a rudimentary pulmonary valve and marked dilation of the right and left pulmonary arteries. The aorta descends to the right of the spine. (**b**) This view of the upper mediastinum shows the gross dilation of the right and left pulmonary arteries as well as the right ventricular outflow tract. (**c**) Use of colour flow Doppler confirms turbulent antegrade flow across the rudimentary pulmonary valve ring. (**d**) Colour flow Doppler confirms retrograde flow from the pulmonary arteries into the right ventricle due to pulmonary valve regurgitation. (**e**) Pulsed Doppler interrogation of this fetus at 17 weeks gestational age confirms the typically increased velocity of antegrade flow and severe pulmonary regurgitation giving a "to / fro" Doppler signal

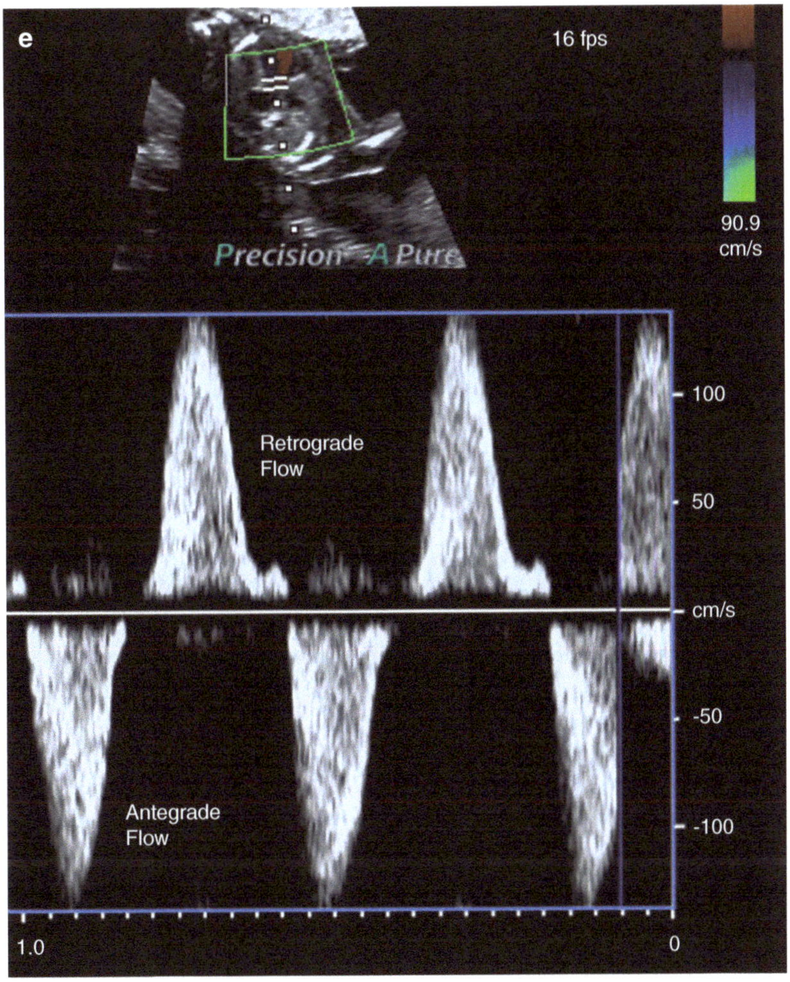

Fig. 8.20 (continued)

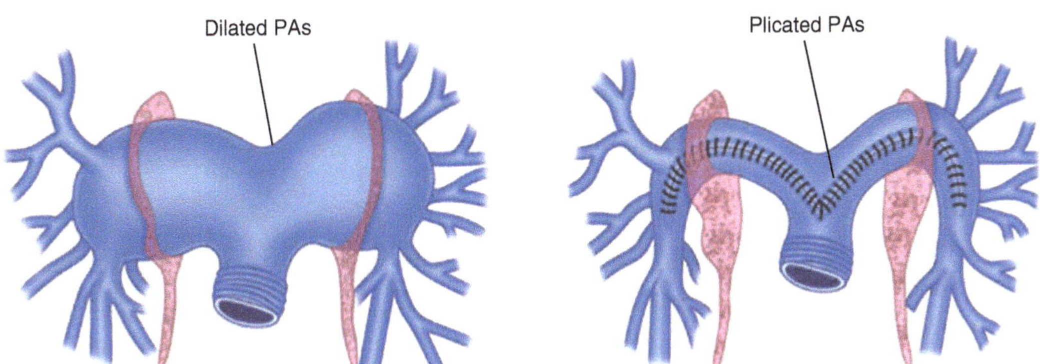

Fig. 8.21 Plication of the pulmonary arteries is an integral part of repair of tetralogy of Fallot with absent pulmonary valve. The surgeons reduce the size of the branch pulmonary arteries by excision of redundant tissue with the aim of reducing compression of adjacent bronchi and lungs

Double Outlet Right Ventricle

Double outlet right ventricle (DORV) is defined as a lesion where both the aorta and pulmonary artery arise either exclusively or predominantly from the right ventricle of the heart. This condition is not a single form of congenital heart disease but has major individual variability. The incidence is approximately 1 per 10,000 live births, accounting for less than 1.5% of all CHD. DORV may occur in the context of major abnormalities of the atrioventricular connections, for example, with mitral atresia, an atrioventricular septal defect or discordant atrioventricular connections. This chapter will focus on where there are normal atrioventricular connections and relatively balanced size of the ventricles. A schematic diagram of DORV is shown in Fig. 8.22.

In virtually all cases there is a ventricular septal defect but the position, size and number of defects is highly variable. Although by definition, the aorta and pulmonary artery arise completely or predominantly from the right ventricle, their relative position is highly variable. In some cases, the aorta is anterior to the pulmonary artery with a parallel arrangement of the arteries whereas in others the great arteries are normally related. There may be associated pulmonary valve or subpulmonary stenosis or, conversely, subaortic stenosis, aortic valve stenosis or coarctation of the aorta. Close examination of the mitral and tricuspid valves is essential because these may be abnormally formed and can straddle the ventricular septum. The details of the anatomy of such cases has a huge impact on the type of repair which can be undertaken after birth (Lagopoulos et al. 2010).

Echocardiographic features

There are no "typical" echocardiographic features of DORV, rather a variability which is summarised in Table 8.7. A systematic assessment of the cardiac connections is essential. The cardiac

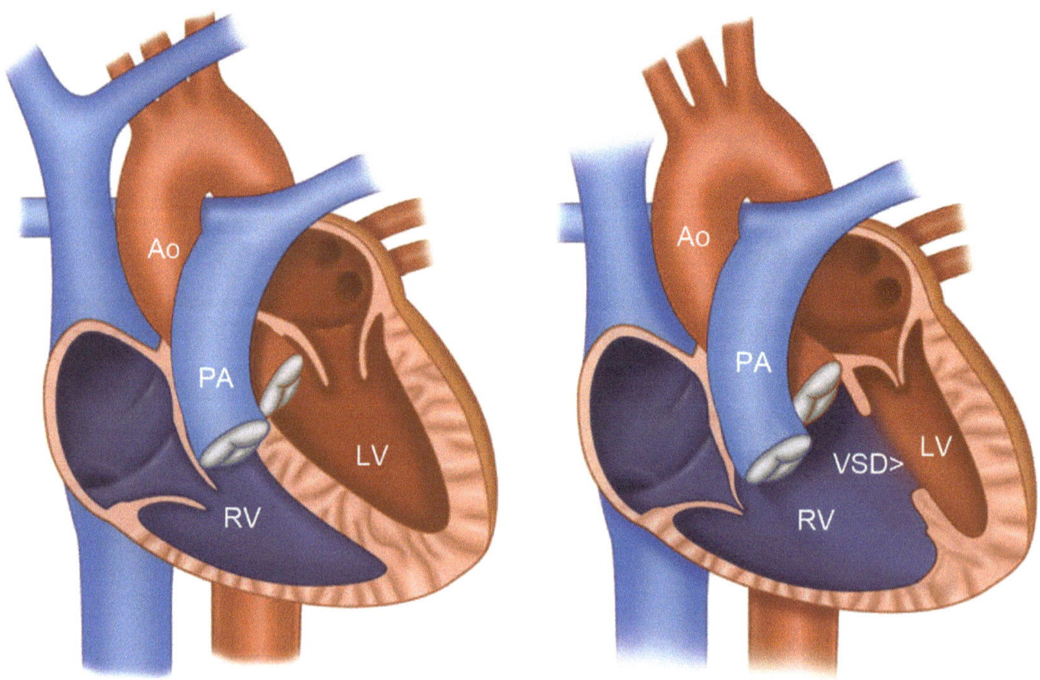

Fig. 8.22 This figure illustrates and example of DORV where both the aorta and the pulmonary artery arise from the right ventricle. The ventricular septal defect accompanying this lesion is also shown

Table 8.7 Summary of echocardiographic features of double outlet right ventricle with normal atrioventricular connections

Feature	Normal heart	Double outlet right ventricle
4 chamber view	Normal	Normal/VSD/ Straddling valves
LVOT	Aorta directed towards right shoulder	Highly variable
Relationship of GA	Aorta and PA cross each other with PA anterior	Highly variable, normally related, transposed
size of great arteries	Aorta similar to PA	Highly variable: equal sized, Aorta larger than PA or vice versa
Three vessel trachea view	Aortic arch and ductal arch meet in a "V" shape	Aortic arch left or right sided

situs should be assessed. Defects of laterality ("isomerism") can be associated with DORV, often with associated lesions such as an atrioventricular septal defect. The four-chamber view may be abnormal (Table 8.7) or normal. The VSD may be visible on the four-chamber view or only visible when scanning towards the outlets of the heart (Fig. 8.23a, Video 8.31). The relationship of the great arteries may be "usual" in which case the aorta is the first great artery seen when scanning cranially from the four-chamber view, and the pulmonary artery crosses in its usual orientation (Fig. 8.23a, b, Video 8.31). Conversely, the great arteries may arise in parallel with the ventricular septal defect in closest relationship to the PA. In this setting the aorta is anterior to the pulmonary artery (Fig. 8.23c, Video 8.32 and 8.33). Doppler interrogation of the aortic and pulmonary flow is essential as well as comparison of size of the vessels. Colour flow Doppler assist in assessing the relationship of the great arteries, position of the VSD and detection of turbulent blood flow suggesting aortic or pulmonary valve stenosis. The size of the aortic arch should be assessed to exclude associated coarctation of the aorta. DORV may be interrogated by 3D imaging modalities including spatio-temporal image correlation (STIC) to assess the individual anatomy to plan the surgical approach (Fig. 8.23d, e, Videos 8.34 and 8.35) (Zidere et al. 2013).

Associations

Double outlet right ventricle may be associated with extra-cardiac or genetic abnormalities including major trisomies, 22q11 and other conditions such as CHARGE syndrome and VACTERL association. In all cases, detailed anomaly scanning is indicated and the option of fetal karyotypic is discussed.

Cardiac Management

The management of DORV is dictated by the underlying anatomy. Assuming that the cardiac situs and venous connections are normal, a reasonable starting point is to examine the four-chamber view. If there is severe imbalance of ventricular size, straddling of atrioventricular valves or atresia of either the tricuspid or mitral valve then management would be towards a single ventricle (Fontan) circulation. This circulation is not regarded as curative and there are longer term complications which are discussed in Chap. 18. The biggest dilemmas in terms of postnatal management relate to cases where there is normal cardiac situs, normal venous connections and a normal four chamber view. In this setting, the crucial features include the size and location of the ventricular septal defect and the relationship of the great arteries.

If the aorta is close to the ventricular septal defect, and the great arteries are normally related, then the surgeon may be able to direct blood flow from the left ventricle to the aorta using a patch. If the pulmonary artery is close to the VSD, then it may be possible for the surgeon to switch the position of the great arteries and redirect flow from the left ventricle to the aorta. In other cases, both great arteries are "remote" from the VSD and it may not be feasible to fully repair the heart and patients may

Fig. 8.23 Double outlet right ventricle. (**a**) The aorta can be seen arising predominantly from the right ventricle and the location of the VSD is evident (*). (**b**) On scanning further cranially the pulmonary artery is also seen to arise from the right ventricle. (**c**) In this different example, the aorta in this arises anterior and to the right of the pulmonary artery. The precise anatomy of the great arteries is highly individual. (**d**) Spatio-temporal image correlation (STIC) can be used to slice through different levels of the heart to assess the relationship of different cardiac structures to predict the type of repair which may be required. (**e**) In this image 3D echocardiography with colour flow Doppler gives the depth of field to visualise the course of the great arteries and the location of the ventricular septal defect. Such imaging can assist in understanding of the anatomy in DORV

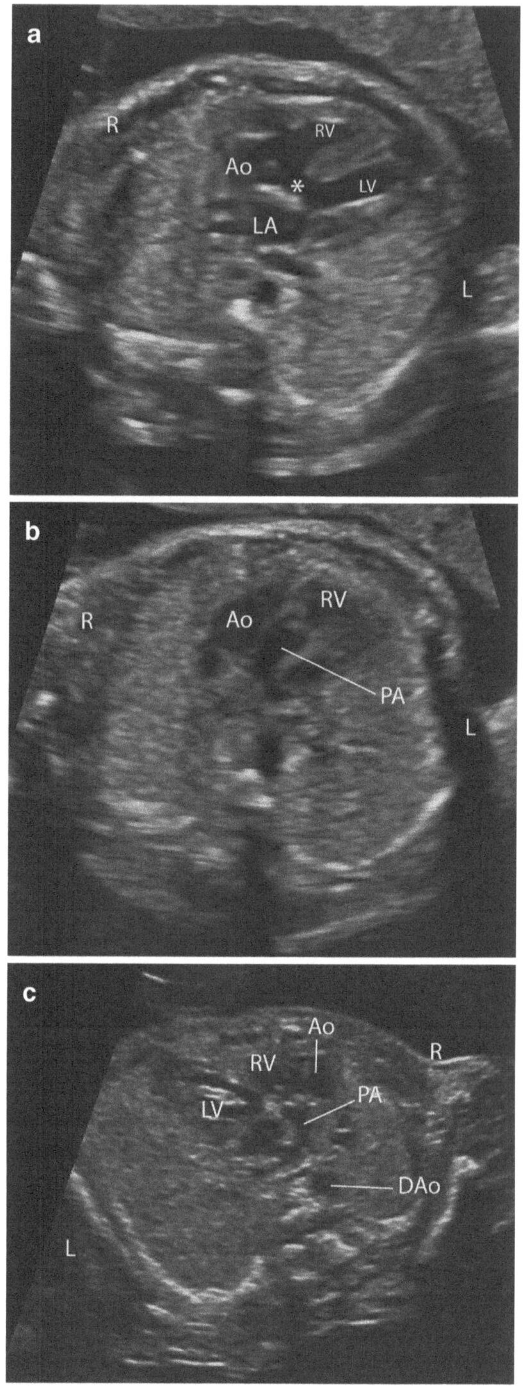

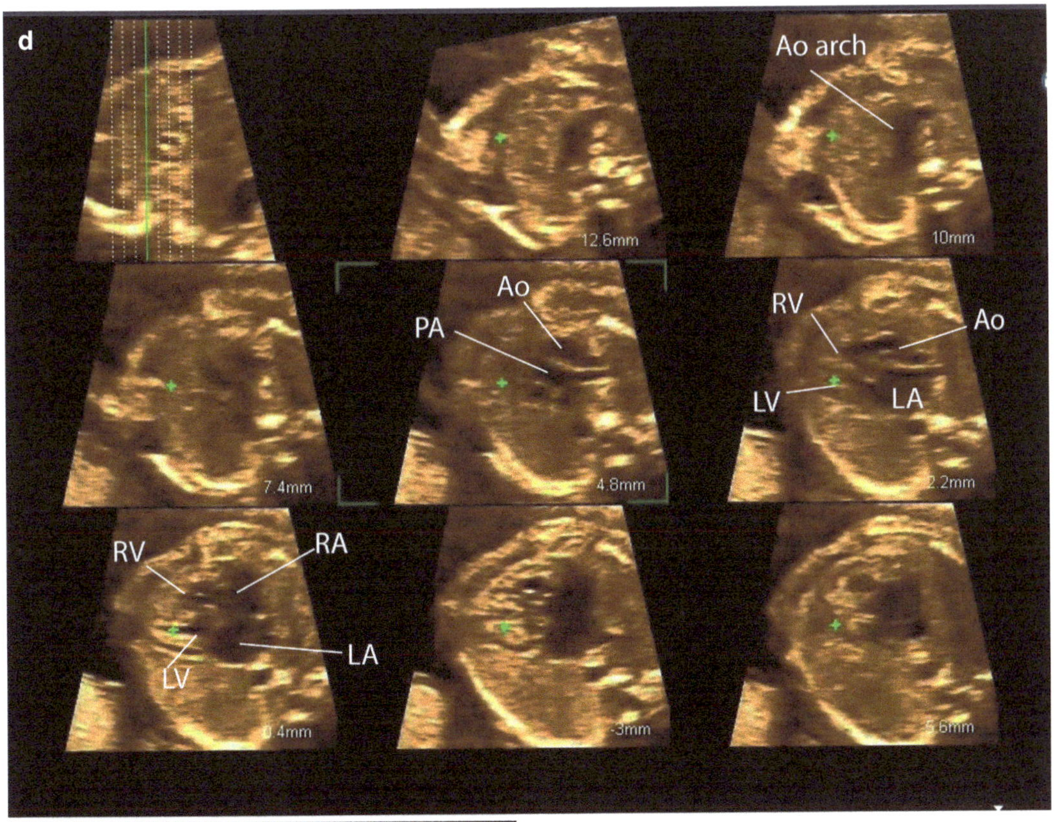

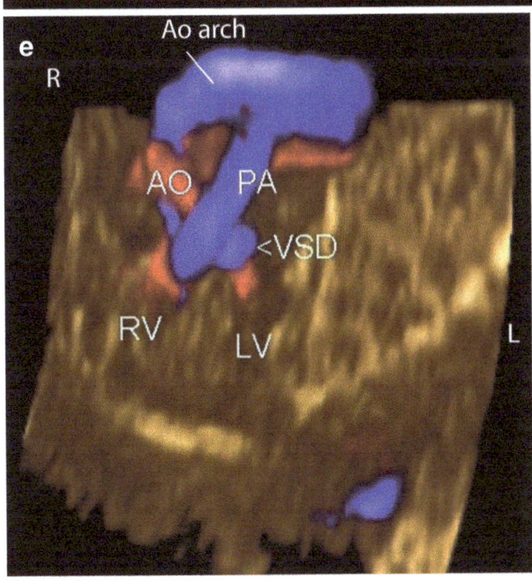

Fig. 8.23 (continued)

be managed down a single ventricle or "Fontan" pathway. For each case there needs to be an individual assessment by a team familiar with the crucial diagnostic information and the types of surgical approach which can be undertaken after birth. Such decision making frequently involves 3D imaging including 3D echocardiography, MRI and 3D printing of the heart.

Aortic Valve Stenosis

Aortic valve stenosis is defined as a narrowing of the aortic valve. Congenital aortic valve stenosis This has an incidence of 3–4/10,000 live births and represents less than 2% of congenital heart defects diagnosed prenatally. A diagram of this lesion is shown in Fig. 8.24. The aortic valve is congenitally abnormal and may have a variable number of leaflets including unicuspid, bicuspid and tricuspid morphology. During fetal life, the morphology of the aortic valve is difficult to visualise with certainty, although in later gestation this is now more feasible. In haemodynamic terms, the severity is variable from a mild

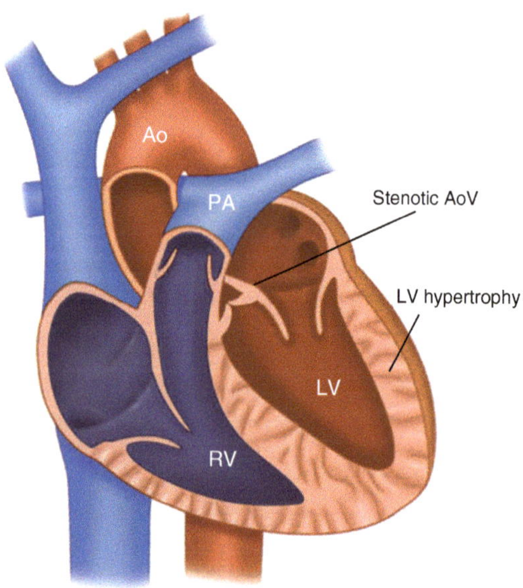

Fig. 8.24 Diagram of aortic valve stenosis. The aortic valve is abnormal and does not open fully during systole, leading to obstruction to blood flow out of the left ventricle. The morphology of the aortic valve is difficult to visualise before birth

degree of narrowing through to critical obstruction of the aortic valve. The sonographic features of the mild versus more severe cases vary widely.

The natural history of aortic valve stenosis during fetal life is of fundamental importance with respect to prognosis after birth (Simpson and Sharland 1997). There is a tendency for this lesion to become progressively more severe with advancing gestational age. Thus, in some cases, screening views of the heart in the midtrimester may be within normal limits. Significant stenosis of the aortic valve impacts all left heart structures, as well as the aortic valve. There is a trend for growth of the mitral valve, left ventricle and aorta to be subnormal in the face of significant aortic valve obstruction. In the worst affected cases, the sonographic appearances are akin to hypoplastic left heart by term. Prognostication based on the sonographic features of aortic valve stenosis, particularly with respect to size and function of the left heart has been the subject of considerable research because of the possibility of prenatal catheter intervention to dilate the aortic valve and prevent / ameliorate the progression of the disease.

Echocardiographic Features

In the mildest cases, the four-chamber view of the fetal heart may be normal with preserved function of the left ventricle of the heart. Such cases are typically detected only if Doppler interrogation of aortic flow is undertaken by pulsed Doppler or if there is aliasing of colour when colour flow Doppler is used to visualise the outflow tracts (Fig. 8.25a). An example of mild aortic valve stenosis is shown in Video 8.36. There is an elevated Doppler velocity across the aortic valve (Fig. 8.25a) and in some cases, dilation of the ascending aorta may be observed (Fig. 8.25b, Video 8.37). Such cases can progress significantly so that later in gestation the appearances can be those of severe aortic valve stenosis (Table 8.8). Until relatively recently, it has not been possible to image the

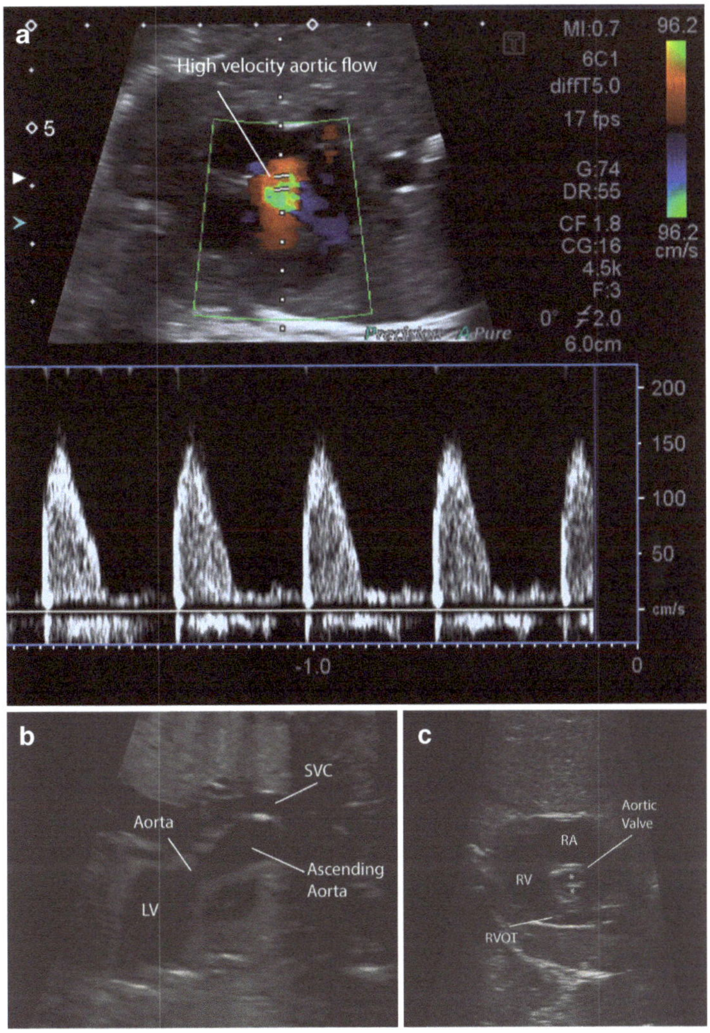

Fig. 8.25 (**a**) Mild to moderate aortic valve stenosis. In this fetus aliasing of colour flow can be seen on interrogation of the aortic valve. The Doppler velocity is elevated at 150 cm/s. (**b**) Post-stenotic dilation of the ascending aorta. This fetus had moderately severe aortic valve stenosis with preserved left ventricular function. In critical aortic stenosis, in contrast, the aorta becomes more hypoplastic with advancing gestational age. (**c**) Bicuspid aortic valve. With improved resolution of ultrasound systems, the morphology of the aortic valve can now be visualised in some fetuses. This short axis image shows a bicuspid aortic valve in a fetus at 30 weeks gestational age. Each of the leaflets is marked by an asterisk (*)

Table 8.8 Summary of echocardiographic features of aortic valve stenosis

Feature	Mild aortic valve stenosis	Severe aortic stenosis	Critical aortic stenosis with hypoplasia of left heart
4 chamber view	LV normal size Normal LV contraction MV motion normal	Echogenic LV Variable LV size Reduced LV contraction MV excursion reduced. Variable MR +/− Enodcardial fibroelastosis	Hypoplastic LV/non apex forming LV non-contractile and echogenic MV excursion reduced/absent Variable MR Endocardial fibroelastosis
MV inflow	Biphasic	Monophasic	Monophasic
Flow at atrial septum	Right to left	Left to right +/− restriction	Left to right +/− restriction
size of great arteries	Ao = PA Post-stenotic dilation of aorta	PA > Ao	PA > > Ao
Three vessel trachea view	Aortic and ductal arch similar size Antegrade flow in aortic arch	Hypoplasia of aortic arch Retrograde flow in aortic arch	Severe hypoplasia of aortic arch Retrograde flow in aortic arch.

morphology of the aortic valve reliably. Currently, this is more feasible with advances in ultrasound technology usually in the late second or third trimester (Fig. 8.25c, Video 8.38).

In more severe cases, the typical finding in the second trimester is of a dilated, echogenic left ventricle with impaired contraction (Fig. 8.26a, Video 8.39). The mitral valve appears restricted in its motion with monophasic inflow and a variable degree of mitral valve regurgitation (Fig. 8.26b, Video 8.40). The shunt at atrial level is reversed due to left heart obstruction (Fig. 8.26c, Video 8.41) and reversal of flow in the aortic arch is observed due to obstruction of blood flow from the left ventricle (Fig. 8.26d, Video 8.42). On pulsed Doppler interrogation of the aortic valve the flow velocity may be elevated (>1 m/s in the second trimester) but may be within the normal range reflecting reduced LV function rather than mild stenosis. Doppler interrogation of inflow to the left ventricle through the mitral valve shows an abnormal monophasic pattern in severe cases (Fig. 8.26e).

With continued obstruction to aortic flow, left heart structures grow poorly so that by the third trimester the sonographic appearances are very similar to those of hypoplastic left heart syndrome with diminutive LV and aorta (Videos 8.43, 8.44, and 8.45).

Over the past decade, there has been a focus on whether prenatal balloon dilation of the aortic valve might promote growth of left heart structures and have a positive impact on postnatal prognosis. Scoring systems have been developed to predict which fetuses will progress to have severe hypoplasia of the left heart by term. Echocardiographic features which suggest such progression include LV dysfunction, monophasic MV inflow, left to right shunt at atrial level and reversal of flow in the transverse aortic arch. This type of score may be supplemented by a separate "threshold" score to determine in which fetuses the left heart may be "salvageable" if balloon dilation of the aortic valve were performed (Moon-Grady et al. 2015; Hunter et al. 2015; Freud and Tworetzky 2016).

Associations

Fetuses with aortic valve stenosis seldom have associated chromosomal abnormalities. A minority have coexisting extracardiac abnormalities. In all cases, our usual practice is for detailed anomaly scanning but in the absence of other sonographic markers or abnormal screening investigations, an abnormality of the fetal karyotype is the exception rather than the rule.

Management

The management of the fetus with aortic valve stenosis is complex and must take account of the potential for disease progression. Thus, all cases of aortic valve stenosis should have sequential follow-up irrespective of the perceived severity when first diagnosed.

Fig. 8.26 A Critical aortic valve stenosis. This four chamber view demonstrates the typical dilation, globular shape and echogenicity of the left ventricle typical of critical aortic valve stenosis. With advancing gestational age, growth of the left ventricle is usually severely impaired, so that by term the RV may be larger than the LV. (**b**) Mitral valve stenosis and/or regurgitation is a frequent accompaniment of critical aortic valve stenosis. In this case, both mitral and tricuspid valve regurgitation are visualised by colour flow Doppler. (**c**) In severe aortic valve stenosis, left to right shunting at atrial level may be evident. Thus, filling of the left ventricle is reduced as a consequence of left ventricular dysfunction +/− stenosis of the mitral valve. (**d**) Reversal of flow in the aortic arch is a sign of severe obstruction to the left ventricular outflow tract. In this example, there was antegrade flow through the arterial duct but blood supply to the head and neck was maintained by blood flowing retrograde from the arterial duct to the cerebral and coronary circulation. (**e**) Abnormal mitral valve Doppler flow patterns are observed in critical aortic valve stenosis with a short monophasic flow pattern across the mitral valve in contrast to the normal biphasic flow pattern. This is one of the sonographic features which has been used to predict progression to hypoplastic left heart

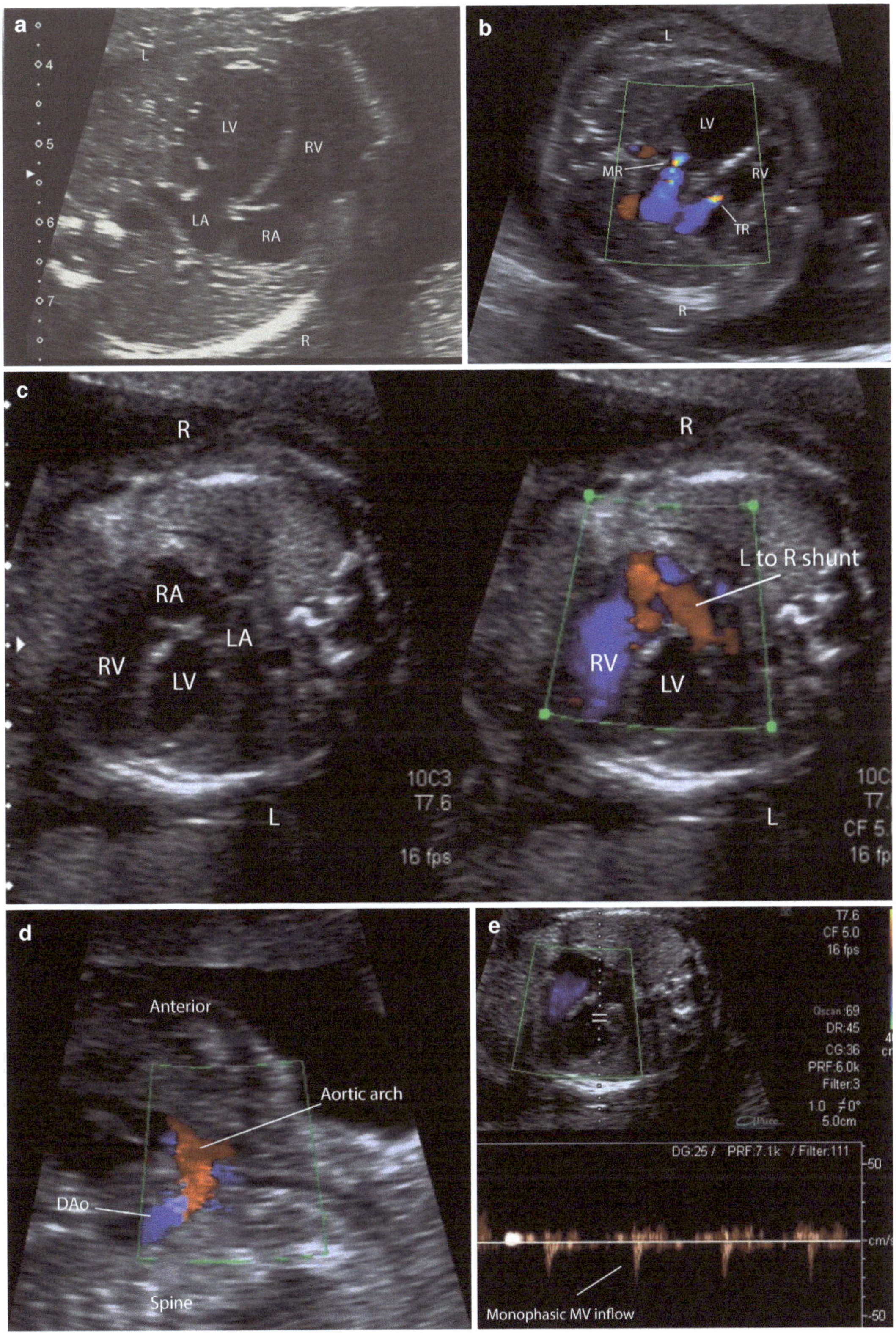
a
L
LV
RV
LA
RA
R
b
L
LV
MR
RV
TR
R
c
R
RA
LA
RV
LV
L
10C3
T7.6
16 fps
R
L to R shunt
RV
LV
L
d
Anterior
Aortic arch
DAo
Spine
e
T7.6
CF 5.0
16 fps
DG:25 / PRF:7.1k / Filter:111
Monophasic MV inflow

For cases where LV function and left heart growth remain good during fetal life then early neonatal assessment is required. If postnatal intervention is indicated this may be done either by surgical valvotomy or by balloon dilation of the aortic valve. The precise approach will vary by institution. All patients require long term postnatal review and repeat surgeries are often necessary as the patient grows.

For moderate to severe cases (see Table 8.8) there is the potential to intervene before birth. This remains highly controversial with respect to the risks versus benefits of prenatal intervention. The judgement to be made is whether the findings will progress during fetal life so that a normal biventricular circulation will not be feasible after birth. There are published criteria to assist with this judgement, which is made on a case by case basis. Even if intervention is considered, there are differing opinions as to whether prenatal intervention is worth the procedural risk and to what extent this improves the postnatal prognosis. International registries have been established to gauge the results and effectiveness of prenatal intervention. Postnatally, if the left heart structures are not sufficiently developed to support the systemic circulation then management is analogous to hypoplastic left heart syndrome with an eventual single ventricle ("Fontan") circulation. The approach to management is covered in more detail in Chap. 18. If the left heart structures are judged suitable to support the systemic arterial circulation then the initial approach is usually balloon dilation of the aortic valve or a surgical valvotomy. Depending on the associated lesions surgery may also be required on the mitral valve and the aortic arch. In some centres, endocardial fibroelastosis may be surgically removed with the aim of making the ventricle less "stiff" and promoting more normal filling and ejection from the left ventricle. This is an important consideration because if the left ventricle relaxes poorly and is stiffer than normal this may lead to elevated left atrial and pulmonary artery pressure (pulmonary hypertension). For many patients the aortic valve may either need to be replaced or the patient's own pulmonary valve placed in the aortic position (Ross operation). The exact approach is considered on a case by case basis, and varies considerably by institution.

Pulmonary Valve Stenosis

Pulmonary valve stenosis (PS) is defined as a narrowing of the pulmonary valve. This has an incidence of 4/10,000 in newborn infants and represents less than 2% of congenital heart defects diagnosed before birth. A diagram of this lesion is shown in Fig. 8.27. In affected

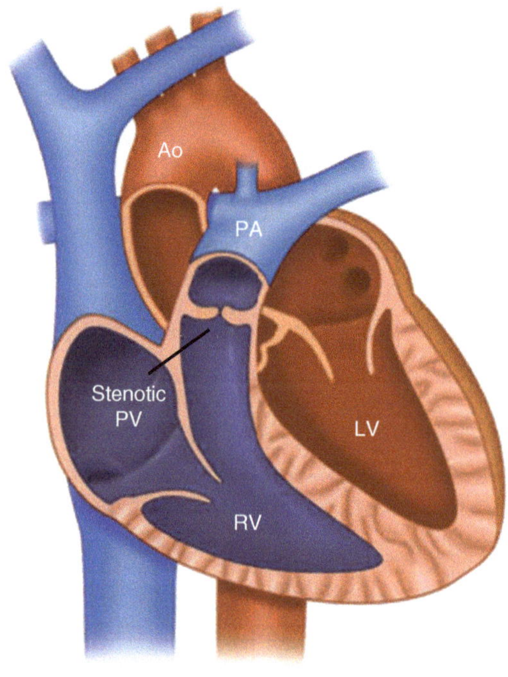

Fig. 8.27 Schematic diagram of pulmonary valve stenosis. The pulmonary valve is congenitally abnormal. In severe cases, there is significant right ventricular hypertrophy and ventricular dysfunction, frequently accompanied by tricuspid valve regurgitation. In severe cases, the ductal flow may be reversed i.e. from the aorta to the pulmonary circulation

cases, the pulmonary valve is congenitally abnormal. The morphology of valve leaflets may be normal but with fusion between them through to bicuspid or unicuspid morphology. The severity of pulmonary valve stenosis is also variable ranging from mild stenosis through to critical pulmonary valve stenosis. There is a bias towards more severe cases being detected during fetal life, because in milder cases screening views may be within normal limits. The sonographic findings in critical pulmonary valve stenosis are very similar to those of pulmonary atresia with intact ventricular septum. In a small minority of cases, critical pulmonary valve stenosis may progress to pulmonary atresia with advancing gestational age.

The echocardiographic features described here relate to isolated PS but stenosis of this valve may be observed in the context of other cardiac lesions, for example, tetralogy of Fallot or transposition of the great arteries and is discussed in those sections. The sonographic features of pulmonary valve stenosis vary according to the severity of the stenosis. In mild pulmonary valve stenosis, the four-chamber view may appear normal with normal size and function of the right ventricle. Such cases may be detected if there is observed to be restriction of motion of the pulmonary valve, aliasing of colour using colour flow Doppler or if an elevated velocity is detected by pulsed or continuous wave Doppler. In some cases, post-stenotic dilation of the main pulmonary artery may also be observed. In mild cases, ductal flow direction is normal. The appearances may progress with advancing gestational age to become more severe.

In severe cases of PS, the four-chamber view is abnormal with a variable degree of hypertrophy and size of the right ventricle (Fig. 8.28a) coupled with reduced ventricular function (Videos 8.46 and 8.47). The size of right heart structures may assist in the prediction of postnatal outcome and the type of approach adopted after birth (Lowenthal et al. 2014). The Doppler inflow through the tricuspid valve may be monophasic and tricuspid valve regurgitation is a frequent accompaniment (Fig. 8.28b, Video 8.47). Doppler interrogation of tricuspid valve regurgitation and across the pulmonary valve may be significantly elevated (often greater the 4 m/s) confirming elevated right ventricular pressure (Fig. 8.28b). Interrogation of such high velocity jets necessitates use of continuous wave Doppler. The pulmonary valve motion is either absent or restricted (Fig. 8.28c, Video 8.48) and the size of the pulmonary valve ranges from normal to severely hypoplastic. Antegrade flow of blood across the pulmonary valve is best interrogated using a combination of colour flow Doppler and pulsed or continuous wave Doppler (Fig. 8.28d, Video 8.49). The direction of flow through the arterial duct is a good marker of severity, with reversal of ductal flow in more severe cases (Fig. 8.28e).

Feature	Mild pulmonary valve stenosis	Severe pulmonary valve stenosis
4 chamber view	RV normal size Normal RV contraction TV motion normal	Echogenic RV Variable RV size Reduced RV contraction TV excursion reduced. Variable TR
TV inflow	Biphasic	Monophasic
Flow at atrial septum	Right to left	Right to left
great arteries	Ao = PA Post-stenotic dilation of PA	Ao > PA Turbulent flow across pulmonary valve
Three vessel trachea view	Antegrade flow in arterial duct Normal sized PA	Retrograde flow in arterial duct PA size variable

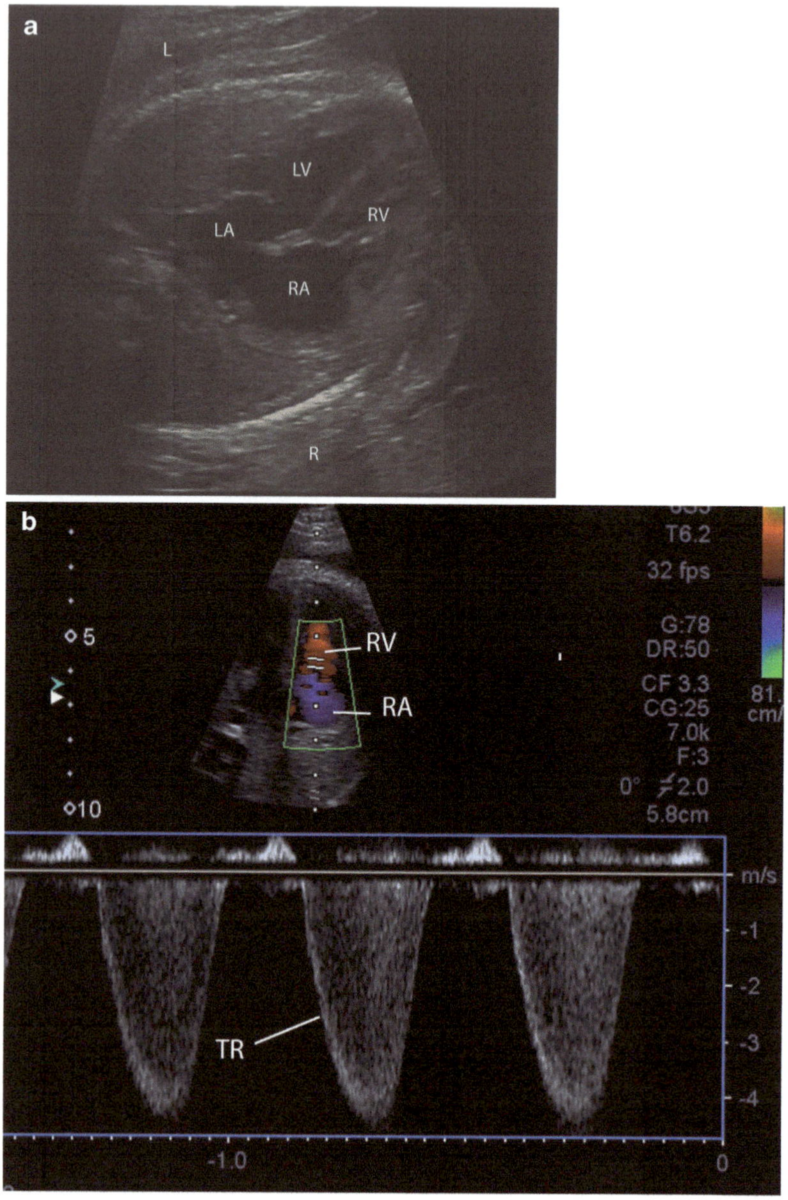

Fig. 8.28 (**a**) The four-chamber view is usually abnormal where this is significant pulmonary valve stenosis but may be normal in milder cases. In this example, the RV is hypertrophied with diminished cavity size. (**b**) Tricuspid valve regurgitation frequently accompanies severe pulmonary valve stenosis. Doppler interrogation confirms an abnormally high tricuspid regurgitant jet velocity of over 4 m/s, confirming elevated right ventricular pressure in response to the stenosis of the PV. (**c**) This image of the pulmonary valve in systole, obtained from a sagittal projection shows "doming" of the pulmonary valve, confirming that it does not open fully as the right ventricle contracts. (**d**) Colour flow Doppler confirms a turbulent jet of blood flow across the PV which had an elevated velocity of 3 m/s. (**e**) Reversal of flow in the arterial duct. The sagittal view of the aortic arch confirms normal flow in the aortic arch but the flow in the arterial duct is reversed (i.e. flow is from the aorta to the pulmonary arteries) as is shown by the blue colour

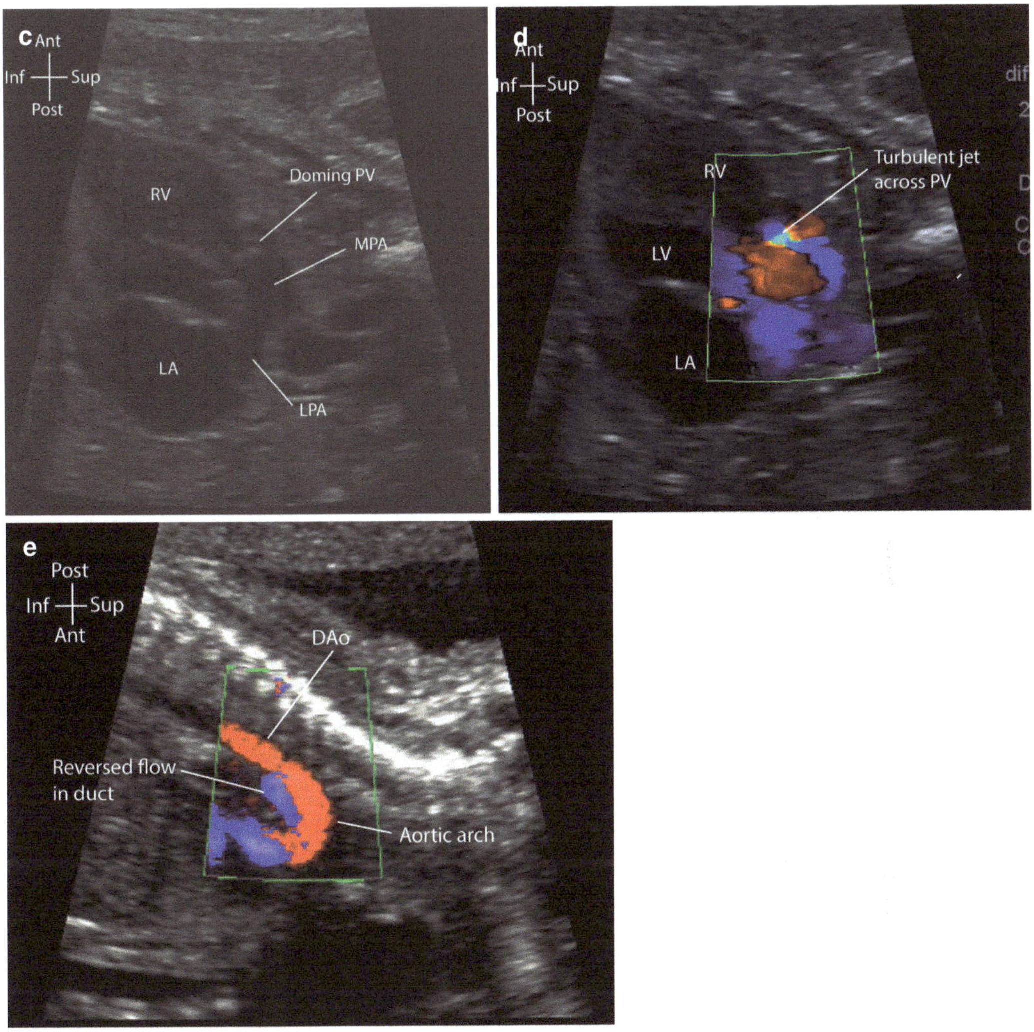

Fig. 8.28 (continued)

Associations

Pulmonary valve stenosis is usually isolated but can be associated with Noonan syndrome. Further pointers towards Noonan syndrome include persistent increase of nuchal translucency and development of hypertrophic cardiomyopathy in the late second or third trimester (Vigneswaran et al. 2017) or after birth. Pulmonary valve stenosis may also be observed in the recipient twin of Twin-Twin transfusion syndrome. In all cases detailed anomaly scanning is offered and fetal karyotyping is discussed.

Management

For mild cases of pulmonary valve stenosis, postnatal review may be all that is required. If pulmonary stenosis progresses after birth then balloon dilation of the pulmonary valve is the most common initial approach. For severe cases, prostaglandin E infusion is indicated after birth to maintain patency of the arterial duct and allow adequate pulmonary blood flow. Balloon dilation of the pulmonary valve is the usual approach after birth. The pulmonary valve in patients with Noonan syndrome is often hard to dilate by balloon valvuloplasty and in those cases surgical valvotomy is frequently necessary. In all cases, ongoing review is indicated through childhood to monitor for restenosis of the pulmonary valve or for the effects of pulmonary valve regurgitation which often occurs after catheter or surgical intervention. In a small minority of cases, the right ventricle may be so hypoplastic that an additional source of pulmonary blood flow such as a Glenn shunt (anastamosis of superior vena cava to pulmonary artery) may be required, or even management by single ventricle approach (Chap. 18).

Pulmonary Atresia with Intact Ventricular Septum

In pulmonary atresia with intact ventricular septum (PATIVS) there is no antegrade flow from the right ventricle to the pulmonary arteries. This can be due to an imperforate pulmonary valve alone (membranous pulmonary atresia) or lack of continuity between the right ventricle and the pulmonary arteries with muscle interposing between the pulmonary arteries and the right ventricle. This condition has an incidence of 4.5 per 100,000 live births and accounts for less than 3% of congenital heart defects detected before birth.

With respect to echocardiographic features, the size of the right ventricle ranges from diminutive to dilated so that the lesion is initially suspected from abnormal appearances of the four-chamber view. Most commonly the RV is hypoplastic, hypertrophied, echogenic and poorly contractile (Fig. 8.29a, Video 8.50). The severity of tricuspid valve regurgitation is highly variable and in a minority of cases there may be apical displacement of the tricuspid valve (Ebstein anomaly). Doppler interrogation of tricuspid valve regurgitation demonstrates high velocity tricuspid valve regurgitation, similar to critical pulmonary valve stenosis (Fig. 8.28b). The pulmonary blood supply is retrograde via the arterial duct (Figs. 8.28e and 8.29b, Video 8.51). In a minority of fetuses there are abnormalities of the coronary circulation, which manifest as abnormal to/fro colour jets over the body of the right ventricle (Video 8.51). This is due to abnormal communications between the right ventricular cavity and the coronary circulation (sinusoids).

Postnatal management is dictated by details of the cardiac anatomy. If the tricuspid valve and right ventricle are severely hypoplastic or if there are major coronary abnormalities, then management is generally towards a functionally single ventricle circulation (Chap. 18) (Lowenthal et al. 2014). However, if there is an imperforate pulmonary valve and the right ventricle is sufficiently developed, then catheter or surgical intervention is used to perforate / open the pulmonary valve to restore the connection between the right ventricle and the pulmonary arteries to achieve a biventricular circulation. The exact approach varies significantly between institutions. Decision-making is normally done on a case by case basis: echocardiographic measurements of the tricuspid valve and right ventricular size may assist in prediction of which fetuses will be suitable for a single ventricle versus biventricular repair. Prenatal cardiac intervention has been used in selected cases to perforate the pulmonary valve before birth to promote growth and development of the right heart, to maximise the chance of a biventricular repair (Moon-Grady et al. 2015). This type of intervention remains controversial given the procedural risks and efficacy versus intervention only after the fetus is delivered. The longer term prognosis is heavily influenced by whether a single ventricle or biventricular circulation is achieved. All patients require life-long follow up by congenital heart disease specialists.

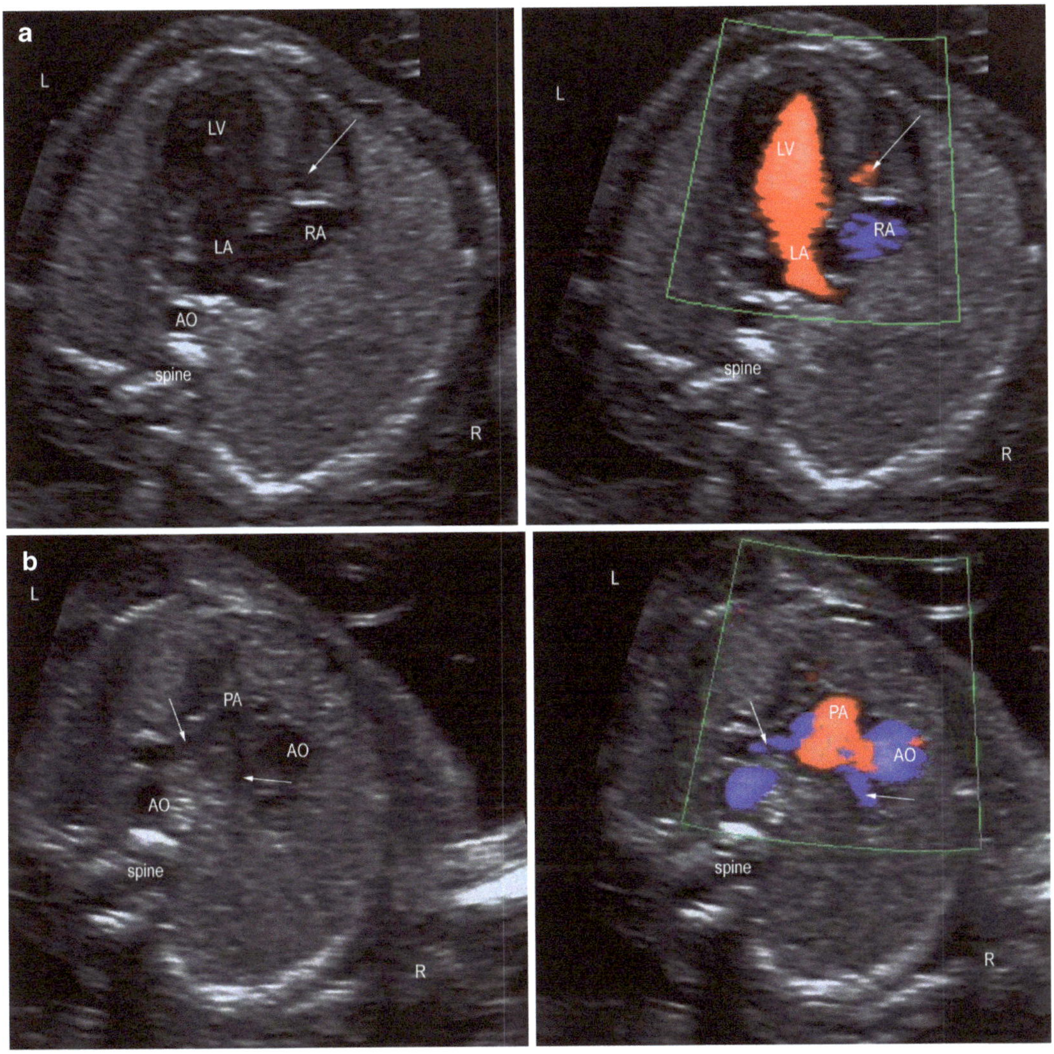

Fig. 8.29 Pulmonary atresia with intact ventricular septum (PATIVS). (**a**) This four-chamber view shows the characteristic features of PATIVS. The left pane shows that the right ventricle is severely hypoplastic and hypertrophied (arrow). The right pane shows a broad jet of flow across the mitral valve but only a tiny flash of antegrade flow across the tricuspid valve (arrowed). (**b**) This view is above the level of the four-chamber view and shows hypoplastic central pulmonary arteries (arrowed). There is retrograde flow into the main pulmonary artery

References

Duke C, Sharland GK, Jones AM, Simpson JM. Echocardiographic features and outcome of truncus arteriosus diagnosed during fetal life. Am J Cardiol. 2001;88:1379–84.

Freud LR, Tworetzky W. Fetal interventions for congenital heart disease. Curr Opin Pediatr. 2016;28:156–62. https://doi.org/10.1097/MOP.0000000000000331.

Gomez O, Soveral I, Bennasar M, Crispi F, Masoller N, Marimon E, Bartrons J, Gratacós E, Martinez JM. Accuracy of fetal echocardiography in the differential diagnosis between truncus arteriosus and pulmonary atresia with ventricular septal defect. Fetal Diagn Ther. 2015;39:90–9. https://doi.org/10.1159/000433430.

Hunter LE, Chubb H, Miller O, Sharland G, Simpson JM. Fetal aortic valve stenosis: a critique of case selection criteria for fetal intervention. Prenat Diagn. 2015. https://doi.org/10.1002/pd.4661.

Lagopoulos ME, Manlhiot C, McCrindle BW, Jaeggi ET, Friedberg MK, Nield LE. Impact of prenatal diagnosis and anatomical subtype on outcome in double outlet right ventricle. Am Heart J. 2010;160:692–700. https://doi.org/10.1016/j.ahj.2010.07.009.

Lowenthal A, Lemley B, Kipps AK, Brook MM, Moon-Grady AJ. Prenatal tricuspid valve size as a predictor of postnatal outcome in patients with severe pulmonary stenosis or pulmonary atresia with intact ventricular septum. Fetal Diagn Ther. 2014;35:101–7. https://doi.org/10.1159/000357429.

Moon-Grady AJ, Morris SA, Belfort M, Chmait R, Dangel J, Devlieger R, Emery S, Frommelt M, Galindo A, Gelehrter S, Gembruch U, Grinenco S, Habli M, Herberg U, Jaeggi E, Kilby M, Kontopoulos E, Marantz P, Miller O, Otaño L, Pedra C, Pedra S, Pruetz J, Quintero R, Ryan G, Sharland G, Simpson J, Vlastos E, Tworetzky W, Wilkins-Haug L, Oepkes D. International Fetal Cardiac Intervention Registry. A worldwide collaborative description and preliminary outcomes. J Am Coll Cardiol. 2015;66:388–99. https://doi.org/10.1016/j.jacc.2015.05.037.

Pascal CJ, Huggon I, Sharland GK, Simpson JM. An echocardiographic study of diagnostic accuracy, prediction of surgical approach, and outcome for fetuses diagnosed with discordant ventriculo-arterial connections. Cardiol Young. 2007;17:528–34. https://doi.org/10.1017/S1047951107000728.

Pepas LP, Savis A, Jones A, Sharland GK, Tulloh RMR, Simpson JM. An echocardiographic study of tetralogy of Fallot in the fetus and infant. Cardiol Young. 2003;13:240–7.

Quartermain MD, Glatz AC, Goldberg DJ, Cohen MS, Elias MD, Tian Z, Rychik J. Pulmonary outflow tract obstruction in fetuses with complex congenital heart disease: predicting the need for neonatal intervention. Ultrasound Obstet Gynecol. 2013;41:47–53. https://doi.org/10.1002/uog.11196.

Razavi RS, Sharland GK, Simpson JM. Prenatal diagnosis by echocardiogram and outcome of absent pulmonary valve syndrome. Am J Cardiol. 2003;91:429–32.

Simpson JM, Sharland GK. Natural history and outcome of aortic stenosis diagnosed prenatally. Heart. 1997;77:205–10.

Swanson TM, Selamet Tierney ES, Tworetzky W, Pigula F, McElhinney DB. Truncus arteriosus: diagnostic accuracy, outcomes, and impact of prenatal diagnosis. Pediatr Cardiol. 2009;30:256–61. https://doi.org/10.1007/s00246-008-9328-7.

Vesel S, Rollings S, Jones A, Callaghan N, Simpson J, Sharland GK. Prenatally diagnosed pulmonary atresia with ventricular septal defect: echocardiography, genetics, associated anomalies and outcome. Heart. 2006;92:1501–5. https://doi.org/10.1136/hrt.2005.083295.

Vigneswaran TV, Kametas NA, Zinevich Y, Bataeva R, Allan LD, Zidere V. Assessment of cardiac angle in fetuses with congenital heart disease at risk of 22q11.2 deletion. Ultrasound Obstet Gynecol. 2015;46:695–9. https://doi.org/10.1002/uog.14832.

Vigneswaran TV, Homfray T, Allan LD, Simpson JM, Zidere V. Persistently elevated nuchal translucency and the fetal heart. J Matern Neonatal Med. 2017:1–5. https://doi.org/10.1080/14767058.2017.1342804.

Wertaschnigg D, Jaeggi M, Chitayat D, Shannon P, Ryan G, Thompson M, Yoo SJ, Jaeggi E. Prenatal diagnosis and outcome of absent pulmonary valve syndrome: contemporary single-center experience and review of the literature. Ultrasound Obstet Gynecol. 2013;41:162–7. https://doi.org/10.1002/uog.11193.

Zidere V, Tsapakis EG, Huggon IC, Allan LD. Right aortic arch in the fetus. Ultrasound Obstet Gynecol. 2006;28:876–81. https://doi.org/10.1002/uog.3841.

Zidere V, Pushparajah K, Allan LD, Simpson JM (2013) Three-dimensional fetal echocardiography for prediction of postnatal surgical approach in double outlet right ventricle: a pilot study. Ultrasound Obstet Gynecol. 42:n/a-n/a. doi: https://doi.org/10.1002/uog.12512.

Aortic Arch Abnormalities

9

Trisha Vigneswaran and Vita Zidere

Abstract

Aortic abnormalities are being diagnosed more frequently during fetal life due to the incorporation of views of the upper mediastinum into screening views of the fetal heart. Morbidity and mortality is reduced when duct-dependent lesions such as coarctation of the aorta are prenatally diagnosed and lesions such as double aortic arch and right aortic arch are of clinical significance because they can cause airway compression. Abnormalities of the aortic arch and an aberrant right subclavian artery can be associated with chromosomal abnormalities. All aortic arch abnormalities can be associated with intracardiac abnormalities so assessment of the intracardiac anatomy is mandatory. This chapter however focuses on isolated abnormalities of the aortic arch and its branches.

Keywords

Vascular anomalies · Coarctation of the aorta · Interrupted aortic arch · Double aortic arch · Right aortic arch · Aberrant right subclavian artery · Vascular ring

Coarctation of the Aorta

Introduction

Coarctation of the aorta is a narrowing of the aortic isthmus, the region of the aorta beyond the origin of the left subclavian artery and proximal to the insertion of the arterial duct. Coarctation can present clinically after birth following constriction of the arterial duct which causes obstruction of blood flow through the aortic arch. Aortic arch narrowing may include hypoplasia of the transverse aortic arch which is the more commonly identified prenatal variant. Isolated coarctation of the aorta constitutes 7–10% of cases of congenital heart disease. The prevalence in liveborn infants is 2/10,000 and is likely to be much higher during fetal life due to its association with genetic abnormalities which may result in miscarriage or termination of pregnancy. Despite the prevalence of coarctation of the aorta and the advancement of fetal echocardiography in the last 25 years this remains a difficult diagnosis to make with confidence in the prenatal period with marked variation in the prenatal detection rate of coarctation of

Electronic Supplementary Material The online version of this chapter (https://doi.org/10.1007/978-3-319-77461-9_9) contains supplementary material, which is available to authorized users.

T. Vigneswaran · V. Zidere (✉)
Evelina London Children's Hospital, Guy's and St Thomas' NHS Foundation Trust, London, UK

King's College Hospital NHS Foundation Trust, London, UK
e-mail: trisha.vigneswaran@gstt.nhs.uk; vita.zidere@gstt.nhs.uk

© Springer International Publishing AG, part of Springer Nature 2018

J. Simpson et al. (eds.), *Fetal Cardiology*, https://doi.org/10.1007/978-3-319-77461-9_9

the aorta and a high false positive rate of diagnosis (Head et al. 2005; Pinto et al. 2012).

Fetal Echocardiogram

Coarctation of the aorta is initially suspected when there is asymmetry of the width of the right and left ventricles on the four-chamber view (Fig. 9.1, Video 9.1). This disproportion favours a larger right ventricular width compared to the left ventricular width. In most cases the left ventricle reaches the apex of the heart unless there is severe hypoplasia of the left ventricle (see Chap. 7). The asymmetry of the ventricles is matched by asymmetry of the great arteries with dominance of the pulmonary artery and ductal arch compared to the aorta and transverse aortic arch. (Figs. 9.2 and 9.3, Video 9.2) Objective measurements of the pulmonary artery and arterial duct dimensions are towards or above the upper limit of normal for gestation and aortic measurements approach, or are below the lower limit of normal for gestation (Vigneswaran et al. 2018a). The mitral valve annulus may be at the lower end of the normal range (Familiari et al. 2016). There is a significant false positive diagnosis rate associated with prenatal diagnosis of coarctation due to the patency of the arterial duct and all prenatal series report significant overlap of measurements between false positive and true positive cases of coarctation of the aorta. Colour flow Doppler assists in the assessment of suspected coarctation. In contrast to classical hypoplastic left heart syndrome, there is antegrade flow across the mitral valve and aortic valve. In most cases, there is antegrade systolic flow in the aortic arch (Fig. 9.4, Video 9.3). In the normal fetus, flow at the foramen ovale is from the right atrium to the left but in the setting of a severe coarctation, the foramen ovale flow direction may be reversed i.e. from the left atrium to the right atrium (Sharland et al. 1994). If retrograde systolic flow in the aortic arch is seen, this indicates that either the aortic valve is atretic or critically narrowed or, that the hypoplasia of the left ventricle is severe. The flow across the mitral valve should show a normal biphasic pattern. It is important to assess the morphology of the mitral valve as abnormalities such as parachute mitral valve or mitral valve stenosis can impact the prognosis. A short axis view of the left ventricle can be obtained from a sagittal view of the fetus. This demonstrates the mitral valve leaflets and the papillary muscle anatomy. Normally, the mitral valve has two papillary muscles but with a parachute mitral valve there is only a single papillary muscle usually accompanied by tethered mitral valve chords and restricted

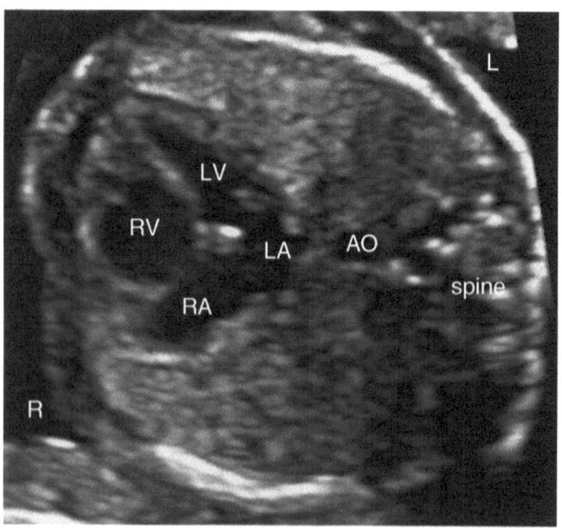

Fig. 9.1 A four-chamber view of the fetal heart taken from a transverse section of the fetal thorax. This demonstrates asymmetry of the right and left sides of the heart. The right atrium and right ventricle are wider than the left atrium and left ventricle, but the left ventricle reaches the apex of the heart

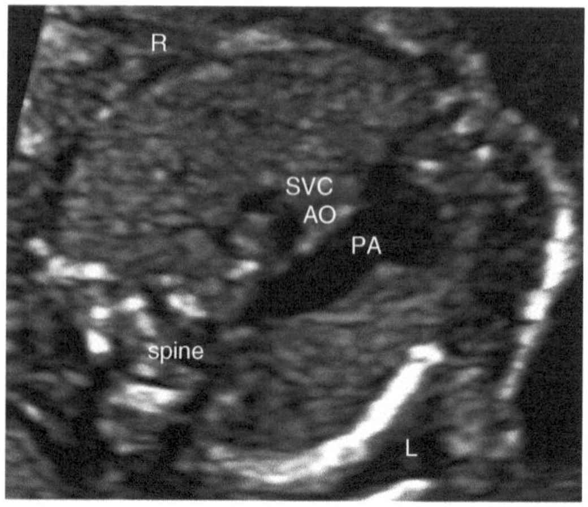

Fig. 9.2 The three vessel view shows disproportion of the pulmonary artery and ascending aorta

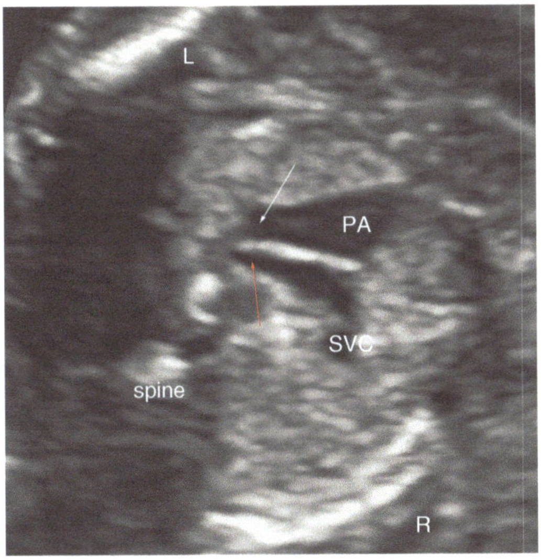

Fig. 9.3 The three vessel and tracheal view shows disproportion of the transverse aortic arch and aortic isthmus (red arrow) and the arterial duct (white arrow). The transverse aortic arch is significantly smaller than the ductal arch

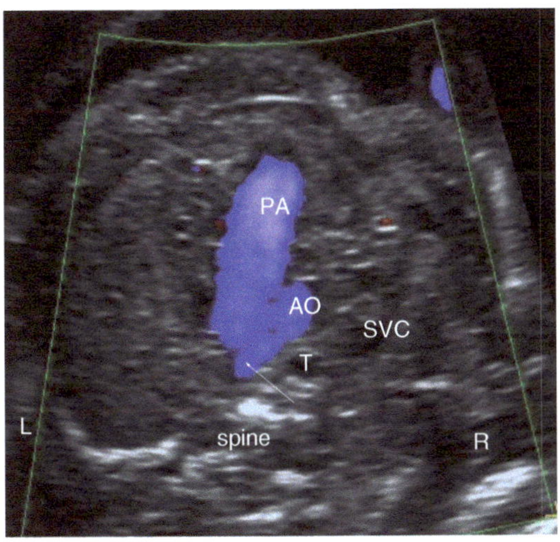

Fig. 9.4 The three vessel and tracheal view with colour Doppler of the upper mediastinum demonstrates disproportion of the pulmonary artery and duct compared to the transverse aortic arch and aortic isthmus (white arrow). There is antegrade flow in the transverse aortic arch

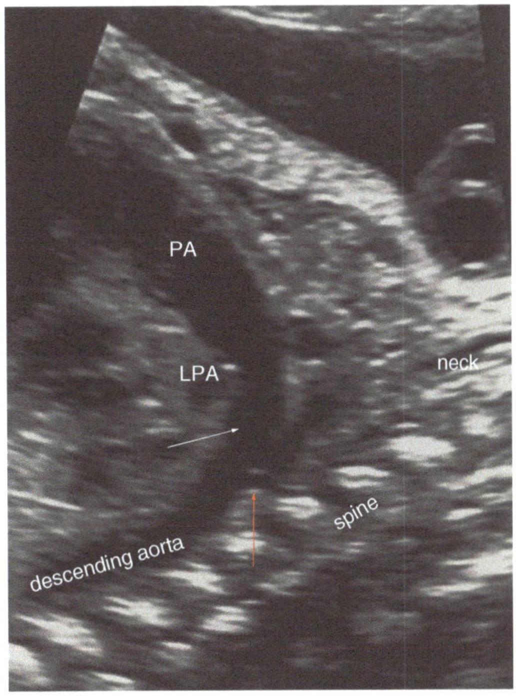

Fig. 9.5 A sagittal view demonstrates the dominant ductal arch (white arrow) and the slender aortic isthmus (red arrow), which inserts almost perpendicular into the arterial duct. The aortic isthmus is diminutive compared to the diameter of the descending aorta

opening of the mitral valve. Although asymmetry of ventricular size is a frequent reason for suspicion of coarctation of the aorta, in some affected cases there is no asymmetry between the size of the ventricles and asymmetry is confined to the great arteries and arch views. This may be seen in association with a ventricular septal defect. Coarctation of the aorta can still occur in the absence of ventricular size discrepancy and more emphasis should be placed on the morphology and size of the ductal and aortic arches.

One of the key views in the assessment of coarctation of the aorta is the comparison of ductal and aortic arch size on the transverse three vessel and tracheal view. However, experienced sonographers may strengthen the diagnosis with sagittal views (Fig. 9.5) of the aortic arch. An increased distance between the origins of the left common carotid artery and left subclavian artery may be appreciated on the sagittal arch views (Fig. 9.6); Furthermore, the sagittal view may show a posterior "shelf" due the aortic isthmus connecting into the side of the ductal arch at an angle (Fig. 9.6). It is important to ensure that the sagittal views of the arterial duct are not confused with those of the aortic isthmus. This is further discussed in Chap. 3 on extended views of the

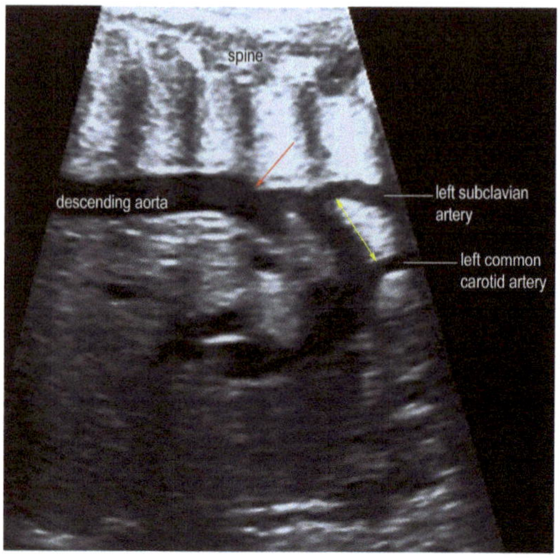

Fig. 9.6 Sagittal view demonstrating an increased distance between the left common carotid and left subclavian artery (yellow arrow). A posterior "shelf" (red arrow) due the slender aortic isthmus connecting into the side of the ductal arch at an angle is seen in this example of coarctation of the aorta

fetal heart. Due to their different planes, the aortic and ductal arches cannot be visualised in the same sagittal sonographic plan—the sonographer has to angulate the transducer from side to side to visualise each arch separately.

The finding of ventricular asymmetry during the third trimester of pregnancy poses particular challenges because dominance of the right ventricle is a normal finding during this period. Aside from the features covered above, comparison of measurements to normal gestation-specific *Z* scores is particularly helpful in this group (Vigneswaran et al. 2018a). In particular confirmation that the aortic isthmus diameter is below the normal range for gestation would favour a diagnosis of coarctation.

Associations

A bicuspid aortic valve is a common association of coarctation of the aorta (over 50%) and with modern ultrasound systems this may sometimes be identified before birth. (Video 9.4) Other associations of coarctation include: hypoplastic left heart syndrome, atrioventricular septal defect, transposition of the great arteries and double inlet left ventricle. Some fetuses show multiple levels of obstruction of the left heart including mitral valve stenosis and aortic valve stenosis. This has been termed "Shone complex" (or syndrome) and emphasises the importance of careful assessment of all left heart structures if coarctation of the aorta is suspected. Some components of the complex, such as a supramitral membrane or subaortic stenosis may only develop after birth. A persistent left superior vena cava can be identified in some fetuses with coarctation of the aorta (Fig. 9.7a, b, Video 9.5). In the setting of asymmetry of the left and right ventricles, a persistent left SVC is seen in just as many false positive as true positive cases of coarctation (Head et al. 2005). Current consensus is to offer repeat fetal echocardiography in the third trimester when bilateral superior vena cava are identified (Gustapane et al. 2016).

In the first trimester there is a high incidence of 45XO, and overall the incidence of chromosomal abnormalities is in the region of 10% (Allan et al. 2009). Monosomy 45XO should be suspected in fetuses with a markedly increased nuchal translucency/cystic hygroma and coarctation. Furthermore, disproportion of the great vessels can be seen with congenital diaphragmatic hernia and aneuploidies and in some cases, coarctation is not evident after birth. Coarctation of the aorta can develop in the donor twin in the setting of twin-to-twin transfusion syndrome.

The aortic isthmus is the watershed area between the left and right ventricular circulations (Fouron 2003). In the setting of intrauterine growth restriction, a 'brain-sparing effect' can be seen which results in cerebral run-off from the aortic arch blood flow towards the fetal brain in diastole. This can manifest as a slender aortic isthmus. On colour flow Doppler there will be reversed flow in diastole in the aortic isthmus and pulse wave Doppler in the aortic isthmus will confirm the timing of the reversed flow (Fig. 9.8a, b). It must be noted that coarctation of the aorta and intrauterine growth retardation can co-exist so a complete fetal assessment must be performed.

Management

As with all major congenital cardiac abnormalities, a detailed fetal medicine review is warranted to

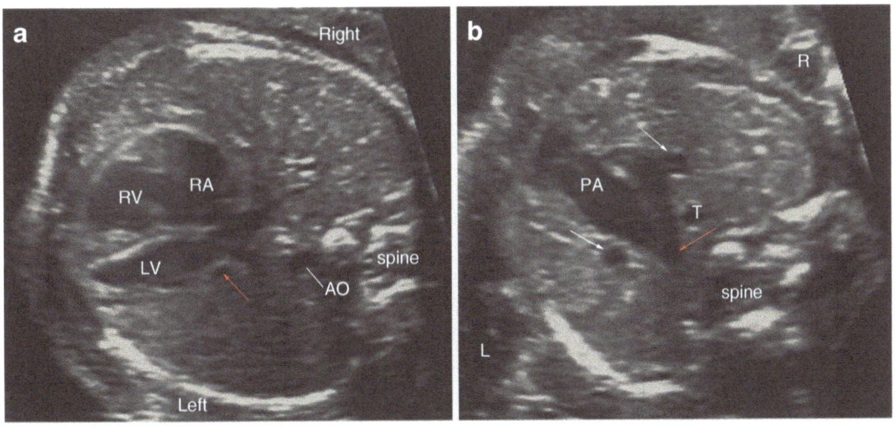

Fig. 9.7 (**a**) Four-chamber view demonstrating a dilated coronary sinus (red arrow). There is also disproportion between the right and left sides of the heart, which can be seen in fetuses with isolated bilateral superior caval veins. (**b**) Three vessel and tracheal view demonstrating bilateral superior vena cava (white arrows) and a slender distal transverse aortic arch (red arrow)

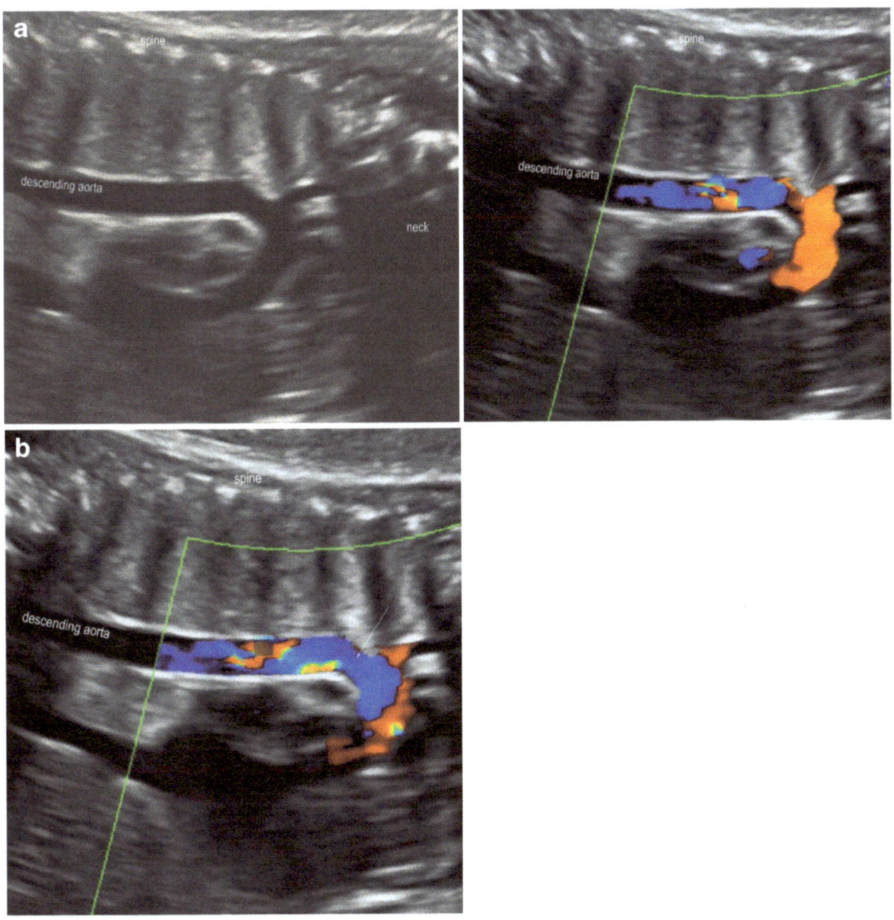

Fig. 9.8 (**a**) Sagittal view of the aortic arch showing antegrade (red) flow in systole (right panel, white arrow). The left-hand panel shows the aortic isthmus is well formed. (**b**) Sagittal view of the aortic arch showing retrograde (blue, white arrow) flow in diastole which represents diastolic run-off to the cerebral circulation which can be seen in intra-uterine growth restriction

exclude extracardiac anomalies and for further genetic testing where appropriate. For fetal coarctation no treatment is required in utero, however cases are recommended for delivery in a specialised unit for early neonatal assessment and commencement of prostaglandin E2 infusion in selected cases to prevent postnatal cardiovascular decompensation with ductal closure. After birth, serial echocardiograms may be required to confirm or refute the diagnosis as the arterial duct constricts in the transition to the postnatal circulation. Once coarctation has been confirmed, the approach to repair is surgical. For discrete coarctation, the approach is usually via a lateral thoracotomy without use of cardiopulmonary bypass. If there is a major degree of aortic arch hypoplasia, more extensive surgery is required on the aortic arch and most surgeons will prefer to approach this via a median sternotomy under cardiopulmonary bypass. In modern practice the vast majority of patients will survive neonatal repair of coarctation of the aorta.

Children with repaired coarctation of the aorta would be expected to have a good quality of life without restriction of activities, but lifelong cardiac surveillance is required. Late complications include recurrent coarctation which is usually amenable to percutaneous balloon dilatation/stent implantation. Even in the absence of recoarctation, there is a risk of premature arterial hypertension, coronary artery disease and increased arterial stiffness in these patients (Vigneswaran et al. 2018c). For those patients with a bicuspid aortic valve, aortic valve stenosis, aortic valve regurgitation and dilation of the aortic root and/or ascending aorta may occur. Depending on severity, this may require intervention later in life.

Interrupted Aortic Arch

Introduction

Interrupted aortic arch is a rare anomaly where there is a lack of luminal continuity of the aortic arch. Thus, in contrast to coarctation of the aorta where the aortic arch is narrowed, in interrupted aortic arch there is a complete break

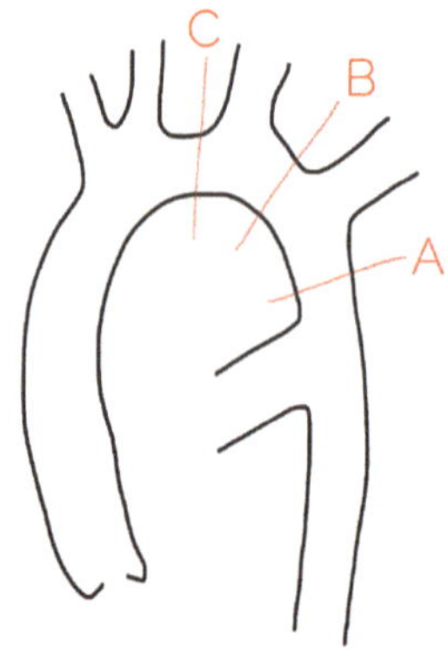

Fig. 9.9 This drawing demonstrates the three types of interruption of the aortic arch. Type B, where the site of interruption is between the left common carotid artery and the left subclavian artery (most common). Type A, interruption is beyond the left subclavian artery origin (severe spectrum of coarctation of the aorta). Type C, interruption is after the innominate artery origin (very rarely seen)

or interruption of the aortic arch. The type of interruption is classified according to it position with respect to the head and neck vessels. The site of interruption (Fig. 9.9) is most commonly between the left common carotid artery and left subclavian artery (type B). Type A interruption is beyond the left subclavian artery origin and is considered on the spectrum of a severe coarctation of the aorta. Type C interruption is after the innominate artery origin and is the least frequent (1%). In virtually all cases, interruption of the aortic arch is associated with a ventricular septal defect.

Fetal Echocardiography

The four-chamber view may be normal, but on sweeping towards the LVOT view, an outlet ventricular septal defect with posterior deviation of the outlet septum (into the left ventricular outflow tract) is seen. On the three vessel and tracheal view, the normal transverse aortic arch either cannot be visualised at all or is hypoplastic. The appearances can be difficult to differentiate from severe coarctation of the aorta on these views. On sagittal views, the ascending aorta appears hypoplastic and directed towards the head. In the most common form, the ascending aorta bifurcates to supply the innominate and left carotid arteries (Figs. 9.9 and 9.10). The arterial duct is continuous with the descending aorta.

Associations

Interrupted aortic arch can be seen in combination with common arterial trunk. Type B interruption is commonly associated with chromosome 22q11 deletion and less frequently, other chromosomal abnormalities. Extracardiac anomalies can co-exist and therefore, a detailed fetal medicine review is recommended.

Management

These cases are recommended for delivery in a tertiary unit for early neonatal assessment with commencement of prostaglandin E2 infusion to prevent cardiovascular decompensation with ductal closure. Surgical repair is performed in the neonatal period by reconstructing the aortic arch and closing the ventricular septal defect. In recent years, the overall survival through initial surgery is over 90–95% (NICOR web portal 2017). In some cases, a two-stage repair may be preferred.

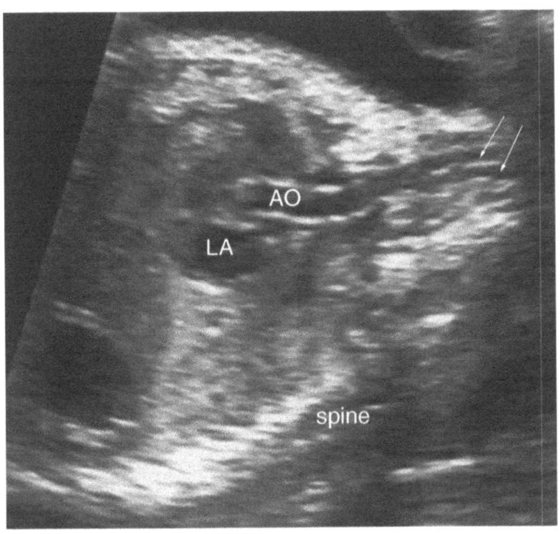

Fig. 9.10 Sagittal view demonstrating the ascending aorta which continues to the neck, branching like a tuning fork into the right subclavian and right common carotid artery (white arrows). A complete aortic arch is not seen

Following repair, lifelong cardiac surveillance is required, but no restrictions are usually placed on activities. Left ventricular outflow tract obstruction may develop either due to muscular obstruction related to posterior deviation of the outlet septum or due to hypoplasia or stenosis of the aortic valve which is frequently bicuspid. This may require further surgical repairs. The site of reconstruction of the aortic arch also merits sequential assessment to check for arch obstruction.

Right Aortic Arch

Introduction

The anatomy of the aortic arch and its branching can be appreciated from an early stage in pregnancy. Abnormalities of the laterality of the aortic arch can coexist with abnormal intracardiac anatomy, but can also be seen in isolation (Zidere et al. 2006). The true prevalence of an isolated right aortic arch is not known, historically it is reported at 0.1%, but this may be an underestimation. There is an increased prenatal detection of right aortic arches, due to incorporation of views of the aortic and ductal arch into screening programs (Vigneswaran et al. 2018b).

Fetal Echocardiography

Prenatally, the diagnosis of a right aortic arch is made when the aortic arch passes to the right of the trachea on the three vessel and tracheal view (Fig. 9.11, Videos 9.6a and 9.6b) It is important to identify the branching pattern of the aortic arch and the position of the arterial duct as it may aid in risk stratification and postnatal management. Previously, a mirror-image of the branching pattern of a left aortic arch was described as the most frequent branching pattern with a right aortic arch. However, in our experience, a right aortic arch is most often seen in combination with an aberrant left subclavian artery. This aberrant vessel can be seen to originate from the descending

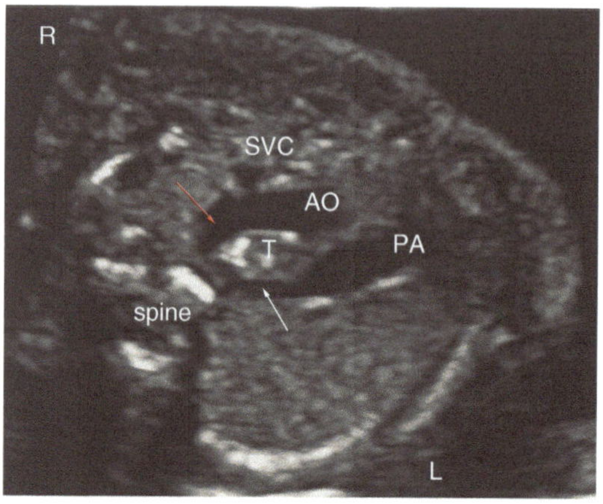

Fig. 9.11 Three vessel and tracheal view demonstrating the aortic arch (red arrow) passing to the right of the trachea. The arterial duct (white arrow) passes to the left of the trachea. The trachea lies between the aortic and ductal arches so there is potential for tracheal compression. The aortic arch and ductal arch meet in a "U" shape

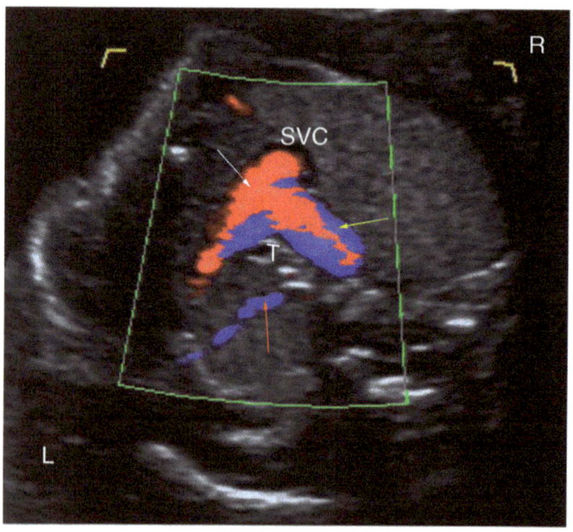

Fig. 9.12 A modified three vessel and tracheal view demonstrating the right aortic arch (yellow arrow). The probe has been tilted in order to identify the aberrant left subclavian artery (red arrow) passing behind the trachea. The innominate vein can be seen passing anterior to the ascending aorta as red Doppler flow (white arrow) which drains into the right superior vena cava

aorta and pass behind the trachea (Fig. 9.12). The arterial duct most frequently passes to the left of trachea. This leads to the appearance of a "U" sign as the right aortic arch meets the left sided arterial duct. However, if left-right orientation is not ascertained, a right arterial duct with right aortic arch will be overlooked prenatally as the normal "V"-formation is present, but on the contralateral side (Fig. 9.13a–c). The association of a right arterial duct with right aortic arch is rarely identified in the fetus either because this occurs less often or because it is more difficult to recognise as abnormal.

The right-sided position of the descending aorta in front of the spine on the situs view can be used as an indicator of presence of the right aortic arch. However, this is not diagnostic and only helps if the descending aorta maintains the right-sided position within the thorax. The descending aorta can cross the midline from right to left at any level within the thorax and thus, if the descending aorta is to the left of the spine on the four-chamber view, this does not exclude a right aortic arch.

Associations

A right aortic arch may be associated with major intracardiac anomalies, for example, tetralogy of Fallot or double outlet right ventricle. These lesions are discussed in Chap. 8. In prenatal life, it can be difficult to exclude a double aortic arch especially if there is atresia of a segment of a smaller left arch.

A right sided aortic arch may be seen in association with extracardiac abnormalities. A recent meta-analysis has reported extracardiac malformations in 15% of feuses with an isolated right aortic arch (D'Antonio et al. 2015). Overall, chromosomal anomalies are seen in 15% of prenatal cases, which includes chromosome 22q11 deletion and trisomy 21. The difficulties in counselling relate to the finding of a right aortic arch in the presence of normal screening investigations and in the absence of associated CHD or extracardiac abnormalities. In this setting the observed incidence of chromosomal abnormalities is lower (6%), but not negligible. (D'Antonio et al. 2015). These associations are observed regardless presence of aberrant subclavian artery and position of the arterial duct.

A right aortic arch is in immediate proximity to the distal trachea and in combination with a left arterial duct and an aberrant left subclavian artery can encase the trachea and oesophagus causing compression. These can cause symptoms

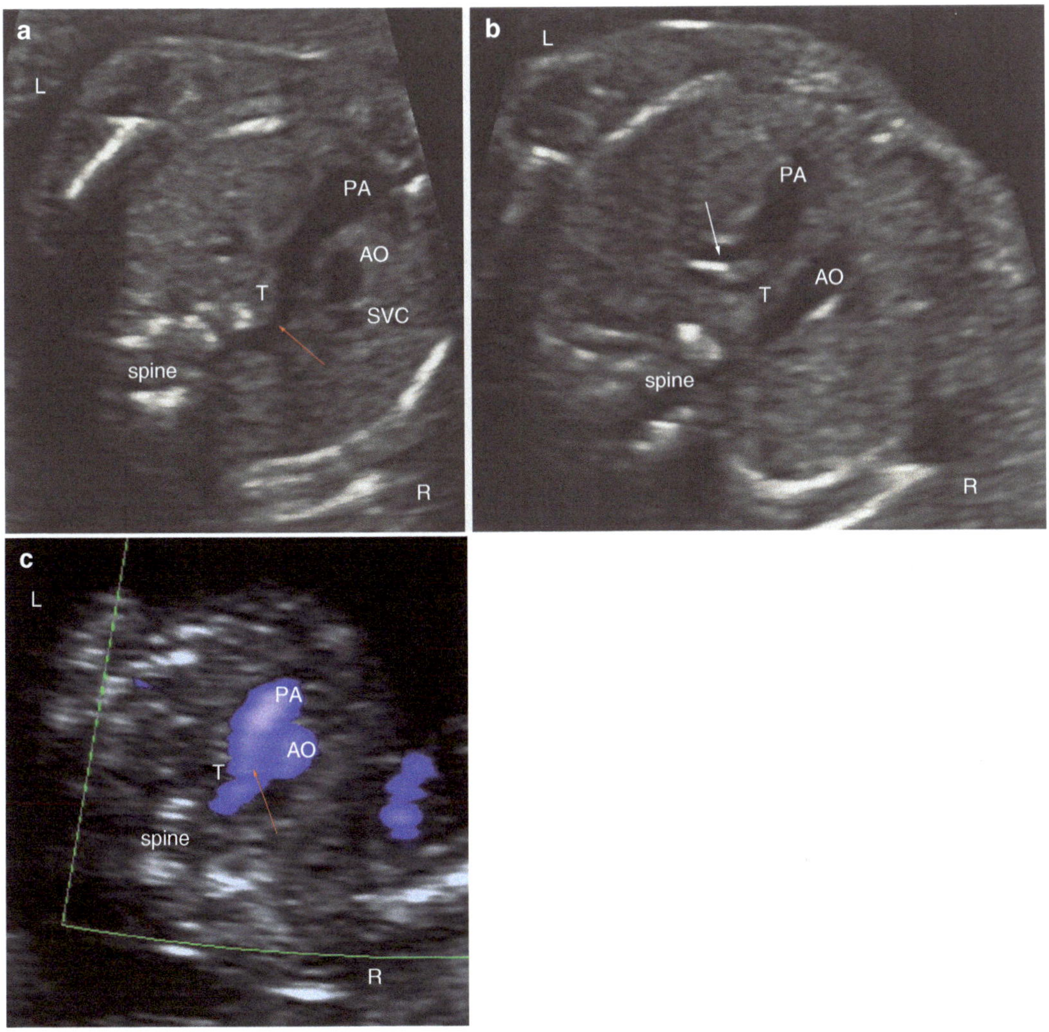

Fig. 9.13 (**a**) The three vessel view shows the arterial duct (red arrow) passes to the right of the trachea. (**b**) The three vessel and tracheal view shows the aortic arch passes to the right of the trachea. The arterial duct cannot be visualised in its expected position to the left of the trachea as it is seen below the right aortic arch in (**a**). (**c**) Colour Doppler demonstrating the right sided aortic arch and right arterial duct (red arrow), forming the "V-sign" on the right side of the trachea

such as recurrent lower respiratory tract infections, recurrent stridor or dysphagia. In symptomatic patients, further investigation is clearly indicated including bronchoscopy and CT/MRI imaging to assess the site and severity of airway compression. Surgical intervention is indicated to relieve significant airways compression. A more controversial issue is the management of patients with RAA who are asymptomatic. Traditionally, such patients are simply observed but in our recent experience we have identified many patients with significant tracheal compression on bronchoscopy who do not have symptoms (Vigneswaran et al. 2018b). In selected cases we have operated on asymptomatic patients to promote normal airways development even in the absence of symptoms.

Management

1. A detailed fetal echocardiogram in order to rule out associated cardiac lesions is warranted in cases of right aortic arch.

2. A specialist fetal medicine assessment to exclude associated extracardiac lesions and discuss genetic testing.
3. Postnatally all cases with a right aortic arch detected prenatally should have cardiac assessment in order to rule out additional minor intracardiac anomalies, confirm the arch anatomy and refute the presence of a double aortic arch.
4. A right aortic arch may cause tracheal compression and if symptoms or signs are present an urgent airways assessment is required. The absence of airways symptoms does not exclude airways compression.
5. If significant pulsatile tracheal compression secondary to the right arch is seen then low risk surgery to release the vascular ring is usually recommended.

Double Aortic Arch

Fetal Echocardiography

Double aortic arch is an abnormality when both a left and right aortic arch are present (Fig. 9.14a, b, Video 9.7). Classically, the right aortic arch is dominant and the left is smaller. In some situations, the smaller arch may have a partially atretic segment with no luminal continuity. This will not be visualised on echocardiography and may therefore appear as a right aortic arch with mirror image branching pattern. With improvements in both ultrasonography and our understanding of the aortic arch morphology, there has been an increase in the number of cases of double aortic arch diagnosed during fetal life.

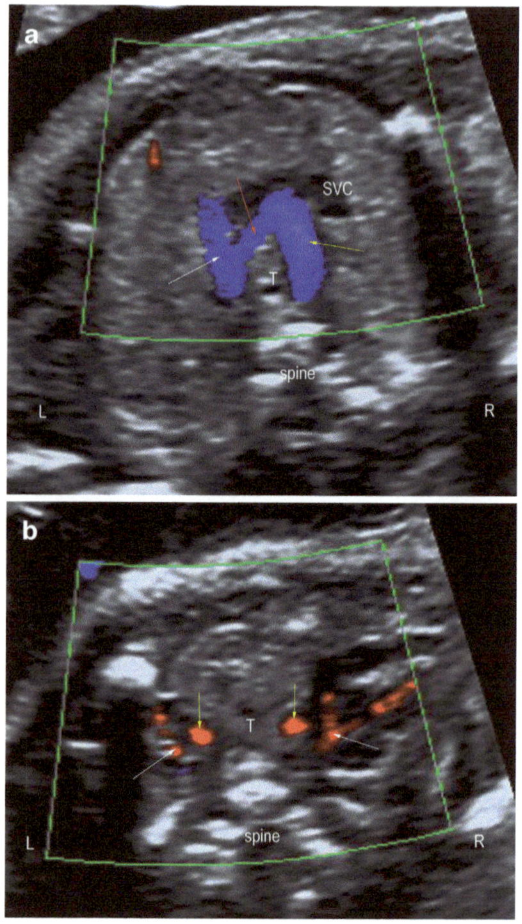

Fig. 9.14 (**a**) A double aortic arch can be seen with a dominant right sided arch (yellow arrow) and a smaller left sided aortic arch (red arrow). The white arrow demonstrates the arterial duct. The usual "V-sign" is not present, instead the vessels form a "Z" shape. (**b**) Colour Doppler demonstrating the branching of the head and neck vessels from both the right and left arches. There is a symmetrical origin of two vessels from each arch. The yellow arrows show the right and left common carotids and the white arrows the subclavian arteries

Associations

A double aortic arch is often seen in isolation, but can be seen in association with intracardiac lesions such as ventricular septal defect and tetralogy Fallot. Genetic associations are as described with a right aortic arch.

Management

Management of a double aortic arch is similar to that of a right aortic arch, however, early assessment is required in these cases as signs of significant airways compression can be seen in the neonatal period. Early involvement of an airway specialist is recommended and should be expedited if symptoms such as stridor or recurrent respiratory tract infections are present. If no symptoms are present, elective investigation with computed tomography (CT) and a free-breathing bronchoscopy without positive airways pressure are recommended due to the high risk of tracheal compression. If significant extrinsic pulsatile tracheal compression is identified low risk surgery to release the vascular ring is performed. This surgery involves division of the non-dominant aortic arch and the arterial duct.

Aberrant Right Subclavian Artery

Introduction

The right subclavian artery typically arises as the first branch from the brachiocephalic artery, arising above the level of the left aortic arch (Video 9.8). With a left sided aortic arch, the right subclavian artery may arise aberrantly from the descending aorta (Fig. 9.15 and Videos 9.9a and 9.9b). The incidence of this normal variant is not known, but it is seen with increasing frequency, estimated at 1% of the normal population.

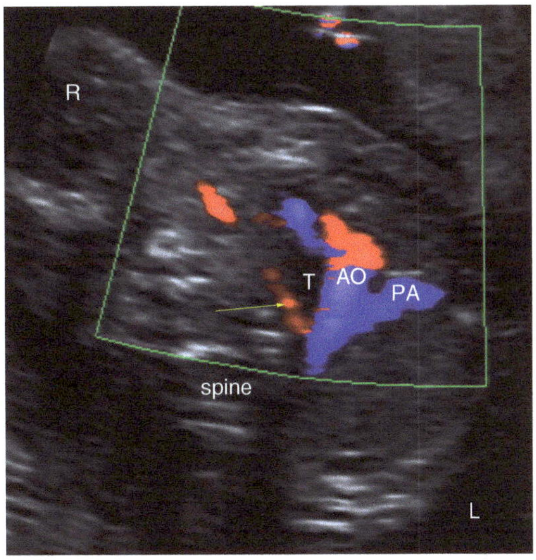

Fig. 9.15 Modified three vessel and tracheal view using colour Doppler which demonstrates a left sided aortic arch with an aberrant right subclavian artery (yellow arrow) passing behind the trachea. In order to obtain the aortic arch and the aberrant right subclavian artery in one view, the probe must be tilted

Fetal Echocardiography

A normal origin of a right subclavian artery can be seen passing anterior to the trachea, coursing towards the right arm on a transverse sweep above the aortic arch. Whereas as an aberrant right subclavian artery arises from the descending aorta behind the trachea and below the transverse aortic arch at the level of the arterial duct (Borenstein et al. 2010). Thus, it cannot be seen in sagittal view in the same plane with the other head and neck vessels.

Associations

An aberrant right subclavian artery can be associated with major intracardiac anomalies for example, with an atrioventricular septal defect, tetralogy of Fallot, hypoplastic left heart syndrome and transposition of the great arteries. These lesions are discussed in Chaps. 7 and 8.

The finding of an isolated aberrant right subclavian artery is associated with an increase to the first trimester screening risk for trisomy 21. Postnatally, in a minority of cases, the aberrant right subclavian artery has been associated with feeding difficulties which relate to compression of the posterior aspect of the oesophagus by the vessel. In even rarer cases, tracheal compression has been observed.

Management

1. Detailed fetal echocardiography to rule out associated cardiac lesions is warranted.
2. A detailed fetal medicine assessment to exclude associated extracardiac lesions and discuss possible genetic associations.
3. In the absence of intracardiac abnormalities, there is no need for postnatal cardiac assessment or alteration of obstetric management.

4. There is no substrate for a complete vascular ring and therefore elective airways investigation is not required after birth unless there are symptoms. However, there should be a low threshold for specialist referral if respiratory or gastro-intestinal symptoms arise. Supplementary material is provided in Figs. 9.16, 9.17a–c and 9.18.

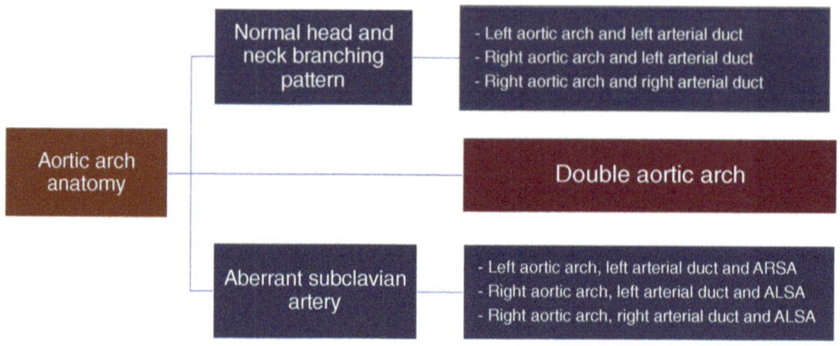

Fig. 9.16 Schematic diagram explaining the variations in aortic arch branching pattern

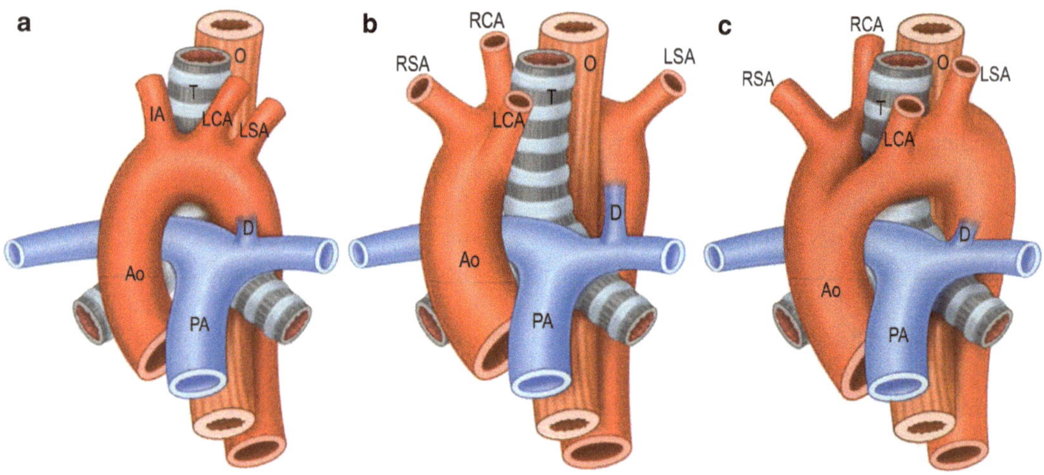

Fig. 9.17 (**a**) Relationship of a left aortic arch with normal branching pattern to the airway and oesophagus. (**b**) Relationship of a right aortic arch with an aberrant left subclavian artery and left arterial duct to the airway and oesophagus. (**c**) Relationship of a double aortic arch to the tracheal and oesophagus

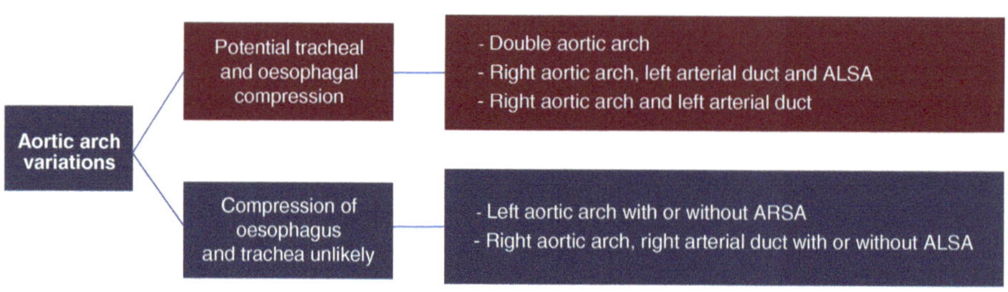

Fig. 9.18 Schematic diagram describing which aortic arch morphologies may be associated with tracheal and/or oesophageal compression after birth

References

Allan LD, Cook AC, Huggon IC. Fetal echocardiography a practical guide. Cambridge: Cambridge University Press; 2009.

Borenstein M, Minekawa R, Zidere V, Nicolaides KH, Allan LD. Aberrant right subclavian artery at 16 to 23 + 6 weeks of gestation: a marker for chromosomal abnormality. Ultrasound Obstet Gynecol. 2010;36:548–52.

D'Antonio F, Khalil A, Zidere V, Carvalho JS. Fetuses with right aortic arch Multicentre cohort study and meta-analysis. Ultrasound Obstet Gynecol. 2015;47(4):423–32.

Familiari A, Morlando M, Khalil AA, Sven-Erik S, Scala C, Rizzo G, Del Sordo G, Vassallo C, Flacco ME, Manzoli L, Lanzone A, Scambia G, Acharya G, D'Antonio F. Risk factors for Coarctation of the aorta on prenatal ultrasound: a systematic review and meta-analysis. Circulation. 2016;135(8):772–85.

Fouron JC. The unrecognized physiological and clinical significance of the fetal aortic isthmus. Ultrasound Obstet Gynecol. 2003;22:441–7.

Gustapane S, Leombroni M, Khalil A, Giacci F, Marrone L, Bascietto F, Rizzo G, Acharya G, Liberati M, D'Antonio F. Systematic review and meta-analysis of persistent left superior vena cava on prenatal ultrasound: associated anomalies, diagnostic accuracy and postnatal outcome. Ultrasound Obstet Gynecol. 2016;48:701–8.

Head CE, Jowett VC, Sharland GK, Simpson JM. Timing of presentation and postnatal outcome of infants suspected of having coarctation of the aorta during fetal life. Heart. 2005;91:1070–4.

NICOR web portal 2017. https://nicor4.nicor.org.uk. Accessed 2 July 2017.

Pinto NM, Keenan HT, Minich LL, Puchalski MD, Heywood M, Botto LD. Barriers to prenatal detection of congenital heart disease: a population-based study. Ultrasound Obstet Gynecol. 2012;40:418–25.

Sharland GK, Chan KY, Allan LD. Coarctation of the aorta: difficulties in prenatal diagnosis. Br Heart J. 1994;71:70–5.

Vigneswaran TV, Akolekar R, Syngelaki A, Charakida M, Allan LD, Nicolaides KH, Zidere V, Simpson JM. Reference Ranges for the Size of the Fetal Cardiac Outflow Tracts From 13 to 36 Weeks Gestation: A Single-Center Study of Over 7000 Cases. Circ Cardiovasc Imaging. 2018;11(7):e007575. https://doi.org/10.1161/CIRCIMAGING.118.007575. PubMed PMID: 30006353.

Vigneswaran TV, Kapravelou E, Bell AJ, Nyman A, Pushparajah K, Simpson JM, Durward A, Zidere V. Correlation of symptoms with bronchoscopic findings in children with a prenatal diagnosis of a right aortic arch and left arterial duct. Pediatr Cardiol. 2018b;39:665–73.

Vigneswaran TV, Sinha MD, Valverde I, Simpson JM, Charakida M. Hypertension in coarctation of the aorta: challenges in diagnosis in children. Pediatr Cardiol. 2018c;39:1–10.

Zidere V, Tsapakis EG, Huggon IC, Allan LD. Right aortic arch in the fetus. Ultrasound Obstet Gynecol. 2006;28:876–81.

Abnormalities of the Systemic and Pulmonary Veins

10

Marietta Charakida and John Simpson

Abstract

Abnormalities of the systemic and pulmonary veins can occur in isolation or in conjunction with other congenital heart defects. When venous anomalies present in isolation it can be particularly difficult to detect them during routine fetal anomaly scans as these are relatively small extra-cardiac structures. However, advances in ultrasound technology with higher resolution on 2D and colour Doppler ultrasound have facilitated and improved prenatal detection. The systemic venous variations and abnormalities, which will be discussed in this chapter include persistent left superior vena cava, interrupted inferior vena cava and agenesis of the ductus venosus. Anomalies of the pulmonary veins including total or partial anomalous pulmonary venous connections may be difficult to diagnose in isolation. Disorders of laterality which can be associated with systemic and/or pulmonary venous abnormalities as well as intracardiac defects will also be addressed.

Electronic Supplementary Material The online version of this chapter (https://doi.org/10.1007/978-3-319-77461-9_10) contains supplementary material, which is available to authorized users.

M. Charakida (✉) · J. Simpson
Evelina London Children's Hospital, Guy's and St Thomas' NHS Foundation Trust, London, UK
e-mail: john.simpson@gstt.nhs.uk

Keywords

Left superior vena cava · Anomalous pulmonary venous connection · Interrupted inferior vena cava · Isomerism · Agenesis of the ductus venosus

Normal Systemic and Pulmonary Venous Drainage

The appearances of the normal systemic and pulmonary veins are covered on screening and extended views of the fetal heart in Chaps. 2 and 3 respectively. With the higher resolution of the latest generation of ultrasound systems, details of the fetal venous system can now be visualised more clearly than was previously the case. The additional normal venous structures, which can now be visualised are included in this chapter along with selected anatomic variations and abnormalities.

When imaging the systemic and pulmonary veins, use of colour flow Doppler is an integral part of the assessment. The settings for colour flow Doppler are different for optimisation of visualisation of venous flow versus arterial flow. Venous flows require a colour scale of around 20–30 cm/s (occasionally lower) as there is a relatively low velocity of blood flow within them. Low wall filter and increase of colour gain just until colour "sprinkle" begins to occur all help to improve visualisation with the colour box size reduced to the minimum necessary to include the

© Springer International Publishing AG, part of Springer Nature 2018

J. Simpson et al. (eds.), *Fetal Cardiology*, https://doi.org/10.1007/978-3-319-77461-9_10

region of interest. New colour Doppler techniques such as directional power Doppler can be very helpful tools in visualizing small venous structures with low flow velocity. Most manufacturers have proprietary colour flow modalities to assist.

Details of the Normal Fetal Venous System

Key images of the normal fetal venous system are shown so that these are not confused with abnormal findings. Some of these structures, notably the normal azygous system are increasingly noted with the latest generation of high-resolution ultrasound systems.

- *Normal azygous vein*

The normal azygous vein can be seen on a transverse view used to determine cardiac situs (Video 10.1) or more superiorly at the level of the four-chamber view (Fig. 10.1). The normal azygous vein is posterior to the aorta, but much smaller than the aorta in size. The finding of an azygous vein of similar size to the descending aorta should raise the suspicion of interruption of the inferior vena cava. In the three-vessel view the normal azygous vein can occasionally be visualised draining into the right superior vena cava (Fig. 10.2).

- *Normal innominate vein*

The innominate vein drains the left jugular and left subclavian veins to the right superior vena cava. This vein is usually visualised just above the aortic arch when angulating cranially from the three-vessel / trachea view (Fig. 10.3). In fetuses with a persistent left superior vena cava the innominate vein may be absent.

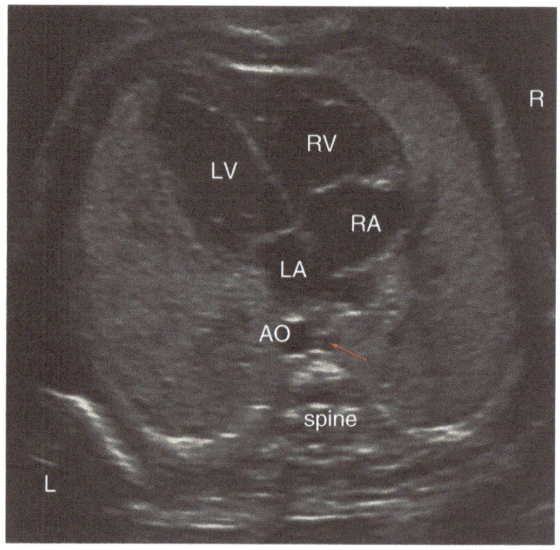

Fig. 10.1 Transverse view of the fetal heart at the level of four-chamber view. The normal azygous vein (red arrow) is seen posterior and to the right of the aorta. Note the small size of the normal azygous vein compared to that of the aorta

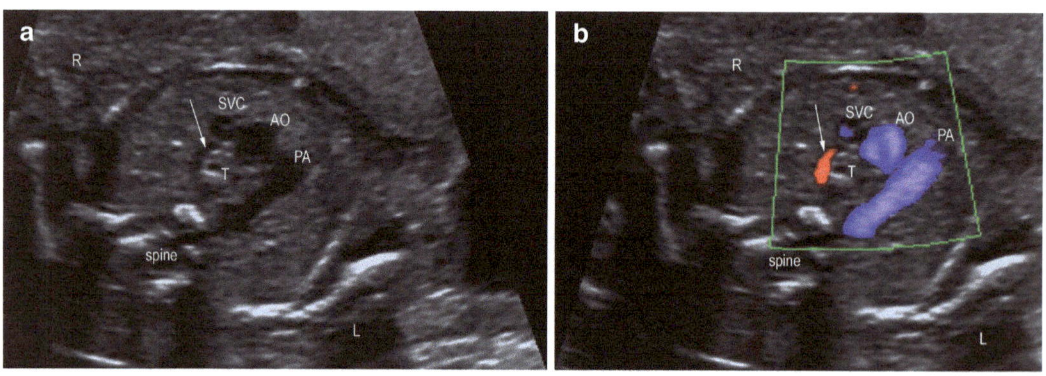

Fig. 10.2 Panel **a**: Transverse view at the level of three-vessel view demonstrating the small azygous vein (white arrow) joining the superior vena cava. Panel **b**: On colour the small azygous vein is visualized with red colour indicating flow from the azygous vein anteriorly into the right superior vena cava (white arrow)

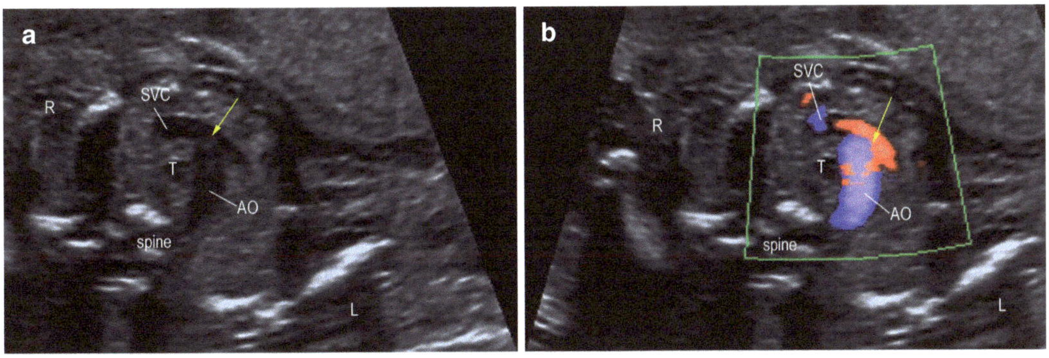

Fig. 10.3 Panel **a**: Transverse view superior to the three-vessel view demonstrating the normal innominate vein (yellow arrow) joining the superior vena cava. Panel **b**: On colour flow Doppler flow the normal innominate vein flow pattern is seen with red colour towards the SVC (yellow arrow)

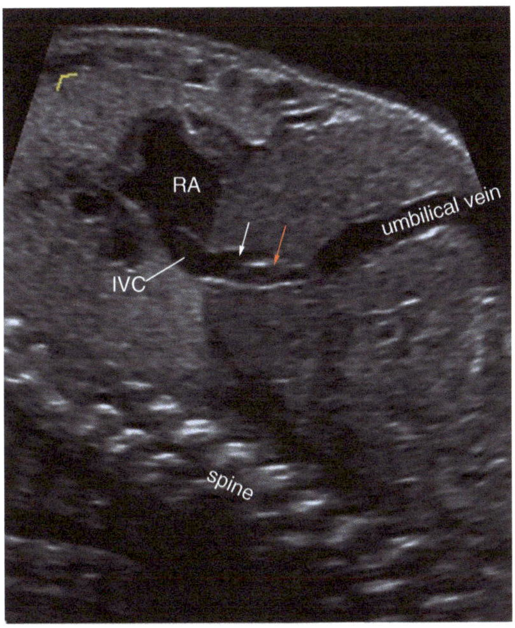

Fig. 10.4 Normal ductus venosus. Parasagittal view demonstrating the normal course of the umbilical vein towards the ductus venosus (red arrow) as it joins the inferior vena cava. A small hepatic vein is also seen (white arrow)

- *Normal ductus venosus*

The ductus venosus is best seen by following the umbilical vein through the abdomen as it passes towards the liver (Fig. 10.4, Video 10.2). Blood flow accelerates in the ductus venosus, which can be seen on colour flow Doppler. Such flow acceleration assists the passage of this highly oxygenated blood from the right atrium to the left atrium across the foramen ovale. The normal appearances of this structure are covered in Chap. 2.

Abnormalities of the Systemic Veins

Persistence of the left superior vena cava and interruption of the inferior vena cava are two systemic venous malformations seen in fetal and postnatal life. Another rare abnormality is agenesis of the ductus venosus which is accompanied by abnormal drainage of the umbilical vein.

Persistent Left Superior Vena Cava

Introduction: The presence of a persistent left superior vena cava (PLSVC) is one of the most common forms of systemic venous variations, which occurs in 0.5% of the general population and in 4–8% of patients with congenital heart disease (Allan et al. 2000a, b). The most common site of drainage of PLSVC is to the coronary sinus which itself drains into the right atrium. In this context the systemic venous return drains appropriately to the right atrium, albeit by a different route from normal. In around 10% of cases, the PLSVC drains directly to the roof of the left atrium. During postnatal life, this results in abnormally low oxygen saturations due to abnormal systemic venous return to the left heart.

The presence of a single left SVC is a rare abnormality. In general, the diagnosis of PLSVC has no clinical impact as the systemic venous blood continues to return to the right atrium. However, a prenatal diagnosis of PLSVC plays an important role in prenatal counseling and management, since it is associated with other cardiac abnormalities and extra-cardiac malformations (Berg et al. 2006, Galindo et al. 2007).

Echocardiography: The presence of a PLSVC is normally suspected because of an abnormal three-vessel/trachea view or because a dilated coronary sinus is noted in the four-chamber view. Dilation of the coronary sinus is best visualized in a transverse transthoracic cross-sectional plane slightly caudal to the apical four-chamber view (Fig. 10.5, Video 10.3). Enlargement of the coronary sinus can impede visualization of the normal crux of the heart leading to an erroneous diagnosis of an atrioventricular septal defect. If the ultrasound transducer is angled cranially, above the coronary sinus, the normal crux of the heart can normally be visualized. It is critical to assess drainage of the pulmonary veins whenever the coronary sinus is dilated to exclude drainage of the pulmonary veins into the coronary sinus rather than into the left atrium.

Although the presence of PLSVC can be suspected in the apical four-chamber view, it must be confirmed in the three-vessel view. PLSVC is easily and accurately diagnosed in the three-vessel view, where four vessels are visualized instead of three, with an extra vessel located to the left of the pulmonary trunk (Fig. 10.6, Video 10.4). Colour flow Doppler can help differentiate PLSVC from the vertical vein commonly found in total anomalous pulmonary venous drainage as the blood flow is towards the heart in PLSVC and in the opposite direction in the ascending vein in total anomalous pulmonary venous drainage. In rare instances of the absence of the right SVC, there are three abnormally arranged vessels in the upper mediastinum. The aortic and ductal arches are in their normal position but the single LSVC is to the left of the pulmonary trunk (Fig. 10.7, Video 10.5).

If the PLSVC drains to the coronary sinus it can be shown in its long axis in a sagittal view of the heart with the transducer angulated towards the left of the fetus (Fig. 10.8). If a

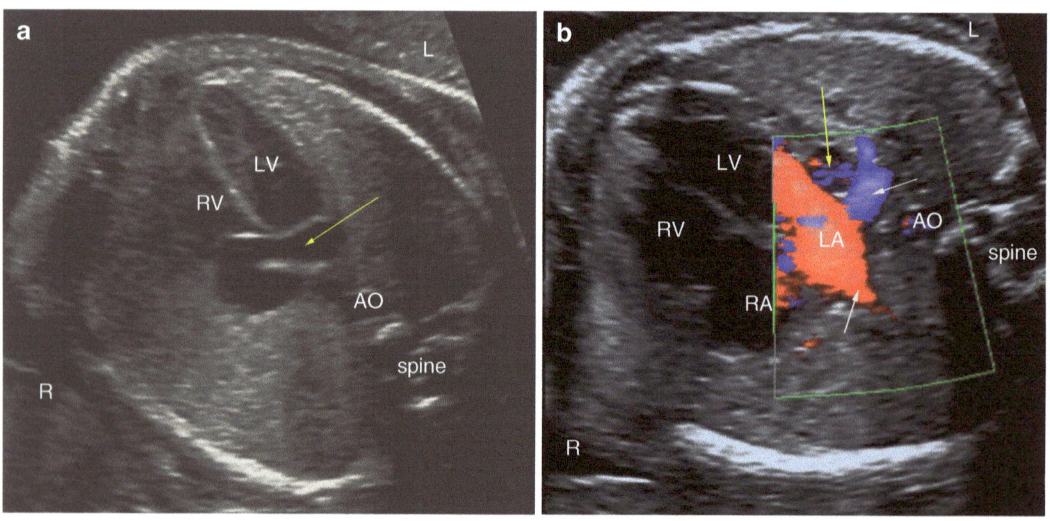

Fig. 10.5 Dilated coronary sinus. (**a**) This view is a plane inferior to the four-chamber view, which demonstrates a dilated coronary sinus (yellow arrow) due to a persisting left superior vena cava draining to the coronary sinus. This finding may be erroneously interpreted as an atrioventricular septal defect due to apparent loss of differential insertion and lack of visualisation of the primum atrial septum. Insonation more superiorly will show normal appearances at the crux of the heart (panel b). (**b**) Transverse view at the level of four chamber view, which demonstrates the dilated coronary sinus in cross section (yellow arrow). This finding is suggestive of the presence of PLSVC when pulmonary veins are seen draining normally to the left atrium (white arrows)

PLSVC is recognized on the three-vessel trachea view and the coronary sinus is not dilated, it is particularly important to assess the site of drainage of the PLSVC. This vessel can drain to the roof of the left atrium rather than to the coronary sinus leading to systemic arterial desaturation during postnatal life.

Associations: As an isolated cardiac defect, PLSVC to coronary sinus is not commonly associated with extracardiac abnormalities. PLSVC is present in 50–70% of cases of laterality disturbance (isomerism or heterotaxy syndromes). Associations with left ventricular tract obstructive defects including aortic coarctation and

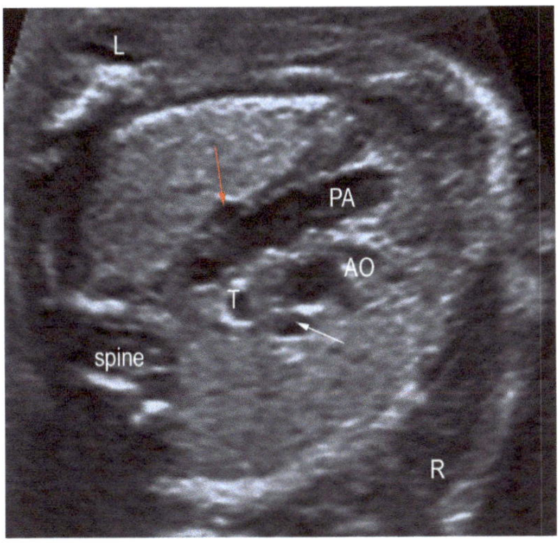

Fig. 10.6 Transverse view at the level of three-vessel view demonstrating the presence of four vessels. The right SVC (white arrow) and the aorta are seen in cross section. The main pulmonary artery and duct are seen longitudinally. The fourth vessel to the left of the pulmonary artery is the persistent left superior vena cava (red arrow)

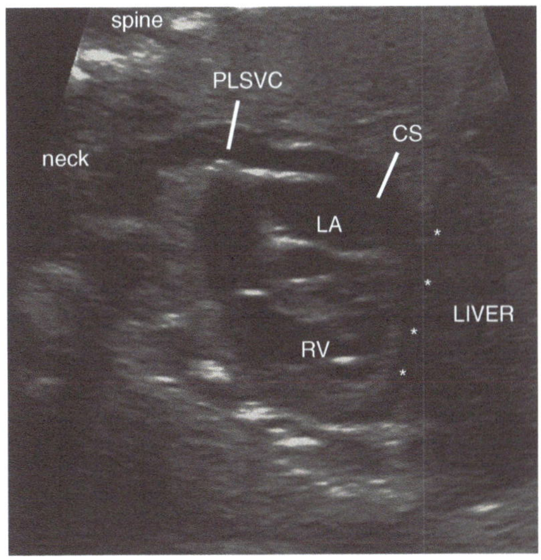

Fig. 10.8 Sagittal view demonstrating the course of the persistent left superior vena cava to the coronary sinus (CS). The right ventricle (RV) is seen in oblique view. Note that the coronary sinus is located inferiorly close to the diaphragm (marked by asterisks)

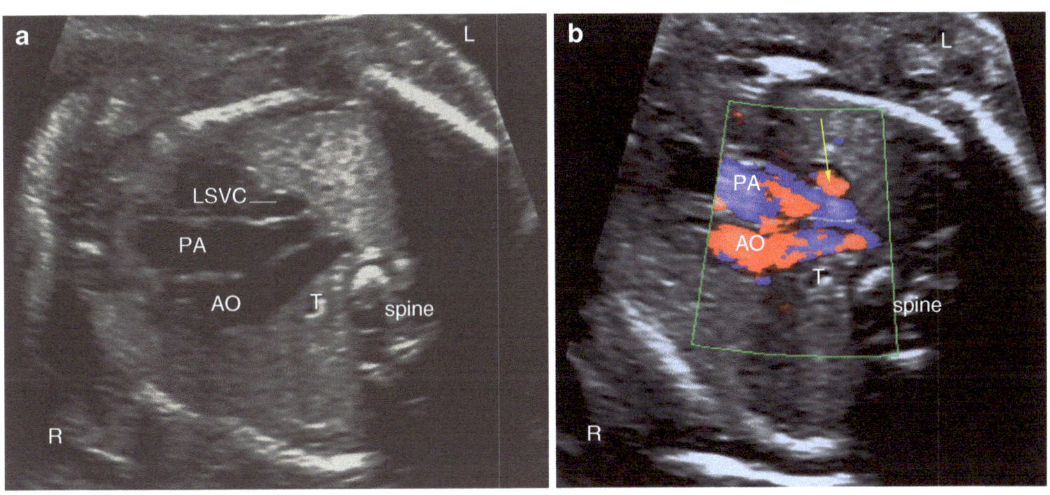

Fig. 10.7 Transverse plane at the level of the three-vessel view demonstrating the presence of a single superior vena cava to the left of the pulmonary artery on 2D (Panel **a**) and colour (Panel **b**). The aorta is seen to the right of the pulmonary artery

conotruncal anomalies have also been reported (Berg et al. 2006). At our centre, all cases of suspected PLSVC have a detailed fetal echocardiogram and anomaly scan to exclude congenital heart disease or other fetal anomalies.

Management: PLSVC to the coronary sinus may occur as an isolated variation with no hemodynamic consequence and does not need treatment. No special precautions in the perinatal management are needed. Given the association with coarctation of the aorta, many advise fetal echocardiography in the third trimester to ensure that growth of the aortic arch is normal. If the PLSVC drains directly to the left atrium, postnatal follow up is indicated to confirm the anatomy and to monitor oxygen saturations. If there is significant desaturation then occlusion or ligation of the left SVC may have to be considered. Some centres will advise postnatal echocardiography of all cases of PLSVC diagnosed during fetal life.

Outcome: The outcome of patients with PLSVC depends on whether there are additional intracardiac or extracardiac abnormalities. In the absence of associated lesion, PLSVC to coronary sinus does not pose any risk to the fetus or infant and medium and long term outcome is excellent. The presence of a single PLSVC may cause difficulties in interventions during later life, such as implantation of a transvenous pacemaker, systemic venous cannulation for cardiopulmonary bypass and placement of a pulmonary artery catheter for intra-operative or intensive care unit monitoring (Goyal and Rosenthal 2005).

Interrupted Inferior Vena Cava

Introduction: Interruption of the inferior vena cava (IVC) is the most common abnormality of the IVC (Allan et al. 2000a, b). Interruption often occurs at the level of the renal arteries and the venous return from the lower body is facilitated via the azygous or hemiazygous veins. These veins drain above the heart to a right or left SVC respectively.

Echocardiography: The diagnosis of interrupted IVC should be suspected in the abdominal situs view by the detection of two vessels of similar size, the aorta and the azygous vein, lying in the posterior thorax behind the heart (Fig. 10.9). The azygous (or hemiazygous) vein lies posterior to the aorta (Fig. 10.10a) in contrast to the normal arrangement of the abdominal vessels where the IVC lies anterior and to the right of the aorta. Interrupted IVC should also be suspected when a sagittal view through the fetal chest and abdomen fails to demonstrate the full length of the IVC. Using colour flow Doppler the pulsatile descending aorta and the more posteriorly located azygous vein may be seen in parallel in a sagittal view (Fig. 10.10b, Video 10.6). The direction of flow in the descending aorta is caudally whereas the azygous vein flow is cranially. In the normal fetus, it is possible to follow the IVC caudally beyond the liver, whereas when the IVC is interrupted only the hepatic veins are seen within the liver.

Associations: An interrupted IVC with direct drainage of the hepatic veins into the atria is found in over 80% of cases of left atrial isomerism (see section "Left Atrial Isomerism").

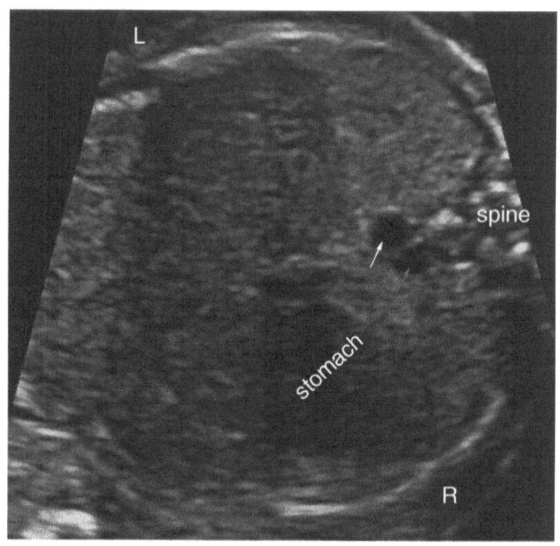

Fig. 10.9 Transverse abdominal view demonstrating the stomach on the right and the liver on the left side. Two vessels of similar size ("double vessel" appearance) are seen in front of the spine. The white arrow demonstrates the aorta and the red arrow the azygous vein. The two vessels are of similar size. The "double vessel" appearance is indicative of the presence of interrupted inferior vena cava and left atrial isomerism

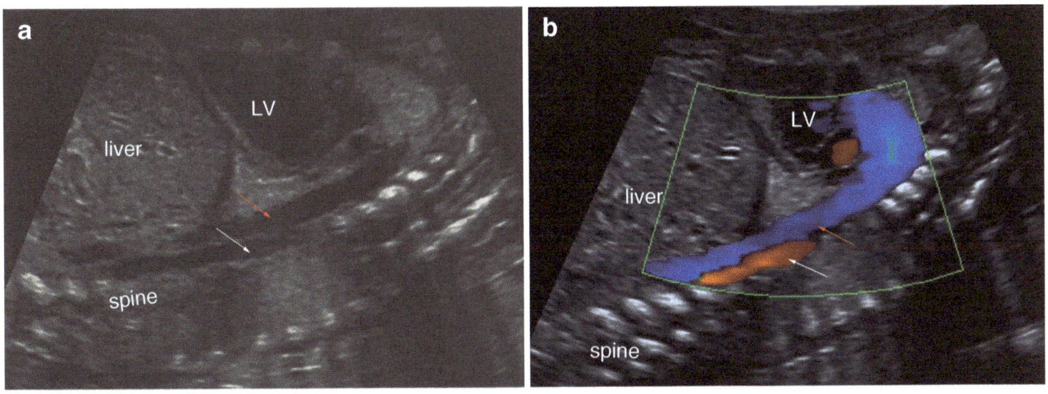

Fig. 10.10 (**a**) Parasagittal view of the fetal thorax and abdomen in a fetus with left atrial isomerism. The aorta and azygous vein are seen in parallel orientation. The dilated azygous vein is posterior to the pulsatile descending aorta. (**b**) Colour flow Doppler demonstrates the different flow directions of the azygous vein (red colour, towards the heart) and the aorta (blue colour, away from the heart)

Management: The presence of interrupted IVC in isolation is usually a benign finding and does not pose any risk to the fetus or infant. No precautions in perinatal management are needed. Due to the strong association with left atrial isomerism, postnatal assessment following prenatal diagnosis is needed. Our normal policy is to advise an abdominal ultrasound scan as a minimum to assess anatomy of the liver and spleens. In rare instances biliary atresia may be associated with interruption of the IVC even in the absence of other intracardiac or extracardiac abnormalities.

Outcome: The outcome of patients with interrupted IVC will depend on the presence of other associated intracardiac or extracardiac abnormalities. As an isolated finding, interrupted IVC does not have any haemodynamic consequence for the infant and the long-term prognosis is excellent. The outcome where interrupted IVC is part of left atrial isomerism is discussed in section "Left Atrial Isomerism".

Agenesis of the Ductus Venosus

Introduction: The ductus venosus (DV) is a key structure in fetal life, which enables the highly oxygenated blood returning from umbilical vein to enter the IVC whilst bypassing the liver. Agenesis of DV is a rare fetal vascular anomaly. It affects approximately 6:1000 of fetuses in a high-risk population. In the absence of DV, three abnormal patterns of (Yagel et al. 2010) umbilical vein (UV) connections have been described:

- it may bypass the liver and then connect to the subdiaphragmatic IVC or to the iliac or renal veins
- it may connect directly to the right or left atrium (Fig. 10.11a, b, Video 10.7)
- it may connect directly to the portal vein.

Echocardiography: The ideal echocardiographic plane to visualize the ductus venosus is the median-sagittal section of the fetal trunk. The origin of the ductus venosus can also be identified through a transverse (slightly oblique) section of the superior part of the fetal abdomen. At the origin of the DV, the blood coming from the umbilical vein accelerates and can be seen as colour flow aliasing in low Doppler velocity settings. Imaging of the DV is easier in the first and second trimester, while it can be technically challenging in the third trimester (Fig. 10.4, Video 10.2).

Associations: Unexplained cardiomegaly is the most common referral reason leading to a diagnosis of agenesis of the ductus venous. The absence of the ductus venosus leads to volume loading of the fetal heart resulting in enlargement of the heart and in some cases development of fetal hydrops. Agenesis of DV can be associated

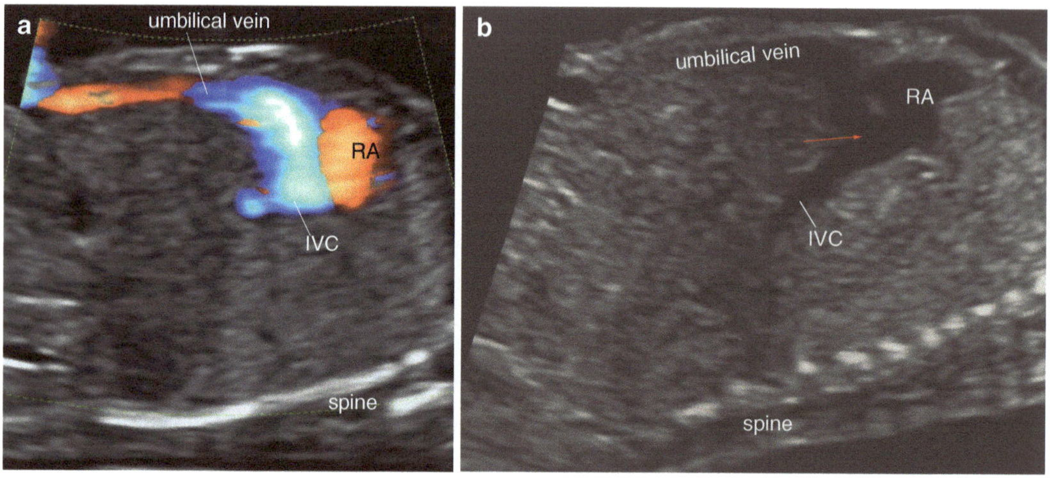

Fig. 10.11 Agenesis of the ductus venosus. (**a**) Sagittal view of the fetal trunk demonstrating a case of agenesis of the ductus venosus with direct drainage of the umbilical vein into the right atrium on colour flow Doppler. (**b**) In this image the red arrow is pointing to the entrance of the umbilical vein into the IVC

with genetic anomalies i.e. Turner syndrome, or Noonan syndrome. Congenital cardiac abnormalities can be found in up to half of cases and these include septal defects, tricuspid atresia, double outlet right ventricle, pulmonary atresia, left atrial isomerism and transposition of the great arteries. Other common extracardiac associated anomalies include duodenal atresia, tracheo-esophageal fistula, bilateral hydronephrosis, ectopic kidney, hemivertebrae and structural anomalies of the radius and ulna (Clerici et al. 2010, Thubert et al. 2012).

Management: In cases where agenesis of DV is suspected, a detailed fetal anatomy scan and echocardiography are indicated (Thomas et al. 2012). In cases where agenesis of DV is an isolated finding, serial echocardiograms are advised to monitor for signs of volume loading of the fetal heart, cardiac failure and hydrops. Postnatal imaging is also required to exclude agenesis of the portal system or portosystemic shunts. In cases where agenesis of ductus venosus is not an isolated finding, monitoring and management will be dictated by the associated clinical conditions. In all cases fetal karyotyping should be considered.

Outcome: Counselling of parents about agenesis of DV is challenging given the complexity of outcomes. Prognosis for the few reported cases of agenesis of DV that are isolated or associated with only minor abnormalities is better when the umbilical vein does not bypass the liver. Extrahepatic umbilical venous drainage produces the worst fetal outcomes as it causes chronic volume overload of the central venous system and the cardiac chambers with associated cardiomegaly and fetal congestive heart failure. The prognosis is determined by the diameter and site of the shunt. If the shunt is narrow, the portal system will have developed normally and this carries good prognosis. In contrast, a wide shunt is associated with underdevelopment or absence of the portal system with poor prognosis. A number of postnatal complications including pulmonary oedema, focal hepatic nodular hyperplasia and hepatic tumours have been reported (Shen et al. 2011).

Abnormalities of the Pulmonary Veins

The abnormalities of the pulmonary veins (PV) may involve abnormal drainage of all pulmonary veins (total anomalous pulmonary venous connection) or abnormal drainage of one or more (but not all) of the pulmonary veins (partial anomalous pulmonary venous connection).

The normal screening views of the PVs are shown in Chap. 2 and extended views in Chap. 3. Currently, most screening guidelines do not include detailed assessment of the pulmonary veins. There are four pulmonary veins, two left sided and two right sided which are in a superior – inferior relationship and drain their respective segments of the lungs. These veins typically enter the left atrium separately and have their own ostium. It is generally difficult to visualize all four pulmonary veins in the fetus but in the four-chamber view the two inferior veins can be visualized.

Total Anomalous Pulmonary Venous Connection

Introduction: Total anomalous pulmonary venous connection (TAPVC) is a condition in which all pulmonary veins drain either directly or indirectly into the right atrium (Allan et al. 2000b). Total anomalous pulmonary venous drainage accounts for 2% of live births with congenital heart disease and occurs in about 0.9 of 10,000 live births.

The diagnosis of isolated TAPVC is difficult in the fetus and most cases have been missed prenatally, even in "expert" hands. Recently, with improvements in ultrasound technology, series and case reports on the accurate detection of anomalous pulmonary venous connections in the fetus either in isolation or as part of heterotaxy syndrome have emerged (Ganesan et al. 2014). New imaging modalities such as fetal CMR can be particularly useful in delineating the anatomy when suspicion of anomalous pulmonary venous drainage exists in fetal echocardiogram.

According to the anatomic site of the anomalous connection, four types of TAPVC exist.

- **Supracardiac type.** This is the most common form of anomalous pulmonary venous connection and accounts for about 45% of cases. The four pulmonary veins merge into a confluence posterior to the left atrium and connect via an ascending vein, usually to the left innominate vein, which in turn drains into the SVC.
- **Cardiac type.** The pulmonary veins connect directly to the coronary sinus, which becomes dilated, or connect directly into the posterior wall of the right atrium.
- **Infracardiac type**. The four pulmonary veins form a confluence behind the atriums. This confluence is connected to an anomalous descending vein that drains through the diaphragm, usually entering the portal venous system. Obstruction of pulmonary venous drainage is the rule rather than the exception in this type.
- **Mixed pattern**. This type is rare and involves a variety of pulmonary venous drainages.

Echocardiography: Total anomalous pulmonary venous drainage is a difficult diagnosis to make during fetal life. The posterior wall of the left atrium is normally immediately adjacent to the descending aorta in the four-chamber view. In TAPVC a venous confluence may be visible behind the left atrium in the four-chamber view plane with no direct connection between the pulmonary veins and the posterior wall of the left atrium (Fig. 10.12, Video 10.8) (Allan and Sharland 2001). In some cases there may be asymmetry of size of the ventricles with dominance of the right heart. The pulmonary artery may also

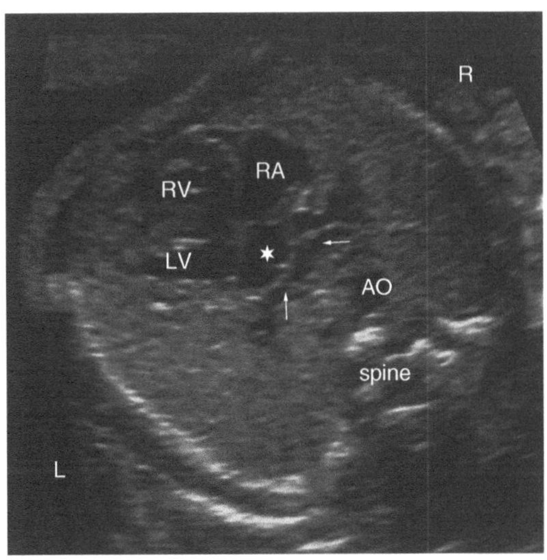

Fig. 10.12 Right atrial isomerism with total anomalous pulmonary venous drainage. The left atrium (white asterisk) has a smooth wall. Two pulmonary veins are seen draining to a confluence behind the left atrium

appear enlarged at the three-vessel view and a vertical vein may be seen. In the three-vessel view, the ascending vein may be visible in circular cross-section, usually to the left of the pulmonary artery. Colour flow Doppler is essential for the evaluation of the connections of the pulmonary veins to the left atrium when TAPVC is suspected. Pulsed Doppler interrogation of the pulmonary veins in TAPVC shows loss of the normal phasic flow pattern, particularly when the draining of the pulmonary venous confluence is obstructed (Fig. 10.13). The four-chamber view may show size discrepancy between the right and left sides of the heart with an enlarged right atrium and ventricle due to increased venous return. The inter-atrial septum bulges into the left atrium, especially in the third trimester of pregnancy, due to increased right to left shunting of blood as all of the pulmonary venous return enters the right atrium.

Supracardiac TAPVC: At the three-vessel view plane, a fourth vessel, the vertical vein can be seen at the same anatomic location as PLSVC (Fig. 10.14, Video 10.9A and Video 10.9B). In contrast to the LSVC, where blood from the left jugular vein continues via the LSVC towards the heart, blood flow in the vertical vein in supracardiac TAPVC goes to the opposite direction toward the upper thorax. Furthermore, the innominate vein is significantly dilated in TAPVC when compared to PLSVC where the innominate vein is small or absent. The SVC can also appear dilated in the three-vessel view when it is receiving more blood than usual in cases of supracardiac TAPVC.

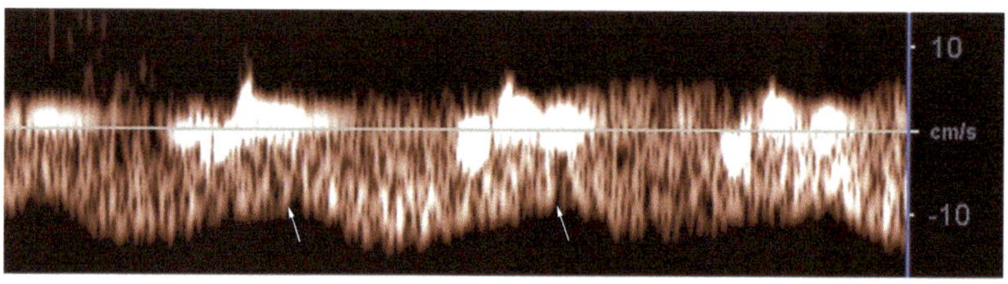

Fig. 10.13 Abnormal pulsed Doppler waveform of the pulmonary venous confluence in a fetus with total anomalous pulmonary vein connection. Note the loss of the normal phasic flow pattern which assists in the confirmation of the diagnosis

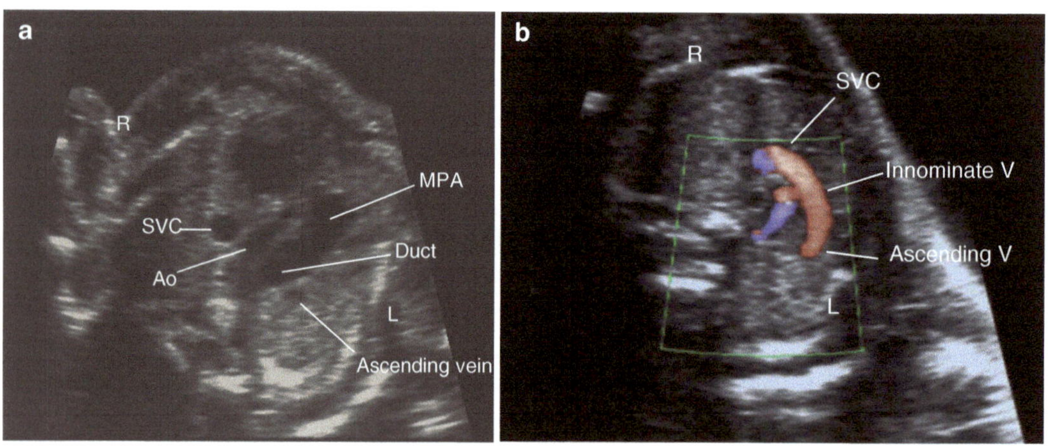

Fig. 10.14 (**a**) Transverse view at three-vessel view demonstrating on the presence of four vessels. The transverse aorta is smaller than the pulmonary artery and duct. The ascending vein from the pulmonary venous confluence to the innominate vein is shown is cross-section to the left of the pulmonary artery. (**b**) At a higher plane to the three-vessel view a dilated innominate vein is demonstrated. The direction of blood in the ascending vein is towards the head (red) in comparison to SVC flow which is towards the heart (blue). This differentiates an ascending vein from PLSVC

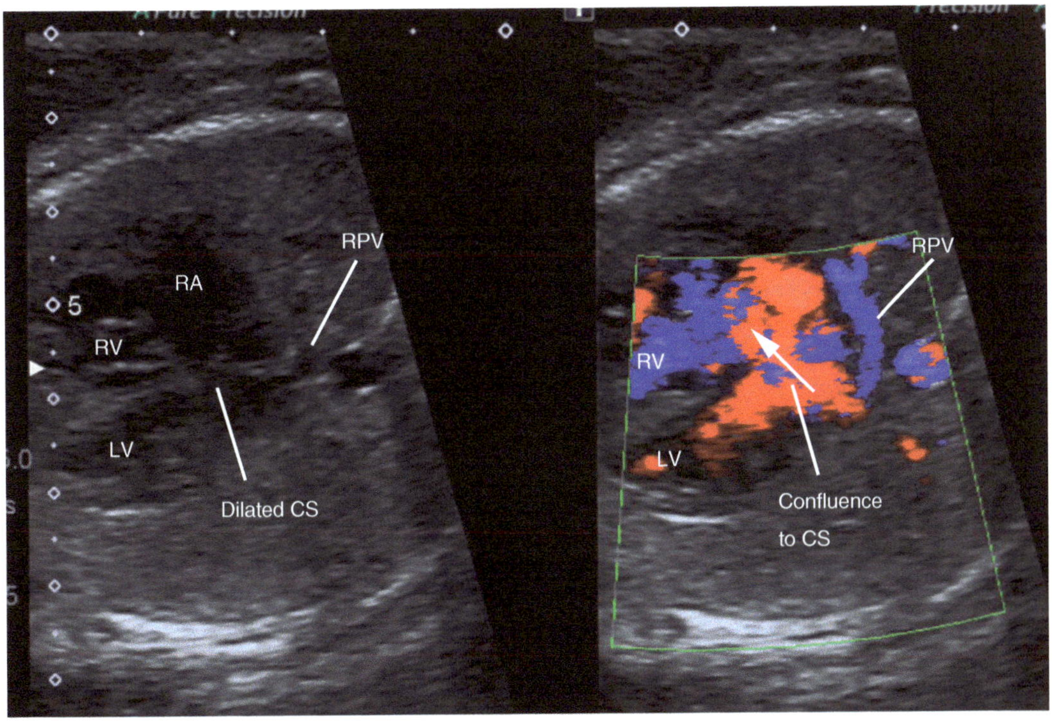

Fig. 10.15 Transverse view at an inferior plane to four chamber view demonstrating on 2D and colour a case of TAPVD to the coronary sinus (intracardiac TAPVD). The right pulmonary vein is seen joining a confluence. The confluence drains to the right atrium via the coronary sinus, which is dilated. The white arrow demonstrates the left to right shunt at the atrial level in contrast to the normal right to left shunt commonly seen at the atrial level

Cardiac TAPVC: When the pulmonary veins connect to the coronary sinus, the coronary sinus becomes dilated (Fig. 10.15, Video 10.10). A dilated coronary sinus in the absence of a LSVC should raise the suspicion of TAPVC. The coronary sinus is best demonstrated in a transverse plane inferior to the four-chamber view. Direct connection of the pulmonary veins to the right atrium can be visualised by high-resolution ultrasound on 2D, colour and pulsed Doppler evaluation.

Infracardiac TAPVC: The confluence and the descending vein are small and difficult to recognize on routine 2D fetal echocardiogram. Sagittal views of the chest and upper abdomen on colour Doppler may demonstrate a small vessel crossing the diaphragm, entering the liver with cranial to caudal flow direction. When the pulmonary veins drain to a confluence, which then drains below the diaphragm, there is an additional vessel passing through the diaphragm with caudal flow in it (Video 10.11). The direction of blood flow in the confluence is in the same direction as the aorta but there is venous flow pattern on Doppler.

Echocardiographic signs of TAPVC in fetal life

- No pulmonary vein flow into the left atrium
- Confluence seen behind the left atrium
- Dilated coronary sinus or presence of an ascending or a descending vein
- Small left atrium
- Dilated right heart relative to the left
- Dilated pulmonary artery relative to the aorta
- Loss of normal phasic flow pattern in the pulmonary veins.

Associations: Total anomalous pulmonary venous connection can be an isolated finding but can also occur in association with other cardiac anomalies (Seale et al. 2012). One of the most common associated cardiac abnormalities is right atrial isomerism (heterotaxy syndrome). Atrial septal defects of the sinus venosus type are associated with TAPVC and PAPVC but are exceedingly difficult to diagnose before birth. Other associated cardiac anomalies include atrioventricular septal defect, coarctation of the aorta and hypoplastic left heart syndrome. Extracardiac associated anomalies are rare outside of heterotaxy syndromes. Associated chromosomal abnormalities are also rare. "Cat eye" syndrome is an abnormality of chromosome 22 and is the most frequent syndrome associated with TAPVC. This can be associated with renal, gut, palate and eye abnormalities.

Management: When a prenatal diagnosis of TAPVC is made, serial evaluation with fetal echocardiography is important to confirm or exclude the development of obstruction to pulmonary venous drainage. The site of obstruction is usually within the vein decompressing the confluence of pulmonary veins. TAPVC with or without pulmonary venous obstruction has significant haemodynamic consequences for the neonate as various degrees of mixing of pulmonary and systemic blood occurs which leads to cyanosis. If there is significant obstruction of the pathway draining the pulmonary venous confluence to the right atrium then severe hypoxia and metabolic acidosis can occur early after birth. TAPVC does not commonly cause cardiovascular compromise in utero but can be associated with high perinatal risk, thus delivery in tertiary centre is advocated when early postnatal cardiology review can be performed. In cases of obstructed TAPVC, urgent cardiac intervention will be needed in the postnatal period, to allow the oxygenated pulmonary venous blood to drain into the heart. If the pulmonary venous drainage is anomalous and obstructed in the context of a "single ventricle" circulation, this has major prognostic implications. This is because the cardiac surgery undertaken depends on low pressures and resistance in the pulmonary circulation. Where the pulmonary venous drainage is obstructed, there may be maldevelopment of the pulmonary circulation so that the resistance in the lungs is too high for surgical repair to be undertaken.

Outcome: The outcome for TAPVC is reported as poor in the prenatal series whereas more favourable outcome is reported in neonatal reports. This discrepancy is mostly related to the higher prevalence of other associated cardiovascular abnormalities in the prenatal series. Infracardiac TAPVC has a worse prognosis than the other types due to a higher association with pulmonary venous obstruction. The overall prognosis for neonates with isolated TAPVC who survive surgical correction is usually good. A minority of survivors may develop recurrent pulmonary venous obstruction, which can prove extremely difficult to treat effectively.

Partial Anomalous Pulmonary Venous Connections

Introduction: In partial anomalous pulmonary venous connections (PAPVC) one, two or three of the pulmonary veins drain directly or indirectly into the right atrium. Anomalous drainage of the right upper pulmonary vein is commonly a component of a sinus venosus atrial septal defect but this is extremely difficult to diagnose before birth. Anomalous drainage of the right lower and middle lobe pulmonary veins in association with right lung hypoplasia is termed as Scimitar syndrome (Valsangiacomo et al. 2003). In such cases, there is an associated aortopulmonary collateral vessel which may require occlusion.

Echocardiography: Partial anomalous pulmonary venous drainage can be extremely difficult to identify prenatally. Scimitar syndrome can be suspected in the four-chamber view due to hypoplasia of the right lung leading to the heart being positioned more towards the right than normal, with the cardiac apex pointing more antero-posterior than normal. The right inferior pulmonary veins drain into the IVC instead of the left atrium, which is best demonstrated in a longitudinal plane.

Associations: Partial anomalous pulmonary venous drainage is commonly associated with a "sinus venosus" type of atrial septal defect which is a superiorly positioned defect beneath the superior vena cava which overrides the atrial septum. This is an exceedingly difficult diagnosis to make during fetal life. Scimitar syndrome is often associated with abnormal arterial supply to the right lung, arising directly from the descending aorta. Other associated cardiac defects include ventricular septal defects, coarctation of the aorta and tetralogy of Fallot. Noonan's syndrome and cat-eye syndrome can be associated with PAPVC.

Management: A patient with one or two anomalous pulmonary veins is usually asymptomatic and may not present until later in childhood or adult life with clinical features of left to right shunt. Surgical management is elective and involves incorporating the anomalous vein into the left atrium. Patients with Scimitar syndrome may present in the neonatal period with respiratory compromise related to lung hypoplasia or with evidence of pulmonary hypertension.

Outcome: An elective repair of partial anomalous pulmonary venous connection has low surgical mortality. The postoperative course will be related to any associated cardiac defects and lung hypoplasia.

Disorders of Laterality

The embryo, as it develops into a fetus, must be able to place organs in their correct position in the body. For example, the liver is normally on the right, stomach / spleen on the left, right atrium on the right and vice versa. This process involves a complex signalling arrangement, which remains relatively poorly understood. A disorder of laterality is a term, which is used to describe abnormal organ arrangement where this process has become disrupted. The overall incidence of laterality anomalies is 1.44 per 10,000 live births in the Baltimore Washington study. From a cardiac perspective, abnormalities of this type disturb cardiac situs. The nomenclature and definitions around this group of conditions are confusing. Terms such as isomerism, visceral heterotaxy, Ivemark syndrome or polysplenia/asplenia syndromes have all been used to describe this constellation of abnormalities. Isomerism is a form of laterality disorder, which is used to describe the situation where paired structures occur as a mirror image of each other, or in duplicate. From a cardiac perspective, this group of conditions can have a major impact on cardiac development. The terms right and left atrial isomerism have been used to describe this group of abnormalities in relation to the anatomic features of the atria. The morphology of the atrial appendages is the most consistent feature used to determine which atrium is of morphologically left type and which is of right type. The left atrium has a long, thin "finger-like" appendage but the right atrium has a broader based appendage. In some patients there are two atria of right atrial type (right atrial isomerism) and in others two appendages of left atrial type (left atrial isomerism). In right atrial isomerism, there is generally over-representation of right-sided structures e.g. bilateral superior vena cavas and under-representation of left sided structures e.g. absence of the spleen. Conversely, in left atrial isomerism there is over-representation of left sided structures e.g. multiple spleens and absence of right sided structures e.g. interruption of the inferior vena cava. The typical echocardiographic features are outlined below, but it should be emphasised that there is huge individual variation. The echocardiographic features and out-

	Usual atrial arrangement	Right atrial isomerism	Left atrial isomerism
Spleen	Left sided	Usually absent	Polysplenia
Bowel	Stomach on left	Malrotation of bowel/Stomach on right	Malrotation of bowel/stomach on right
Liver	Right sided	Midline/left	Midline
IVC	Right sided	Same side as aorta Left or right sided	Interrupted
SVCs	Right sided	Bilateral SVC	Variable
Pulmonary veins	To Left atrium	Anomalous PVC	Usually normal
Intracardiac anatomy	Normal Apex to left	AVSD PS/ Pat TGA Double outlet RV Apex to left or right	Variable Left heart obstruction Apex to left or right.
Rhythm	Sinus	Normal	CHB. Slow sinus

Abbreviations: *SVC* superior vena cava, *AVSD* atrioventricular septal defect, *CHB* complete heart block, *PS* pulmonary stenosis, *Pat* pulmonary atresia, *PVC* pulmonary venous connection, *RV* right ventricle, *TGA* transposition of the great arteries.

come of fetuses with laterality disturbances has been reported recently (Vigneswaran et al. 2018).

Right Atrial Isomerism

Introduction: In right atrial isomerism, both atrial appendages are of right morphology. Fetal cases with right atrial isomerism are often detected in the routine fetal ultrasound, due to abnormal position of the stomach or heart, or because the four-chamber view is abnormal.

Echocardiography: The most common reasons for referral of affected cases are abnormal screening views of the fetal heart particularly suspected atrioventricular septal defect or the heart and stomach on opposite sides of the body. Most commonly the diagnosis of right atrial isomerism can be confirmed in the abdominal situs transverse view and involves juxtaposition of the abdominal aorta and IVC (Fig. 10.16). Typically in right atrial isomerism, the position of the IVC is anterior and on the same side of the descending aorta. The apex of the heart is often to the right but can be to the left or midline. Intracardiac anomalies are present in nearly all cases of right atrial isomerism. In the four-chamber view, the most common cardiac finding is that of an unbalanced atrioventricular septal defect. The pulmonary venous connection should be also carefully examined as by definition it is always anomalous because there is no true left atrium for the veins to connect to.

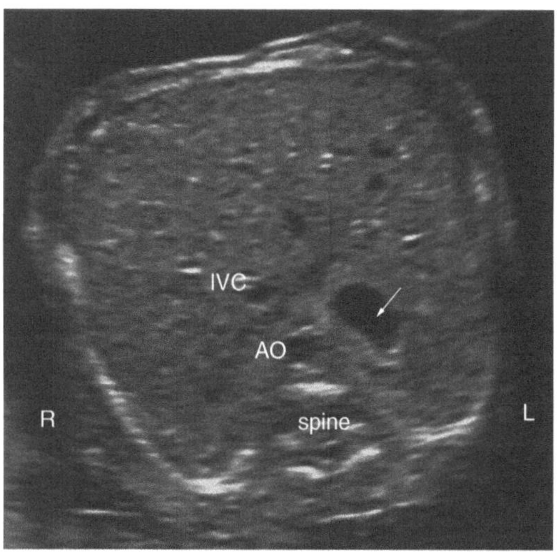

Fig. 10.16 Transverse view of the fetal abdomen identifying the stomach (white arrow) to the left of the spine, whilst the aorta and inferior vena cava are to the right of the spine. The finding of the aorta and IVC on the same side is consistent with right atrial isomerism, but other abnormal features of the cardiac anatomy should be sought to confirm. The finding of a right sided descending aorta and IVC is seen in same cases of isolated right aortic arch

Echocardiographic features of right atrial isomerism in fetal life

- Stomach and heart on opposite sides of the body
- Inferior vena cava is anterior to the aorta and lies on the same side of spine
- Associated with complex intracardiac abnormalities (commonly unbalanced atrioventricular septal defect)
- Anomalous pulmonary venous drainage
- Bilateral superior vena cavas.

Associations: Right atrial isomerism is associated with atrioventricular septal defect and most commonly unbalanced atrioventricular septal defect in up to 80–90% of cases. Bilateral superior vena cava veins are seen in 61% of cases. The pulmonary venous connections are by definition abnormal as there is no morphological left atrium present. Malformation of the atrioventricular connections and right ventricular outflow obstruction are also commonly reported in cases of right atrial isomerism. There are almost always extracardiac abnormalities associated with this condition. In the upper abdomen, a midline large liver with a right-sided stomach is a common finding. Asplenia can be found in about 75% of cases and malrotation of the gut in over 50% of cases. Chromosomal abnormalities rarely coexist with right atrial isomerism.

Management: The management of fetuses with right atrial isomerism will be influenced by the presence and severity of associated lesions. In the presence of right ventricular outflow obstruction, affected babies in the neonatal period may be cyanotic and require administration of prostaglandin to maintain the patency of arterial duct. In addition, in fetuses with right atrial isomerism there is always TAPVC. The presence of obstruction in the pulmonary venous connections is an adverse prognostic feature. In the majority of cases, the heart cannot be truly repaired. Management is more often towards a single ventricle or "Fontan" type of repair (Chap. 17).

The delivery of fetuses with prenatal diagnosis of right atrial isomerism is advised to occur in a tertiary unit where prostaglandin infusion can be initiated in the presence of cyanosis and early cardiology review can be organized. In cases of asplenia, prophylactic penicillin is administered lifelong and surgical repair of malrotation of the bowel may also be required.

Outcome: Fetal compromise in foetuses with right atrial isomerism is rare despite the association with complex intracardiac and extracardiac abnormalities. If there is severe atrioventricular valve regurgitation, in utero cardiac failure may occur. The presence of TAPVC, particularly when there is also obstruction to pulmonary arterial flow is associated with a worse prognosis in infancy and childhood. The prognosis of the single ventricle "Fontan" circulation is discussed in Chap. 17.

Left Atrial Isomerism

Introduction: In left atrial isomerism the atrial appendages are both of left morphology (Allan et al. 2000a). The presence of fetal bradycardia, increased nuchal translucency in the first trimester screening as well as discordant position between the stomach and the heart (Pepes et al. 2009) are the most common reasons for referral for fetal echocardiogram in the presence of left atrial isomerism.

Echocardiography: Abnormal abdominal situs may be the first indication of the presence of left atrial isomerism (Fig. 10.8). Two vessels are seen posteriorly in the transverse abdominal situs view. The most posterior vessel is the azygous continuation of the interrupted IVC. A parasagittal view of the abdomen and chest can also demonstrate the azygos vein posterior to the descending aorta and colour Doppler can demonstrate flow in the opposite direction in each vessel (Fig. 10.10, Video 10.6). The azygos vein can be visualised draining into the SVC in the three-vessel view and in the sagittal view of the chest (Video 10.12). The hepatic veins may connect directly into the right atrium in the absence of an inferior vena cava. The orientation of the fetal heart is commonly abnormal with the apex lying more leftwards or centrally in the chest. If there is complete heart block, there is often cardiomegaly and biventricular hypertrophy.

Echocardiographic features of left atrial isomerism in fetal life

- Interrupted IVC
- Hepatic veins drain directly to the atrial mass
- Two abdominal vessels (aorta and azygous vein) are seen behind the heart (Video 10.13)
- Cardiac axis can be more leftward or more central than normal
- May have associated complete heart block
- May have associated atrioventricular septal defect.

Associations: Left atrial isomerism can exist with normal intracardiac anatomy. When a cardiac anomaly is present, it is most commonly an unbalanced atrioventricular septal defect or simple ventricular septal defect. The origin of the great vessels is generally concordant. Double outlet right ventricle can occur in combination with a ventricular septal defect or atrioventricular septal defect. Left and right-sided outflow tract obstructions have been reported in association with left atrial isomerism. PLSVC is found in 50–60% of the cases. Cardiomegaly especially in the setting of complete heart block is common. Other extracardiac abnormalities include malrotation of the bowel, atresia of the upper gastrointestinal tract (duodenal or jejunal atresia), a symmetric left sided or midline liver and rarely absence of the gallbladder. The presence of multiple spleens has been reported in up to 96% of infants with left isomerism but antenatal diagnosis of polysplenia is not reliable on ultrasound. Chromosomal abnormalities are extremely rare but a case of microdeletion of chromosome 22 in association with left atrial isomerism has been reported (Yates et al.

1996). Biliary atresia is a well-recognised association, which cannot be reliably diagnosed before birth.

Management: The management of fetuses with left atrial isomerism will be influenced by the presence of associated lesions. In the presence of normal intracardiac anatomy and no evidence of fetal arrhythmia, there is no indication to alter the delivery plan. However cardiology follow up will be needed to identify late presentation of complete heart block. In the presence of complex intracardiac abnormality or significant arrhythmia delivery in a tertiary centre where early cardiology review can occur is advised.

Outcome: The presence of complete heart block with a complex cardiac malformation in fetal cases with left atrial isomerism may often lead to cardiac failure and fetal hydrops in more than 30% of cases and is responsible for the high rate of in utero demise.

Although morbidity and mortality in the neonatal period are determined mainly by the cardiac defects, the visceral anomalies may affect the long-term outcome of these patients. Biliary atresia is found in up to 10% of surviving infants.

References

Allan LD, et al. Heterotaxy syndromes/isomerism of the atrial appendages textbook of fetal cardiology. London: Greenwich Medical Media Limited; 2000a. p. 335–46.

Allan LD, et al. Abnormalities of the systemic and pulmonary venous connection. Textbook of fetal cardiology. London: Greenwich Medical Media Limited; 2000b. p. 105–14.

Allan LD, Sharland GK. The echocardiographic diagnosis of totally anomalous pulmonary venous connections in the fetus. Heart. 2001;85:433–7.

Berg C, Knüppel M, Geipel A, et al. Prenatal diagnosis of persistent left superior vena cava and its associated congenital anomalies. Ultrasound Obstet Gynecol. 2006;27:274–80.

Clerici G, Rosati A, Di Renzo GC. Absent ductus venosus associated with skeletal anomalies of the ulna and radius. Prenat Diagn. 2010;30:83–5.

Galindo A, Gutiérrez-Larraya F, Escribano D, Arbues J, Velasco J. Clinical significance of persistent left superior vena cava diagnosed in fetal life. Ultrasound Obstet Gynecol. 2007;30(2):152–61.

Ganesan S, et al. Prenatal findings in total anomalous pulmonary venous return: a diagnostic road map starts with obstetric screening views. J Ultrasound Med. 2014;33(7):1193–207.

Goyal S, Rosenthal L. Persistent left superior vena cava-inferior vena caval communication complicating implantation of an implantable cardioverter defibrillator. Pacing Clin Electrophysiol. 2005;28:1245–6.

Pepes S, Zidere V, Allan LD. Prenatal diagnosis of left atrial isomerism. Heart. 2009;95(24):1974–7.

Seale AN, et al. Total anomalous pulmonary venous connection: impact of prenatal diagnosis. Ultrasound Obstet Gynecol. 2012;40(3):310–8.

Shen O, et al. Shunt diameter in agenesis of the ductus venosus with extrahepatic portosystemic shunt impacts on prognosis. Ultrasound Obstet Gynecol. 2011;37:184–90.

Thomas JT, et al. Absent ductus venosus-outcomes and implications from a tertiary centre. Prenat Diagn. 2012;32:686–91.

Thubert T, et al. Agenesis of the ductus venosus: three-dimensional power Doppler reconstruction. Ultrasound Obstet Gynecol. 2012;39:118–20.

Valsangiacomo ER, et al. Partial and total anomalous pulmonary venous connection in the fetus: two dimensional and Doppler echocardiographic findings. Ultrasound Obstet Gynecol. 2003;22(3): 257–63.

Vigneswaran TV, et al. Effect of prenatal laterality disturbance and its accompanying anomalies on survival. The American Journal of Cardiology. 2018;122(4):663–671.

Yagel S, Kivilevitch Z, Cohen SM, et al. The fetal venous system, Part II: ultrasound evaluation of the fetus with congenital venous system malformation or developing circulatory compromise. Ultrasound Obstet Gynecol. 2010;36:93–11.

Yates RW, Raymond FL, Cook A, Sharland GK. Isomerism of the atrial appendages associated with 22q11 deletion in a fetus. Heart. 1996;76:548–9.

Vigneswaran TV, Jones CB, Zidere V, Charakida M, Miller OI, Simpson JM, Sharland GK. Effect of prenatal laterality disturbance and its accompanying anomalies on survival. Am J Cardiol. 2018;122(4):663–71.

Fetal Arrhythmias

11

Trisha Vigneswaran and John Simpson

Abstract

Pathological heart rhythm disturbances in the fetus are uncommon, however, being able to correctly diagnose the type of arrhythmia and instigate the appropriate treatment is crucial for a good fetal outcome. In contrast to postnatal life, the diagnosis is usually made using ultrasound rather than electrocardiographic techniques. Tachycardias, bradycardias and irregular fetal heart rhythms are discussed including the approach to diagnosis and management.

Keywords

Arrhythmia · Fetus · Fetal heart · Bradycardia · Tachycardia · Ectopic beats · Echocardiography

Electronic Supplementary Material The online version of this chapter (https://doi.org/10.1007/978-3-319-77461-9_11) contains supplementary material, which is available to authorized users.

T. Vigneswaran
Evelina London Children's Hospital, Guy's and St Thomas' NHS Foundation Trust, London, UK

King's College Hospital NHS Foundation Trust, London, UK
e-mail: trisha.vigneswaran@gstt.nhs.uk

J. Simpson (✉)
Evelina London Children's Hospital, Guy's and St Thomas' NHS Foundation Trust, London, UK
e-mail: john.simpson@gstt.nhs.uk

Assessment of Fetal Cardiac Rhythm

The normal fetal ventricular rate is typically between 110 and 160 beats per minute and is related to the gestational age of the fetus (Fig. 11.1). At a practical level fetal arrhythmias can be broadly divided into three major categories:

i. Irregular fetal heart rhythms
ii. Fetal tachycardias—heart rate > 200 beats per minute
iii. Fetal bradycardias—heart rate < 100 beats per minute

Assessment of cardiac rhythm in childhood is performed using an electrocardiogram, however, application of this technique to the fetus is challenging due to movement, insulation of the fetus by vernix caseosa and the low intensity of the fetal ECG compared to the mother (Simpson 2006). Magnetocardiography measures the magnetic field related to the electrical impulses within the heart and can permit detailed evaluation of heart rhythm and time intervals such as the QT interval. However, this technique is relatively costly and usually requires a magnetically shielded room so its application is limited. Ultrasound is by far the most widely used technique to evaluate the fetal heart rhythm. This uses mechanical events to ascertain the temporal relationship between atrial and ventricular contractions. The different

© Springer International Publishing AG, part of Springer Nature 2018
J. Simpson et al. (eds.), *Fetal Cardiology*, https://doi.org/10.1007/978-3-319-77461-9_11

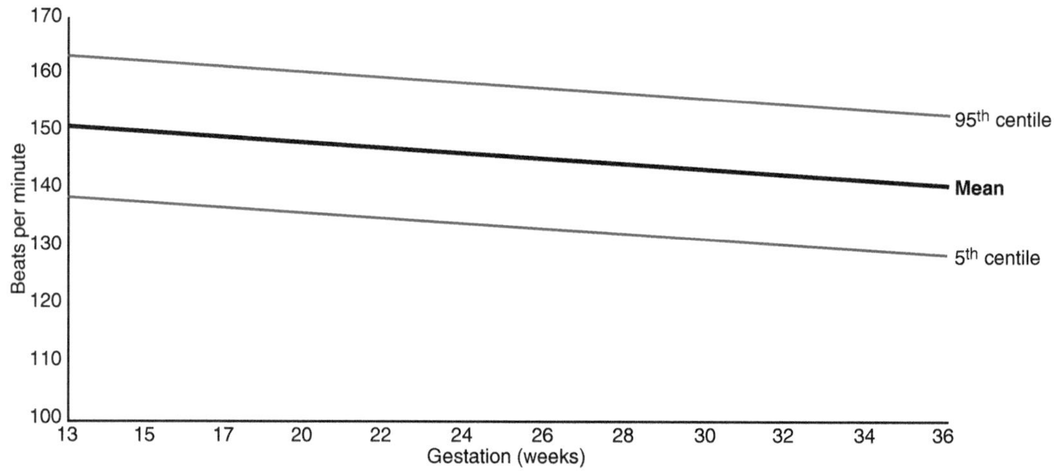

Fig. 11.1 Reference range for fetal heart rate based on over 7000 fetuses from our centre (unpublished data)

ultrasound modalities used include M-mode, pulsed Doppler and tissue Doppler methods.

Techniques

M-mode

The M-mode cursor can be placed through the heart at a near perpendicular angle to both the atrial and ventricular walls. Optimal magnification of the heart to allow for the visualisation of small movements is vital. Care should be taken to sample the atrial contraction and not the pericardial movement in this region. The rate and relationship of the atrial and ventricular contractions can then be ascertained (Fig. 11.2).

Doppler Interrogation

Pulsed wave Doppler can be used to assist in the diagnosis of some types of fetal arrhythmia. Simultaneous Doppler sampling of mitral valve inflow and outflow of the heart can be used (Fig. 11.3). Normally there is a biphasic inflow pattern but at high fetal heart rates these become fused so that the E waves and A waves cannot be seen separately, which limits its use in the context of fetal tachycardias. Alternative techniques include measurement of spectral Doppler and direction of blood flow simultaneously in the pulmonary vein-branch pulmonary artery (Fig. 11.3b) or superior vena cava with ascending aorta (Fig. 11.3c) (Carvalho et al. 2007). The latter two techniques are used most commonly to differentiate different types of supraventricular tachycardia. To ascertain both signals simultaneously, the pulsed wave Doppler cursor is placed across the region of interest with an increased sample gate of 3–5 mm. To assess the mitral inflow and aortic outflow the sample gate should be placed in the left ventricular outflow tract. To interrogate a pulmonary vein and branch pulmonary artery the Doppler cursor should be placed over a portion of the pulmonary vein and pulmonary artery within the lung parenchyma using colour flow Doppler for localisation of these structures. For simultaneous assessment of the superior vena cava and ascending aorta, a near sagittal view is preferred. The relationship of the atrial and ventricular contraction can also be sought using this pulse wave Doppler method.

Tissue Doppler Imaging

Tissue Doppler measures myocardial velocity. There are two major tissue Doppler modalities. The first is colour tissue Doppler where the velocity of myocardial motion is colour encoded according to the mean velocity. The direction of motion is coded red (towards the ultrasound probe) or blue (away from the ultrasound probe) using the same convention as blood pool Doppler. The entire heart can be sampled or only a portion. During analysis, the motion of the atriums and ventricles can be assessed to provide information about the timing of myocardial events such as

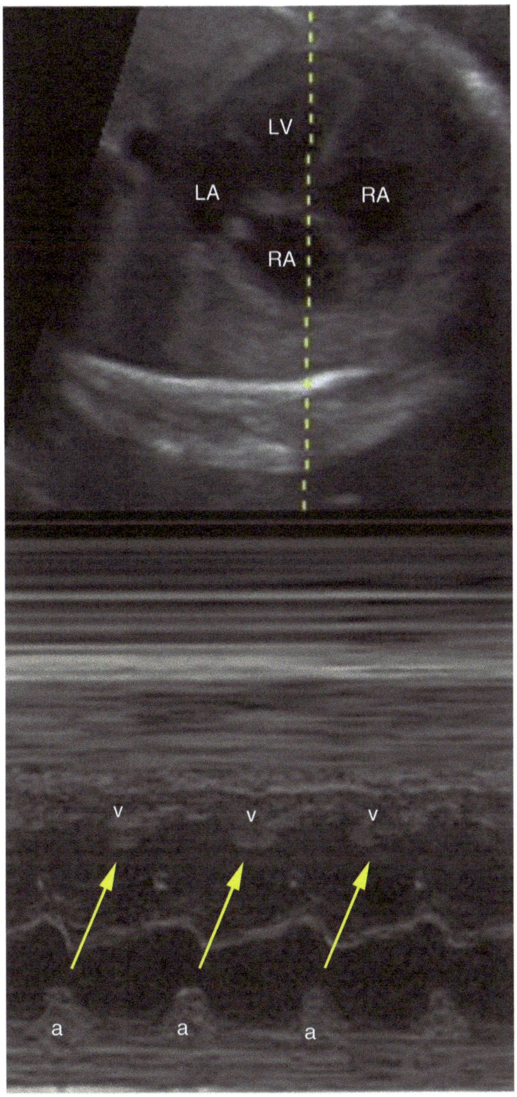

Fig. 11.2 M mode with measurement of atrial and ventricular rate. A cursor is placed at a near perpendicular angle to the ventricular and atrial septum to demonstrate the atrial (a) and ventricular (v) contractions

atrial and ventricular contraction. This technique is usually applied in a research setting due to the need to post-process images.

The alternative technique is pulsed wave Tissue Doppler where the Doppler cursor is placed in the region of interest. For the assessment of fetal arrhythmias the cursor can be placed at either the mitral or tricuspid valve annulus, the junction between the atriums and ventricles, so that both atrial and ventricular signals are detected on the same trace. Tissue Doppler may not be an option on many ultrasound systems which use curvilinear probes so the technique remains largely a research modality for fetal arrhythmias.

Magnetocardiography

Magnetocardiography detects the magnetic field associated with the electrical signals within the fetal heart. This technique provides novel insights because of its ability to measure features such as QRS morphology and QT interval which cannot be assessed by ultrasound techniques. The technique is relatively expensive and normally requires a magnetically shielded room so its use remains restricted to a few specialist centres.

Irregular Heart Rhythm

Atrial Extrasystoles

An irregular fetal heart rhythm, usually detected during routine auscultation, is the commonest form of fetal arrhythmia, particularly in the third trimester. On auscultation, this is often reported as “extra beats” or “missed beats”. The most frequent explanation for the observed irregularity is atrial extrasystoles (atrial ectopic beats) Video 11.1. In most instances, the overall fetal ventricular rate is within normal limits. If the heart rate is faster than normal and irregular, then assessment for fetal tachycardia should be performed. Atrial extrasysoles are usually followed by a compensatory pause as the heart repolarises which is appreciated as a delayed or “missed” beat (Fig. 11.4). In some fetuses, there can be multiple atrial ectopic beats which are not conducted to the ventricles i.e. the impulses are “blocked”. In this scenario, the overall ventricular rate can be subnormal and detailed assessment is required to differentiate this rhythm from complete heart block.

The sonographic findings of atrial extrasystoles are shown in Fig. 11.4a–d. Once confirmed using ultrasound techniques, no treatment is generally required although some units advise maternal abstinence from caffeine. The natural history is for such ectopic beats to resolve without ill effect. In a small proportion of fetuses (less than 2–3%) a fetal tachycardia may develop which may require treatment. Thus, our general

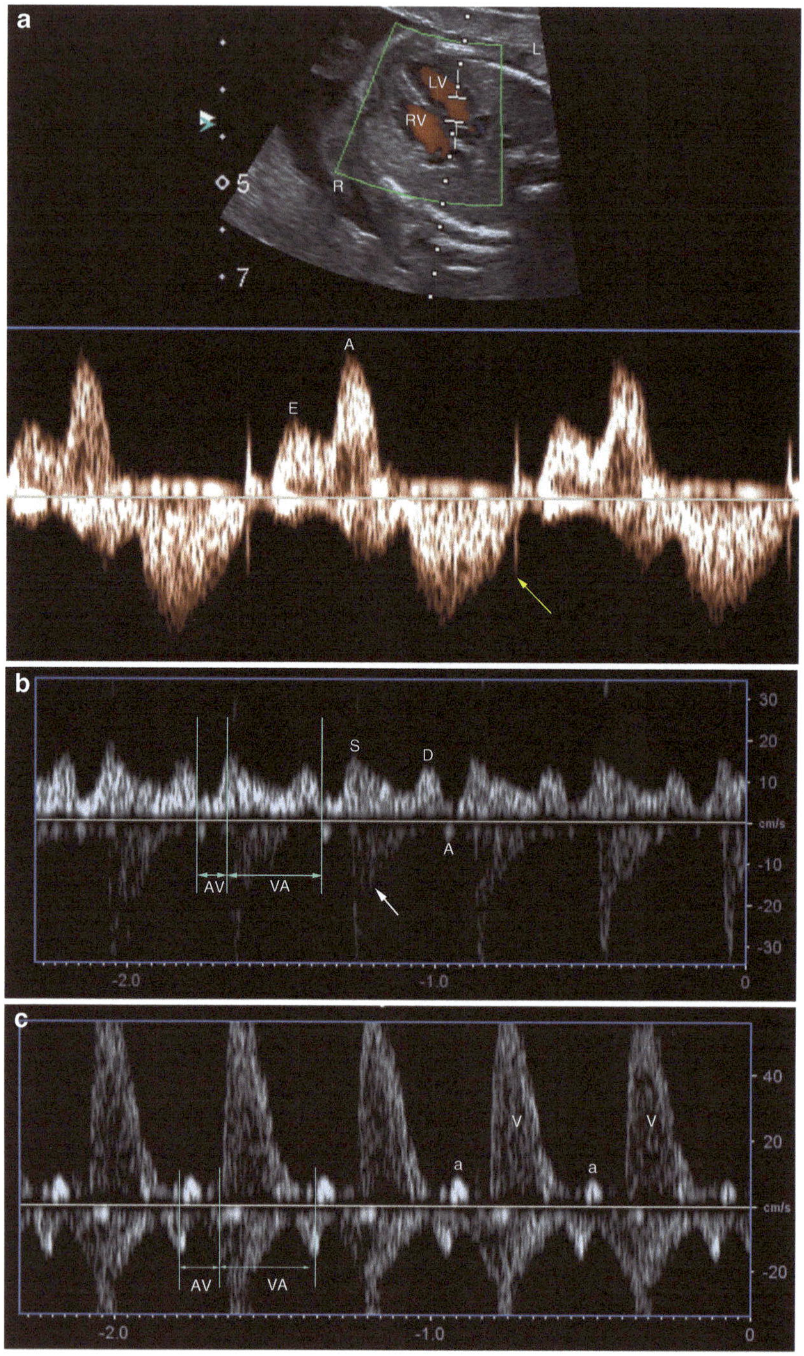

Fig. 11.3 (**a**) Mitral valve inflow-aortic outflow. The E wave of early atrial filling and the A wave of atrial contraction across the mitral valve inflow are seen. Below the baseline the aortic Doppler is seen with aortic valve closure clicks (yellow arrow). (**b**) Pulmonary vein-pulmonary artery Doppler: The normal phasic pattern of the S and D waves of the pulmonary venous Doppler are seen above the baseline. The A wave corresponding to reversed flow into the pulmonary veins with atrial contraction is seen below the line as is the pulsatile trace of the accompanying branch pulmonary artery (white arrow). The onset of the branch pulmonary artery flow marks the onset of ventricular systole (V) and the reversal of flow or reduction of velocity to near zero marks atrial contraction (A) This permits measurement of the AV and VA time intervals. (**c**) Superior vena cava—aortic Doppler. The normal phasic pattern of the S and D waves of the superior vena cava Doppler are seen below the line. The A wave corresponding to reversed flow into the superior vena cava with atrial contraction is seen above the line as is the pulsatile trace of the neighbouring aorta

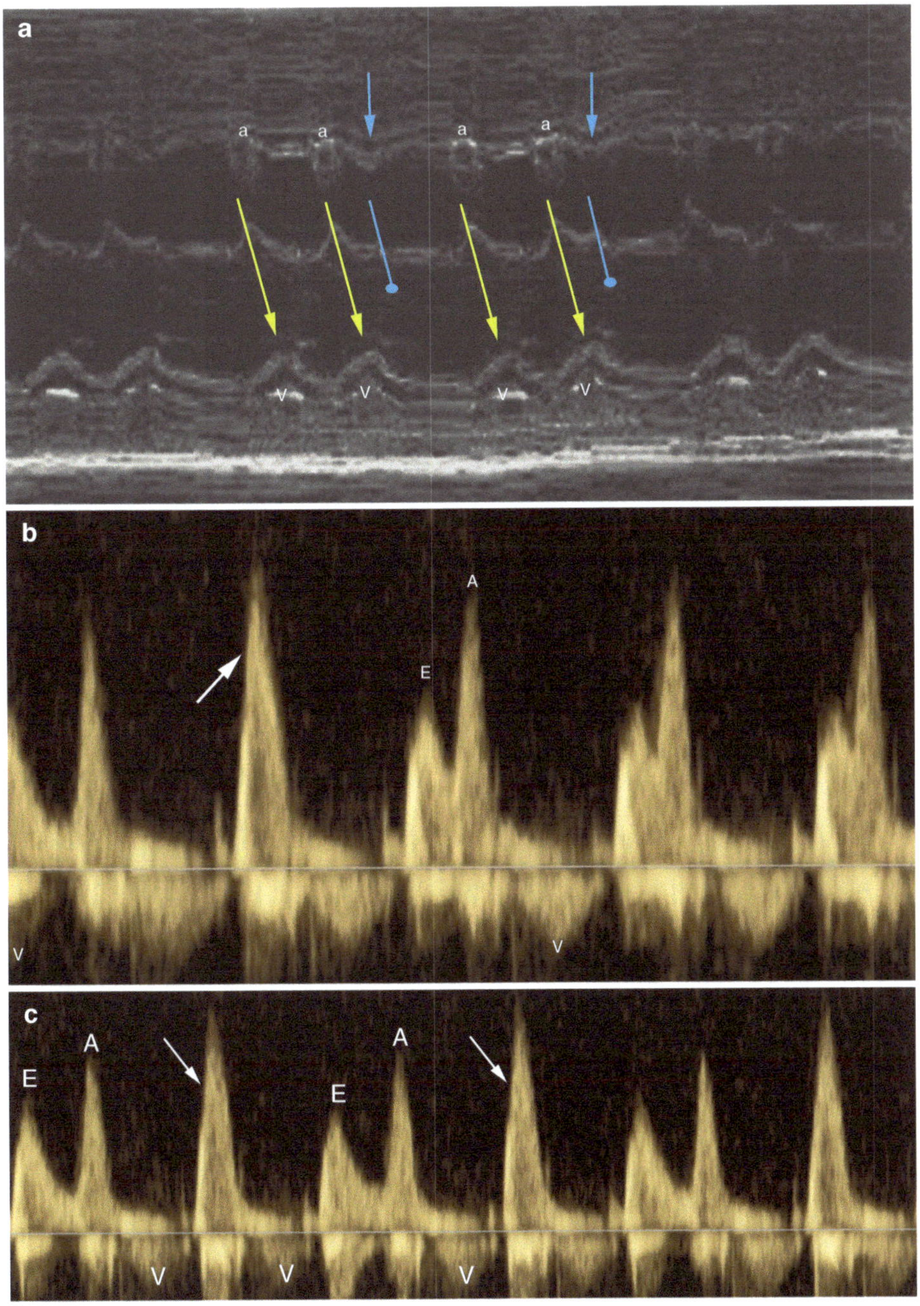

Fig. 11.4 (**a**) M Mode demonstrating blocked atrial ectopics. The normal atrial contractions (a) are conducted to the ventricles (v) (yellow arrows) whereas the atrial extrasystoles (blue arrow) which occur after every two sinus beats are not conducted to the ventricles (blue line). There is a consistent pause between the non-conducted atrial ectopic and the subsequent normal atrial contractions. (**b**) Single atrial ectopic beat (white arrow) demonstrated on pulsed wave Doppler across the mitral valve. Normal flow across the aortic valve is shown by the trace below baseline. Flow across the aortic valve during ventricular systole is denoted by V. (**c**) Mitral valve inflow Doppler demonstrating atrial bigeminy with alternating normal E/A inflow followed by a single-peaked inflow from the atrial ectopic beat (white arrow) which is conducted to the ventricles (V). To confirm the diagnosis M mode should be used as a complementary technique. (**d**) Aortic valve Doppler in a fetus with atrial bigeminy. The normal beat (V) is followed by early ejection of the ventricle (yellow arrow) due to a conducted atrial ectopic beat. There is a pause as the heart repolarises for the next normal contraction. If this type of trace is identified, an M mode must be performed to assess the atrial contractions and their relationship to ventricular contraction to confirm the diagnosis. (**e**) M mode demonstrating ventricular ectopic beats (v) which occur prior to the atrial contraction (**a**)

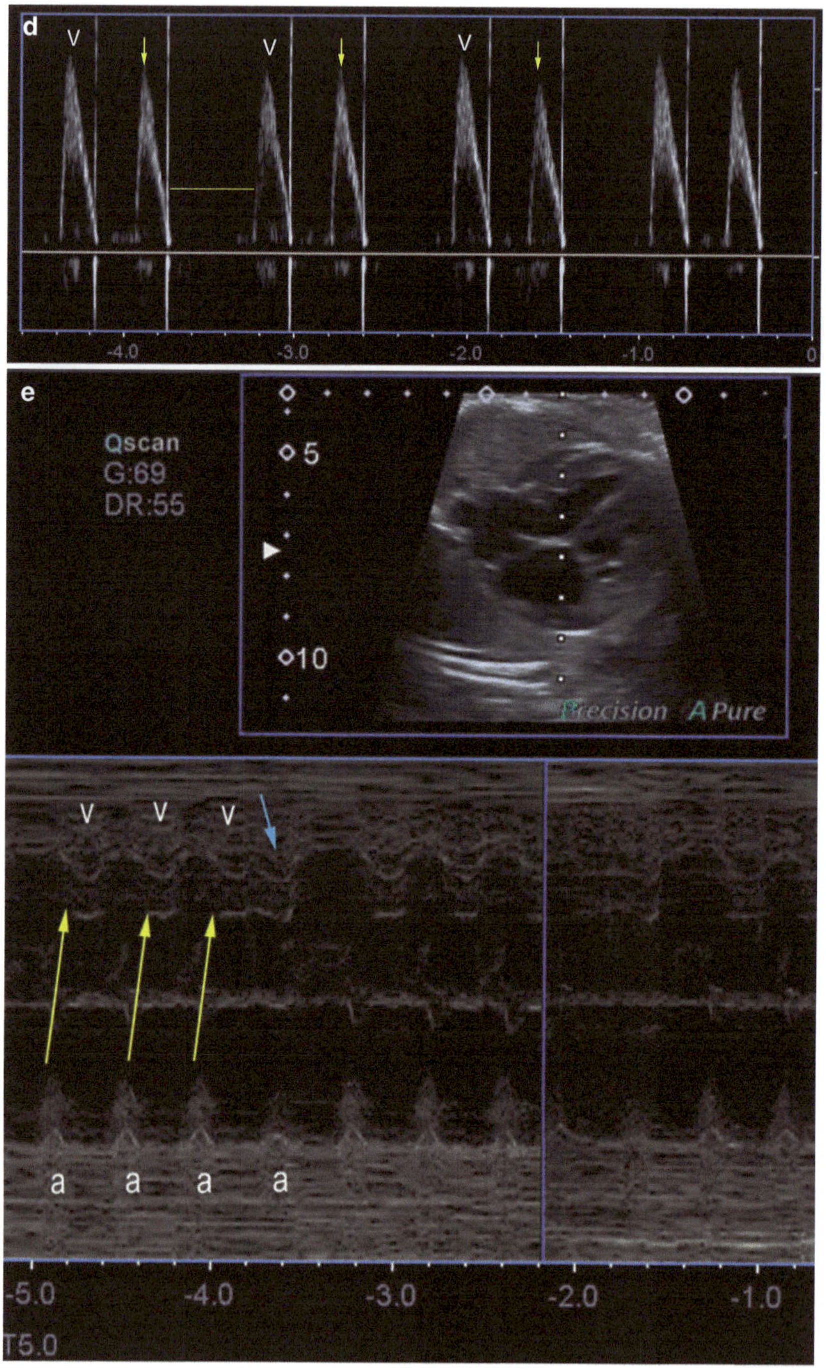

Fig. 11.4 (continued)

approach is for auscultation of the heart rate at the local obstetric unit every 1–2 weeks if more than one ectopic beat occurs for every 10 sinus beats. In our own experience, less frequent ectopic beats have not been associated with adverse outcome. In our setting, many obstetric units will manage irregular fetal heart rhythms without specialist referral but others value cardiology assessment, particularly if there are persistent ectopic beats or if the ventricular rate is low due to multiple blocked atrial ectopic beats. Frequent extrasystoles can make intrapartum cardiotocographic monitoring of fetal heart rate difficult and therefore, the obstetric team needs to be warned that this form of monitoring may be unreliable. If the heart rate irregularity has not resolved prior to delivery, we generally advise that a postnatal ECG is obtained to check the nature of the ectopic beats and to look for any markers of a re-entry pathway such as a Wolff-Parkinson-White (WPW) type of pattern on the ECG which can be identified by a short PR interval with a "delta" wave on the QRS complex. It is good practice to make parents aware of the signs and symptoms of supraventricular tachycardia in infancy in the unlikely event that this were to supervene. Patients with a WPW pattern on their ECG are typically followed up to monitor for any signs of tachycardia.

Ventricular Extrasystoles

Ventricular ectopic beats are rarer than atrial ectopic beats and can be identified on M mode echocardiography by identifying an early ventricular contraction which has not been preceded by an atrial contraction (Fig. 11.4e). Multiple ventricular ectopic beats would warrant a period of postnatal heart rate monitoring to ensure that they are infrequent and that there are no episodes of sustained ventricular arrhythmias. In our experience, the overwhelming majority of ventricular ectopic beats resolve spontaneously without treatment.

Fetal Tachycardias

Sinus Tachycardia

The definition of a fetal tachycardia is a ventricular rate above that expected for the gestation-specific normal range. Fetal sinus tachycardia can be seen with maternal fever, fetal distress, anaemia and thyrotoxicosis. If the main structures of the heart are normal, this does not warrant specialist echocardiography. Most physiological tachycardias do not exceed 200 beats per minute and there is usually variability in the heart rate.

Supraventricular Tachycardias

During fetal life, the term "supraventricular tachycardia" is typically applied to pathological tachycardias where there is a 1:1 ratio of the atrial to ventricular (A:V) rate. However, a variety of different types of tachycardia can have a 1:1 A:V ratio. This is illustrated in Fig. 11.5. The importance of differentiating the different mechanisms is that the choice of drug therapy may be impacted by such an assessment. The fetal heart rate is frequently greater than 220 bpm, most commonly around 240 beats per minute. Fetal supraventricular tachycardia (SVT) is a treatable arrhythmia, but if untreated, fetal SVT can lead to fetal hydrops with a significant risk of fetal demise.

The most common mechanism underlying fetal SVT is the presence of an accessory electrical pathway between the atriums and the ventricles. The exact location of this pathway cannot be determined by fetal echocardiography. A rapid onset and offset of tachycardia may be observed and provides strong evidence of a re-entry electrical pathway. The first step is to assess the relationship of the atrial to ventricular contraction (Fig. 11.1). In SVT there is a 1:1 A:V conduction ratio (Fig. 11.6). The mechanism of tachycardia can be further refined by measurement of the time between atrial contraction and ventricular contraction (A-V time) and the time between ventricular contraction and the next atrial contraction (V-A time). A variety of methods have been described to measure these time intervals including M-mode, pulsed wave Doppler and tissue Doppler techniques.

Short V-A Tachycardia

In the majority of cases of SVT diagnosed before birth the V-A interval is shorter than the A-V interval (short V-A tachycardia). This is a result of an accessory pathway (atrioventricular re-entry tachycardia) where there is rapid conduction from the ventricle back into the atrium. Conduction from the atrium to the ventricle is slower because of the delay introduced at the atrioventricular node. It is important to recognise that this form of SVT is not the only type of tachycardia which can present during fetal life with a short V-A interval (Figs. 11.7 and 11.8, Videos 11.2 and 11.3). Other

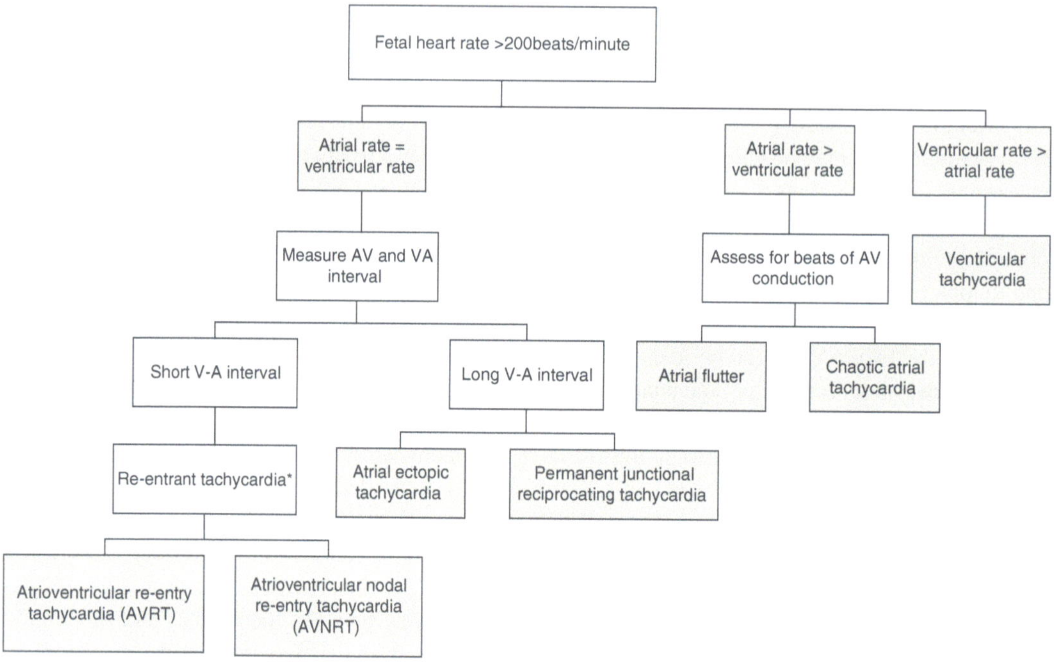

Fig. 11.5 Algorithm for differentiation of tachycardias. The * indicates that the subtypes of re-entrant tachycardias can only be differentiated with an electrocardiogram. (Taken from Vigneswaran et al. 2014)

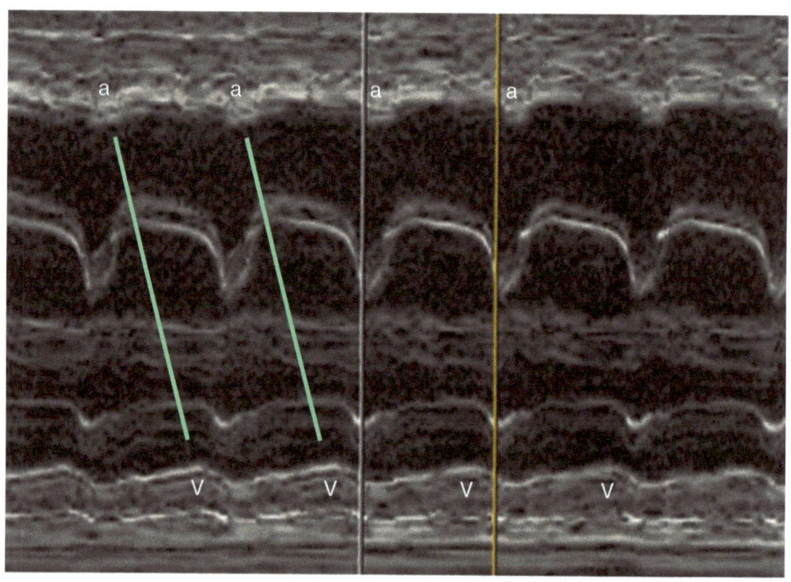

Fig. 11.6 M Mode showing 1:1 atrial:ventricular ratio with a heart rate of 267 beats per minute. The green lines represent the atrial followed by ventricular contractions. The vertical lines are used to calculate the heart rate

types, notably atrioventricular nodal re-entry tachycardia (where the re-entry circuit is within the AV node itself) may present in this way but this is an extremely rare mechanism during fetal life. Accessory pathways can be seen in Ebstein's anomaly of the tricuspid valve so exclusion of congenital heart disease is part of the assessment of all fetuses with pathological arrhythmias.

Long V-A Tachycardia

A long V-A tachycardia is defined as a tachycardia where there is 1:1 conduction between the

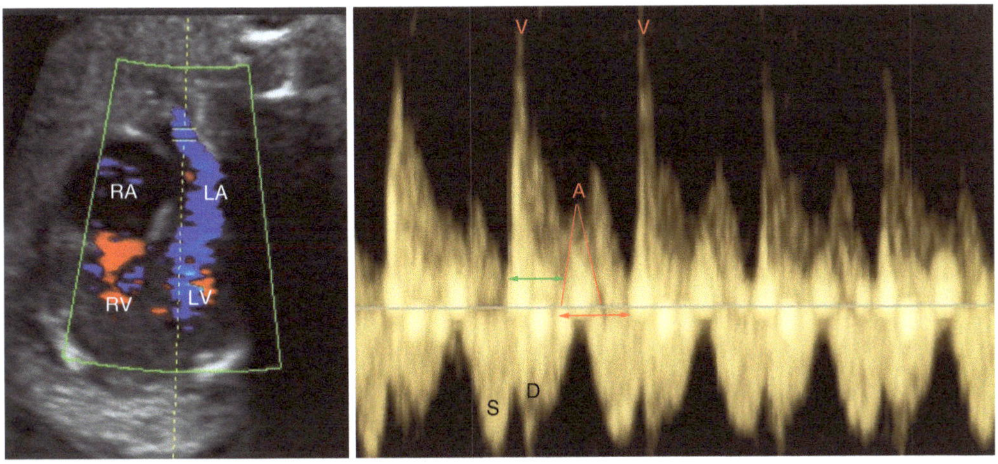

Fig. 11.7 Pulmonary vein–artery Doppler demonstrating a short V-A tachycardia. The pulmonary vein S and D waves are seen below the baseline and the A waves reversal (A) and branch pulmonary arterial trace (V) are seen above the line. The red arrow shows the A-V interval and the green arrow shows the V-A interval

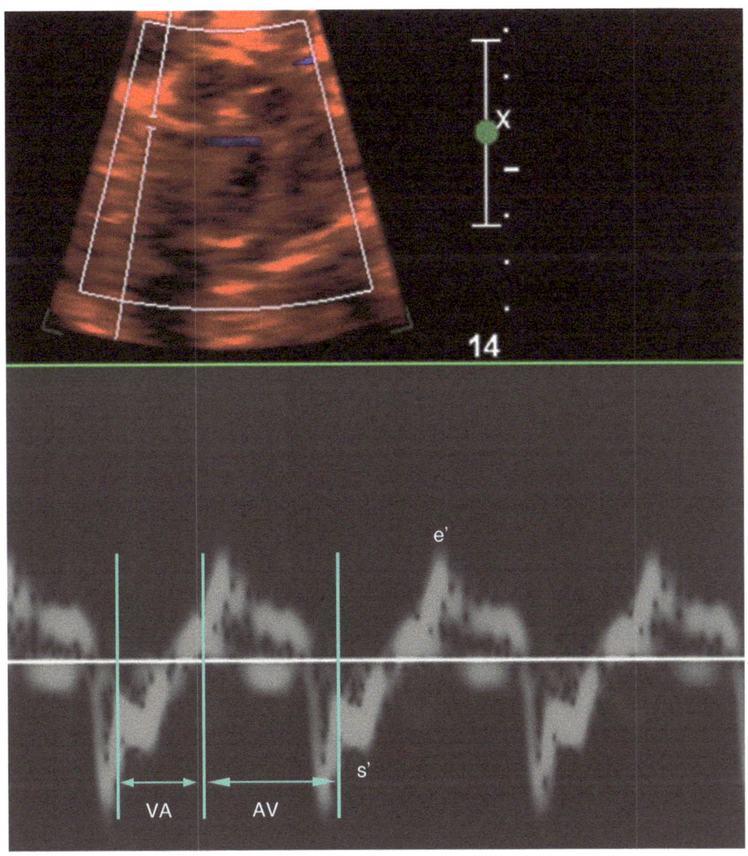

Fig. 11.8 Pulsed tissue Doppler of short VA tachycardia. Using tissue Doppler imaging the cursor is placed on tricuspid valve annulus giving the e', a' and s' waves which can be used to measure the A-V and V-A intervals. In this example, the VA time interval is shorter than the AV interval indicating a short VA tachycardia

atriums and ventricles, but the V-A time is longer than the A-V time. This is usually due to either an atrial ectopic tachycardia, where there is an abnormally fast electrical focus within the atriums which is still conducted to the ventricles or, permanent junctional reciprocating tachycardia (PJRT) where antegrade conduction is through the AV node and the retrograde conduction pathway is also slow accounting for the long V-A time. Long V-A tachycardias are much less common than short V-A tachycardias. Initial clues to the presence of a long V-A tachycardia can include: a slightly slower heart rate than short V-A tachycardias (typically 190–220 beats per minute) and the incessant nature of PJRT. These tachycardias can be more difficult to control in the fetal and postnatal period. The importance of differentiating the different mechanisms relates to the potential selection of different types of antiarrhythmic drugs to control each type of tachycardia.

Atrial Flutter, Chaotic Atrial Tachycardia and Atrial Fibrillation

Atrial flutter, chaotic atrial tachycardia and atrial fibrillation are characterised by an atrial rate which is much faster than the ventricular rate. The atrial rate is usually between 350 and 500 beats per minute, but the atrioventricular node cannot conduct electrical impulses to the ventricles at such a high rate so the resulting ventricular rate is much lower (Fig. 11.9, Video 11.4). As with other types of tachycardia, cardiac failure and fetal hydrops can develop. In most cases the structure of the fetal heart is normal but atrial flutter can be seen in the setting of a stretched right atrium such as with severe tricuspid regurgitation in Ebstein's malformation.

In atrial flutter, the atrial rate is typically fast and regular, giving rise to a "saw tooth" pattern (Fig. 11.9). With chaotic atrial tachycardia and atrial fibrillation the atrial rate is more irregular than in atrial flutter.

Ventricular Tachycardia

Ventricular tachycardia is an exceedingly rare arrhythmia in fetuses. By far the most frequent context in which it is seen is in fetuses with long QT syndrome. Fetuses with long QT syndrome may show a slightly slow sinus rate during fetal life (typically 90–110 beats per minute) interspersed with periods of exceedingly fast ventricular rate with a normal atrial rate. The QT interval can also be prolonged in fetuses with immune -mediated congenital complete heart block where it can occasionally give rise to ventricular tachycardia (Simpson et al. 2009). Cardiac tumours and non-compaction of the myocardium are other rare causes of ventricular tachycardia during fetal life.

The diagnosis of ventricular tachycardia can be made by M-mode where the ventricular rate is faster than the atrial rate (Fig. 11.10, Video 11.5). Assessment of the fetal QT interval is not possible by echocardiography but is feasible by magnetocardiography. If fetal long QT syndrome is

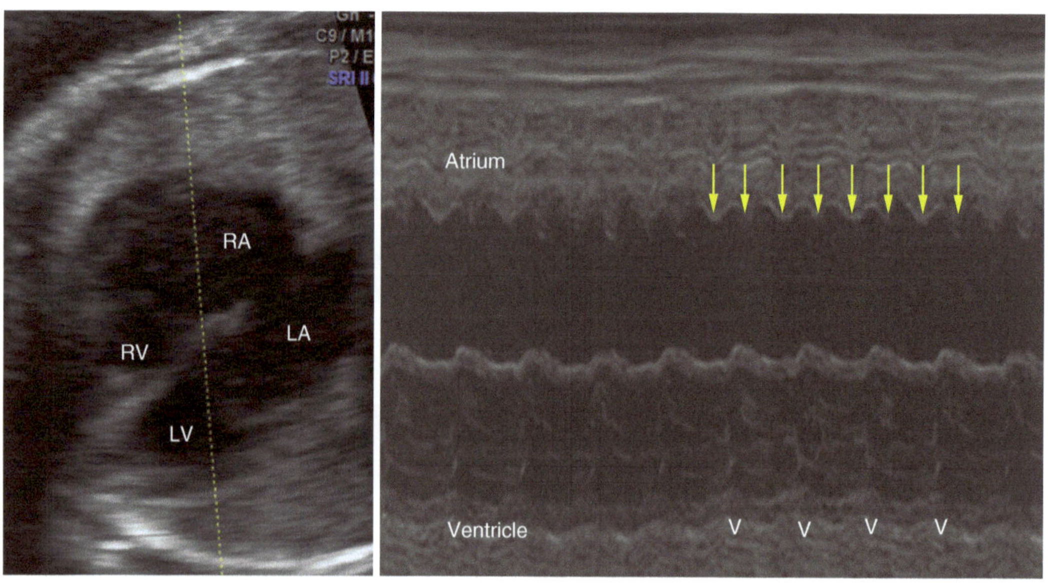

Fig. 11.9 M mode demonstrating atrial flutter. The atrial contractions demonstrate the typical 'sawtooth' pattern of atrial flutter (yellow arrows). Alternate flutter waves are conducted to the ventricles (V) giving 2:1 block. The atrial rate is 474 beats per minute

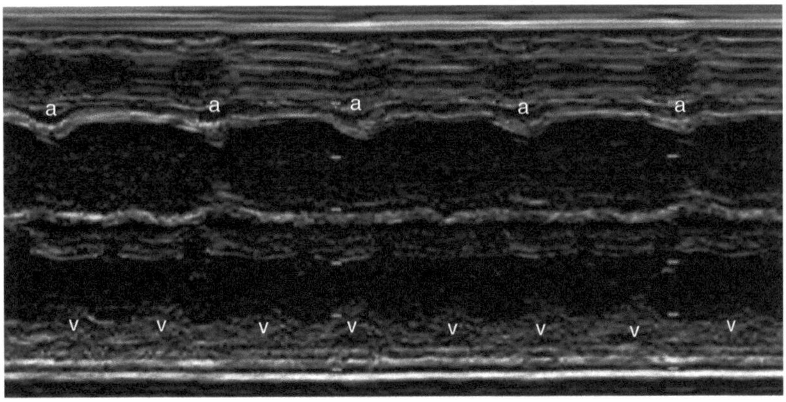

Fig. 11.10 M Mode demonstrating with ventricular tachycardia. The atrial rate (a) is slow and the ventricular rate (v) is faster

suspected, parental ECGs may be valuable as this is a dominantly inherited condition. In some cases the parents may be unaware they have the condition whereas in others there is a new mutation causing the condition in the fetus and the parents are unaffected.

General Approach to Management of Pathological Fetal Tachycardias

Previous reports of fetal supraventricular tachycardia indicated a high mortality, however with effective treatment, this has reduced (Simpson and Sharland 1998; Vigneswaran et al. 2014). There are several options which are open to those treating fetal tachycardias which can be generically applied rather than to a specific type of arrhythmia. These options include:

1. **Observation of the arrhythmia without treatment**
   This might be favoured for short-lived episodes of tachycardia in a fetus near term.
2. **Delivery of the fetus for postnatal therapy**
   In some settings, this might be favoured, for example if a fetus has atrial flutter near term. This can be rapidly treated with DC cardioversion after birth, which is not an option during fetal life.
3. **Transplacental therapy**
   Many anti-arrhythmic drugs cross the placenta, therefore administration to the mother leads to fetal therapy by proxy. The ability of drugs to cross the placenta varies by drug type and presence of hydrops which can reduce placental transfer. This impacts upon the choice of therapy.
4. **Direct fetal therapy**
   Anti-arrhythmic drugs may be administered directly to the fetus. A variety of routes have been used including intravenous, intraperitoneal and intramuscular administration. This avoids the problem of placental transfer of drug from the mother to the fetus but carries procedural risk. Furthermore, the mother will normally need to be loaded with the drug in question to avoid redistribution of drug to the mother.

Management of Tachycardias

The management of fetal tachycardias varies with each centre and drug therapy is typically based on published case series, institutional experience, the presence of fetal hydrops and gestational age (Jaeggi et al. 2011; Simpson and Sharland 1998). The optimal outcome is to convert the tachycardia prenatally so that the infant is delivered in sinus rhythm at full-term, without hydrops or other signs of congestive cardiac failure. Prior to commencing anti-arrhythmic therapy, a maternal history is taken and a baseline maternal 12-lead ECG is performed. Some units will also perform a maternal echocardiogram and check electrolytes. Given the potential complications of administration of anti-arrhythmic therapy to both the mother and fetus, management needs to be under the supervision of a cardiologist who has experience of the drugs being used and potential effects to both the mother and fetus. Table 11.1

Table 11.1 Anti-arrhythmic agents with potential uses and monitoring

Drug	Uses	Dosing	Reviews	Monitoring	Side effects
Digoxin	Non-hydropic short V-A tachycardia Atrial flutter Atrial fibrillation Chaotic atrial tachycardia	• Oral 250 mcg tds • Adjust dose depending on maternal plasma concentration and fetal response	• Outpatient management • Review after 7 days • Thereafter depending on response	• Baseline 12 lead maternal ECG before commencing • Check plasma concentration after 5 days of treatment (6 h pre-dose) • Therapeutic concentration: 0.9–2 ng/ml • 12 lead maternal ECG with each visit: upsloping ST segment	Nausea, vomiting, diarrhoea, dizziness, conduction disturbances
Flecainide	Rapid cardioversion Hydropic short V-A tachycardia Long V-A tachycardia May be used in combination with digoxin for atrial flutter and other atrial tachycardias	• Oral 100 mg tds • Adjust dose with maternal plasma concentration and fetal response—can increase to 150 mg three times a day or 100 mg four times daily	• Outpatient management • Review after 3 days • Thereafter depending on response	• Baseline 12 lead maternal ECG before commencing • Check plasma concentration after 3 days of treatment (trough, pre-dose) • Trough therapeutic concentration: 200–700 mcg/l • 12 lead maternal ECG with each visit—QRS duration, PR interval, QTc will prolong with treatment	Blurred vision, paraesthesia, headaches, nausea, vomiting, conduction disturbance
Sotalol	Short V-A tachycardia Long V-A tachycardia Atrial flutter and other atrial tachycardias	Oral 80 mg bd for 48 h Increase to 160 mg bd If no response after 5 days then 240 mg bd	• Outpatient management • Review 48 h after starting • Thereafter depending on response	• Baseline 12 lead maternal ECG before commencing • 12 lead maternal ECG with each visit—QTc assessment	Maternal bradycardia, Conduction disorders: prolongation of QT interval, peripheral vasoconstriction, bronchospasm
Amiodarone	Short V-A tachycardia Long V-A tachycardia Atrial flutter in refractory cases	• Oral loading to mother 1.8–2.4 g/day for 2–7 days • 800 mg/day for 1 week • 200–400 mg/day maintenance dose [single oral doses not to exceed 800 mg]	• Inpatient management for initial loading doses	• Daily maternal 12 lead ECG during loading dose • Allow 2 day drug-free period (to washout other medications)	Nausea, vomiting, taste disturbance, thyroid dysfunction, liver dysfunction, corneal deposits, QTc prolongation

Table 11.1 (continued)

Magnesium	Ventricular tachycardia	Infusion at 3–4 g/h		• Adjust according to maternal serum magnesium levels (aim for level >1 mmol/l)	
Propranolol	Prevention of VT in LQTS	Oral 2–3 mg/kg/day		• Absorption is variable	
Dexamethasone	Immune-mediated complete heart block with hydrops Immune-mediated second degree heart block	Oral 4 mg daily	• Weekly review		Maternal: Immune suppression, psychosis, loss of glycaemic control, adrenal suppression Fetus: possible IUGR, abnormal brain development Oligohydramnios Alteration in the hypothalamic-pituitary axis, possible effects on myocardial development
Slow release salbutamol	Complete heart block with HR <50 bpm	Oral up to 8 mg bd	• Weekly review	• Baseline serum potassium • Weekly serum potassium	Tremor, tachycardia, arrhythmias, hypokalemia, peripartum pulmonary oedema

The doses indicated reflect our practice, however, local policies will vary
bd twice daily, *tds* three times a day, *bpm* beats per minute, *IUGR* intrauterine growth restriction

summarises the types of drugs, doses, side effects and monitoring of drugs which have been administered for fetal tachycardias. It should be emphasised that practice differs greatly between centres and this information serves only as a general guide. At our centre, the drugs used are normally orally administered to the mother. Initially patients are followed up at least weekly to assess the fetal response and to check for any side effects. Assessment of the maternal ECG and measurement of maternal blood/serum drug concentrations are routinely obtained. In combination these factors assist in tailoring the dosage of medication.

Short V-A Tachycardia

For short V-A tachycardia, treatments described in the literature include transplacental digoxin, sotalol or flecainide therapy (Table 11.1). In the presence of fetal hydrops the placental membranes are oedematous and therefore adequate placental transfer of some drugs, notably digoxin, does not occur and therefore, alternative agents such as flecainide, which have better placental transfer, may be favoured. If the fetus remains in tachycardia after loading doses are given, the maternal serum drug concentration is usually checked and adjusted to achieve the therapeutic range. The maternal 12 lead ECG is also repeated to look for drug induced changes.

After birth, our policy is to continue anti-arrhythmic treatment for at least 6 months. However, some units will only continue therapy if there is proven recurrence of tachycardia after birth. If fetal treatment was successful in reverting to sinus rhythm, this medication can either be continued in the infant or an alternative because the issue of placental transfer is no longer an issue after delivery. Approximately 90% of infants are free from further episodes of tachycardia after the first year, but late recurrence is well described.

Long V-A Tachycardias

This type can be more difficult to control, often requiring a number of anti-arrhythmic agents (Table 11.1). As for short V-A tachycardias, postnatal treatment is generally continued.

Atrial Flutter

This arrhythmia is often treated with a combination of medications. Some units use a combination of flecainide and digoxin whereas others prefer sotalol in place of flecainide. Digoxin monotherapy may be limited by placental transfer of the drug, particularly when the fetus is hydropic, and the fact that digoxin does not have an impact on atrial flutter itself but only on conduction at the atrioventricular node. Flecainide alone may be effective but there have been postnatal reports that it may precipitate 1:1 atrioventricular conduction as a result of slowing of the atrial rate. This has a paradoxical effect of increasing the ventricular rate. Therefore, in many institutions, if flecainide is used, an additional drug such as digoxin is administered to slow atrio-ventricular conduction.

Atrial flutter may be difficult to control prenatally, but after birth it can be managed effectively with a synchronised DC shock. In the majority of cases this treatment is definitive. In the rare cases where it recurs in the neonatal period, longer term anti-arrhythmic therapy may be required.

Ventricular Tachycardia

This is a rare finding in fetuses and thus treatment is based on case reports. Flecainide, amiodarone, propranolol and intravenous magnesium have all been used to control ventricular tachycardia (Simpson et al. 2009). There is a very high incidence of long QT syndrome in this patient group. Beta blockers have been used prenatally to prevent recurrence of tachycardia but with limited success.

Direct Therapy

If cardioversion does not occur with transplacental treatment, fetal hydrops persists and fetal gestation is too early to consider delivery, then direct fetal therapy may be considered (Table 11.2). The risks of cord access in these sick fetuses is much higher than for other indications and therefore, this direct approach involves a considered discussion amongst the multidisciplinary team of obstetricians, fetal medicine specialists, electrophysiologists and fetal cardiologists. Drugs which have not controlled the arrhythmia may need to be discontinued prior to the procedure. If a drug is to be administered directly, the mother

Table 11.2 Direct fetal anti-arrhythmic therapies. These are considered for refractory cases and administered directly into the fetal circulation. Doses provided are those reported in the literature, but local policies must be consulted

Drug	Uses	Dose	Comment/side effects
Adenosine	Diagnostic purposes	• 100–200 mcg/kg of estimated fetal weight	Short half time (<30 s)
Digoxin	Hydropic, refractory SVT	• 10–15 mcg/kg of estimated fetal weight	
Propafenone	Refractory SVT	• 6 mg/kg of estimated fetal weight	
Amiodarone	Refractory cases of SVT and VT	• 2.5 mg/kg of estimated fetal weight administered as slow injection	Fetal bradycardia—may require adrenaline

will need to be loaded with the same drug to prevent any drugs administered direct into the fetal circulation from simply redistributing into the maternal circulation. Multiple different routes have been used, including intravenous (umbilical vein), intramuscular and intraperitoneal.

Fetal Bradycardias

Sinus Bradycardia

The obstetric definition of fetal bradycardia is heart rate less than 110 beats per minute (American College of Obstetricians and Gynecologists 2009). However, evidence shows that heart rate less than the 3rd centile should be considered for detailed investigation (Mitchell et al. 2012). Ascertainment of 1:1 atrial to ventricular conduction will confirm the rhythm to be sinus bradycardia. Causes of sinus bradycardia include:

- Preterminal event in a sick fetus
- Excessive application of pressure to the fetus during the ultrasound examination
- Left atrial isomerism
- Long QT syndrome

Fetal bradycardia can be seen when there is significant fetal distress such as hypoxia which can represent a preterminal event. This does not require input from a cardiac specialist. The most common cause of intermittent fetal sinus bradycardia is due to compression of the fetal head by excessive application of pressure during ultrasonography. Removal of this pressure should lead to rapid recovery of the heart rate.

In the setting of left atrial isomerism, the sino-atrial node (a right atrial structure) is absent. An alternate area within the atriums may act as the pacemaker region, but the atrial rate is lower than that of the sino-atrial node so the heart rate will be slower. Thus, in the context of an interrupted inferior vena cava and sinus bradycardia, left atrial isomerism should be suspected. This may evolve to complete heart block. Persistent fetal sinus bradycardia less that the 3rd percentile for gestation has been described in long QT syndrome. This is an ion channelopathy which predisposes to ventricular tachycardia and is associated with sudden cardiac death. The fetal QT interval cannot be calculated using ultrasound, however, periods of ventricular tachycardia may be identified. Prenatal management of persistent sinus bradycardia includes parental ECG to investigate for familial long QT syndrome. Normal parental ECGs do not exclude long QT syndrome in the fetus and hence, these fetuses should be followed up after birth with a 12 lead ECG. Prenatal counselling should include the possibility of long QT syndrome and its implications. If a parent is found to have long QT syndrome, referrals to a specialist cardiologist and/or clinical genetics are appropriate.

Irregular Bradycardia

Blocked atrial ectopic beats can also present as intermittent bradycardia. In this situation, the atrial ectopic beat is sufficiently early that it cannot be conducted to the ventricles. Following the blocked atrial ectopic beat there is a compensatory pause so that there is a delay to the subsequent beat and therefore, this appears as an irregular bradycardia. M-mode and Doppler echocardiography can be used to assess the timing of atrial and ventricular contractions. Atrial ectopic beats are not usually harmful for the fetus, however, they need to be highlighted to the obstetric team as intrapartum cardiotocographic monitoring for assessment of fetal distress will not be reliable. The implications and management are described in section “Atrial Extrasystoles”.

Heart Block

Classification of Heart Block

Heart block refers to either prolongation of conduction time, or failure to conduct impulses from the atrium to the ventricles and requires assessment using both M mode and Doppler echocardiography.

First Degree Heart Block

First degree heart block is a prolongation of the time taken for atrial beats to be conducted to the ventricles. M Mode echocardiography will demonstrate a 1:1 conduction of atrial to ventricular beats. The prolongation of the A:V conduction time is best appreciated using the mitral valve inflow with aortic outflow Doppler tracing which will show an increased A:V conduction time for gestation (Nii et al. 2006) (Fig. 11.11). This time interval between the onset of atrial contraction (A wave) and the onset of ventricular contraction (V wave) provides a mechanical surrogate of the PR interval.

Second Degree Heart Block

In second degree heart block, some (but not all) atrial impulses are conducted to the ventricles, thus there is a 2:1 or 3:1 relationship of the atrial to ventricular contractions. A Wenckebach pattern can be seen as a progressive lengthening of the atrio-ventricular contraction time interval followed by an atrial beat which is not followed by a ventricular beat (dropped beat).

Third Degree Heart Block

In third degree heart block (complete heart block), no impulses at all are conducted from the atriums to the ventricles—thus, atrial and ventricular contractions are completely dissociated from each other. The diagnosis of 3rd degree heart block is made when there is no temporal relationship between the atrial and ventricular contractions. This can be identified most readily on M mode (Fig. 11.12, Videos 11.6 and 11.7). The ventricular escape rate is usually between 45 and 70 beats per minute and the atrial rate is usually within normal limits. If the atrial rate is low this may indicate left atrial isomerism. Assessment of the umbilical vein Doppler may show notching during ventricular systole and the ductus venosus

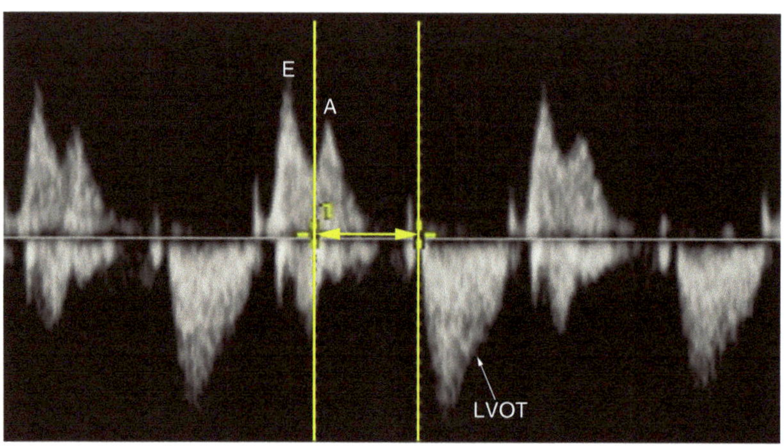

Fig. 11.11 Prolongation of the A:V conduction time as seen on colour Doppler. The Doppler gate is increased and placed to cover both the mitral inflow and the left ventricular outflow. The time interval from the onset of the mitral valve A wave to the onset of the aortic flow (V) is 230 ms (double headed arrow) which is increased according to the gestation-related normal range

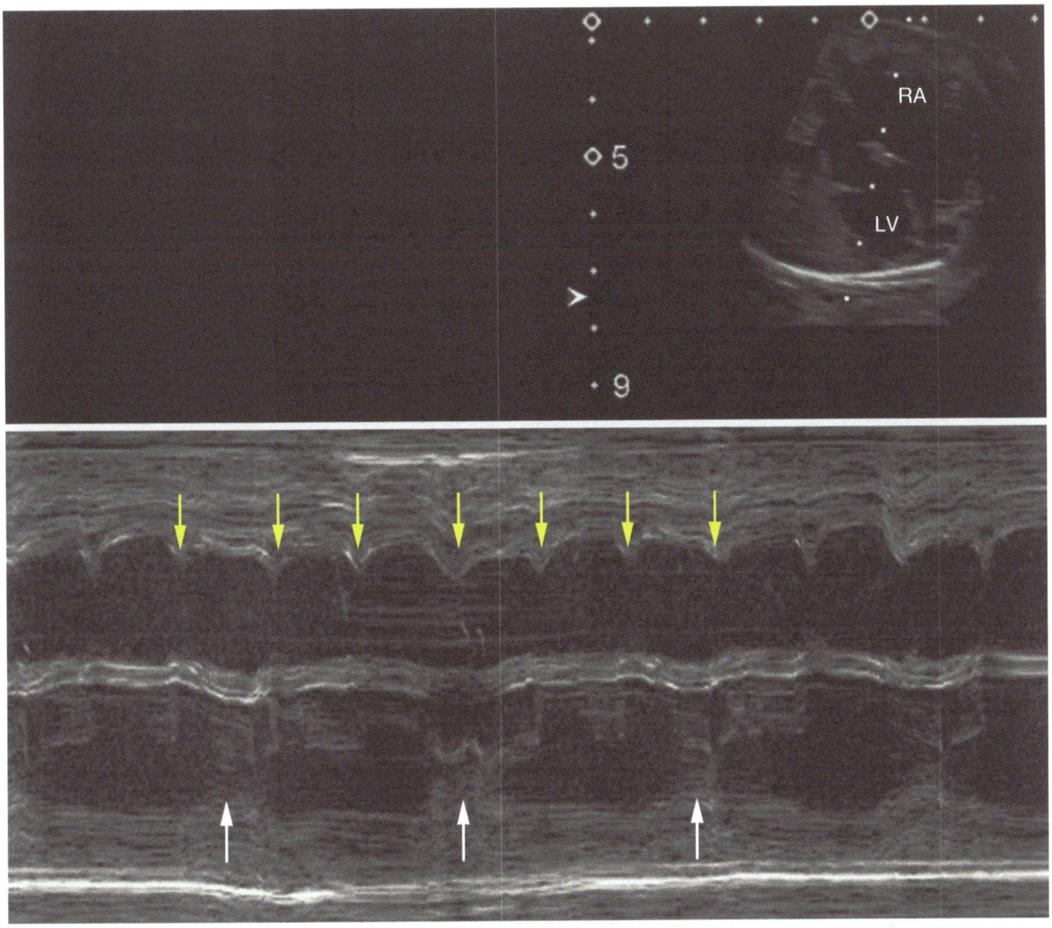

Fig. 11.12 M mode demonstrating complete heart block. There is no association between the atrial contractions (yellow arrows) and the ventricular contractions (white arrows). The atrial rate continues as dictated by the sino-atrial node. Due to block at the atrioventricular node, the ventricular rate is slower reflecting its escape rate

Doppler will demonstrate large a wave reversal due to atrial contraction against a closed tricuspid valve, similar to the cannon a waves which can be seen in the central veins after birth. (Fig. 11.13a, b) There may be associated fetal hydrops.

Complete heart block can occur in the setting of:

- Left atrial isomerism
- Discordant atrioventricular connections i.e. left atrium connected to morphologic right ventricle and vice versa
- Maternal anti-Ro and anti-La (SS-A and SS-B) antibodies

Once complete heart block is confirmed, detailed fetal echocardiography is required as these forms of congenital heart disease can be subtle and the prognosis is poor in these groups when complete heart block is present. Maternal testing for anti-Ro and anti-LA antibodies must be performed.

Auto-immune Mediated Complete Heart Block

In the presence of maternal anti-Ro antibodies, the incidence of fetal complete heart block is 2% and this increases to 20% following one affected pregnancy (Hunter and Simpson 2015). Lesser degrees of heart block can also be seen. Anti-Ro and anti-La antibodies can be identified in maternal systemic lupus erythematosus, Sjogren's syndrome or rheumatoid arthritis, but in many cases fetal complete heart block is the

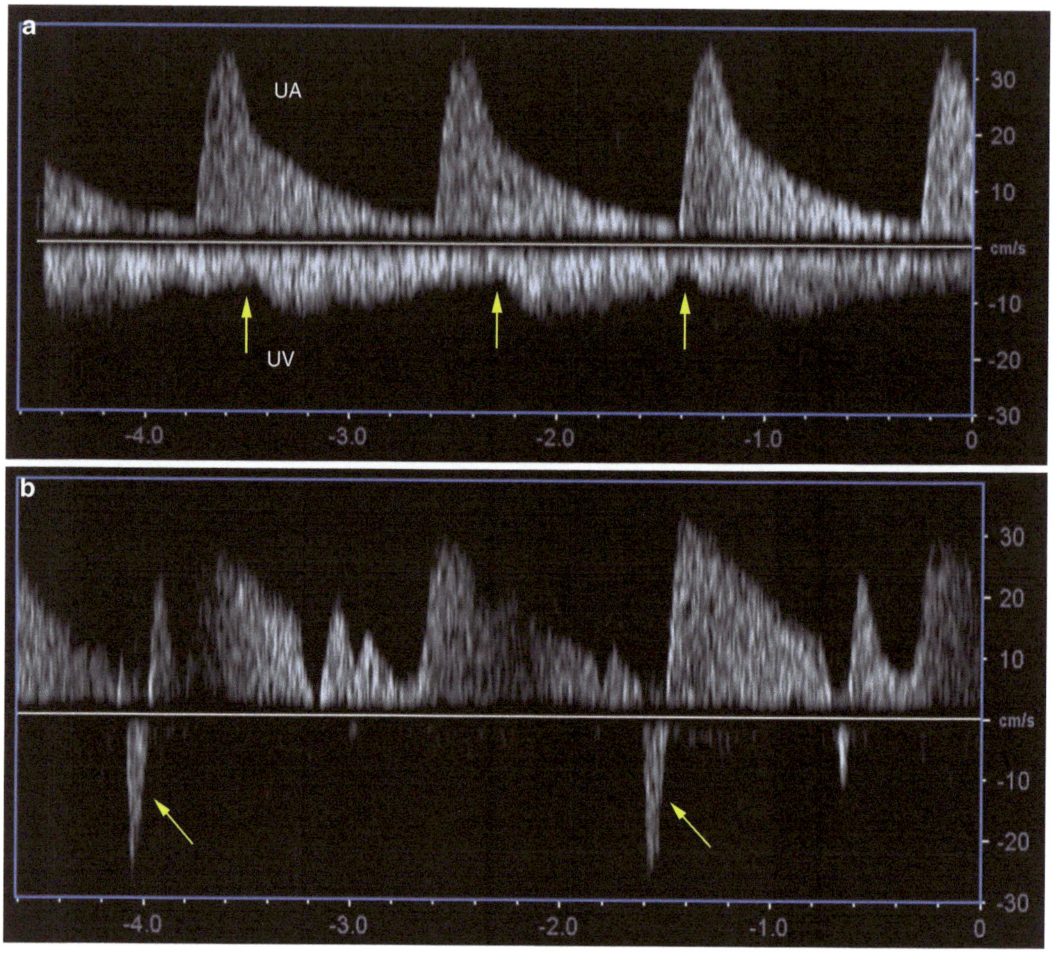

Fig. 11.13 (**a**) Umbilical Dopplers in complete heart block. Spectral Doppler showing the umbilical artery Doppler (above the baseline) appears normal, whereas the umbilical vein Doppler (below the baseline) demonstrates notching (yellow arrows) which are coincident with ventricular systole. (**b**) Ductus venosus flow in complete heart block. This shows a wave reversal (yellow arrows) which reflects atrial contraction against a closed tricuspid valve (cannon wave) giving rise to backflow of blood in the ductus venosus. Thus, the ductus venosus Doppler cannot be used as a marker of fetal wellbeing in the setting of complete heart block

first sign that the mother carries auto-antibodies. Anti-Ro and anti-La antibodies can cross the placenta from 16 weeks gestation onwards causing inflammation of the conduction system and myocardium and therefore screening is offered in these cases.

Fetal Echocardiography Screening

Varying degrees of heart block can be identified with anti-Ro antibodies. The atrial and ventricular rates must be measured. When there is 1:1 atrioventricular conduction, assessment of conduction times can be performed using pulsed wave Doppler of an inflow-outflow. Assessment of the degree of heart block is important as this determines the management options which are discussed below.

In addition to rhythm disturbances, inflammation of the heart can also occur, which is seen as echogenicity of the atrioventricular groove or endocardial fibroelastosis (Video 11.8). Cardiomyopathy can develop as a result of myocardial fibrosis and necrosis. The pulmonary and aortic valve Doppler velocities may be increased reflecting increased stroke volume. If there is a major discrepancy between the Doppler velocities across the aortic and pulmonary valves then valve stenosis or reduced ventricular function should be excluded.

Treatment of First Degree Heart Block

It should be emphasised that fetuses with first degree heart block have a normal ventricular rate and are only detected by measurement of the AV time interval. There are a few reported cases of first degree heart block due to maternal anti-Ro antibodies in which the A-V prolongation has normalised following administration of steroids. However, the A-V interval may "normalise" spontaneously without therapy and furthermore, first degree heart block has not been shown to progress or be predictive of higher degrees of heart block (Friedman et al. 2008). Some units would offer treatment with maternal steroids with the hypothesis that this would reduce ongoing inflammation, however, this is based on limited evidence of improvement in long term outcome. Our current approach is to simply to monitor such fetuses.

Treatment of Second Degree Heart Block

In some fetuses, second degree heart block may be evident at presentation, where some atrial beats are conducted to the ventricles and others are not. Treatment with corticosteroids has been associated with conversion back to sinus rhythm in some cases, but this is not always sustained and only studies with small sample sizes have assessed the effect of maternal steroids to revert to sinus rhythm (Lopes et al. 2008). In our practice, we would consider a trial of dexamethasone therapy with the aim of conversion back to sinus rhythm, but this is not continued if there is no fetal response.

Treatment of Complete Heart Block

The treatment of immune-mediated complete heart block is controversial as there is no randomised control trial data to support treatments. Therapies which are commonly tried include: maternal steroids and beta-2-agonists (Jaeggi et al. 2004), but an improved outcome has not been universally demonstrated (Eliasson et al. 2011; Rosenthal et al. 2005). Immune-modulators such as intravenous immunoglobulin, hydroxychloroquine, B cell depletion, azathioprine, cyclophosphamide and plasmapheresis have also been used. There is considerable institutional variation in practice. Our own approach is to monitor fetuses with complete heart block who are not hydropic and whose ventricular function is good. Dexamethasone is reserved for fetuses with hydrops or significant impairment of ventricular function. The proposed benefits of therapy need to be balanced against the risk of side effects (Table 11.1). In the presence of fetal hydrops or cardiomyopathy, a course of oral maternal steroids may prove beneficial to reduce hydrops and improve myocardial function. If the heart rate is very slow (for example, less than 50 beats per minute), a beta-agonist such as salbutamol may be used. Cases where intractable hydrops has developed or where premature delivery has occurred have a poor prognosis (Ho et al. 2015). Therefore, our aim is to balance the risks of intra-uterine death and of preterm delivery such that delivery occurs at the most favourable time. After birth these babies may require ventilatory support and a beta-agonist such as intravenous isoprenaline to maintain an adequate heart rate and circulation. Pacemaker insertion is required in infancy in the majority of cases. Long term follow up is required both of cardiac rhythm and cardiac function because late cardiomyopathy has been described. Recent data from our unit described 77% survival at 30 years following live-birth with improving results in recent years (Ho et al. 2015).

Prophylaxis

If anti-Ro antibodies have been detected as a result of investigation for fetal complete heart block, without a pre-existing maternal diagnosis, a referral to a rheumatological specialist for investigation and counselling should be instituted. The treatment of future pregnancies varies by institution but may include drugs such as hydroxychloroquine with the aim of reducing the incidence of complete heart block.

In our unit mothers who are positive for anti-Ro/La antibodies are assessed 2–3 times between 18 and 30 weeks gestation. Risk stratification of expectant mothers using anti-Ro and anti-La titres may aid identification of patients who are more likely to develop heart block and this approach is followed by some units. Mothers with anti Ro levels >100 IU/l or high titres of anti-La have a high risk of developing fetal complete heart block, whereas anti-Ro levels <50 IU/L are considered low risk. The rationale for risk stratification is when protocols utilise treatment with steroids or immunoglobulins to treat fetuses with incomplete heart block or endocardial fibroelastosis (Kan et al. 2017).

References

American College of Obstetricians and Gynaecologists. ACOG Practice Bulletin No. 106: intrapartum fetal heart rate monitoring: nomenclature, interpretation, and general management principles. Obstet Gynecol. 2009;114:192–202.

Lopes LM, Tavares GM, Damiano AP, Lopes MA, Aiello VD, Schultz R, et al. Perinatal outcome of fetal atrioventricular block: one-hundred-sixteen cases from a single institution. Circulation. 2008;118(12):1268–75.

Carvalho JS, Prefumo F, Ciardelli V, Sairam S, Bhide A, Shinebourne EA. Evaluation of fetal arrhythmias from simultaneous pulsed wave Doppler in pulmonary artery and vein. Heart. 2007;93:1448–53.

Eliasson H, Sonesson SE, Sharland G, Granath F, Simpson JM, Carvalho JS, Jicinska H, Tomek V, Dangel J, Zielinsky P, Respondek-Liberska M, Freund MW, Mellander M, Bartrons J, Gardiner HM, Fetal Working Group of the European Association of Pediatric Cardiology. Isolated atrioventricular block in the fetus: a retrospective, multinational, multicenter study of 175 patients. Circulation. 2011;124:1919–26.

Friedman DM, Kim MY, Copel JA, Davis C, Phoon CK, Glickstein JS, Buyon JP, Pride Investigators. Utility of cardiac monitoring in fetuses at risk for congenital heart block: the PR Interval and Dexamethasone Evaluation (PRIDE) prospective study. Circulation. 2008;117:485–93.

Ho A, Gordon P, Rosenthal E, Simpson J, Miller O, Sharland G. Isolated complete heart block in the fetus. Am J Cardiol. 2015;116:142–7.

Hunter LE, Simpson JM. Atrioventricular block during fetal life. J Saudi Heart Assoc. 2015;27:164–78.

Jaeggi ET, Carvalho JS, De Groot E, Api O, Clur SA, Rammeloo L, Mccrindle BW, Ryan G, Manlhiot C, Blom NA. Comparison of transplacental treatment of fetal supraventricular tachyarrhythmias with digoxin, flecainide, and sotalol: results of a nonrandomized multicenter study. Circulation. 2011;124:1747–54.

Jaeggi ET, Fouron JC, Silverman ED, Ryan G, Smallhorn J, Hornberger LK. Transplacental fetal treatment improves the outcome of prenatally diagnosed complete atrioventricular block without structural heart disease. Circulation. 2004;110:1542–8.

Kan N, Silverman ED, Kingdom J, Dutil N, Laskin C, Jaeggi E. Serial echocardiography for immune-mediated heart disease in the fetus: results of a risk-based prospective surveillance strategy. Prenat Diagn. 2017;37(4):375–82.

Mitchell JL, Cuneo BF, Etheridge SP, Horigome H, Weng HY, Benson DW. Fetal heart rate predictors of long QT syndrome. Circulation. 2012;126:2688–95.

Nii M, Hamilton RM, Fenwick L, Kingdom JC, Roman KS, Jaeggi ET. Assessment of fetal atrioventricular time intervals by tissue Doppler and pulse Doppler echocardiography: normal values and correlation with fetal electrocardiography. Heart. 2006;92:1831–7.

Rosenthal E, Gordon PA, Simpson JM, Sharland GK. Letter regarding article by Jaeggi et al, "transplacental fetal treatment improves the outcome of prenatally diagnosed complete atrioventricular block without structural heart disease". Circulation. 2005;111:e287–8. author reply e287–8

Simpson JM. Fetal arrhythmias. Ultrasound Obstet Gynecol. 2006;27:599–606.

Simpson JM, Maxwell D, ROSENTHAL E, GILL H. Fetal ventricular tachycardia secondary to long QT syndrome treated with maternal intravenous magnesium: case report and review of the literature. Ultrasound Obstet Gynecol. 2009;34:475–80.

Simpson JM, Sharland GK. Fetal tachycardias: management and outcome of 127 consecutive cases. Heart. 1998;79:576–81.

Vigneswaran TV, Callaghan N, Andrews RE, Miller O, Rosenthal E, Sharland GK, Simpson JM. Correlation of maternal flecainide concentrations and therapeutic effect in fetal supraventricular tachycardia. Heart Rhythm. 2014;11:2047–53.

Role of Fetal Cardiac Magnetic Resonance Imaging

12

Kuberan Pushparajah and David F.A. Lloyd

Abstract

Cardiac magnetic resonance imaging (CMR) is widely used in the diagnosis and assessment of congenital heart disease (CHD) in postnatal life. However, technical constraints have historically limited its application in fetal cardiology where echocardiography remains the major diagnostic imaging modality. Recent technological advances in CMR have led to its use as an adjunct in the diagnosis of structural fetal cardiac defects. Quantification of flow and oxygen content by CMR allows assessment of changes in the fetal circulation in the setting of structural heart disease in the third trimester. It has an additive role in diagnosing associated extracardiac abnormalities, such as co-existing lung pathology, laterality disorders and brain lesions. These major advances currently serve as research tools but already demonstrate potential to form part of mainstream clinical care in the coming years.

Keywords

Cardiac magnetic resonance imaging · Fetal · Morphology · Vascular · Intracardiac · Extracardiac · Flow · Haemodynamics

Basics of CMR in Congenital Heart Disease

Cardiac magnetic resonance imaging (CMR) is an established imaging tool in the multimodality assessment of CHD in early postnatal life through to adulthood. It permits detailed assessment of cardiac anatomy and cardiovascular haemodynamics. This includes static and dynamic, 2D and 3D imaging of cardiac structures. Quantification of ventricular volumes and flow across major vessels permit the assessment of cardiac function and haemodynamics. Tissue characterization defines myocardial characteristics including fibrosis and scar. Some angiographic and tissue characterisation sequences require intravenous administration of gadolinium-based contrast agents.

Most CMR imaging sequences in postnatal life require ECG-gating and are susceptible to motion artifact and as such requires a patient to remain still, often with breath-holds to reduce motion. Free breathing sequences can be employed and require some form of image averaging and navigator sequences that track the diaphragm to compensate for respiratory motion.

Electronic Supplementary Material The online version of this chapter (https://doi.org/10.1007/978-3-319-77461-9_12) contains supplementary material, which is available to authorized users.

K. Pushparajah · D. F.A. Lloyd (✉)
King's College London, London, UK

Evelina London Children's Hospital, Guys and St Thomas' NHS Foundation Trust, London, UK
e-mail: kuberan.pushparajah@kcl.ac.uk; david.lloyd@kcl.ac.uk

© Springer International Publishing AG, part of Springer Nature 2018
J. Simpson et al. (eds.), *Fetal Cardiology*, https://doi.org/10.1007/978-3-319-77461-9_12

There are established recommendations for an approach to imaging in CHD (Fratz et al. 2013) however, no guidelines exist for fetal CMR.

Technical Challenges in Fetal CMR

Imaging in the fetus is challenged by unpredictable fetal motion in all dimensions, maternal bulk motion, and respiratory motion in both the mother and fetus. The fetal heart is also small and beats at high heart rates, thereby challenging the limits of spatial and temporal resolution of conventional CMR without an available ECG trigger. An ECG trigger is also essential in phase contrast CMR sequences for flow quantification. There are currently no reliable means of obtaining an actual fetal ECG signal during CMR. Intravenous contrast is generally avoided in pregnancy and has no role in fetal CMR. Sedation of the fetus is also avoided due to safety concerns.

Imaging Capabilities in Fetal CMR

Critical elements of fetal CMR include maintaining comfort of the mother during the scan, and safety of the mother and fetus. Fetal CMR has been shown to be safe, but attention needs to be paid to minimise the generation of heat and noise.

Current fetal CMR imaging protocols are published and available for review (Lloyd et al. 2016b, Prsa et al. 2014).These include single-shot fast spin-echo ('SSFSE') where the blood-pool and vessels appear black against the bright, fluid filled lungs and balanced steady-state free precession ('bSSFP') gradient echo sequences where the blood-pool appears white with better visualisation of the myocardium. These sequences offer the best signal contrast and spatiotemporal resolution. Coverage consists of multi-slice imaging to provide whole heart coverage using parallel overlapping slices or single-slice imaging in targeted scan planes where dynamic imaging is needed.

The standard approach to fetal MR imaging is to acquire a sequence of contiguous 2D dimensional images as a "stack" in pre-determined orthogonal planes relative the fetal thorax. To manage fetal motion, this acquisition phase will usually require some flexibility from the operator, with adjustment to the field of view, acquisition plane, number of slices, and repeated sequences when needed, with off-line analysis of acquired data.

Flow assessment is now available mainly through the incorporation of metric optimised gating techniques, which utilises 'oversampled data' and retrospectively reconstructs the data in an iterative manner according to a hypothetical ECG waveform until an image metric is optimized. This technique has been validated in phase contrast flow quantification and cine imaging in the fetus (Jansz et al. 2010). Measurements of oxygen saturation by means of T2 mapping in large vessels when combined with phase contrast flows allow for assessment of oxygen delivery and consumption in the fetal circulation (Sun et al. 2015).

Indications for Fetal CMR and Added Value

Fetal echocardiography is widely accepted as the imaging modality of choice in the prenatal assessment of congenital heart disease. However, there are inherent limitations with its diagnostic accuracy particularly in some forms of congenital heart disease (Bensemlali et al. 2016) creating a need to identify other means of imaging to improve this. Fetal CMR is appealing in that it allows for acquisition of a 3D dataset to identify complex structural lesions, along with quantification of flow to assess changes in the fetal circulation with congenital heart disease. The current capabilities of fetal CMR are explained in the following section.

Morphological Assessment

Intracardiac Anatomy

Balanced steady state free precession (bSSFP) can be used to generate a limited assessment of general intracardiac morphology, such a ventricular asymmetry, cardiac diverticulums or aneurysms, and intracardiac masses (Fig. 12.1a–c). bSSFP sequences can be planned as either as

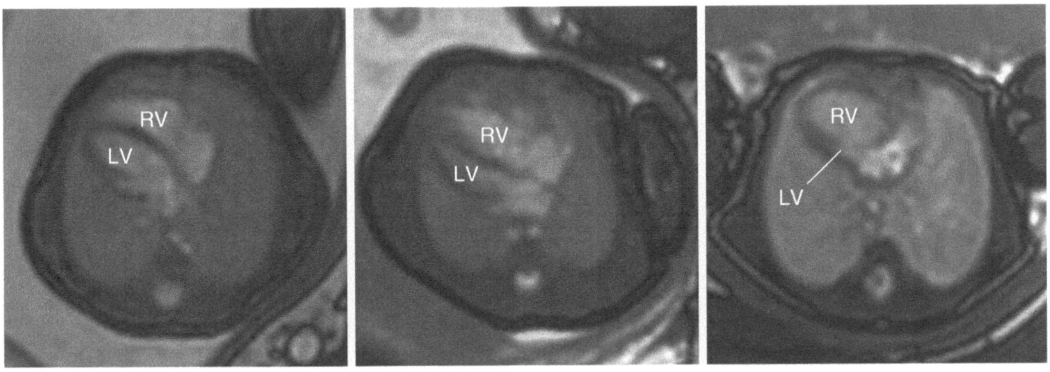

Fig. 12.1 Transverse axial plane bSSFP cine imaging in a normal fetus (left panel), a fetus with left ventricular hypoplasia associated with coarctation of the aorta (middle panel) and a fetus with hypoplastic left heart syndrome (right panel). *LV* left ventricle, *RV* right ventricle

stack of single two-dimensional (2D) slices or a single slice "cine" sequence for dynamic imaging. Blurring and motion artefacts are common in the presence of excessive fetal motion. Despite this, there may be additive value in cases where echocardiography has been limited by late presentation or maternal habitus. When used in combination with fast spin echo sequences, it allows for limited tissue characterisation of intracardiac masses (Lloyd et al. 2016b).

Vascular Assessment

Major vessels are more static over short periods than the beating heart, and as such can generally be imaged more effectively with CMR. Single shot fast spin echo (SSFSE) sequences produce high contrast between the vessels are surrounding structures in the thorax. bSSFP, while less robust to motion, also generate contrast between intraluminal blood and the vessel wall, which may be useful over SSFE sequences for vessels in close proximity either to each other or to the base of the heart.

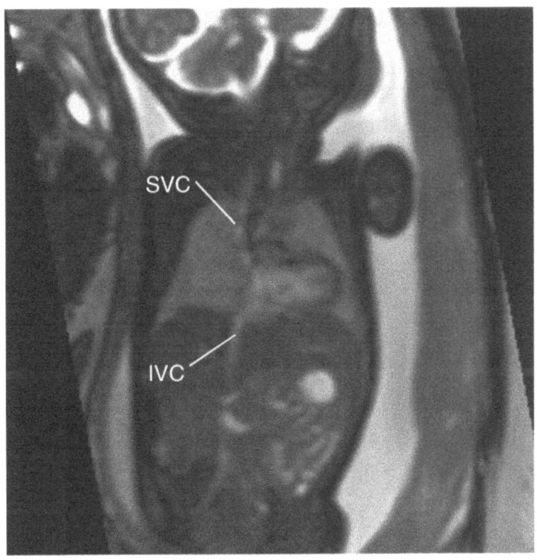

Fig. 12.2 Bicaval view with single right superior vena cava (SVC) and inferior vena cava (IVC) to right atrium (bSSFP)

Systemic and Pulmonary Venous Drainage

The larger field of view in fetal CMR may provide useful anatomical information of systemic and pulmonary venous connections, which may be difficult to obtain using echocardiography alone (Figs. 12.2 and 12.3). Anomalies of pulmonary venous drainage are best seen on SSFE sequences where the surrounding lung provides good contrast against the pulmonary veins (Figs. 12.4 and 12.5).

Pulmonary Arteries

CMR may have an adjunctive role in cases where identifying the source of pulmonary blood supply is challenging to define by echocardiography, such as cases of pulmonary atresia associated with major aortopulmonary collaterals (MAPCAs) and common arterial trunk (Fig. 12.6).

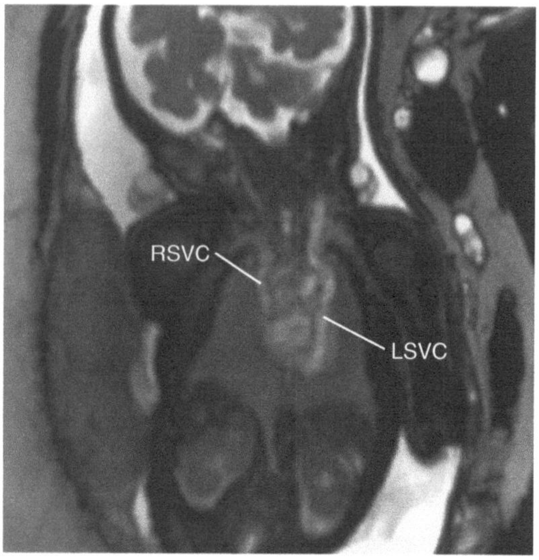

Fig. 12.3 Bilateral superior vena cavas (SVCs), with the right SVC (RSVC) draining to the right atrium and the left SVC (LSVC) draining to the coronary sinus with no bridging vein (bSSFP)

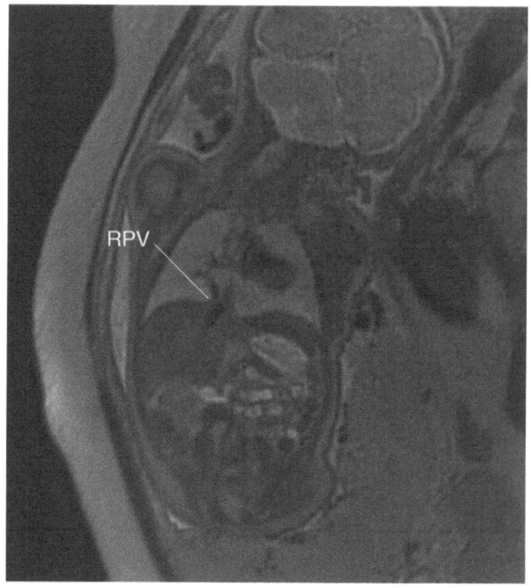

Fig. 12.5 Partial anomalous pulmonary venous drainage of right pulmonary veins to the IVC (SSFSE). *RPV* right pulmonary veins

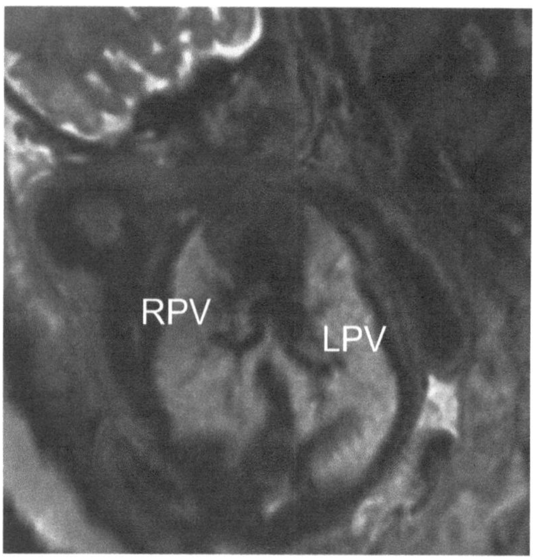

Fig. 12.4 Abnormal pulmonary venous drainage with tortuous pulmonary veins in a patient with hypoplastic left heart syndrome (SSFSE) (*RPV* right pulmonary veins, *LPV* left pulmonary veins)

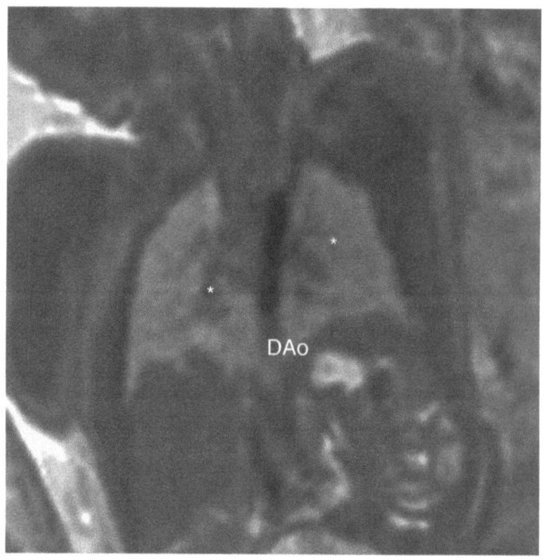

Fig. 12.6 Coronal projection of the descending aorta (DAo) giving rise to major aortopulmonary collateral arteries (marked with asterisks; SSFSE)

Aortic Arch Anomalies

CMR provides excellent characterisation of the vascular anatomy of the aortic arch and its branching pattern particularly in cases of suspected vascular rings, offering not just a view of the arch but its relationship with the trachea (Figs. 12.7, 12.8, and 12.9).

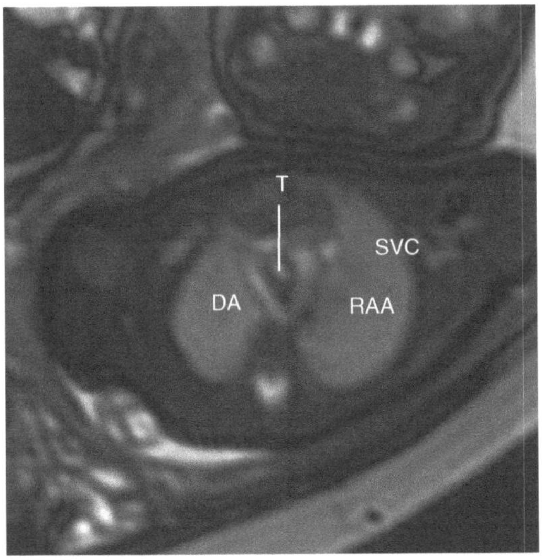

Fig. 12.7 Axial plane of right aortic arch (bSSFP). *DA* arterial duct, *T* trachea, *RAA* right aortic arch, *SVC* superior vena cava

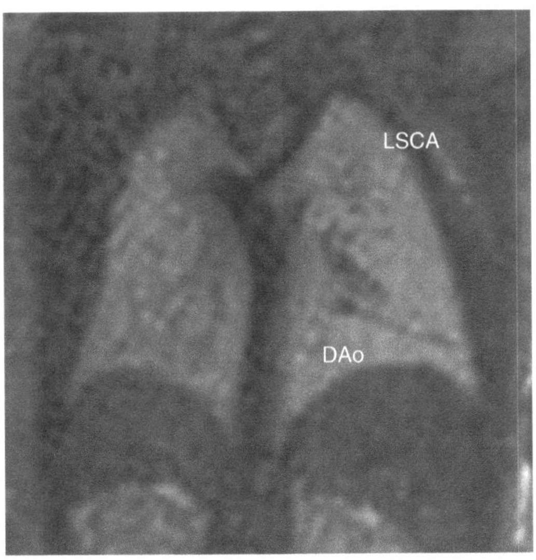

Fig. 12.8 Right arch with aberrant left subclavian artery (LSCA) (SSFSE). *DAo* descending aorta

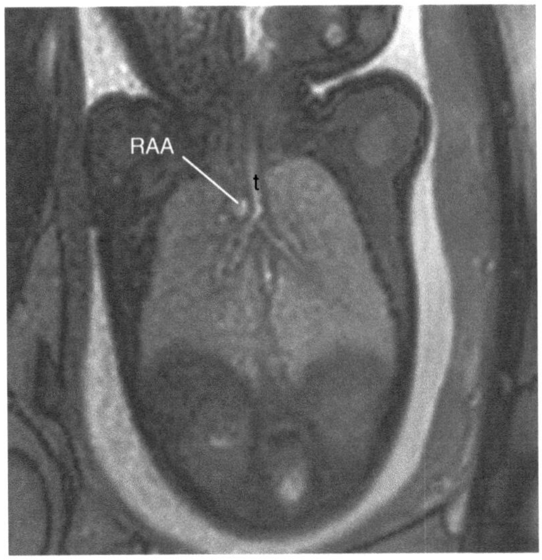

Fig. 12.9 The normal trachea (t) with a mild indentation of the distal trachea from a right aortic arch (RAA)

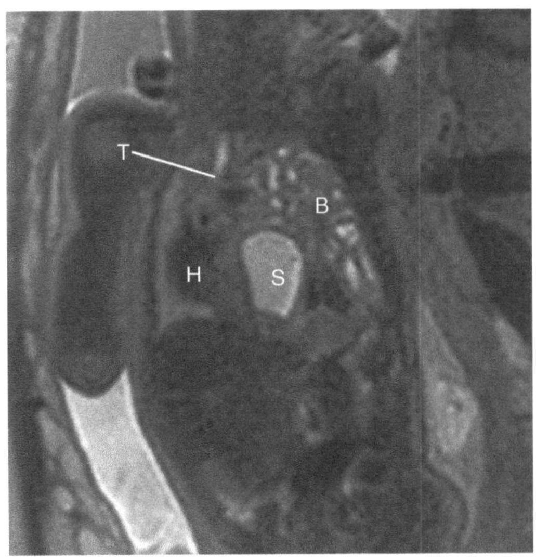

Fig. 12.10 Large left sided congenital diaphragmatic hernia. The stomach (S) and bowel (B) are in the left chest, with tracheal deviation (T) and dextroposition of the heart (H)

Extracardiac Structures

CMR has a larger field of view compared to echocardiography. Contiguous 2D sequences covering the abdomen and thorax can provide useful information such as the position of the liver, stomach and spleen in suspected laterality disorders, such as left or right isomerism. These can provide complementary information in extracardiac conditions with strong associations with CHD, such as congenital diaphragmatic hernia (CDH), pulmonary agenesis, and/or tracheal abnormalities (Figs. 12.9 and 12.10).

Characterisation of lung parenchyma has an important bearing on further investigations,

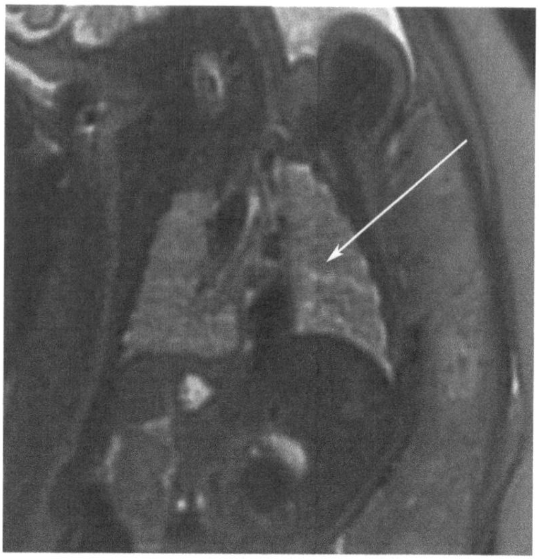

Fig. 12.11 Prominent interlobular septal thickening (arrowed) and enhanced T2 signal in pulmonary lymphangiectasia in a fetus with hypoplastic left heart syndrome

long-term prognosis and antenatal counselling for patients with some forms of CHD. Fetal CMR can identify patients at high risk of early postnatal airway obstruction due to external compression from massive pulmonary arteries in absent pulmonary valve syndrome, and pulmonary lymphangiectasia in patients with pulmonary venous obstruction or intact atrial septum in hypoplastic left heart syndrome (HLHS) (Saul et al. 2015) (Fig. 12.11).

Measuring Flow and Haemodynamics

Flow quantification by CMR in major vessels of the fetal circulation is now possible using techniques as previously described. This has led to in-vivo assessment and mapping of the distribution of blood flow in the fetus (Prsa et al. 2014) (Fig. 12.12). Methods of estimating fetal weight

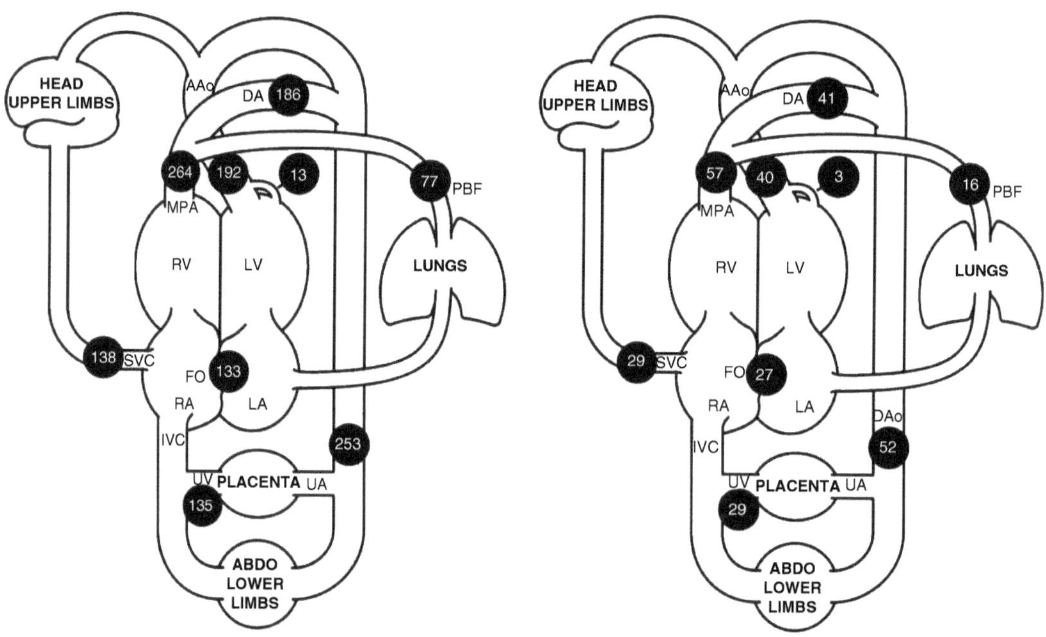

Fig. 12.12 Distribution of the normal human fetal circulation measured by phase-contrast MRI in 40 late-gestation foetuses, expressed as mean flows (**left**) and converted to modelled mean percentages of the combined ventricular output (**right**). *AAo* ascending aorta, *DA* ductus arteriosus, *DAo* descending aorta, *FO* foramen ovale, *LA* left atrium, *LV* left ventricle, *MPA* main pulmonary artery, *PBF* pulmonary blood ow, *RA* right atrium, *RV* right ventricle, *SVC* superior vena cava, *UA* umbilical artery, and *UV* umbilical vein (Prsa et al. 2014). Figure courtesy of Mike Seed, Chris Macgown, Luke Itani, The Hospital for Sick Children, Toronto, Canada, reprinted with permission from circimaging.ahajournals.org/content/7/4/663

from CMR now allow for indexing of flow values to fetal weight. Patterns of blood flow have now been described in the normal fetus and in a spectrum of CHD such as obstructive left heart disease, right heart obstruction and common mixing lesions (Sun et al. 2015).

This is now providing major insights not only to the physiological disruptions to the fetal circulation in CHD, but also the effects on blood flow to the developing fetal brain. When combined with other advanced CMR techniques, such as the T1 and T2 mapping, they may be used to non-invasively estimate intravascular oxygen content as well as end-organ oxygen delivery and consumption. These will provide further insights on the impact of the fetal circulation in CHD on normal fetal growth and neurodevelopment. They can also be applied to assess the effects of interventions such as maternal hyperoxygenation on the placental and fetal circulation.

Future Directions

Computational motion corrected slice-to-volume registration algorithms are now being applied to the multi-slice imaging datasets to reduce motion artefacts. These static 3D datasets can then be interrogated by means of multiplanar reconstruction (MPR) techniques (Fig. 12.13) or volume rendering to create a 3D image of a the heart and its vascular connections with promising results (Fig. 12.14) (Lloyd et al. 2016a).

Using similar techniques, oversampled single-slice imaging of the fetal heart in motion has also been shown to be feasible (van Amerom et al. 2017) producing high temporal resolution 2D images of the fetal heart in motion, comparable to echocardiography (Online Video 12.1). This will improve CMR visualisation of intracardiac structures, and in combination with 3D registration techniques, has the potential for detailed functional and volumetric analysis similar to postnatal CMR.

The role for CMR is currently mainly limited to a research environment, but is already showing promise as a clinical tool. Once these techniques are fully validated, faster scanning protocols and automation of post-processing algorithms will enable its application into mainstream clinical practice with the aim of improving clinical decision making and outcomes.

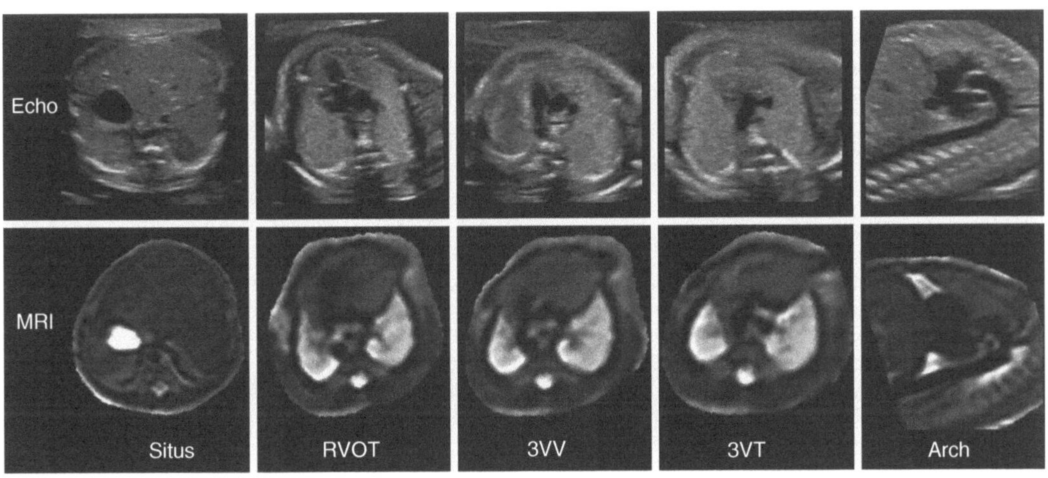

Fig. 12.13 Multiplanar reformatted images from MRI to demonstrate post- processing interrogation of a reconstructed 3D dataset. *RVOT* right ventricular outflow tract; *3VV* three vessel view, *3VT* three vessel and trachea view, *Arch* sagittal view of aortic arch

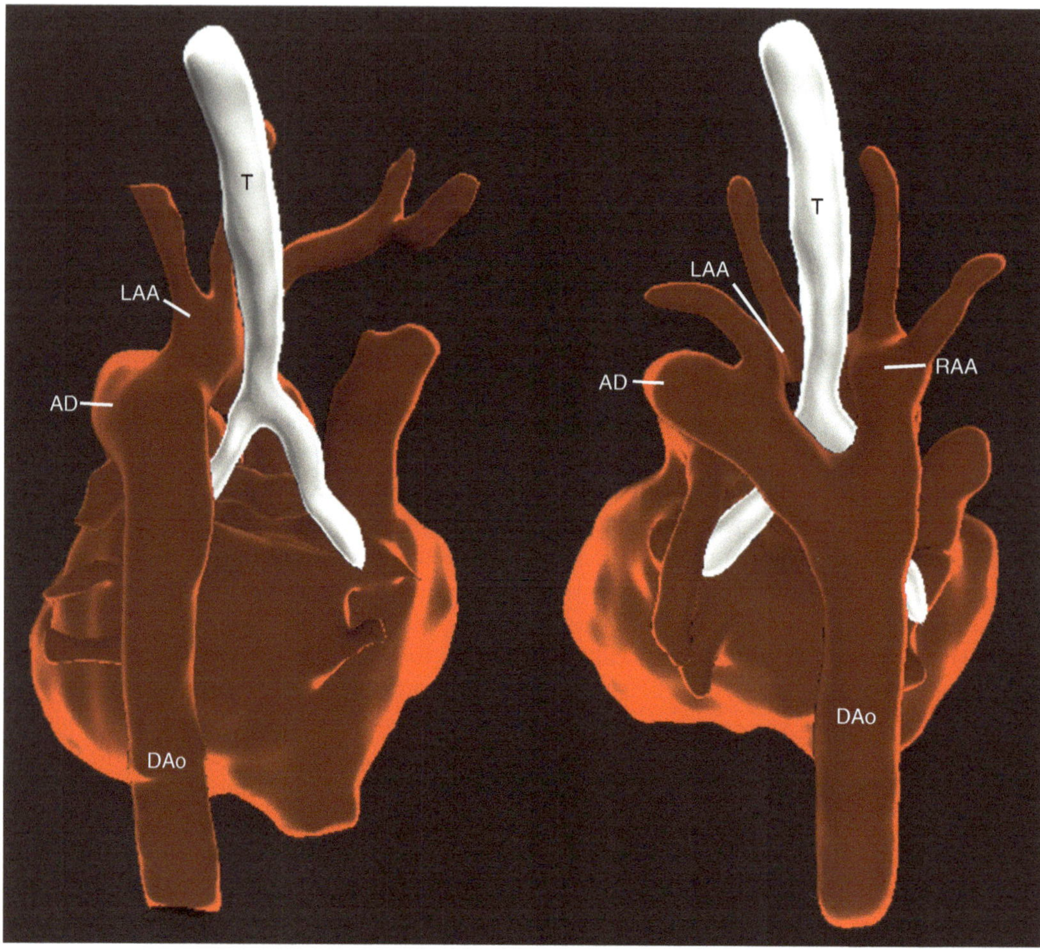

Fig. 12.14 Normal fetal heart at 38 weeks (left) and fetal heart with double aortic arch at 32 weeks (right), both generated from segmentations of motion corrected fetal MRI. Note how the double aortic arch produces a "vascular ring" encompassing the trachea (T). *AD* arterial duct, *LAA* left aortic arch, *RAA* right aortic arch, *DAo* descending aorta

References

Bensemlali M, Stirnemann J, Le Bidois J, Lévy M, Raimondi F, Hery E, Stos B, Bessières B, Boudjemline Y, Bonnet D. Discordances between pre-natal and post-natal diagnoses of congenital heart diseases and impact on care strategies. J Am Coll Cardiol. 2016;68(9):921–30.

Fratz S, Chung T, Greil GF, Samyn MM, Taylor AM, Valsangiacomo Buechel ER, Yoo S-J, Powell AJ. Guidelines and protocols for cardiovascular magnetic resonance in children and adults with congenital heart disease: SCMR expert consensus group on congenital heart disease. J Cardiovasc Magn Reson. 2013;15:51.

Jansz MS, Seed M, van Amerom JFP, Wong D, Grosse-Wortmann L, Yoo S-J, Macgowan CK. Metric optimized gating for fetal cardiac MRI. Magn Reson Med. 2010;64(5):1304–14.

Lloyd D, Kainz B, van Amerom JF, Lohezic M, Pushparajah K, Simpson JM, Malamateniou C, Hajnal JV, Rutherford M, Razavi R. Prenatal MRI visualisation of the aortic arch and fetal vasculature using motion-corrected slice-to-volume reconstruction. J Cardiovasc Magn Reson. 2016a;18(Suppl 1):P180.

Lloyd DFA, van Amerom JFP, Pushparajah K, Simpson JM, Zidere V, Miller O, Sharland G, Allsop J, Fox M, Lohezic M, Murgasova M, Malamateniou C, Hajnal JV, Rutherford M, Razavi R. An exploration of the potential utility of fetal cardiovascular MRI as an adjunct to fetal echocardiography. Prenat Diagn. 2016b;36(10):916–25.

Prsa M, Sun L, van Amerom J, Yoo S-J, Grosse-Wortmann L, Jaeggi E, Macgowan C, Seed M. Reference ranges of blood flow in the major vessels of the normal human fetal circulation at term by phase-contrast magnetic resonance imaging. Circ Cardiovasc Imaging. 2014;7(4):663–70.

Saul D, Degenhardt K, Iyoob SD, Surrey LF, Johnson AM, Johnson MP, Rychik J, Victoria T. Hypoplastic left heart syndrome and the nutmeg lung pattern in utero: a cause and effect relationship or prognostic indicator? Pediatr Radiol. 2015;46(4):483–9.

Sun L, Macgowan CK, Sled JG, Yoo S-J, Manlhiot C, Porayette P, Grosse-Wortmann L, Jaeggi E, McCrindle BW, Kingdom J, Hickey E, Miller S, Seed M. Reduced fetal cerebral oxygen consumption is associated with smaller brain size in fetuses with congenital heart disease. Circulation. 2015;131(15):1313–23.

van Amerom JFP, Lloyd DFA, Price AN, Kuklisova Murgasova M, Aljabar P, Malik SJ, Lohezic M, Rutherford MA, Pushparajah K, Razavi R, Hajnal JV. Fetal cardiac cine imaging using highly accelerated dynamic MRI with retrospective motion correction and outlier rejection. Magn Reson Med. 2017;39:322.

Counselling Following a Prenatal Diagnosis of Congenital Heart Disease

13

Judith Tenenbaum

Abstract
Counselling and support of parents following a prenatal diagnosis of congenital heart disease (CHD) is a complex process. This chapter outlines the general approach which is adopted at our unit to provide explanation and support following diagnosis of CHD during fetal life. There is an emphasis on the practical considerations including the impact of referral indication, the ultrasound examination itself and the provision of information and support both at the time of diagnosis and during follow-up.

Keywords
Prenatal diagnosis · Counselling · Support · Congenital heart disease

Introduction

The purpose of this chapter is to discuss the approach to counselling and support following prenatal diagnosis of congenital heart disease (CHD). Years of development and research in fetal echocardiography have enabled practitioners to diagnose a wide variety of different forms of CHD during fetal life. There are large published series confirming a high degree of diagnostic accuracy in experienced hands. At the same time methods of counselling have been identified, but unlike the diagnostic portion of the fetal scans, research into the most effective way of counselling is in its early stages. This chapter will take a practical approach to this subject, largely based on the experience at a large tertiary fetal cardiology centre. The inclusion of factors which impact on parental reaction to fetal diagnosis of CHD prior to referral, during the ultrasound scanning process itself as well as after the diagnosis has been confirmed will all be addressed.

Impact of Referral Indication

Ultrasound scanning takes place throughout pregnancy with frequency and rationale for scanning depending on sonographic findings, fetal growth and historic risk factors. It is also affected by the compliance of the mother in attending appointments, the accessibility of pre-natal care for the patient, and the adequate provision by the mother (and father) of pertinent medical history. Broadly speaking, the reasons for fetal echocardiography can be divided into those which are known prior to conception, such as maternal diabetes mellitus or a family history of congenital

J. Tenenbaum
Evelina London Children's Hospital, Guy's and St Thomas' NHS Foundation Trust, London, UK

Children's Heart Center, Mount Sinai Health System, New York, NY, USA
e-mail: judith.tenenbaumevans@mountsinai.org

© Springer International Publishing AG, part of Springer Nature 2018
J. Simpson et al. (eds.), *Fetal Cardiology*, https://doi.org/10.1007/978-3-319-77461-9_13

heart disease, and fetal risk factors such as increased nuchal translucency or suspected congenital heart disease. These referral indications are covered extensively in Chap. 1 of this book.

For most pre-existing factors, the vast majority of fetuses will prove to have a normal heart and in most cases fetal echocardiography will provide reassurance of normality. This process remains stressful for parents particularly for those with prior experience of severe congenital heart disease in a previous child who may be returning to the same centre where the child (or parent) was managed. In this setting, there is huge value in being able to reassure expectant parents who are understandably anxious.

Given this background, the diagnosis of CHD in pregnancies where fetal echocardiography was expected to provide reassurance, is particularly distressing because the parents may be relatively unprepared for the news. This makes explanation of the newly diagnosed CHD particularly difficult because parents may be too upset to absorb relevant information. It is important that those undergoing detailed assessment know why they have been referred and that there is a possibility that congenital heart disease might be identified. Parents are unlikely to be familiar with the indications for detailed fetal echocardiography and some may not know what the scan entails or the implications. It is vital that all those involved with the screening and referral process provide patient education and information so that parental expectations are set appropriately. If the information is provided in a thoughtful and informative manner the patient will be more prepared for the scan and the potential findings.

In contrast to the groups above, if a referral is made because of a major fetal risk factor such as raised nuchal translucency or suspected CHD then the parents are generally far more aware of the potential for a diagnosis of CHD. Some may have undergone prior testing such as chorionic villous sampling or amniocentesis. Most parents in this setting are acutely aware that an abnormality might be confirmed. Although many specialists referring mothers for details cardiac assessment are accurate in the diagnosis of specific cardiac lesions, in our experience, being too precise about the exact nature of the lesion, prior to detailed assessment may be counterproductive. We have encountered some parents who have done extensive reading about the wrong diagnosis prior to attendance. Counselling in this situation may have to start with revising a previous diagnosis, which complicates understanding and trust in a significant way. In most circumstances, it is probably best if parents are aware of the findings which have prompted referral i.e. a suspicion of CHD without being too detailed about the exact nature of the lesion.

The Ultrasound Scan

Parents are advised to come for the scan accompanied by their partner, a relative or a friend for support. Fetal cardiology sonographers will be familiar with the indications for referral in addition to the specific technical training required to complete the scan. The sonographer will also need to observe any non-verbal communication that indicates the patient's level of anxiety. It is vital that all staff know the specific referral indication prior to beginning the scan. If a pregnancy is being assessed because of a recent history of major CHD in a previous baby, then it is entirely understandable that parents will be very anxious. Most specialist fetal cardiology services, whether part of a CHD service or practising within a fetal medicine service, are based in a teaching hospital environment. This raises some practical issues with respect to the approach. From patient feedback, the number of people present in the scanning room can be an issue. In our own setting, consent is routinely taken for the examination and a "running commentary" on the scan is not undertaken in the room. It may be difficult to discuss differential diagnoses in front of the patient until a definite diagnosis has been made. At our centre, discussions by the operator as the scan progresses is led by senior staff and needs to be handled sensitively. The use of a separate room for reviewing scans in depth may be of value. If normality of the heart is confirmed, then the result is conveyed to the parents rapidly once the scan is complete. Following detection of an abnormality, our preference is to explain the findings in a room separate from the ultrasound room itself. If friends or relatives have accompanied the parents, the parents make the decision on who should join the conversation. The cardiologist provides the initial counselling and our practice is for a fetal cardiology clinical nurse specialist to participate in the initial discussion as well as ongoing follow-up consultations.

Approach to Explanation of CHD

Prenatal counselling, after a diagnosis of CHD has been detected, is a detailed and emotional process. In a short amount of time, the professionals involved need to establish a relationship with the parents based on frankness, openness and honesty (Allan and Huggon 2004; Bratt et al. 2015; Carlsson et al. 2015). An appreciation and respect for the individual beliefs and backgrounds of the parents must be established. Professionals assigned the responsibility of providing information to patients must remember that they will be using the 'language of medicine', which may be unfamiliar to that family.

The exact approach followed will vary between units but in general the approach, which we adopt, is as follows:

Description of the Normal Heart and the Abnormality

Before providing an explanation of the findings of the heart scans, a drawing of the normal heart and how it works is provided. Differences between the circulations before and after birth are addressed, if relevant to the CHD diagnosed. This diagram is then compared to one of the heart lesion with an explanation of the impact of the abnormalities. Feedback from parents has indicated that they appreciate this individual approach. As professionals we are familiar and confident in the anatomy, physiology and methods of treating CHD. For families, however, it is like hearing a foreign language for the first time, which has vital information and implications for their unborn child. Even if a parent has a background in science, they are a novice in comprehending and reacting to a fetal diagnosis of CHD. It may take time and follow up consultations for parents to take on board the implications of the cardiac defect, but many parents will quite rapidly become familiar with the medical 'jargon' and the use of metaphors can be helpful. Explaining the physiology of the human heart can be explained in an alternative way, for example to explain the narrowing of a blood vessel, "if you step on a garden hose the water will find it difficult to get through." During the explanation of the cardiac lesion, the parents will need to understand which aspects are certain and any areas of diagnostic doubt. For example, in a fetus with suspected coarctation of the aorta, it may not be clear during fetal life whether surgery will be required after birth, or the exact approach, which might be taken.

Implications of the Diagnosis

Once the nature of the cardiac lesion has been explained, then an explanation of the implications of the diagnosis typically follows. From a medical perspective, this may include the nature of any surgery and attendant risks, as well as short, medium, and longer-term survival chances. This poses particular challenges because for many types of CHD the therapeutic approach will have evolved over time and the long term prognosis may not be known with certainty. The quality of life is a frequent cause for concern for expectant parents, which is explored further below.

Potential Associations of the Cardiac Lesion

Some forms of congenital heart disease are strongly associated with extra-cardiac abnormalities including aneuploidies and structural malformations. Parents need to be informed of such associations and the means of investigation such as amniocentesis which may clarify the overall picture. This will involve liaison with fetal medicine specialists and others to arrange appropriate investigations and for their input into management.

Parental Options

Following the explanation of the findings and postnatal management strategy, the options for parents are explained. These include options of further investigation such as fetal karyotyping or further anomaly scanning. It is well recognised that verbal information provided to distressed parents may not be readily absorbed. The role of the professionals includes provision of printed information which pertains to the individual situation, coupled with an explanation of such information. Published, recognised information booklets on CHD should be provided as well as information and contact detail for support groups, where appropriate. This should be identified as an option for families, but they will have a personal choice as to whether they will value this type of support. The provision of such information should complement, and not substitute for, ongoing contact and support. The parents may consider the option of termination of pregnancy depending on the severity of the cardiac lesion and associated abnormalities based on the prognosis (Menahem and Grimwade 2003). The options available vary between countries according to local laws and religious practices. Parents should be allowed 'time and space' to absorb and react to the cardiac diagnosis and other information. If parents are considering termination of pregnancy, honest, factual information is crucial because in some countries the options are linked to the gestational age of the fetus as well as the severity of the fetal abnormalities. In all circumstances, it is the parents who make the final decision about how they wish to proceed.

Support for Parents Through the Decision-Making Process

The brief overview outlined above does not address many important aspects of decision-making. The decision-making process begins at the first meeting. To support the parents with all the information they are receiving, a temporal sequence is advised. A temporal sequence is facilitated by a 'step by step' approach. The parent, or parents, must begin to process information at a very emotional time. They will innately start to use previous coping mechanisms to life changing events in their past. They may react on an individual basis or on their experience as a couple. Feedback from parents and previous work (Menahem and Grimwade 2005) has shown that "parents are particularly concerned, not so much about the detail of the abnormality, but rather about specific issues relating to the pregnancy and perinatal care, and the subsequent impact on the well being of the infant/child/adolescent and to adulthood." This presents a challenge to provide a 'camera into the future.' During pregnancy parents wonder, 'what will my child be like?' Will they be sporty or musical? They will hope and dream for a positive future for their child. At the point of a fetal cardiac diagnosis they must adjust to a new reality. The excitement towards bringing a child into the world is empowering, but for many couples absorbing the information of a heart defect weakens them and many feel powerless. A parent once told me that when they left our department and walked to the train station he realised that the 'rest of the world would just keep spinning.' He saw people getting angry on the train platform because the scheduled train was cancelled. The parent felt invisible, that no one else could, or would, be able to understand what had happened to them, to the news that they heard and the decisions that they now had to make.

It is important to identify this sort of emotional reaction even if the parent does not disclose it. An emotion may be identified that the parent may not see himself or herself. In the midtrimester, when most CHD is diagnosed, the mother and her partner/husband will have told friends and family of their pregnancy. They will have started making plans for their new arrival, but this excitement evaporates when they are informed that their baby has something wrong with their heart. Mixed with the awakening grief, there is often denial and disbelief, suppressed or overt anger and in some cases an attempt to question your expertise.

Parents are faced with a private decision to make which can be lonely and isolating for each parent individually, or as a couple. They are faced with a life-changing decision whilst at the same time having to deal with the ongoing responsibilities of daily life, which can include other family and work. Developing resilience to this situation during pregnancy will help them cope with caring for a child with CHD, or for the bereavement associated with the termination of their pregnancy. One of the aims of specialist support is to avoid feelings of guilt and blame. If one parent is affected with CHD they may blame themselves for recurrence and possible attribution of CHD to some drugs may also lead to self-recrimination.

Parents will often ask, "What would you do in this situation?" or "What do you advise?" to the health professionals involved and will often seek validation of their decision. In this situation, it is imperative to be objective and recognise that although professionals are providing the information and support, they have not been in the same position as the parents, so the decision-making process remains with the parents. In our practice, we guide parents to take ownership of their decision. They may want to seek support from families and/or friends but ultimately the decision is theirs.

Use of Diagrams and Flowcharts

Many parents have reported that they value some visual presentation of decision-making and ongoing care. In our practice we have found such an approach helpful and an example is shown in Fig. 13.1. For the professional, this flow chart or 'mind map' will also assist in the formation of an algorithm of what to say and the order in which information is given. Prenatal counselling is not a mathematical problem, but it does require logical and clear steps to ensure parental understanding. There is also a benefit to the professional in having an algorithm, or structure, to follow to ensure that all aspects of counselling are provided in a consistent manner.

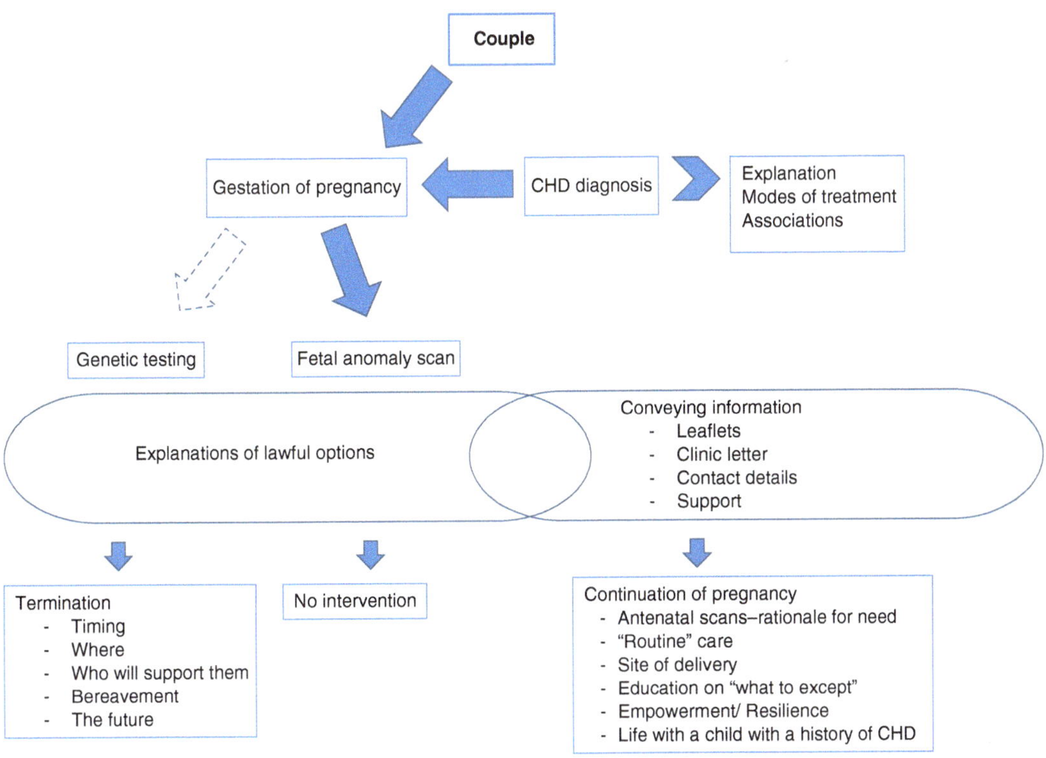

Fig. 13.1 Flow chart outlining the approach to prenatal diagnosis of CHD

Parents themselves and/or relations may turn to the Internet for more information on the CHD diagnosis of their unborn baby. The practitioner cannot deny the parents' choice to seek alternative forms of information. Our own approach is to volunteer links to reliable sources and to ensure that this is pertinent to the individual situation. There are also occasions when a family may request a second opinion from a different specialist centre. Some parents value having the opinions of more than one centre as part of the exploration of their options. In our own practice, we support and facilitate their request by contacting another tertiary centre and by a written referral letter. Parents may either have a view as to which unit they wish to be referred to, or else ask for suggestions as to which units may be able to meet this request.

Assisting Families Understand the Future for Their Baby

Families will be hoping for a normal lifespan and quality of life for their child. It is important that they understand the limitations of medical knowledge in this respect and the challenge in fully predicting lifelong morbidity and impact of life span for many forms of CHD. It is often the case that parents will feel better able to cope with uncertainty by the provision of statistics on success of the operative procedure that they may expect for their baby. Direct, honest and knowledgeable responses are required. For example, explaining that the arterial switch procedure has been performed for less than 40 years, indicating the age of the oldest survivor provides parents with some sense of perspective. In situations where there is evidence of improving techniques and outcome, provision of such information may bring a degree of comfort and security to the parents. Yet, we must also be honest in explaining why only a minority of major operations or cardiac interventions have a 100% success rate, and what the considerations are with respect to longer term follow-up. There may also be aspects of care for example, future neurological development, functional status, or behavioural issues, where concerns may remain and where a candid discussion with expectant parents is vital (Lafranchi and Lincoln 2015). Explaining the course of treatment including surgery, intensive care and risks are part of the counselling, as well as the longer-term prognosis as far as this can be determined. The provision of several consultations during the pregnancy both with senior medical staff and ongoing specialist nursing support aim to address this requirement. Providing information on family support groups at the first counselling session is essential. Parents may choose to seek guidance from these groups on an individual basis. It is our responsibility to explain the benefits of talking to other parents who have been in similar situations, yet remembering for some parents, for personal reasons, this may not be a choice they will pursue following diagnosis or following delivery.

The Legality of Decision-Making

As previously mentioned, parents deal with the information presented from both their intelligence and emotions, and are faced with making a life-changing decision they never thought would ever be a reality. As one parent said, "I was hopeful that someone would wake me up, was I dreaming, was this all really happening to us?"

It is imperative that all lawful options are explained to parents which varies between countries and frequently between regions in the same country. This may affect treatment options as well as the option of termination of pregnancy. As emphasised above, the final decision on continuation of pregnancy or termination rests with the parents. Feedback from couples has shown appreciation of the honest advice that the decision 'belonged to them.' With the initial impact of detection of CHD, it is important for parents to realise that they do not have to make the decision at the initial meeting and the option to return for further discussion should be provided. In addition to prenatal decisions, in certain circumstances there may be the option of non-intervention after birth depending on the prognosis of the cardiac lesion and/or associated anomalies. In our own practice, for example, some parents may not request postnatal surgery in severe forms of hypoplastic left heart syndrome. Guidance around such decision-making will vary in different countries and in such circumstances it is critical that there is a wide discussion between clinicians in advance of delivery. The involvement of palliative care specialists is invaluable so that a plan is agreed between the parents and clinicians in advance of delivery.

Concluding the Counselling Session

A written report of the findings of the fetal cardiac scan and summary of the conversation that took place with the parents should be provided rapidly. This is facilitated by written and electronic communication with parents and other involved healthcare professionals. To promote empowerment and confidence in the parents, they need to know that all teams involved will be "talking to each other". In addition to the written report, other written material should be offered; information on the specific heart diagnosis, hospital prepared leaflets and support leaflets for termination if appropriate. In our department, a direct contact number for the Fetal Cardiology Clinical Nurse Specialist is also provided.

Once their decision is made regarding the pregnancy, the ability to get in touch with someone from the fetal cardiology department is empowering:. "It was important to tell you our decision, it made it feel real, that this was a reality that we were dealing with." Parents also felt comforted that someone was going to put the process in motion, either the continuation or termination of the pregnancy.

Continuation of the Pregnancy

During the first counselling session, an outline of events that will take place during the pregnancy are explained. Specifically, further fetal heart scans accompanied by discussion, support and explanation of the CHD diagnosis and the implications is provided. Accurate information is vital. For diagnosis of duct dependent lesions with a predicted need for intervention in the first days after birth, a discussion of the need for the transfer of delivery to/or near a tertiary heart centre is required. Parents will need to feel confident that the transfer of care is a coordinated process with relevant support in place. Parents find it reassuring that they will need to continue with all their local midwifery and consultant care as they had envisaged when they their pregnancy was confirmed. Collaboration with referring teams is vital. Once the referral to the tertiary fetal medicine department and midwifery group is established, the multi-disciplinary approach will ensure that communication takes place between the groups to provide optimal patient care and meet the needs of both the mother and the unborn baby. Parents will often ask if the mode of delivery needs to be altered. The mode and timing of delivery will need to be discussed by the cardiac and obstetric teams to ensure that information is consistent. The use of named lead specialists in each area assists parents in ensuring that the management plan is consistent and deliverable. For those heart defects that are not duct dependent and who are predicted not to need intervention in the first week of life, local delivery can be organised with the collaboration between the referring hospital and the tertiary centre. What is vital in this circumstance is that the plan for assessment and follow up for the baby is established and that the parents are 'partners' in this process.

In our practice, once parents have made their decision we support their choice and this impacts on the perspective taken in follow-up planning and appointments. A continued and organised provision of information and knowledge is carried out and adapted to the diverse needs of our patients. In our practice, "Antenatal Information Days" are organised so that parents can familiarise themselves with the delivery suite and the intensive care units. They are also given an opportunity to speak with parents who have personal experience of having a child with CHD who has undergone neonatal surgery. Feedback from this approach has proved extremely positive.

An important area for the fetal cardiology team, particularly clinical nurse specialists has proved to be the transition from the "antenatal" to the "postnatal" phase. Following delivery, parents meet a whole range of new teams including intensive care specialists, cardiac surgeons and cardiac interventionalists who may not have been involved with care before birth. There is published evidence of the clear impact birth of a baby with CHD may have on parental mood, particularly stress and depression, even when the diagnosis has been made before birth (Bevilacqua et al. 2013). It is important to educate and prepare parents for what they may experience following delivery. This includes information on what they will see when their baby is in intensive care, an orientation to the structure and policies of the hospital, what they will be able to do for their baby, policies on breastfeeding and storage of breast milk, visiting hours and where they will be staying. In our practice, we have a written hospital information leaflet for parents to improve understanding. Preparation provides the development of self-confidence, which is necessary in caring for a baby with CHD. The continued involvement of those staff who have been involved prenatally has met with favourable feedback and gives parents "a familiar face" and promotes consistency between plans and parental expectations.

For those fetal patients who can deliver at their local hospital in the knowledge that their baby will be discharged home prior to any surgery-taking place, support will need to include both parental education and ensuring that there is a robust plan for review of the child after birth and that local teams are aware of the plans. Liaison should include ensuring that parents are able to meet local paediatricians and other specialists in advance of delivery. This type of liaison is critical in virtually all cases because of the possibility of preterm delivery when delivery will be to the local hospital irrespective of where and when delivery was planned. In our own practice fetal nurse specialists provide guidance on what life at home will be like. In the case of infants with a CHD diagnosis that may develop symptoms of heart failure, information on relevant signs and symptoms should be provided. The goal is for parents to be prepared but not frightened. When this goal is met, parents will be confident in their abilities, which will in turn have an impact on the improvement of patient outcome. Clear parental information on how parents can contact the fetal cardiology service and their local teams is essential.

Looking Towards the Future

If a pregnancy has been affected by CHD, parents will often ask if there is the potential for CHD to recur in future pregnancies. Advice in this regard will need to be individualised depending on the family history and nature of the cardiac lesion. The genetics of CHD, including recurrence risks, is covered in the genetics chapter in this book. It is important for all professionals to ensure that advice in this regard is correct. For future pregnancies, our approach has been to offer early fetal echocardiography where a severe diagnosis has been made. Fetal echocardiography may be offered from around 13–14 weeks gestational age to exclude recurrence of major lesions—this frequently provides early reassurance to parents who have prior experience of a child affected by CHD.

If pregnancy ends in stillbirth or termination then parents will require bereavement support and should have the offer of further contact with the professionals involved. Feedback from our patient group confirmed that this is both necessary and highly appreciated.

For professionals involved in the diagnosis of CHD it is critical to remain up to date with new techniques both in prenatal diagnosis and in postnatal management so that parents are counselled in a manner which reflects current practice. To date, there is no "breakthrough" which can reduce the risk of recurrence of CHD other than folate supplementation which is routine in developed countries in any event. There are several advances in "disease-modification" including the role of maternal hyperoxygenation both with respect to neurological development and altering the natural history of CHD. Keeping abreast of such advances will be necessary to provide some evidence of progress whilst tempering what may be unrealistic expectations of any new therapy.

This chapter provides information on the support which can be given to patients when a fetal diagnosis of CHD is made. It is intended as an outline but the exact approach will vary between departments and professionals according to local practice. Lastly, should we as professionals be better supported? It should be emphasised that for all professionals involved this is also a difficult sub-specialty. Professionals involved should be able to express how this responsibility makes them feel, and to seek advice on how they can improve their methods for the benefit of the patient. Research and analysis of our methods should be encouraged with the involvement of feedback from the patients themselves.

References

Allan LD, Huggon IC. Counselling following a diagnosis of congenital heart disease. Prenat Diagn. 2004;24:1136–42.

Bevilacqua F, Palatta S, Mirante N, Cuttini M, Seganti G, Dotta A, Piersigilli F. Birth of a child with congenital heart disease: emotional reactions of mothers and fathers according to time of diagnosis. J Matern Fetal Neonatal Med. 2013;26(12):1249–53. https://doi.org/10.3109/14767058.2013.776536; Epub 2013 Mar 13.

Bratt EL, Järvholm S, Ekman-Joelsson BM, Mattson LÅ, Mellander M. Parent's experiences of counselling and their need for support following a prenatal diagnosis of congenital heart disease—a qualitative study in a Swedish context. BMC Pregnancy Childbirth. 2015;15:171. https://doi.org/10.1186/s12884-015-0610-4.

Carlsson T, Bergman G, Maritala UM, et al. Information following a diagnosis of congenital heart defect: experiences among parents to prenatally diagnosed children. PLoS One. 2015;10(2):e0117995. https://doi.org/10.1371/journal.pone.0117995.

Hunter LE, Simpson JM. Prenatal screening for structural congenital heart disease. Nat Rev Cardiol. 2014;11:323–34.

Lafranchi T, Lincoln P. 2015. Prenatal counseling and care for single-ventricle heart disease: one center's model for care. Crit Care Nurse. 2015;35(5):53–61. https://doi.org/10.4037/ccn2015247.

Menahem S, Grimwade J. Pregnancy termination following prenatal diagnosis of serious heart disease in the fetus. Early Hum Dev. 2003;73:71–8.

Menahem S, Grimwade J. Pre-natal counselling—helping couples make decisions following the diagnosis of severe heart disease. Early Hum Dev. 2005;81:601–7.

14 Fetal Abnormalities Associated with Congenital Heart Defects

Elena Greco and Sarah Bower

Abstract

Extra-cardiac abnormalities (ECAs) are associated with congenital heart disease (CHD) in up to 70% of fetuses. Characteristic patterns of association may suggest an underlying genetic condition. Alternative aetiologies include maternal metabolic disorders, infections, exposure to drugs and teratogens. The co-existence of ECAs and CHD may profoundly affect prognosis leading to significant morbidity and mortality within this group. If CHD is detected it is crucial to perform a detailed fetal anatomy survey searching for ECAs. Recognition of associated abnormalities and knowledge of underlying causes is important to allow targeted investigations and karyotyping and appropriate counselling. The aim of this chapter is to support the reader in daily practice by reviewing, with wide use of images, the most common aetiologies that must be considered for the diagnostic work-up of fetuses affected by CHD and ECAs.

E. Greco
The Royal London Hospital, London, UK

Fetal Medicine Research Institute, Kings College Hospital, London, UK
e-mail: Elena.Greco@bartshealth.nhs.uk

S. Bower (✉)
Fetal Medicine Research Institute, Kings College Hospital, London, UK
e-mail: Sarah.Bower@nhs.net

Keywords

CHD · Birth defects · Associated anomalies · Aneuploidies · Syndromes · Metabolic disorders · Infections

Overview

There is a well-established, strong association between extra-cardiac fetal abnormalities (ECAs) and congenital heart disease (CHD). The rate of ECAs associated with CHD is highly variable, ranging from 0 up to 70% depending upon defects considered, population studied (inclusion/exclusion of post-mortem findings) and variable prenatal detection rates across different centres (Stoll et al. 2015b; Tegnander et al. 2006). Spontaneous intrauterine loss and elective termination of affected pregnancies account for the lower incidence of such pathologies in live births.

The proportion of fetuses with CHD and ECAs depends on three elements:

1. *Gestational age:* if the cardiac diagnosis is made at an early gestation, the chances of gross, multiple ECAs are higher. Diagnoses made at a later gestational age have a greater association with late-onset anomalies such as fetal growth restriction (FGR) and polyhydramnios.
2. *Severity of CHD:* Severe CHD has a stronger association with ECAs. Referral bias for

© Springer International Publishing AG, part of Springer Nature 2018

J. Simpson et al. (eds.), *Fetal Cardiology*, https://doi.org/10.1007/978-3-319-77461-9_14

Table 14.1 Incidence of extra-cardiac anomalies (ECAs) without or with chromosomal abnormalities in fetuses with congenital heart defects (CHD)

Type of CHD	Toronto study (2009)	Berlin study (1999)	ISPC (1999)	BWIS study (1985)
	Incidence % without and [with] chromosomal abnormalities			
AVSD	15.4 [27.7]	19.1 [61.9]	13.8 [47.1]	24.5
AO stenosis	7.7 [7.7]	- [20]	13 [17.4]	9
TAPVD	– [–]	NA	NA	21
CoA	20 [20]	57.1 [42.9]	12.5 [20.8]	3.5
DORV	25 [33.3]	40 [33.3]	19.3 [45.2]	28
Heterotaxy	44.2 [–]	NA	NA	NA
HLHS	26.3 [3.9]	28.6 [9.5]	10.9 [4.2]	9.1
PS/PA with IVS	13.3 [6.7]	– [–]	25.9 [3.7]	6.8
TGA	16.7 [–]	20 [–]	25.6 [2.6]	7.8
cCTGA	– [–]	NA	5.6 [–]	NA
TOF	26.8 [24.4]	25 [50]	25 [26.7]	22.5
TV atresia	30 [10]	50 [0]	34.4 [8.6]	9.1
CAT	18.2 [36.4]	50 [25]	21.4 [28.6]	39.6
TV dysplasia	17.6 [5.9]	NA	6.25 [6.25]	16
Single ventricle circulation	38.9 [0]	– [–]	17.8 [6.7]	NA

Modified from Song et al. (2009)

detailed anatomy survey in fetuses with gross CHD and chromosomal abnormalities may contribute to this association.

3. *Type of CHD:* it is well recognised that specific cardiac defects carry a greater association with ECAs with or without an underlying genetic abnormality (Table 14.1). Central nervous system, gastro-intestinal, renal and skeletal anomalies are the commonest ECAs found in most prenatal studies (Stoll et al. 2015b).

The co-existence of ECA and CHD may profoundly affect prognosis and perinatal management with mortality rates as high as 70% in this group (Oepkes and Haak 2014). If a cardiac defect is identified, it is therefore crucial to perform a detailed fetal anatomy survey searching for ECAs and to understand patterns of association as well as possible underlying aetiologies, so that targeted investigations and karyotyping are undertaken.

The aim of this chapter is to describe which fetal abnormalities should alert the sonographer to the need for fetal echocardiography, which combination of abnormalities suggest underlying genetic defects and which fetal and maternal conditions are particularly associated with CHD.

First Trimester Abnormalities

Increased Nuchal Translucency

Nuchal translucency (NT) measurement in the first trimester is an effective and established screening method for chromosome abnormality, particularly when used in combination with maternal serum biochemistry (Fig. 14.1). Increased NT is also associated with rare genetic syndromes and structural abnormalities including major CHD. Syngelaki et al. (2011) reported NT measurements greater than the 95th percentile in 34% of such cases. A meta-analysis of chromosomally normal fetuses with major CHD found a NT above the 95th and above the 99th centile in 44% and 20% of fetuses, respectively. However, the authors commented on heterogeneity across the studies as a source of bias (Sotiriadis et al. 2013).

The risk of major CHD increases exponentially with increasing NT with a reported prevalence of about 6% for NT >3.5 mm (Atzei et al. 2005). A NT >3.5 mm should prompt detailed echocardiography in the first trimester or, if this is unavailable, at the time of anomaly scan.

The cause of the increased NT does not appear to be related to the structural cardiac defect as

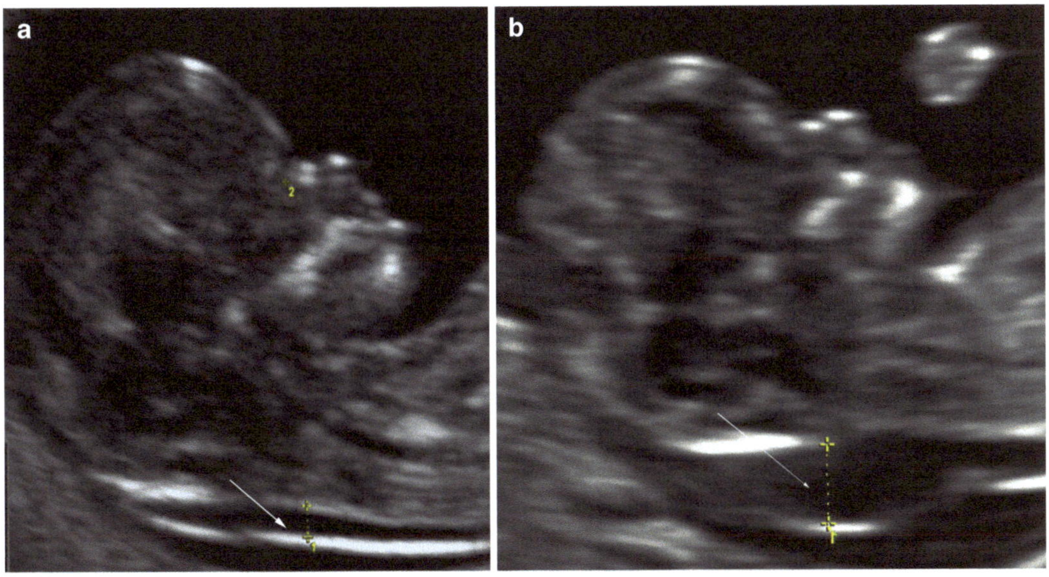

Fig. 14.1 (**a**) Mid-sagittal views of the fetal face demonstrating normal nuchal translucency (NT) thickness and normal nasal bone at 11^{+0} to 13^{+6} weeks scan. The white arrow shows the NT that is the black fluid-filled space outlined by the two white lines corresponding to the occipital bone and the skin. The NT measurement is shown by the yellow caliper (1). The presence of the nasal bone is demonstrated by three echogenic lines visible, representing the tip of the nose, the nasal bridge and the nasal bone (*yellow caliper 2*). (**b**) Mid-sagittal views of the fetal face demonstrating increased nuchal translucency (NT) thickness and absent nasal bone at 11^{+0} to 13^{+6} weeks scan. The white arrow shows increased NT with the measurement shown by the yellow caliper (1). The nasal bone is absent as demonstrated by only two echogenic lines seen (tip of the nose and skin)

several different abnormalities with variable haemodynamics are associated with increased NT. It may result from a temporary impairment of cardiac function early in pregnancy.

Other First Trimester Defects

Some ECAs often associated with CHD can be detected at the time of the first trimester scan (11–13^{+6} weeks' gestation) and should therefore prompt early fetal echocardiography. These include congenital diaphragmatic hernia (CDH), exomphalos, holoprosencephaly, megacystis, encephalocele, cleft lip and palate (Fig. 14.2). Vascular anomalies, such as agenesis of the ductus venosus (DV), can also be detected when examining ductal flow as part of first trimester screening for chromosome abnormalities.

Detection rates for fetal anomalies in the first trimester depend upon the type of defect, skills and training of the operator and the time allocated for a detailed anatomy survey in early pregnancy (Syngelaki et al. 2011).

Hydrops Fetalis

Definition: Hydrops fetalis (HF) is defined as excessive accumulation of fluid in 2 or more serous cavities or body tissues (i.e. pleural effusion, pericardial effusion, ascites and skin oedema) (Fig. 14.3). HF is easily identified by ultrasound at any gestational age. However, HF has a number of primary or secondary cardiac causes as well as other aetiologies (Tables 14.2, 14.3, and 14.4). Thus, determining the underlying cause may be challenging.

Pathophysiology: The accumulation of interstitial fluid in HF results from an imbalance between intravascular and extravascular fluid. The difference between the capillary pressure and the interstitial fluid colloid oncotic pressure governs the movement of fluid out of the

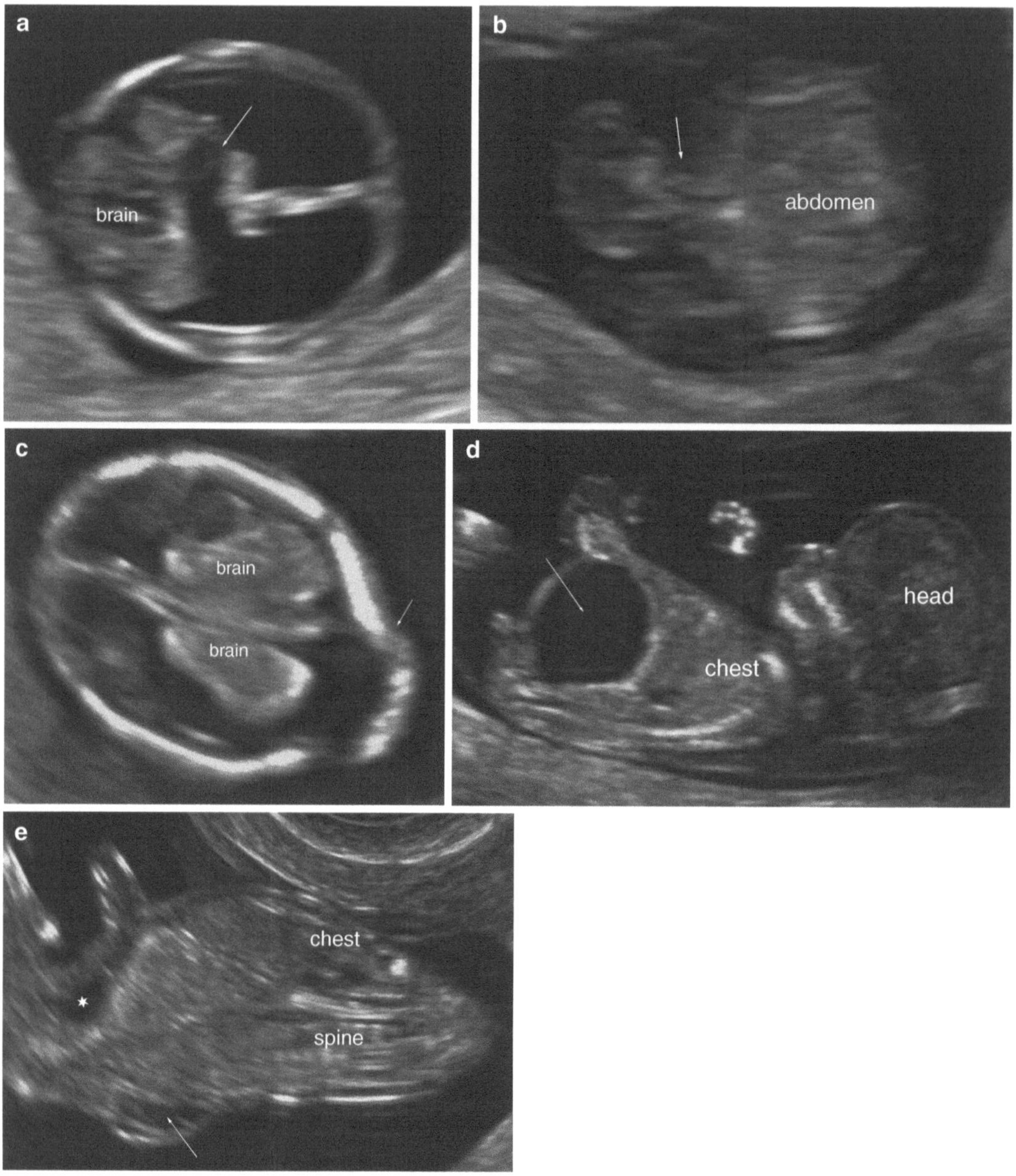

Fig. 14.2 (**a**) Transverse section of the fetal head in a fetus at 12 weeks with holoprosencephaly. The white arrow shows abnormal cleavage of the posterior aspect of the brain. (**b**) Transverse section of the fetal abdomen in a fetus at 12 weeks with exomphalos. The white arrow shows protrusion of echogenic bowel loops within the umbilical cord insertion. (**c**) Transverse section of the fetal head in a fetus at 12 weeks with encephalocele. The white arrow shows loss of continuity in the posterior aspect of the fetal skull with herniation of meninges in the amniotic fluid (meningocele). (**d**) Sagittal section of a 12 weeks fetus with megacystis. The white arrow shows an enlarged bladder extending from the pelvis to the diaphragm. (**e**) Sagittal section of a 12 weeks fetus with spina bifida. The white arrow shows loss of continuity of the skin covering the fetal spine with herniation of meninges and neural tissue (lumbo-sacral spina bifida)

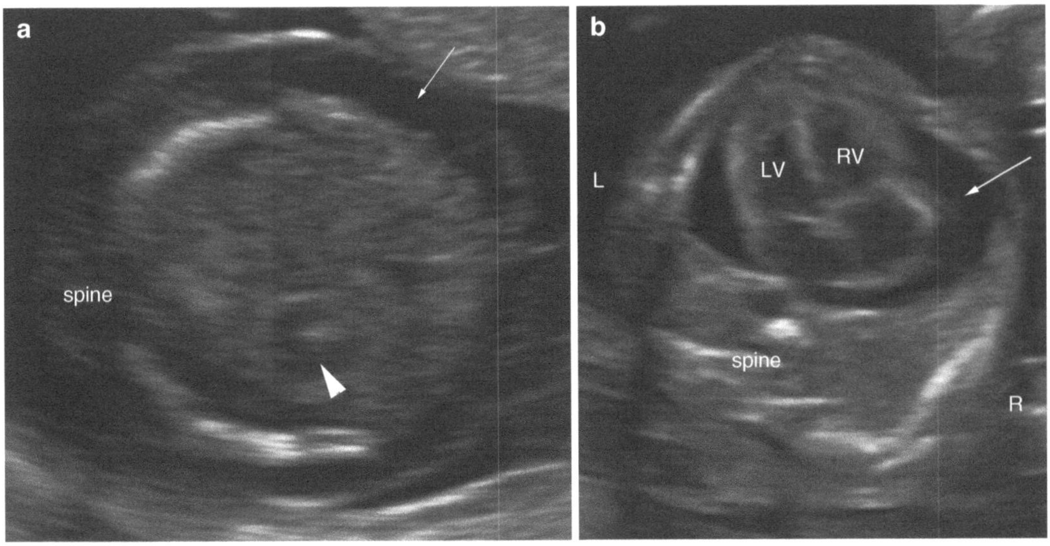

Fig. 14.3 (**a**) Transverse section of the fetal abdomen in a fetus at 12 weeks with hydrops fetalis. The white arrow shows marked accumulation of fluid in the subcutaneous tissue. The arrowhead indicates the stomach bubble. (**b**) Transverse section of the fetal thorax in a fetus at 12 weeks with hydrops fetalis. The white arrow shows marked, bilateral accumulation of fluid in the pericardium

Table 14.2 Primary cardiac causes of fetal hydrops

Category of CHD	Type of CHD
Arrhythmias	– Bradycardias: CHB – Tachycardias: SVT, AF (See Chap. 11)
Structural defects	– AVSD with severe AV valve regurgitation – LAI with CHB – Tricuspid dysplasia or Ebsteins' anomaly of tricuspid valve with severe tricuspid valve regurgitation – Severe obstruction of RVOT: PS/PAT with premature closure of arterial duct or premature closure of FO – Severe obstruction of the LVOT: critical AS or HLHS with severe restriction or closure of FO
Cardiac tumors	– Rhabdomyomas, teratoma, fibroma, hamartomas, haemangiomas
Cardiomyopathy	– Dilated: infection with CMV, Congenital Syphilis, Rubella, Coxsackie and Parvovirus – Hypertrophic: poorly controlled maternal DM – Genetic causes: Barth syndrome, Noonan syndrome.

AVSD atrio-ventricular septal defect, *CHB* congenital heart block, *CMV* cytomegalovirus, *DA*: ductus arteriosus, *DM* Diabetes mellitus, *FO* foramen ovale, *HLHS* Hypoplastic left heart syndrome, *LAI* left atrial isomerism, *LVOT* left-ventricular outflow tract, *PAT* pulmonary atresia, *PS* pulmonary stenosis, *RVOT* right ventricular outflow tract, *SVT* supra-ventricular tachycardia, *TSC* tuberous sclerosis complex

Table 14.3 Secondary cardiac causes of Hydrops Fetalis

Etiology	Underlying disease
Fetal anaemia	– Red cell incompatibility (e.g. Rhesus, Kell, ABO) – Fetal haemorrhage – Fetal infection (e.g. Parvovirus, CMV) – Inherited anaemia (e.g. alpha thalassemia) – Aplastic Anaemia (e.g. Blackfan-Diamond) – Red Cell enzyme disorders (e.g. Pyruvate Kinase deficiency)
Complications in MC twins	– TTTS – TRAP
Fetal thyrotoxicosis	– Goitre – FGR – Tachycardia
AV Malformations	– Vein of Galen malformation
Placental tumours	– Chorioangioma
Fetal tumours	– Sacrococcygeal teratoma

AV arterio-venous, *CMV* cytomegalovirus, *FGR* fetal growth restriction, *TRAP* twin reversed arterial perfusion sequence, *TTTS* twin-to-twin transfusion syndrome

Table 14.4 Non-cardiac causes of Hydrops Fetalis

Etiology	Underlying disease
Infection	– CMV, Toxoplasmosis, Parvovirus, Coxachie, Syphilis
Metabolic disorder	– Lysosomal storage disease, cardiac glycogen storage disease – Congenital disorders of glycosylation – Carnitine deficiency – Hereditary Haemochromatosis
Thorax masses	– CPAM – CDH
Chromosomes	– Trisomies – Microdeletions/microduplications
Single gene disorders	– Congenital myopathy, Kabuki, SMA – Skeletal dysplasia (e.g. Short rib polydactyly)
Musculoskeletal/Fetal Akinesia	– Primary musculo-skeletal – Primary metabolic disorder – Primary neurological disorder
Lymphatic system	– Lymphatic dysplasias

CMV cytomegalovirus, *CDH* congenital diaphragmatic hernia, *CPAM* congenital pulmonary airways malformation, *SMA* spinal muscular atrophy

intravascular space. In fetal life colloid oncotic pressure difference has less effect than in adult life because of the increased permeability of fetal capillaries and increased compliance of fetal tissues. This leads to an increased loss of vascular fluid before the interstitial colloid oncotic pressure rises to check the flux. The lymphatic system returns fluid and oncotic active proteins to the vascular space and basal lymph flow rates are more active in the fetus than the adult. Clearance of lymph depends on central venous pressure and there is a delicate relationship between the two. If negative pressure is not maintained lymph flow is reduced, leading to accumulation of interstitial fluid and development of HF. A rise in central venous pressure is the most important pathogenic mechanism for the development of HF and is the final common pathway for many conditions, including high output cardiac failure, venous obstruction and low output cardiac failure. Increased capillary permeability, reduced plasma oncotic pressure and lymphatic obstruction also contribute to interstitial fluid accumulation.

Aetiology: The aetiology of HF depends on the gestation at which it is identified:

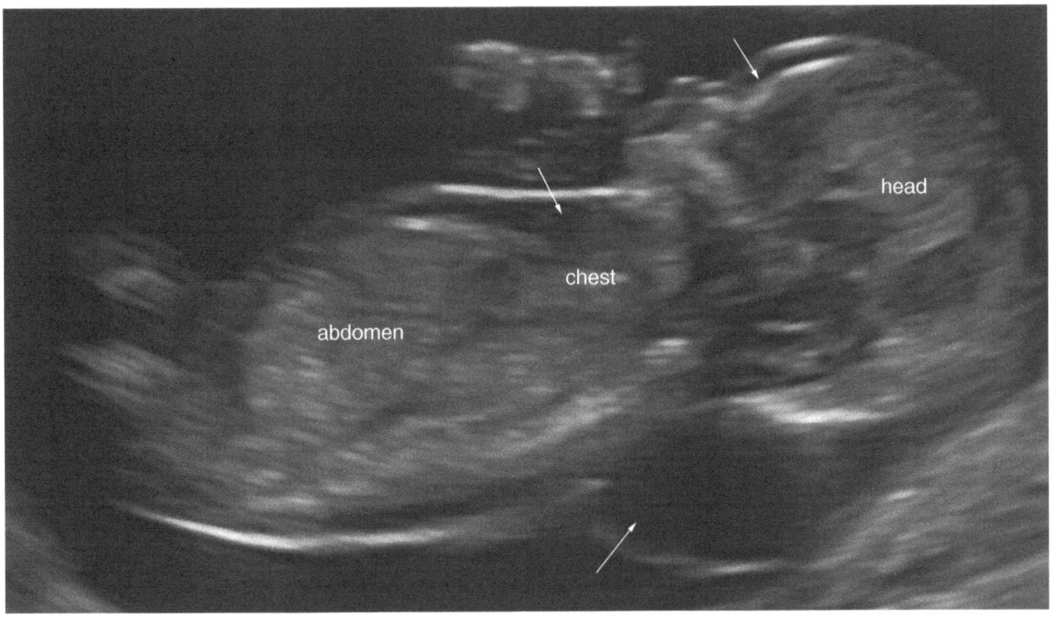

Fig. 14.4 Sagittal section of a fetus at 12 weeks with 45X0 and hydrops fetalis. The white arrows show marked accumulation of fluid in the nuchal area (cystic hygroma) and diffusely elsewhere in the subcutaneous tissue

- *First trimester:* In the first trimester the commonest cause of HF is an underlying chromosome abnormality, such as 45XO (Sect. "Chromosomal Syndromes") and it is usually an indicator of imminent intrauterine death (Fig. 14.4).
- *Second trimester:* Below 20 weeks the commonest cause of HF is chromosomal abnormality. However, the introduction of first trimester combined screening with NT measurement and maternal serum biochemistry has resulted in early identification and termination of pregnancies with major chromosome abnormalities. This has led to a significant reduction in the number of cases with HF secondary to aneuploidies in both the second and third trimesters.
- *Third trimester:* Cardiovascular causes including anaemia-related and primary and secondary cardiac conditions are the commonest aetiologies in the third trimester although a significant proportion remains unexplained.
- Historically, HF was distinguished into immune and non-immune with fetal anaemia secondary to Rhesus isoimmunisation being the commonest underlying cause. The introduction of Anti-D has made red cell incompatibility-related anaemia uncommon compared to other causes.
- Primary cardiac causes of HF include arrhythmias and cardiac defects (Table 14.2). Fetal bradycardia is most commonly due to complete heart block and is strongly associated with maternal anti-Ro/La antibodies. Tachycardias are usually supraventricular and sustained in cases of HF, but more subtle intermittent tachycardias may also cause HF. This diagnosis should be considered for unexplained HF in the third trimester and repeated ultrasound examinations may be required. CHD may be part of a multiple malformation syndrome with HF being due to the underlying condition rather than the cardiac defect.
- Secondary cardiac causes comprise a number of non-cardiac conditions leading to HF through cardiac failure (Table 14.3). These include space-occupying lesions within the chest such as CDH and congenital pulmonary airway malformations (CPAM), which can cause an increase in CVP thus leading to HF. However, many of these, such as CDH may also have associated CHD.

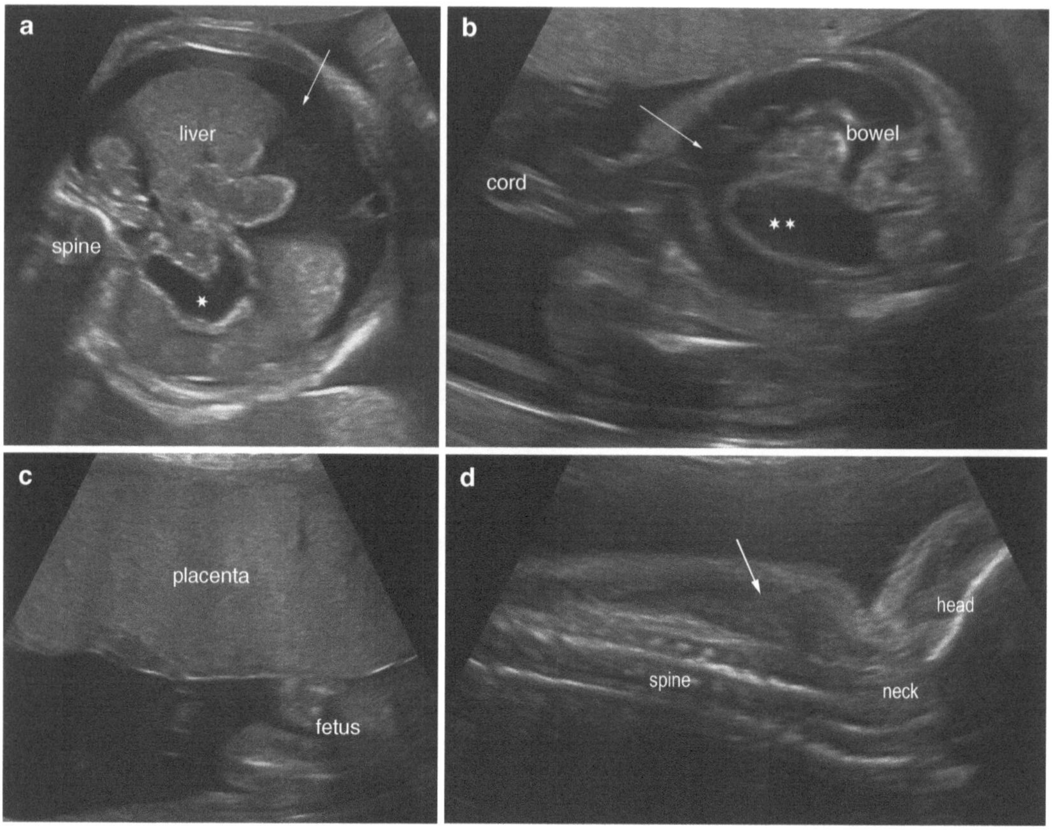

Fig. 14.5 (**a**) Transverse section of the abdomen in a fetus at 22 weeks' gestation with severe anemia due to acute Parvovirus infection. Liver, stomach (*asterisk*) and bowel are floating within ascitic fluid (*white arrow*). (**b**) Transverse section of the lower abdomen and pelvis in a fetus at 22 weeks' gestation with severe anemia due to acute Parvovirus infection. Both bladder (*double asterisk*) and small bowel loops float within the ascitic fluid (*white arrow*). (**c**) Evidence of placentitis in a pregnancy at 22 weeks' gestation complicated by severe anemia due to acute Parvovirus infection. The placenta is thickened and echogenic. Note the size of placenta as compared to the fetus. (**d**) Sagittal back-up view of a fetus at 22 weeks' gestation with severe anemia due to acute Parvovirus infection. The white arrow shows marked subcutaneous oedema in the region of the fetal neck

- Abnormal development of the lymphatic system has also been implicated in a significant proportion of cases of unexplained HF and delayed development of the thoracic duct is associated with increased NT in the first trimester.

Ultrasound findings: Once HF has been identified, it is important to ensure that the fetus is not anaemic as this requires urgent treatment with blood transfusion. Ultrasound features strongly suggestive of fetal anaemia include pericardial effusion and ascites, less commonly skin oedema and pleural effusions. Doppler interrogation of the fetal Middle Cerebral Artery (MCA) demonstrating a peak systolic velocity (PSV) greater than 1.5 SDs above the mean for gestation has a high sensitivity for fetal anaemia (Fig. 14.5). A detailed structural survey should be undertaken looking for specific cardiac and extra-cardiac anomalies to understand the aetiology of the HF. In metabolic conditions hepatosplenomegaly may be seen.

Investigations: Investigations will be driven by the ultrasound findings and maternal history. These include:

- *Fetal tests:*
  - Fetal chromosome analysis including array comparative genome hybridization (a-CGH)
  - Full blood count (fetal blood)

- Fetal thyroid function (fetal blood)
  - PCR for infection if CMV suspected (amniotic fluid)
  - Metabolic investigations (amniotic fluid storage)
  - Genetic investigations (DNA storage)
- *Maternal tests*
  - Infection screen in unexplained cases.
  - Thyroid function tests (TFTs)
  - Anti-Ro, anti-La antibodies
  - Acetylcholine receptors and DNA analysis for myotonic dystrophy if ultrasound features of fetal akinesia

Management: This depends on the underlying condition and includes:

- *Fetal blood transfusion* for fetal anaemia
- *Maternal anti-thyroid drugs* to treat fetal thyrotoxicosis
- *Maternal steroids* for congenital heart block secondary to SLE
- *Maternal anti-arrhythmic drugs* for fetal tachycardia
- *Shunting of pleural effusions* if HF secondary to primary hydrothorax
- *Laser ablation* of feeding vessels in placental or fetal tumours.

Fetal hydrops has many causes and associations and a systematic approach is required, including detailed fetal anatomical survey and echocardiography, to determine the likely aetiology and to advise parents of appropriate management. Sadly the prognosis is often poor, but there are some conditions where effective treatment is available. Unfortunately an explanation for the HF is not always identified either before or after birth.

Anomalies Related to Fetal Growth Restriction

Definition: FGR refers to the inability of the fetus to reach its genetic growth potential. Diagnosis is made by serial ultrasound examinations showing slow or static growth. Percentiles are often used to define FGR and the most common is estimated fetal weight (EFW) less than the 5th centile for gestation. FGR is associated with significant morbidity and mortality in perinatal and adult life.

Aetiology: FGR has a number of different causes and differential diagnosis may be challenging (Table 14.5). However, in this section we will focus on cardiac and extra-cardiac ultrasound features of FGR related to placental dysfunction as those related to both genetic and infective causes are discussed elsewhere in this chapter.

Pathophysiology: In FGR related to placental dysfunction, critical changes in partial pressure of O_2 and CO_2 trigger specific alterations in peripheral vascular resistance aimed at maximizing delivery of oxygen and nutrients to vital organs. These circulatory changes are known as the "brain sparing effect" and lead to preferential blood supply to the brain, myocardium and adrenals and reduced flow to the kidneys, gastrointestinal tract and lower extremities. As a result, the fetus shows asymmetrical fetal growth, with relatively maintained head size and reduced or static increment of the abdomen and long bones. Cardiac changes related to FGR include reduced LV afterload due to cerebral vasodilation and increased RV afterload due to systemic and pulmonary vasoconstriction. Fetal hypoxaemia may impair cardiac contractility both via a direct effect on the myocardium and through polycythaemia and increased blood viscosity. However the benefits from cerebral vasodilation are limited as this reaches its peak about 2 weeks before fetal cardiac decompensation occurs. In deteriorating FGR there is a steady decline in cardiac function as cardiac output gradually worsens leading to compromised cardiac filling.

Ultrasound features:

- *Cardiac appearances:* Three distinct cardiac morphological appearances have been described in FGR (Rodríguez-López et al. 2016) including *globular*, *elongated* and *hypertrophic*. The *globular* and *elongated* appearances account for most cases and are associated with late-onset FGR. Both feature a

Table 14.5 Aetiologies and ultrasound features of Fetal Growth Restriction (FGR)

	Non-cardiac features	Cardiac features
Placental insufficiency	*Early-onset* – Asymmetrical FGR (FL, AC < 5th ctl; HC/FL > 95th ctl) – Oligohydramnios – Dyshomogeneous, thickened haemorrhagic or thin placenta – Raised PI Uterine artery Doppler – Raised PI UA, absent/reversed a-wave DV) – Echogenic bowel – Hypospadia (male fetuses)	– Hypertrophic appearance: myocardial hypertrophy, cardiomegaly, systolic and diastolic dysfunction
	Late-onset – Asymmetrical FGR (FL, AC < 5th ctl; HC/FL > 95th ctl) – Oligohydramnios/normal amniotic fluid – Dyshomogeneous, thickened or thin placenta – Raised PI Uterine artery Doppler – Brain sparing effect (raised PI UA, reduced PI MCA) – Reduced fetal movements	– Globular appearance: mild cardiomegaly and hypertrophy, spherical geometry of both ventricles, mild systolic and dystolic dysfunction – Elongated appearance: mild cardiomegaly and hypertrophy, elongated LV, mild systolic and dystolic dysfunction
Chromosomal and genetic anomalies	*Early-onset* – Symmetrical FGR (HC, FL, AC < 5th ctl) – Normal amniotic fluid, polyhydramnios – Normal or dyshomogeneous placenta – Normal or raised PI Uterine artery Doppler – Normal or abnormal UA, DV Dopplers – Often ECAs and hydrops	– CHD – Ventricular disproportion – Relative cardiomegaly (if small chest)
Infections	– Variable onset – FL, HC <5th centile and normal AC – Oligohydramnios or polyhydramnios – Hepatosplenomegaly, abdominal calcifications – Brain abnormalities (e.g. ventriculomegaly, calcifications) – Thickened and hyperechogenic placenta – Usually normal uterine artery Doppler – Other features infection-specific	– Cardiomegaly Rubella: CHD CMV: thick myocardium often with punctuate calcifications

AC abdominal circumference, *CMV* cytomegalovirus, *ctl* centile, *DV* ductus venosus, *FGR* fetal growth restriction, *FL* femur length, *HC* head circumference, *MCA* middle cerebral artery, *PI* pulsatility index, *UA* umbilical artery

mild, but significant increase in cardiac dimensions and thickness and subtle systolic and diastolic dysfunction. However, the *globular* appearance is characterised by a spherical geometry of both ventricles, whereas in the *elongated* the longitudinal diameter of LV is predominantly affected. The *hypertrophic* appearance is characterised by extensive myocardial hypertrophy, cardiomegaly, a spherical shape and systolic and diastolic dysfunction. This morphology is associated with early onset FGR and worse perinatal outcomes (Fig. 14.6).

- The association between CHD, low birth weight and intra-uterine death is well known, but the specific reasons for this are unclear. More recently, a higher rate of pre-eclampsia, as well as FGR and stillbirth, have been reported in pregnancies complicated by CHD. It has been hypothesised that the same unbalance of angiogenic-antiangiogenic factors underlying placental insufficiency may also lead to CHD (Ruiz et al. 2015)
- *Associated extra-cardiac features:* Non-cardiac features of placental insufficiency are listed in Table 14.5. These include biometrical

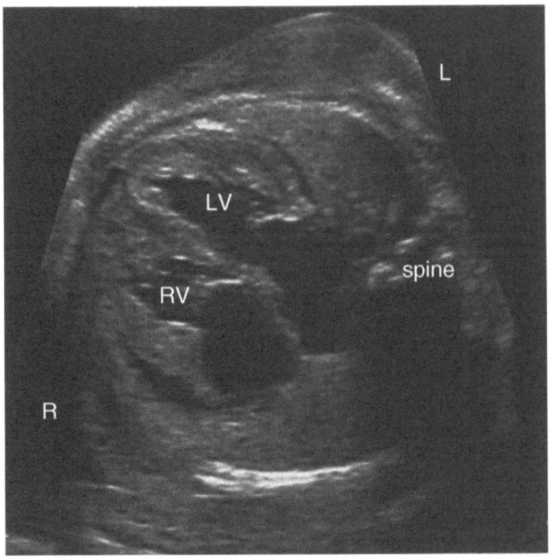

Fig. 14.6 Transverse section of the fetal thorax in a growth restricted fetus at 21 weeks showing increased CT ratio due to cardiomegaly and biventricular hypertrophy

parameters indicating asymmetrical growth, echogenic bowel, hypospadias in male fetuses, amniotic fluid, placental and Doppler abnormalities (Fig. 14.7).

Anomalies in Twin Pregnancies

Structural abnormalities are known to be more common in twin pregnancies and CHD accounts for two-thirds of all defects (Sperling et al. 2007).

In *dizygotic twins* (derived from two fertilized eggs) the excess risk of fetal abnormalities is likely to be due to there being two fetuses each with the same risk of abnormality as a singleton.

In each *monozygotic twin* (derived from the splitting of a single fertilized egg) the risk of defects is two to three times greater than a singleton. This

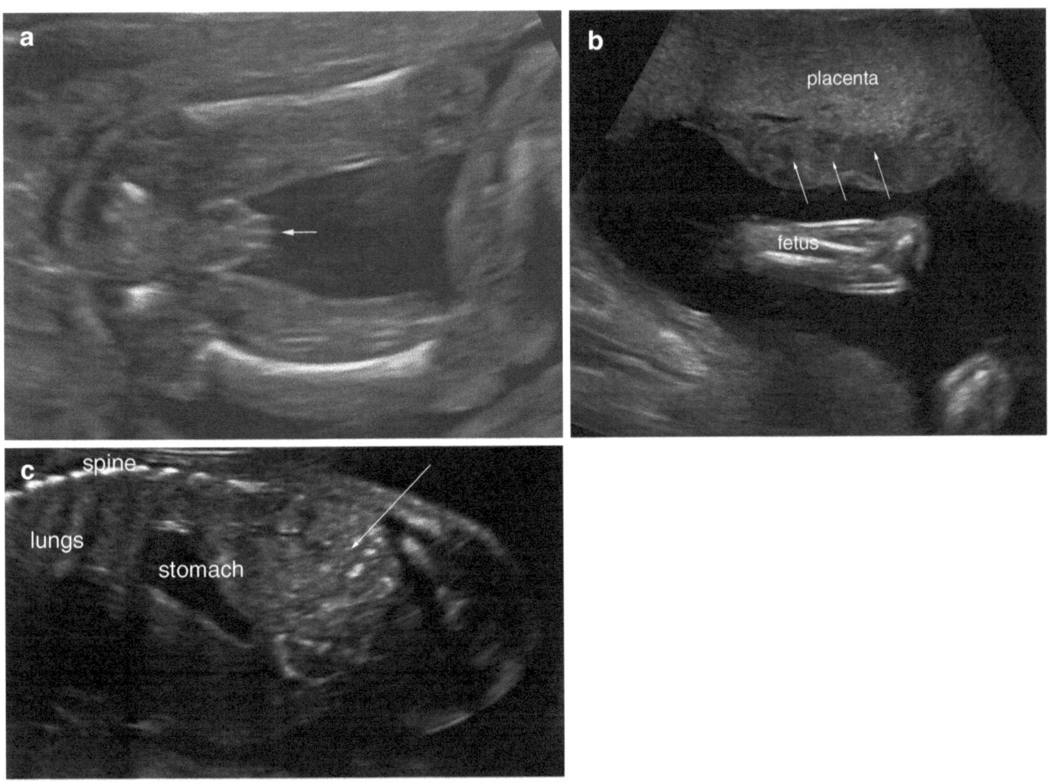

Fig. 14.7 (**a**) Transverse section of the pelvic area in a growth restricted fetus at 24 weeks of gestation. The white arrow shows significant hypospadias. (**b**) Multiple white arrows outline extensive area of placental bleeding (jelly-like placenta) in a growth restricted fetus at 24 weeks of gestation. (**c**) Parasagittal section of a growth restricted fetus at 24 weeks of gestation. The white arrow shows discrete hyperechogenic spots in the fetal abdomen (*white arrow*) below the stomach bubble

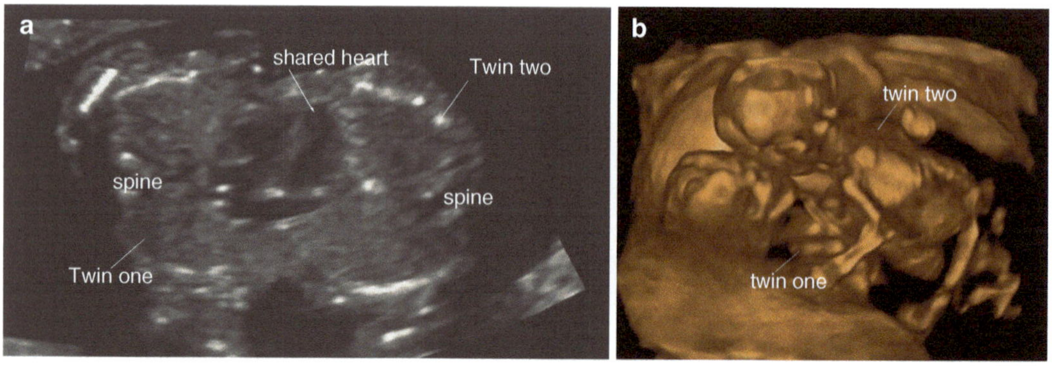

Fig. 14.8 (**a**) Tranverse section at the 4-chamber view demonstrating a shared heart in conjoined thoracopagus twins at 20 weeks of gestation. (**b**) Three-dimensional reconstruction of conjoined thoracopagus twins

holds true particularly in mono-chorionic (sharing a single placenta) pairs, di-amniotic (single placenta, two amniotic sacs) and more so in mono-amniotic (single placenta, single amniotic sac) twins, where the rate of defects is as high as 1 in 5. Conjoined twins are a very rare type of mono-amniotic twins resulting from a late incomplete split of the embryonic disc. These twins are abnormal by definition, as they are joined at different sites, but most often at the thorax, with conjoined hearts (Fig. 14.8).

In spite of being genetically identical, monozygotic twins are typically discordant for abnormalities and it is likely that placental vascular factors affecting haemodynamics either early or later in the pregnancy play a role in the pathophysiology (Springer et al. 2014; Pettit et al. 2013).

The incidence of CHD in MCDA twins is reported as 5–7.5%. A wide spectrum of discordant cardiac defects have been described in MC twins with ventricular septal defects and anomalies of outflow tracts being the most common lesions (Springer et al. 2014). However, abnormalities such as cardiomyopathy or functional pulmonary valve stenosis may also develop as part of the complications related to placental vascular connections.

Twin-to-Twin Transfusion Syndrome (TTTS): TTTS complicates 1 in 10 MC pregnancies and usually occurs between 16 and 26 weeks' gestation. It is characterised by oligohydramnios, small or empty bladder in a volume depleted, oliguric donor and polyhydramnios and a distended bladder in a volume overloaded recipient (Fig. 14.9). TTTS is always associated with unbalanced blood flow through vascular anastomoses, but the detailed mechanisms that lead to the cardiovascular and renal disturbances are unclear. However, as there is continuous blood exchange, vasoactive hormones produced in the donor may be implicated in the hypertension and cardiomyopathy seen in the recipient. The recipient often has signs of RV dysfunction with cardiomegaly due to an increase in myocardial thickness, tricuspid regurgitation and right ventricular outflow obstruction (Van Mieghem et al. 2010).

Selective Fetal Growth Restriction (s-FGR) is defined by the presence of ultrasound features of FGR in one twin (EFW or AC < 5th centile) and >25% size discordance. S-FGR is due to unequal placental sharing and also affects 1 in 10 MCDA pregnancies (Fig. 14.10). Cardiac features associated with TTTS may also be seen in MCDA twins with s-FGR.

Twin-Reversed-Arterial-Perfusion Sequence (TRAP) is a rare complication of MC twins where blood flows from the umbilical artery of a healthy pump twin into the umbilical artery of the parasite co-twin via large artero-arterial anastomoses and usually returns via a veno-venous anastomoses. The perfused twin does not have any cardiac activity of its own and is described as acardiac twin. The pump twin is at high risk of high out-put cardiac failure and

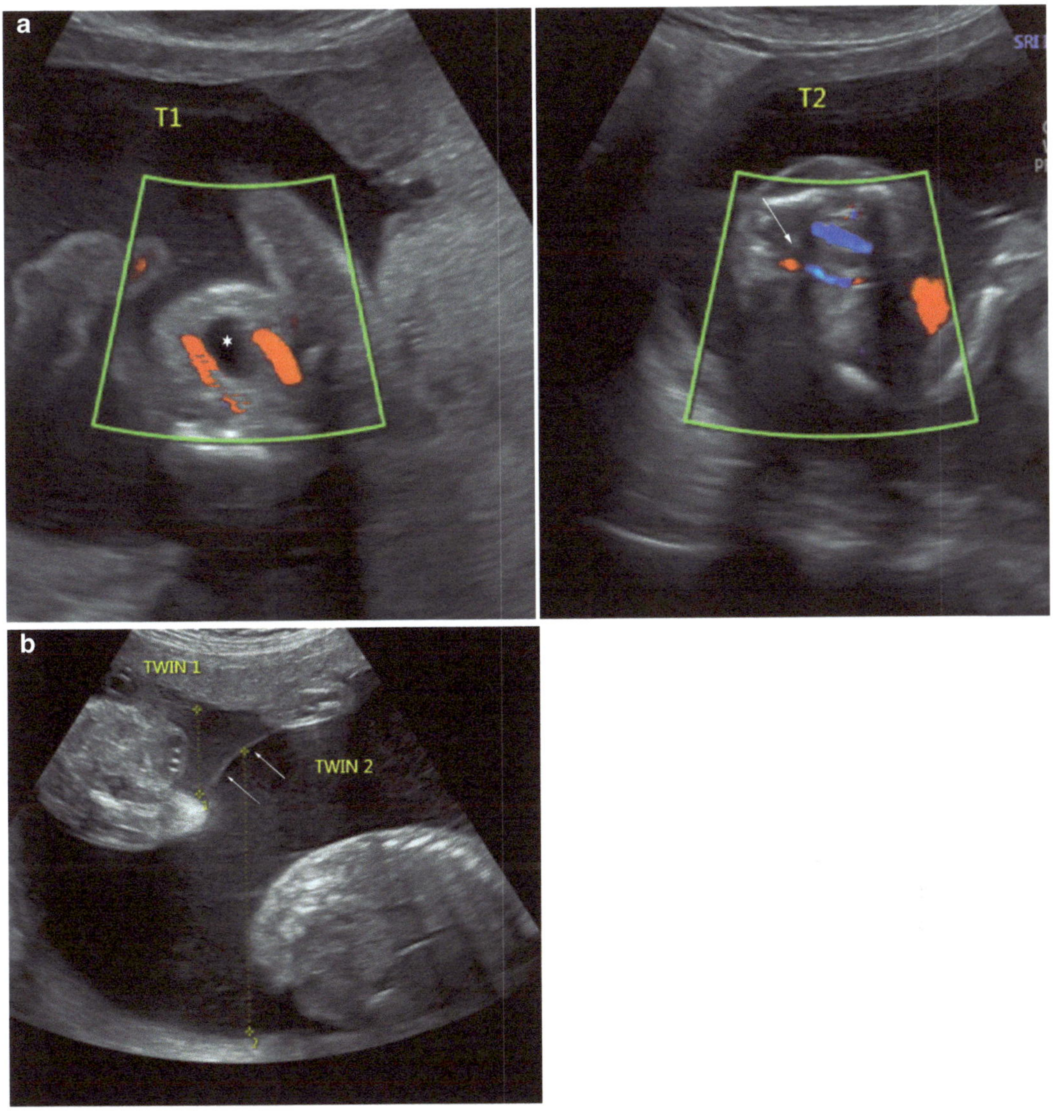

Fig. 14.9 (**a**) Transverse sections of the pelvises in mono-chorionic diamniotic twins with severe TTTS at 18 weeks showing discordant bladder filling. A regular bladder (*asterisk*) outlined by umbilical arteries is demonstrated in the recipient twin (T1) while minimal/no bladder filling (*white arrow*) is seen in the donor co-twin (T2). (**b**) Multiple white arrows show the intertwin membrane and discrepant measurements (*yellow calipers*) in the pool of fluids between the two fetuses in a mono-chorionic diamniotic twin pregnancy complicated by severe TTTS at 18 weeks of gestation. Significant discrepancy in fluid and discrepant bladder filling are required for a diagnosis of severe TTTS

intrauterine death. Outcome may be improved by stopping the circulation in the acardiac twin and this may be done either in the first trimester or at 16 weeks.

Laser separation of the placental circulations is the optimal treatment for TTTS. After treatment the cardiac function in the recipient may normalise within 1 month although 8% of recipient twins will have pulmonary stenosis at birth (Herberg et al. 2006). Functional heart problems may only become apparent in the third trimester. Therefore it is important to continue to monitor the cardiac appearances throughout pregnancy.

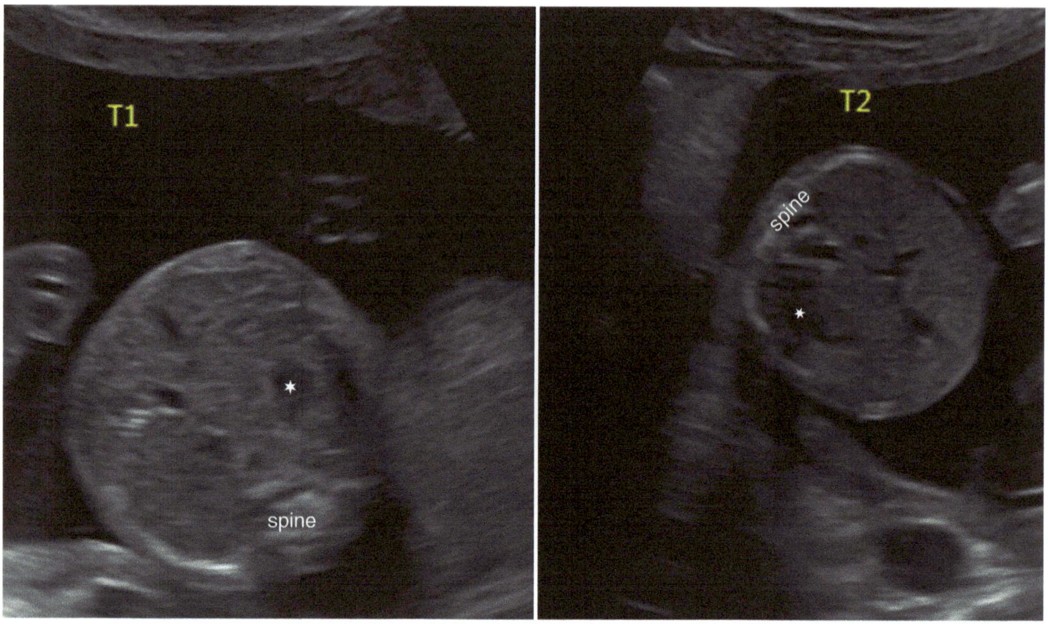

Fig. 14.10 Transverse sections of the fetal abdomens in mono-chorionic diamniotic twin pregnancy complicated by sFGR at 20 weeks of gestation showing marked inter-twin discrepancy in size. A diagnosis of sFGR implies a discrepancy in size of at least 25% with the smaller twin being plotted below the 5th centile for gestational age

Multiple Malformation Syndromes

The rate of chromosomal and non-chromosomal anomalies in the context of multiple malformation syndromes including CHD and ECAs is as high as 20% (Stoll et al. 2015a, b).

Knowledge of the ultrasound features characterizing the most common multiple malformation syndromes will determine when invasive prenatal diagnosis should be offered and assist in counselling the parents regarding postnatal management and prognosis.

Chromosomal Syndromes

Trisomy 21

Definition: Trisomy 21 (T21) or Down syndrome is the most prevalent genetic cause of intellectual disability in humans.

Epidemiology: The risk of T21 increases with advancing maternal age (especially after 35 years) and reduces with gestation (due to increased rate of miscarriages and intrauterine deaths). In the last few decades, the impact of prenatal diagnosis and advancing maternal age has profoundly changed the epidemiology of T21 with recent European data reporting the live birth prevalence to be decreased to 10.2 per 10,000 (Stoll et al. 2015a).

Pathogenesis: T21 is due to an extra copy of chromosome 21. Ninety-five percent of the affected individuals show a full trisomy 21, mostly resulting from a *de novo* nondisjunction error during maternal meiosis. In the remaining 5% of patients, the phenotype results from a Robertsonian translocation (which may be inherited) and mosaicisms of variable degree.

Screening: Screening for aneuploidies has profoundly evolved throughout the past 50 years from using maternal age only in the 1970s, through second trimester serum placental biomarkers in the 1980s, to first trimester screening the 1990s using a combination of maternal age, NT and two serum biomarkers (ß-hCG, free- ß-human chorionic gonadotrophin and PAPP-A, pregnancy associated plasma protein A) between 11^{+0} and 13^{+6}

weeks' gestation. In the last decade, the introduction of non-invasive testing on maternal blood by cell-free fetal DNA (cf-DNA) has represented a major breakthrough in screening for aneuploidies with detection rate for T21 as high as 99.2% for a false positive rate of 0.09% (Gil et al. 2015).

Ultrasound diagnosis: T21 has a well-defined syndromal pattern of major abnormalities and minor defects detectable by prenatal ultrasound (Table 14.6).

- *Cardiac anomalies:* Congenital heart disease is the most common abnormality found in fetuses with T21 and it has significant impact on prognosis. About 40% of fetuses are affected with major CHD such as AVSD and ToF (Mogra et al. 2011).
- *Extra-cardiac anomalies*: About 50% of T21 fetuses show one or more major structural anomalies mostly involving the gastro-intestinal or genito-urinary tracts, the skeletal and central nervous systems. Figure 14.11 shows an overview of the commonest ultrasound abnormalities in T21 fetuses.
- *Minor defects or markers:* In addition to the described major defects, there are a number of signs known as *markers* that are observed more commonly in fetuses with T21 than in euploid fetuses (Fig. 14.12). These are not defects and they have minor or no clinical significance in the context of a normal karyotype. However, the presence or absence of such signs may be used to increase or reduce the background (*a-priori*) risk for T21. The estimated prevalence of the most common markers in T21 and euploid fetuses and the positive and negative likelihood ratios for T21 are reported in Table 14.7. A recent meta-analysis of second trimester markers for T21 has shown that most isolated markers exert only a small effect on modifying the odds for T21. However, ventriculomegaly, thickened nuchal fold and ARSA increase by three to fourfold the *a-priori* risk and hypoplastic nasal bone by six to sevenfold (Agathokleous et al. 2013).

Table 14.6 Ultrasound features and biochemical markers of Trisomy 21

	Serum screening	Ultrasound markers	Fetal defects
First trimester (11^{+0}–13^{+6} weeks)	*Combined test* • β-hCG: ≈2.0 MoM • PAPP-A: ≈0.5 MoM *Triple test* • uE3: low • hCG: high • AFP: low	• Increased NT • Absent NB • Normal FHR • Reversed DV • TR	• Cystic hygroma • Abnormal 4Chv • Omphalocele
Second trimester–third trimester	*Quadruple test* • uE3: low • hCG: low • AFP: high • Inhibin A: low	• Hypoplastic NB • ARSA • Thickened NF • Short humerus • Short femur • Prenasal oedema • Echogenic intracardiac focus • Ventriculomegaly • Pyelectasis • Hyperechogenic bowel • Clinodactyly • Macroglossia • Small ears • Sandal gap	• Cardiac defects (AVSD, VSD, ToF, CoA) • Duodenal atresia • Tracheo-esophageal atresia • FGR • Polyhydramnios

AFP alpha-fetoprotein, *ARSA* aberrant right subclavian artery, *AVSD* atrio-ventricular septal defect, *β-hCG* human chorionic gonadotropin, *CoA* aortic coarctation, *FGR* fetal growth restriction, *FHR* fetal heart rate, *NB* nasal bone, *NF* nuchal fold, *NT* nuchal translucency, *PAPP-A* pregnancy-associated plasma protein A, *Rev DV* reversed a-wave in ductus venosus, *ToF* tetralogy of Fallot, *TR* tricuspid regurgitation, *uE3* unconjugated estriol, *VSD* ventricular septal defect, *4ChV* four chamber view

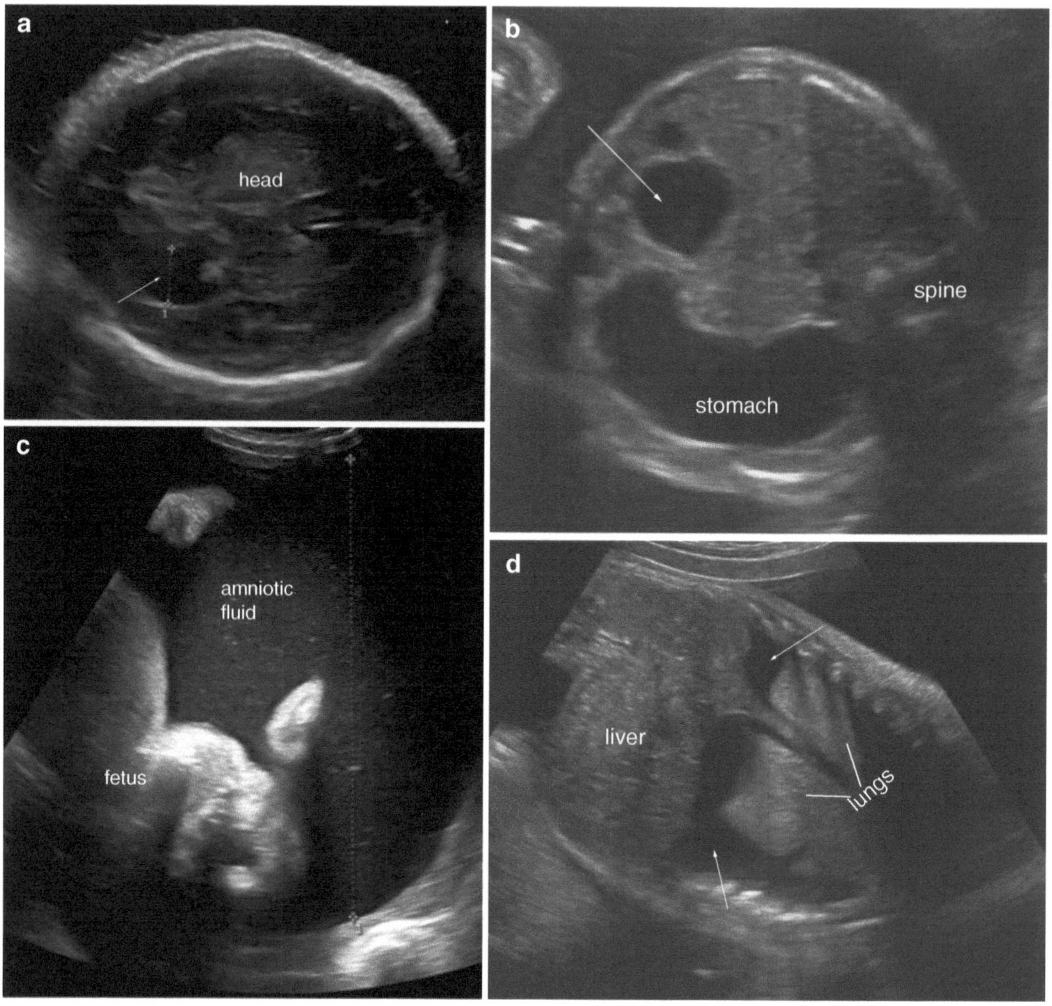

Fig. 14.11 (**a**) Axial, transventricular section of the head demonstrating ventriculomegaly in a fetus at 28 weeks with confirmed postnatal diagnosis of Trisomy 21. The arrow shows dilatation of the posterior horn of the lateral cerebral ventricle (ventriculomegaly) measured with the yellow calipers. (**b**) Transverse section of the abdomen demonstrating duodenal atresia in a fetus at 28 weeks with confirmed postnatal diagnosis of Trisomy 21. The larger bubble represents the stomach, which is separated by a small hyperechogenic area (atretic segment) by a second bubble (*white arrow*), which represents the dilated duodenum. (**c**) Same fetus at 28 weeks with confirmed postnatal diagnosis of Trisomy 21. In view of obstruction of the upper gastrointestinal tract, the amniotic fluid is increased, as shown by the deepest vertical pool measured with yellow calipers as 15 cm (normal value <8 cm) in this fetus. Polyhydramnios increases intrauterine pressure and may lead to premature shortening of the uterine cervix and premature birth. (**d**, **e**) Parasagittal and transverse section of the fetal thorax showing moderate bilateral pleural effusions (*white arrows*) in a fetus at 28 weeks with confirmed postnatal diagnosis of Trisomy 21. The etiology of pleural effusions in Trisomy 21 is unknown. (**f**) Three-dimensional reconstruction of the fetal face showing up-slanting palpebral fissures and depressed nasal bridge in a fetus at 28 weeks with confirmed postnatal diagnosis of Trisomy 21

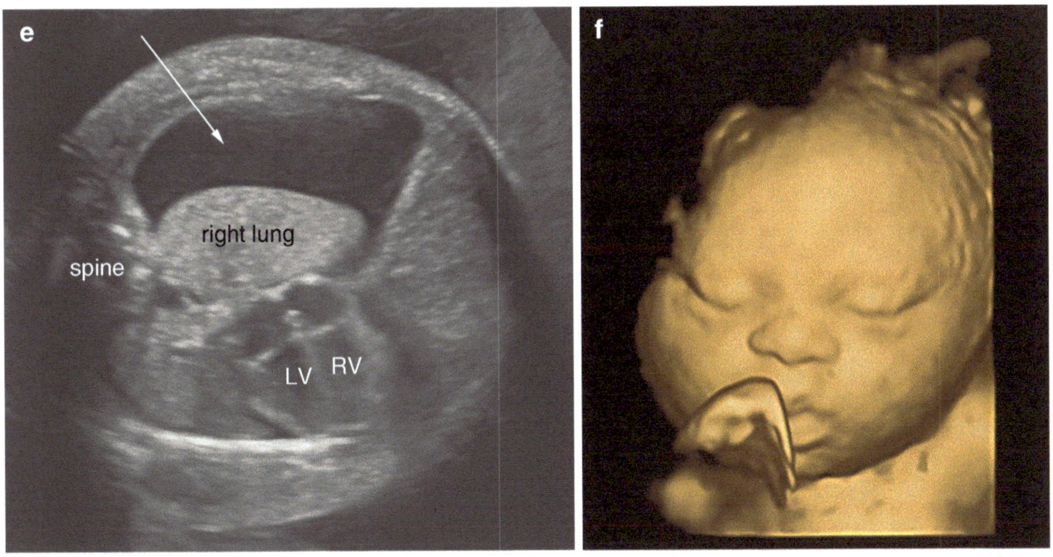

Fig. 14.11 (continued)

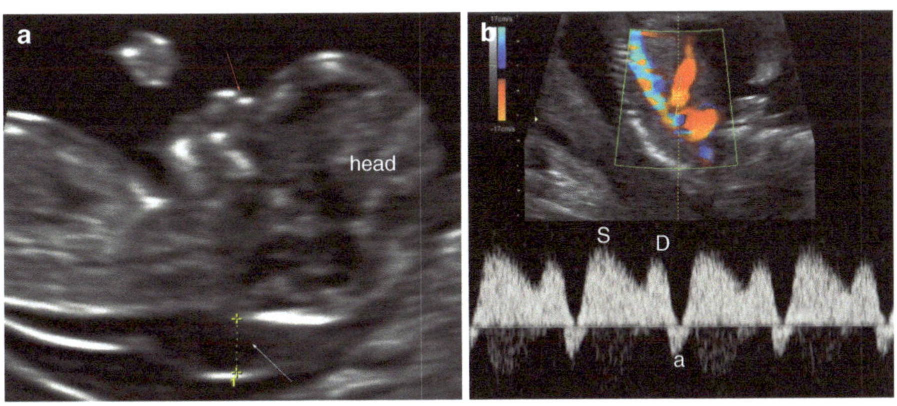

Fig. 14.12 (**a**) Mid-sagittal view of the fetal face at 12 weeks showing absence of the nasal bone. The nose shows only two echogenic lines representing the tip of the nose and the skin covering the nasal bridge (*red arrow*). In the fetus the NT (*white arrow*) was also increased (see normal nasal bone for comparison in Fig. 14.1a). (**b**) Mid-sagittal view of the fetal trunk demonstrating insonation of the ductus venosus of a fetus at 12 weeks with reversed a-wave (A). (**c**) Transverse cut at the four-chamber view demonstrating tricuspid valve regurgitation (*white arrows*) using Pulsed wave Doppler in a fetus at 12 weeks of gestation. (**d**) Transverse section of the fetal thorax at the four-chamber view demonstrating hyperechogenic focus in the left ventricle (*white arrow*) in a fetus at 20 weeks of gestation. (**e**) Coronal section of the fetal trunk showing bilaterally mild dilation of the renal pelvises (*white arrows*) in a fetus at 20 weeks of gestation. (**f**) Transverse section of the fetal thorax demonstrating an aberrant course of the right subclavian artery (*white arrow*) in a fetus at 20 weeks of gestation. (**g**) Para-sagittal section of the fetal abdomen showing below the stomach (*asterisk*) loops of bowel (*white arrow*) of echogenicity similar or greater than the bone (bowel echogenicity). (**h**) Mid-sagittal view of fetal face demonstrating normal echogenicity of the nasal bone (*yellow arrow*) in a fetus at 24 weeks of gestation. The yellow calipers show normal length of the nasal bone (normal value: >5 mm). (**i**) Mid-sagittal view of fetal face demonstrating absent nasal bone (*white arrow*) in a fetus at 24 weeks of gestation

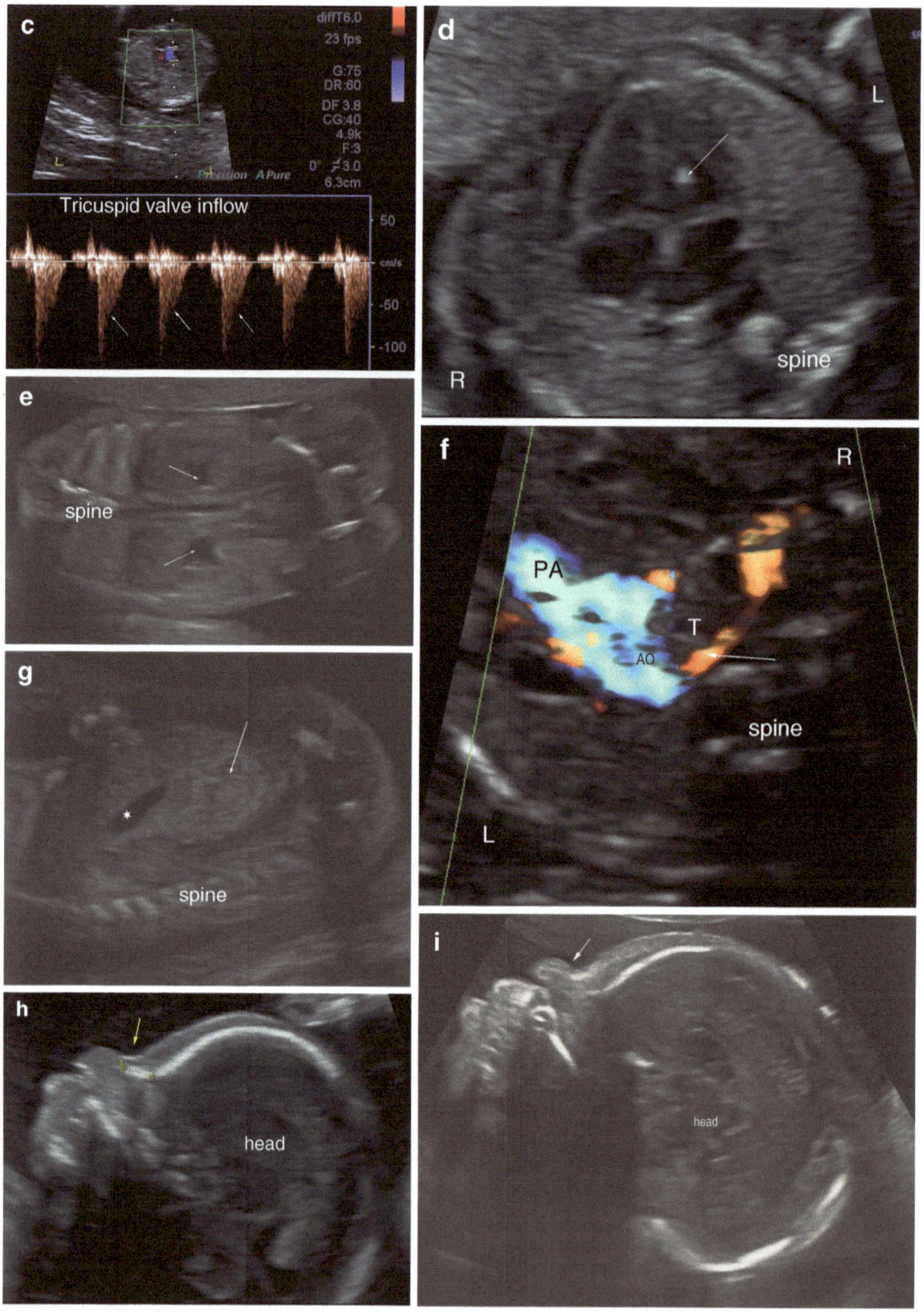

Fig. 14.12 (continued)

Table 14.7 Estimated prevalence, positive and negative likelihood ratios of common second trimester ultrasound markers in Trisomy 21

Marker	DR	FPR	+LR	−LR	LR (isolated)
Intracardiac echogenic focus	24.4	3.9	5.85	0.8	0.95
Ventriculomegaly					
Increased NF	7.5	0.3	25.78	0.94	3.57
Echogenic bowel	26.2	1.2	19.1	0.8	3.12
Mild hydronephrosis	16.7	1.1	11.44	0.92	1.1
Short humerus	13.7	1.4	7.77	0.92	1.1
Short femur	30.3	4.6	4.81	0.74	0.78
ARSA	27.7	6.4	3.72	0.8	0.61
Absent/hypoplastic NB	30.7	1.5	21.48	0.71	3.94
	59.8	2.8	23.26	0.46	6.58

If a defect/marker is present the a priori risk is increased by the positive likelihood ratio and when it is absent the risk is reduced by the negative likelihood ratio. For example, if the a priori risk is 1:300 and the 22-weeks scan demonstrates an aberrant right subclavian artery (ARSA) the risk is increased by a factor of 21.48 to become 21.8:300 or 1:14. If in response to the finding of ARSA a detailed search is carried out for each one of the defects/markers in the table and they are all demonstrated to be absent then the a priori risk should be multiplied by the positive likelihood ratio for the ARSA (Å~21.48) and the negative likelihood ratio for each one of the other defects/markers and therefore the risk of 1:300 is increased by 3.94 to 1:76, rather than 1:14. This approach assumes that each defect/marker is independent of every other marker

From Coady A, Bower S. Twining Textbook of fetal abnormalities—Ed. Churchill Livingston, 2014

ARSA aberrant right subclavian artery, *DR* detection rate, *FPR* false positive rate, *+LR* positive likelihood ratio, *−LR* negative likelihood ratio, *NB* nasal bone, *NF* nuchal fold

Prenatal diagnosis: It is possible by QF-PCR or conventional karyotyping using chorionic villi (chorionic villus sampling-CVS), amniocytes (amniocentesis) and peripheral leukocytes (fetal blood sampling).

Prognosis: Variable, mostly dependent upon the cardiac and extra-cardiac associated abnormalities. Life expectancy has markedly increased in the last 20 years (median age at death 58 years). Individuals with T21 are at high risk of medical problems including hypothyroidism, leukaemia and early-onset dementia.

Recurrence risk: Empirically estimated at less than 1% (0.8%) for women <39 years and age-related risk thereafter. After two consecutive affected pregnancies, the risk is greater than 10% and parental mosaicism should be considered.

Trisomy 18

Definition: Trisomy 18 (T18) or Edward syndrome is the second most common autosomal aneuploidy. The genetic defect leads to multisystem anomalies of the cardio-vascular, nervous, renal, gastro-intestinal, respiratory and musculoskeletal system with very poor prognosis (50% chances of survival beyond 1 week and <10% chances of survival beyond 1 year of life).

Epidemiology and risk factors: The estimated incidence ranges from 1 in 3000 and 1 in 8000 live birth, with a predilection for females. The incidence increases with maternal age, but paternal age also plays a role.

Pathogenesis: In most cases, the extra copy of the chromosome 18 is the result of a nondisjunction during maternal meiosis II or, rarely, due to a post-fertilization paternal error. In approximately 2% of cases, the phenotype is due to a partial trisomy resulting from an inherited balanced translocation/inversion or different degrees of mosaicism.

Screening: The same ultrasound and serum markers used in the first and second trimester for screening for T21 may be used for screening T18. Screening for T18 by cf-DNA on maternal blood is possible but with a lower detection rate than T21 (DR 96.3% FPR 0.13%) (Gil et al. 2015).

Ultrasound diagnosis: T18 has a well-defined pattern of minor and major abnormalities detectable by prenatal ultrasound (Table 14.8).

Table 14.8 Ultrasound features and biochemical markers of Trisomy 18

	Serum screening	Ultrasound markers	Fetal defects
First trimester (11^{+0}–13^{+6} weeks)	*Combined test* • β-hCG: ≈0.2 MoM • PAPP-A: ≈0.2 MoM *Triple test* • uE3: low • hCG: very low • AFP: low	• Increased NT • Rev DV • TR • SUA • Low FHR	• Cystic hygroma • Early onset FGR • Exomphalos • Megacystis • Clubbed hands • Abnormal 4Chv
Second trimester (14^{+0}–26^{+0} weeks)	*Quadruple test* • uE3: low • hCG: very low • AFP: low • Inhibin A: low	• Increased NF • Strawberry shaped skull • Choroid plexus cyst • Clenched hands • Rocker bottom feet	• Cardiac defects: most characteristic is malalignment VSD; occasionally seen: AVSD, HLHS, ToF, CAT, DORV CoA, Asymmetry of the heart, TV dysplasia • Skeleton: polydactyly, syndactyly limb reduction, talipes • Central nervous system: ventriculomegaly, microcephaly, spina bifida • Digestive system: esophageal atresia, congenital diaphragmatic hernia • Uro-genital system: hydronephrosis, renal dyspasia, horse-shoe kidney, hypospadias, ambiguous genitalia • FGR
Third trimester ($>26^{+1}$ weeks)			• Defects as above • FGR • Polyhydramnios

AFP alpha-fetoprotein, *AoV* aortic valve, *AVSD* atrio-ventricular septal defect, *β-hCG* human chorionic gonadotropin, *CoA* coarctation of the aorta, *FGR* fetal growth restriction, *FHR* fetal heart rate, *HLHS* hypoplastic left heart syndrome, *NB* nasal bone, *NF* nuchal fold, *NT* nuchal translucency, *PAPP-A* pregnancy-associated plasma protein A, *PV* pulmonary valve, *Rev DV* reversed a-wave in ductus venosus, *SUA* single umbilical artery, *SV* single ventricle, *CAT* common arterial trunk, *TAPVC* total anomalous pulmonary venous connection, *TGA* transposition of the great arteries, *ToF* tetralogy of fallot, *TR* tricuspid regurgitation, *TV* tricuspid valve, *uE3* unconjugated estriol, *VSD* ventricular septal defect

- *Cardiac anomalies:* CHD is found in 80% of fetuses with T18 with a predilection for females. The most common CHD in T18 is VSD (Springett et al. 2015).
- *Extra-cardiac anomalies:* ECAs are described in over 50% of fetuses with T18 and are summarised in Table 14.8 and Fig. 14.13. Some of these defects may be detected as early as in the first trimester of pregnancy (omphalocele, megacystis, abnormal hand posturing, abnormal four chambers view, single umbilical artery) while others may be late onset (FGR, polyhydramnios).

Prenatal diagnosis: QF-PCR or conventional karyotyping on chorionic villi, amniocytes, and peripheral leukocytes is indicated to confirm the diagnosis.

Prognosis: In view of the multisystem anomalies usually present in fetuses affected by T18, this diagnosis was widely considered lethal in the past with very limited interventions employed. However, in recent times, this view has been challenged by the introduction of aggressive neonatal resuscitation and palliative surgery to improve survival. The influence and the importance of such interventions remain controversial owing to ethical issues arising from treating a multi-systemic disorder with severe developmental delay and dismal survival rate beyond 1 year of age.

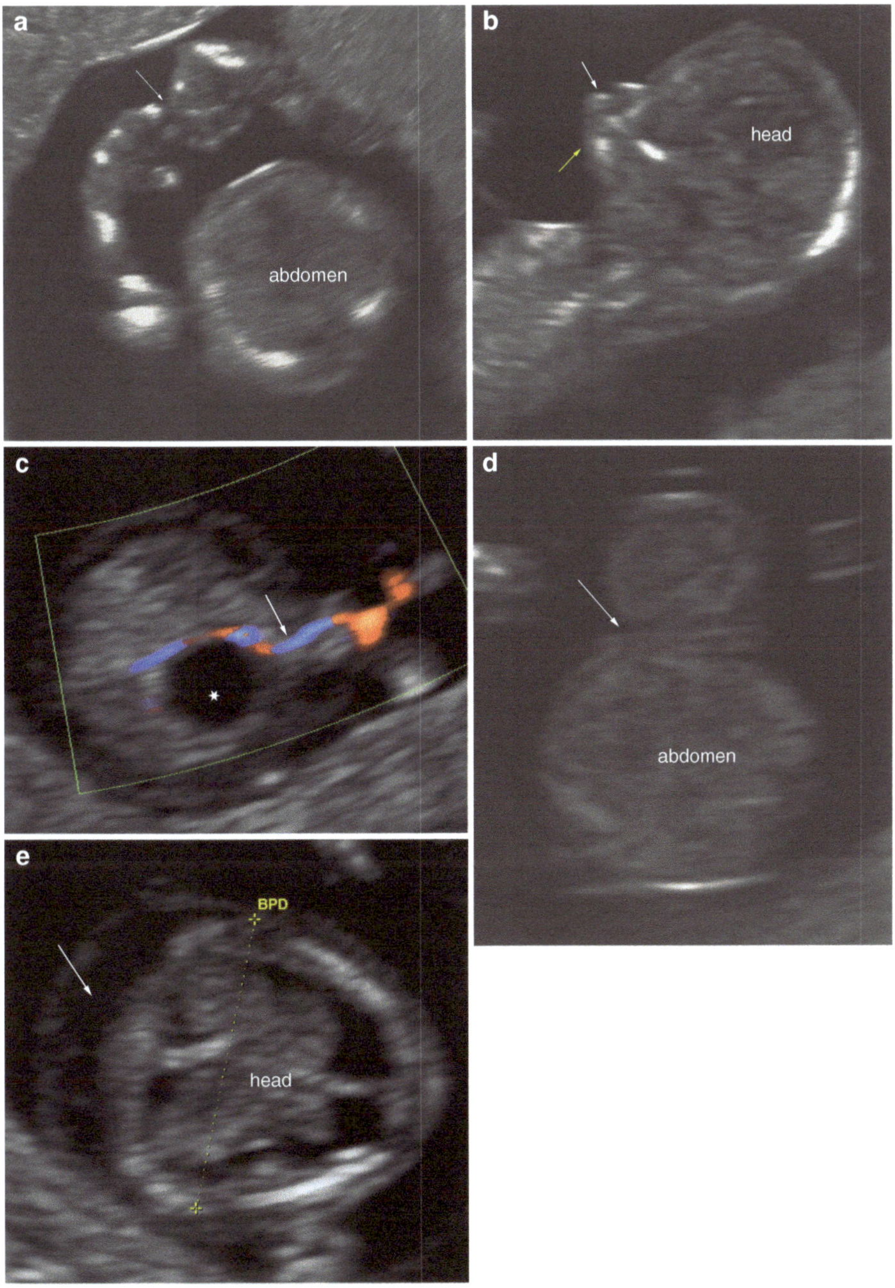

Fig. 14.13 (**a**) Transverse section at the level of the fetal abdomen demonstrating upper limbs extended in front of the body with bilateral abnormal wrists (white arrow) in a 12 weeks fetus with prenatal diagnosis of Trisomy 18. (**b**) Mid-sagittal view of the fetal face demonstrating a small chin (white arrow) and the pre-maxillary protrusion (white arrow) suggestive of median cleft lip palate in a 12 weeks fetus with prenatal diagnosis of Trisomy 18. (**c**) Transverse section of the pelvis with Colour flow investigation showing a moderately enlarged bladder (asterisk) outlined by a single umbilical artery in a 12 weeks fetus with prenatal diagnosis of Trisomy 18. (**d**) Transverse section of the fetal abdomen showing a large defect of the anterior abdominal wall (white arrow) with herniation of viscera covered by peritoneal and amniotic membranes (exomphalos) in a 12 weeks fetus with prenatal diagnosis of Trisomy 18. (**e**) Transverse section of the fetal head showing strawberry-shaped skull and increased NT (white arrow) in a 12 weeks fetus with prenatal diagnosis of Trisomy 18

Recurrence risk: Empirically estimated at 1%.

Trisomy 13

Definition: Trisomy 13 (T13) or Patau syndrome is the third most common autosomal aneuploidy. The genetic defect leads to an almost invariably lethal phenotype comprising multiple anomalies including CHD, oro-facial cleft, abdominal wall, limbs and central nervous system defects.

Epidemiology and risk factors: The estimated incidence ranges from 1 in 5000 to 1 in 20,000 live births. There is a positive correlation with advancing maternal age.

Pathogenesis: T13 is due to an extra copy of chromosome 13. A free trisomy is responsible for 75% of cases (usually due to non-disjunctional error at maternal meiosis II). In the remaining 25%, a Robertsonian translocation is found. Rare cases of mosaicisms with extreme phenotypic variability (depending upon percentage of trisomic cell lines) have also been reported.

Screening: The same algorithm used in the first and second trimester for screening of T21 may be used also for the screening for T13. Screening for T13 by cf-DNA on maternal blood has the worst performance (DR 91.0% FPR 0.13%) amongst autosomic trisomies (Gil et al. 2015).

Ultrasound diagnosis: The spectrum of anomalies associated with T13 is listed in Table 14.9.

- *Cardiac anomalies:* CHD is found in about 60% of fetuses with T13. The most common CHD is VSD (Springett et al. 2015)
- *Extra-cardiac anomalies:* Over 50% of fetuses with T13 have ECAs including central nervous system, facial abnormalities, limb and abdominal wall defects (Fig. 14.14).

Table 14.9 Ultrasound features and biochemical markers of Trisomy 13

	Serum screening	Ultrasound markers	Fetal defects
First trimester (11^{+0}–13^{+6} weeks)	*Combined test* • β-hCG: ≈0.5 MoM • PAPP-A: ≈0.3 MoM *Triple test* • uE3: low • hCG: low • AFP: low	• Increased NT • Rev DV • TR • High FHR	• Cystic hygroma • Holoprosencephaly • Facial abnormalities (proboscis, cleft palate) • Abnormal 4Chv • Omphalocele • Megacystis • Post-axial polydactyly
Second trimester–third trimester	*Quadruple test* • uE3: low • hCG: low • AFP: low • Inhibin A: low		• Cardiac defects: VSD, AVSD, HLHS, ToF, DORV, CoA • Oro-facial: cleft lip-palate, micrognathia • Central nervous system: holoprosencephaly/arhinencephaly, micro-anophtalmos, congenital cataract, microcephaly, ventriculomegaly, encephalocele, spina bifida • Uro-genital system: hydronephrosis, renal dysplasia • Skeleton: polydactyly, syndactyly limb reduction, talipes • Digestive system: anal atresia, congenital diaphragmatic hernia • Abdominal wall defects: omphalocele • FGR

AFP alpha-fetoprotein, *AVSD* atrio-ventricular septal defect, *β-hCG* human chorionic gonadotropin, *CoA* coarctation of the aorta, *FGR* fetal growth restriction, *FHR* fetal heart rate, *NT* nuchal translucency, *PAPP-A* pregnancy-associated plasma protein A, *PAtr* pulmonary atresia, *PS* pulmonary stenosis, *Rev DV* reversed a-wave in ductus venosus, *CAT* common arterial trunk, *ToF* tetralogy of fallot, *TR* tricuspid regurgitation, *uE3* unconjugated estriol, *VSD* ventricular septal defect

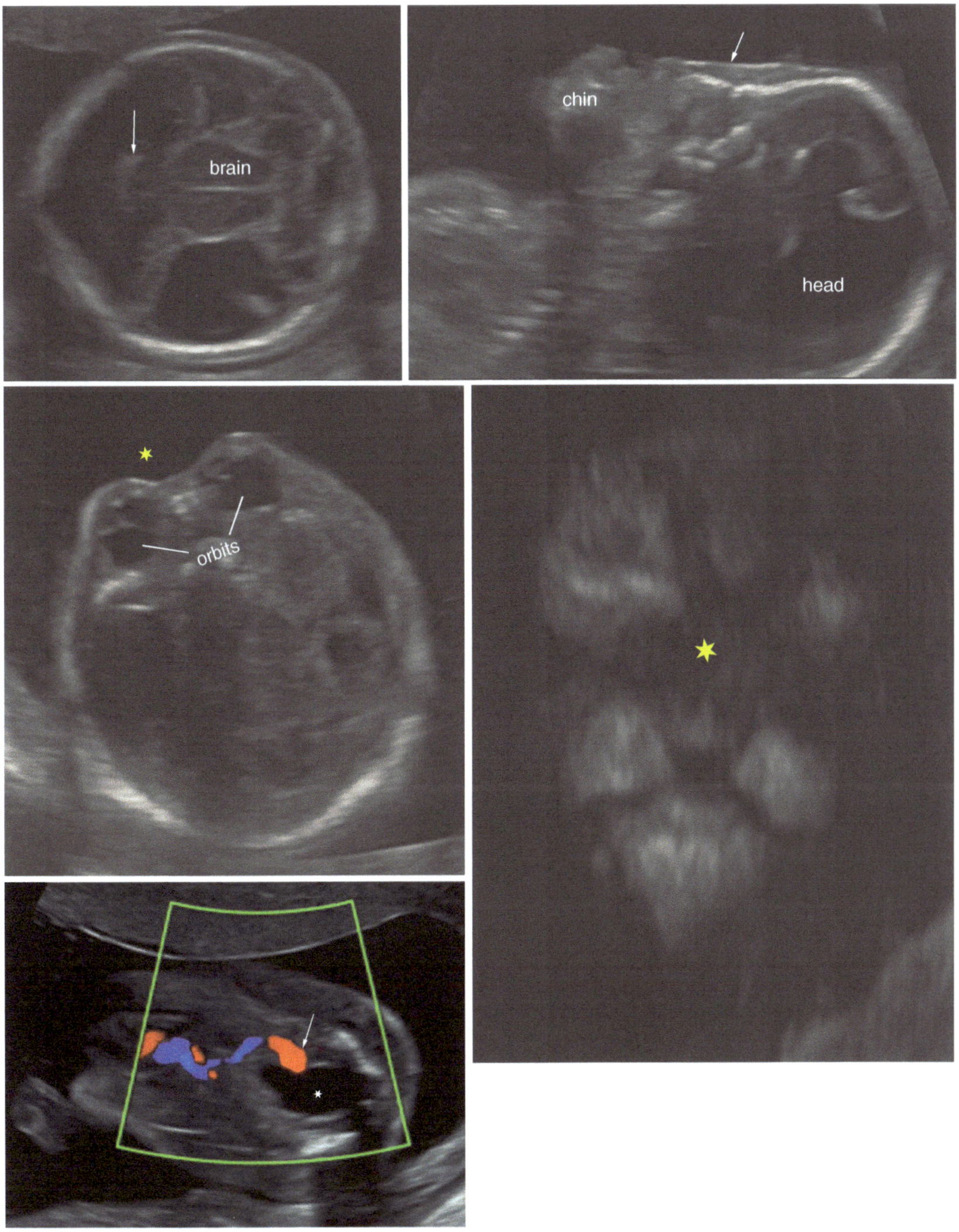

Fig. 14.14 (**a**) Transverse section of the fetal head showing abnormal cleavage of the forebrain with a single large fluid filled cavity (*white arrow*) and fused talami (holoprosencephaly) in this fetus at 20 weeks of gestation with confirmed Trisomy 13. (**b**) Mid-sagittal view of the fetal face demonstrating absence of the nose (*white arrow*) "arrhynia" and marked prognathism in this fetus at 20 weeks of gestation with confirmed Trisomy 13. (**c**) Transverse section of the fetal head at the level of the orbits showing marked hypertelorism and absence of the nose (*asterisk*) in this fetus at 20 weeks of gestation with confirmed Trisomy 13. (**d**) Coronal view of the fetal face showing midline facial defect (*asterisk*) in this fetus at 20 weeks of gestation with confirmed Trisomy 13. The asterisk shows the missing central area including both upper lip and the alveolar ridge. (**e**) Transverse section of the pelvis with Colour flow demonstrating a normal size bladder (*asterisk*) outlined by a single umbilical artery in this fetus at 20 weeks of gestation with confirmed Trisomy 13

Prenatal diagnosis: QF-PCR or conventional karyotyping on chorionic villi, amniocytes, and peripheral leukocytes are indicated to confirm the diagnosis.

Prognosis: Very poor. Approximately half of the pregnancies with a prenatal diagnosis of T13 will result in an intrauterine death. For those born alive approximately 80% die on day 1, and over 95% within 1 week of life. Rare cases with no severe anomalies survive the first year of life.

Recurrence risk: Empirically estimated at 1%. Cases with the typical syndromal pattern of T13 and normal karyotype (pseudo-trisomy 13) have a much higher recurrence risk (25%).

Monosomy X (45X0)

Definition: Monosomy X (45X0) or Turner syndrome is a chromosomal abnormality found in females with diverse clinical features, including short stature, infertility and cardiac and renal anomalies.

Epidemiology and risk factors: The incidence of 45X0 syndrome is estimated at 1 in 2500 live female births and it is unrelated to maternal age.

Pathogenesis: This syndrome is caused by the absence of (full monosomy X), or structural abnormalities in the second X chromosome in all or some of the body cell lines (mosaicism 45X0/46XX). Different genotypes are associated with variable presentations along the syndrome phenotype spectrum, with full monosomy (75%) typically having the most severe.

Screening: Many cases of 45X0 are detected at the time of first trimester screening due to increased NT. Screening for 45X0 is possible by cf-DNA on maternal blood with DR 90.3% and FPR 0.23% (Gil et al. 2015)

Ultrasound features:

- *Cardiac anomalies:* CHD are found in about 30% of fetuses with 45X0 with the most common being ventricular and great arteries asymmetry suggesting the possibility of coarctation after birth.
- *Extra-cardiac anomalies:* About 50% of fetuses with 45X0 have ECA detectable antenatally as reported in Table 14.10. The most common finding is a large, usually septate cystic hygroma in the first trimester (Fig. 14.15), often associated with a general malformation of the lymphatic system and HF (Fig. 14.4). In non-lethal cases, cystic hygroma may persist throughout gestation and be visible at birth as *pterygium*.

Table 14.10 Fetal defects in 45X0

• Lymphatic system: Cystic hygroma, pleural effusions and fetal hydrops
• Cardio-vascular system: aortic arch hypoplasia/CoA, HLHS
• Genito-urinary system: horseshoe kidney, renal dysplasia

CoA coarctation of the aorta, *HLHS* hypoplastic left heart syndrome

Prenatal diagnosis: QF-PCR or conventional karyotyping on chorionic villi, amniocytes, and peripheral leukocytes are indicated to confirm the diagnosis.

Prognosis: In most cases (75%) diagnosed prenatally with full monosomy 45X0 the severity of the phenotype leads to spontaneous demise in the first or second trimester. In the survivors, the prognosis is generally benign and mostly dependent on severity of any CHD. Intelligence is usually normal. All 45X0 females are infertile and most require hormonal treatment to develop and maintain secondary sexual characteristics. Affected individuals are also at increased risk of autoimmune disorders and hearing loss. In cases where mosaic 45X0 is diagnosed counselling is challenging as the spectrum of outcomes ranges from phenotypically normal to completely affected depending on the extent of mosaicism (Chap. 15).

Recurrence risk: Unmodified as compared to the normal population.

Triploidy

Definition: Triploidy is a lethal chromosomal abnormality due to a complete extra set of haploid chromosomes and characterized by severe early-onset FGR, placental and multi-system anomalies.

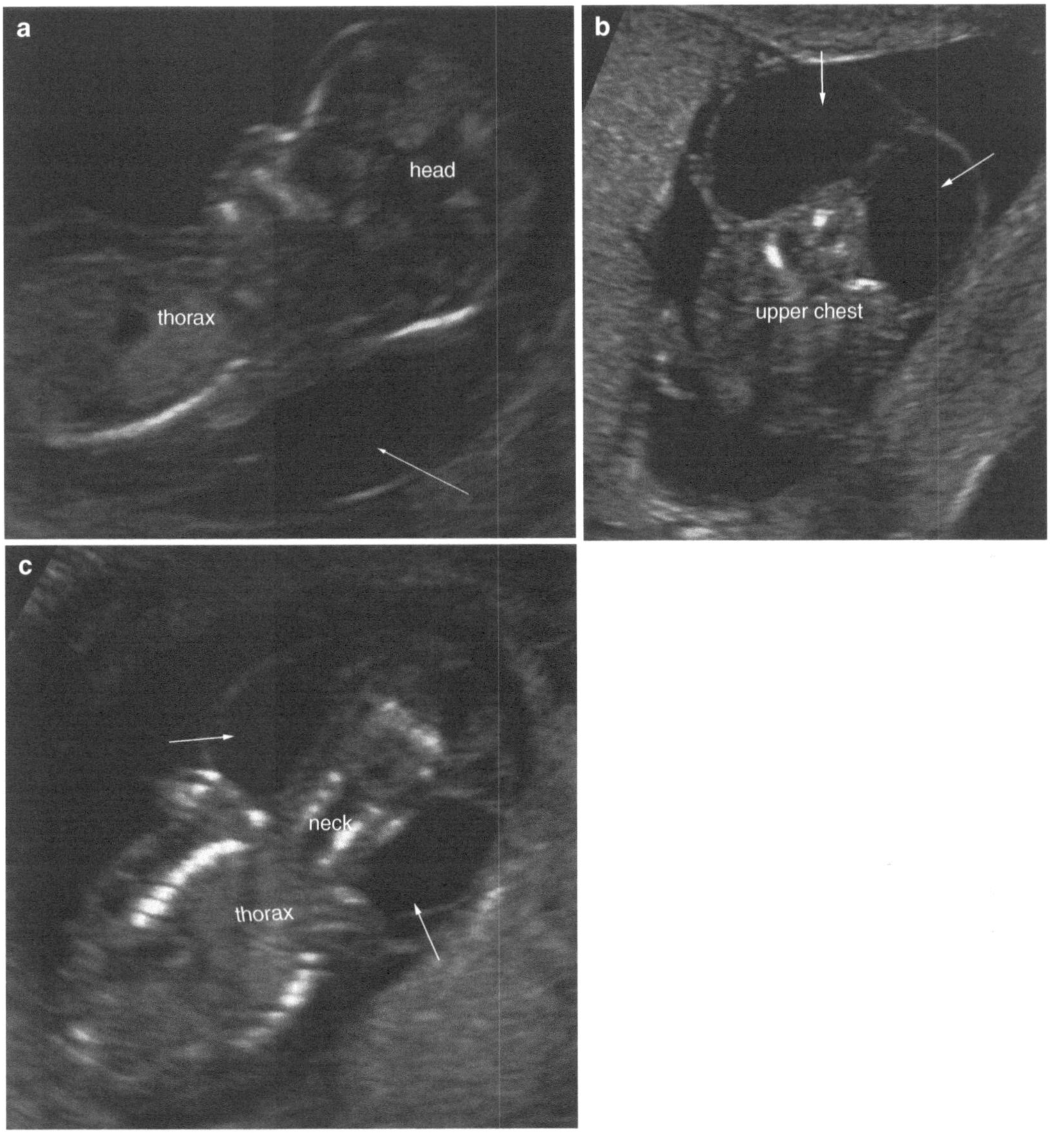

Fig. 14.15 (**a**) Mid-sagittal view of the nuchal area showing a large, septated cystic hygroma (*white arrow*) in a 12 weeks fetus with prenatal diagnosis of 45X0. (**b**) Transverse view of the nuchal area showing a large, septated cystic hygroma (*white arrows*) in a 12 weeks fetus with prenatal diagnosis of 45X0. (**c**) Coronal view of the nuchal area showing a large, septated cystic hygroma (*white arrows*) in a 12 weeks fetus with prenatal diagnosis of 45X0

Epidemiology and risk factors: The incidence at 12 weeks is 1:2500–5000, whereas the incidence at birth is about 1:10,000 as most triploid fetuses undergo spontaneous demise before 20 weeks' gestation. There is no relationship with advancing maternal age.

Pathogenesis: The extra set of haploid chromosomes in triploidy can be of either maternal (digynic) or paternal (diandric) origin with the different karyotypes resulting in markedly different phenotypes.

Screening: Use of the combined algorithm for T21 identifies about 85% of fetuses with triploidy. While non-invasive prenatal testing by cf-fetal DNA can accurately identify additional fetal haplotypes (Nicolaides et al. 2014) the specificity of the test is still too low to distinguish between different underlying aetiologies such as vanishing or unrecognized twins and triploid pregnancies. At present, confirmation with invasive testing is mandatory.

Ultrasound diagnosis: Diagnosis can be suspected in the first trimester for early onset FGR and placental abnormalities, with each karyotype presenting characteristic features (Fig. 14.16). Additional anomalies supporting the diagnosis and common to both types may become apparent in the second trimester (Table 14.11).

Prenatal diagnosis: Prenatal diagnosis is feasible by G-banding of chromosomes on chorionic villi, amniocytes, and peripheral leukocytes.

Prognosis: The vast majority of cases spontaneously demise by the second trimester of pregnancy. Rare cases reaching term survive for only a few hours after birth. Triploidy has been associated with maternal complications during pregnancy and birth, such as varying degrees of pre-eclampsia, persistent trophoblastic disease and emergency operative delivery owing to fetal distress.

Recurrence risk: Unmodified as compared with the normal population.

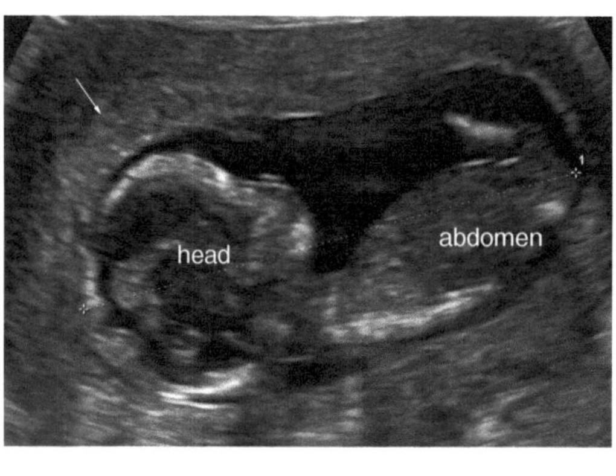

Fig. 14.16 Mid-sagittal view of a fetus at 12 weeks showing gross disproportion between a large head and a diminutive body. Notably, the fetal head appears disproportionally large as compared to the body and the placenta (white arrow) is very thinned

Table 14.11 Fetal defects in Triploidy

First trimester	
Diandric triploidy	*Digynic triploidy*
• FGR: moderate, symmetrical • Placenta: hyperplastic, partial molar changes • Increased NT • Increased β-hCG	• FGR: severe, asymmetrical (small trunk and limbs; normal or large head) • Placenta: small, thin, non-molar • Normal NT • Low β-hCG and PAPP-A
Second trimester	
• CNS: Ventriculomegaly, agenesis of the corpus callosum, Dandy-Walker malformation, holoprosencephaly, meningomyelocele • Cranio-facial: Hypertelorism, microphthalmia, micrognathia • Cardiac defect: VSD • Abdominal wall: Omphalocele • Genito-urinary: Hydronephrosis, renal dysplasia, hypospadia • Limbs: Syndactyly of the third and fourth fingers, talipes • Amniotic fluid: Oligohydramnios	

β-hCG human chorionic gonadotropin, *CNS* central nervous system, *FGR* fetal growth restriction, *NT* nuchal translucency, *PAPP-A* pregnancy-associated plasma protein A, *VSD* ventricular septal defect

Non-chromosomal Syndromes

22q11.2 Deletion

Definition: 22q11.2 deletion is characterized by a highly variable phenotype including CHD, facial dysmorphism, developmental delay, and an array of early- and later-onset medical and psychiatric disorders. 22q11.2 deletion comprises a number of clinical syndromes originally thought to be distinct (e.g. DiGeorge syndrome, velocardiofacial syndrome) before the discovery of a common underlying microdeletion on chromosome 22q11.2.

Epidemiology and risk factors: 22q11.2 deletion is the most common microdeletion syndrome in humans, with an estimated incidence varying between 1 in 1000 and 1 in 6000 across different studies.

Pathogenesis: 22q11.2 deletion is caused by deletion of chromosome 22q11.2, which occurs *de novo* in over 90% of cases. In the remaining

10% either the deletion results from an unbalanced translocation inherited from a parent with a balanced translocation or it is inherited in an autosomal dominant (AD) pattern from an affected parent. Duplications in the same region may lead to a similar phenotype. The genetic defect leads to arrest in the development and migration of neural crest cells toward the pharyngeal arches. Indeed, structural abnormalities in 22q11.2 deletion typically involve anatomic structures developing from the third and the fourth pharyngeal arches. These include abnormalities of the cardiac outflow tracts, thymus and parathyroid hypoplasia/aplasia, palatal anomalies and minor craniofacial anomalies. There is no known association with parental age or any other factor.

Screening: Early diagnosis of 22q11.2 deletion may result in decreased morbidity and mortality. In particular, prompt recognition of hypocalcemia may lead to reduced incidence of seizures thus improving the neurodevelopmental outcome. At present, screening for 22q11.2 deletion is not well established. The association with increased NT in the first trimester is weak. Preliminary data on cf-DNA screening for 22q11.2 deletion appear promising (Gross et al. 2016). However, clinical validation studies including investigation of false-positive results in large populations are needed before screening can be recommended. Such studies may prove difficult to conduct as the true prevalence of this condition is unknown and testing of fetuses and newborns with negative cf-DNA screening results is not generally performed.

Ultrasound features:

- *Cardiac anomalies:* About 40–75% of 22q11.2 deletion individuals have CHD of variable severity ranging from severe to subtle. Cardiac defects such as common arterial trunk, tetralogy of Fallot, absent pulmonary valve syndrome and interrupted aortic arch type B are highly prevalent. More recently, anomalies of aortic arch laterality or branching have been reported.
- *Extra-cardiac anomalies:* Additional ECAs occasionally detectable on prenatal ultrasound include FGR, micrognathia, renal defects and thymus hypoplasia or aplasia (Fig. 14.17). However, the reliability of fetal thymus measurements in predicting del22q11.2 deletion is debatable (Bataeva et al. 2013). One recent study reported dilation of the cavum septum pellucidum in 67.5% of second trimester fetuses with 22q11.2 deletion (Chaoui et al. 2016). Of note, minor facial dysmorphism and cleft palate in 22q11.2 deletion, which usually involves the posterior soft palate, are generally not detectable on prenatal ultrasound. Table 14.12 presents an overview of CHD and ECAs in 22q11.2 deletion.

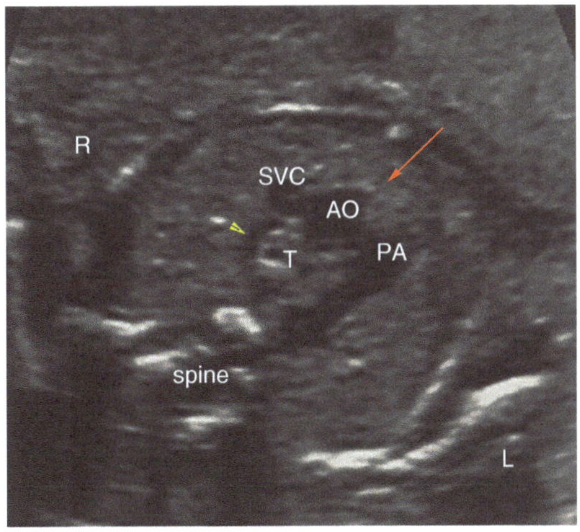

Fig. 14.17 Transverse section of the fetal thorax at 20 weeks demonstrating a normal thymus (*red arrow*) in front of the three-vessel and trachea view. A normal thymus on prenatal ultrasound does not exclude 22q11.2 deletion

Prenatal diagnosis: It is usually made in the second trimester as the discovery of an abnormality of the cardiac outflow tracts prompts invasive diagnosis. 22q11.2 deletion is rarely visible on G-banded chromosomes in a standard karyotype. Historically, fluorescence in situ hybridization (FISH) has been used to identify the deletion. Currently, a-CGH should be preferred as it can detect the classic deletion as well as atypical smaller deletions that are also clinically significant.

Prognosis: The prognosis of individuals diagnosed with the 22q11.2 deletion depends

Table 14.12 Fetal defects in 22q11.2 deletion

Ultrasound findings
• Cardiac defect (ToF, CAT, IAA type B, VSD, RAA)
• Thymus hypoplasia/aplasia
• Microcephaly
• Micrognathia
• Dilated cavum septum pellucidi (CSP)
• Thickened nuchal translucency
• Short long-bones
• FGR
Occasional findings
• Other brain abnormalities
• Renal defects (uni/bilateral hydronephrosis)
• Facial cleft
• Umbilical hernia
• Cryptorchidism
• Hypospadias

ALSA aberrant left subclavian artery, *CSP* cavum septum pellucidi, *FGR* fetal growth restriction, *IAA* interrupted aortic arch, *RAA* right aortic arch, *CAT* common arterial trunk, *ToF* tetralogy of fallot, *VSD* ventricular septal defect

on the phenotypic expression of the syndrome, on the severity of the associated CHD, and on the presence or absence of associated abnormalities. Immunodeficiency related to thymic hypoplasia/aplasia and hypocalcemia secondary to hypoplasia of the parathyroid glands need prompt medical treatment. Most affected individuals have borderline IQ or mild intellectual disability whereas more severe intellectual disability is less common. Learning difficulties and psychosocial problems related to the autism spectrum are also often present. Schizophrenia develops in about 1 in 4 individuals with 22q11.2 deletion, thus making the risk 20-fold higher than the general population (Bassett et al. 2017).

Recurrence risk: In *de novo* mutations the risk of recurrence is low. In the cases of an inherited mutation, the recurrence risk is 50% (autosomal dominant inheritance) and notably the phenotype of the affected parent does not predict that of their offspring.

Noonan Syndrome

Definition: Noonan syndrome (NS) is an autosomal dominant disorder characterized by facial dysmorphism, short stature, webbed neck, cardiac anomalies and variable degree of neurodevelopmental delay. The most frequent cardiac abnormalities are pulmonary valve stenosis and hypetrophic cardiomyopathy.

Epidemiology and risk factors: The estimated incidence of NS ranges from 1 in 1000 to 1 in 2500. It is likely that mild cases are overlooked, and the cardiac features may not be evident until the third trimester. There is an association with advanced paternal age.

Pathogenesis: NS shows significant genetic heterogeneity (Chap. 14). Although traditionally considered an autosomal dominant syndrome, in more than 50% of cases the mutation occurs *de novo*, in families with no prior history. Mutations at the 12q24.1 locus (a gene coding for the non-receptor protein tyrosine phosphate [SHP-2]) have been implicated in about 50% of cases. A significant correlation has been found between the presence/absence of the PTPN11 mutation and the type of CHD: in patients with the mutation pulmonary stenosis is more prevalent, whereas cardiomyopathy is more prevalent in those with different mutations.

Ultrasound features: NS is usually diagnosed on clinical grounds after birth. Prenatally, the diagnosis may be suspected in the first trimester in the presence of increased NT/cystic hygroma and a normal karyotype. In NS, nuchal thickening may persist into the second and third trimesters (Fig. 14.18) and present at birth as webbed neck. Late-onset CHD (50–80%) and further progression of lymphatic anomalies to pleural effusions, and skin edema may further support the diagnosis (Vigneswaran et al. 2017). Occasionally, fully blown HF may develop leading to an increased risk of intrauterine death and perinatal mortality (Table 14.13).

Prenatal diagnosis: Prenatal diagnosis was traditionally limited to the 50% cases with known PTPN11 mutation. At present, complex, expensive molecular genetic testing (multi-gene panel, serial single-gene testing and genome sequencing) may identify up to 75% of the known mutations leading to NS phenotype.

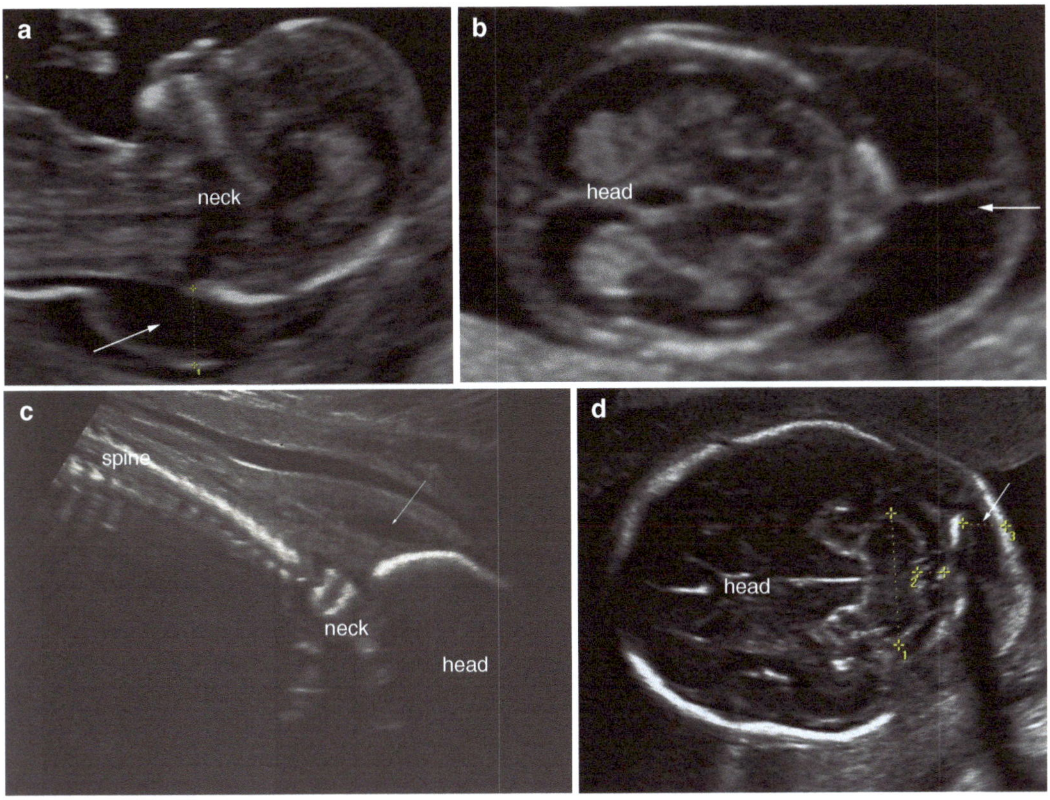

Fig. 14.18 (**a**) Mid-sagittal section of the head and upper chest showing accumulation of fluid confined to the nuchal area (cystic hygroma, *white arrow*) in a fetus at 12 weeks with a postnatal diagnosis of Noonan's. (**b**) Transverse section of the head showing accumulation of fluid in the nuchal area (cystic hygroma, *white arrow*) in a fetus at 12 weeks with a postnatal diagnosis of Noonan's (same fetus as in **a**). A septum is clearly visible within the cystic mass. (**c**) Mid-sagittal back-up view of the head and upper chest showing accumulation of fluid in the subcutaneous tissue of the nuchal area (*white arrow*) in a fetus at 22 weeks with persistent increased nuchal fold and postnatal diagnosis of Noonan's. (**d**) Transverse section of the head showing accumulation of fluid in the nuchal area (*white arrow*) in a fetus at 22 weeks with persistent increased nuchal fold and postnatal diagnosis of Noonan's (same fetus as in **a**). Such collection of fluid is measured as nuchal fold (*yellow calipers*)

Table 14.13 Fetal defects in Noonan syndrome

First trimester
• Cystic hygroma with normal karyotype • Agenesis of ductus venosus and other abnormalities of porto-umbilical system
Second/third trimester
• Persistent nuchal oedema with normal karyotype • Cardiac defect: – pulmonary stenosis, cardiomyopathy, VSD • Pleural effusion, ascites, hydrops (rare) • Renal abnormalities • Polyhydramnios

Prognosis: Individuals with NS may have a normal life expectancy. Prognosticators of poor outcome include HF or cardiomyopathy with severe cardiac dysfunction at birth. Mild to moderate intellectual disability is present in up to 1 in 4 affected individual. There is a tendency towards coagulation and bleeding abnormalities as well as complications related to abnormal lymphatics such as chylothorax.

Recurrence risk: In *de novo* mutations the risk of recurrence is low. In the cases of an inherited mutation, the recurrence risk is 50% (autosomal dominant inheritance).

VACTER/VACTERL

Definition: VACTER/VACTERL association is an acronym for a non-random pattern of abnormalities including Vertebral defects,

Table 14.14 Fetal defects in VACTER/VACTERL

Vertebral anomalies
Hemivertebrae and other vertebral anomalies
Anal atresia
Congenital heart disease:
VSD, ToF, CAT
Tracheo-oesophageal fistula
Oesophageal atresia
Renal anomalies
Unilateral renal agenesis, renal ectopia, horseshoe kidney, cystic dysplasia, hydronephrosis
Limbs
Radial aplasia and hypoplasia, radio-ulnar synostosis
Thumb hypoplasia, syndactyly, pre-axial polydactyly
Occasional:
• Single umbilical artery
• Genital defects

Anal atresia, CHD, Tracheo-Esophageal fistula, esophageal atresia and Renal dysplasias. In addition, VACTERL variant includes Limb defects.

Epidemiology and risk factors: It is very rare. There is a significant association with maternal diabetes.

Pathogenesis: The aetiology and heredity pattern of this condition are unknown.

Ultrasound features: These include abnormalities of spine, kidneys, heart, and limbs and other occasional defects (Table 14.14). There is a wide variation in number, type and severity of defects and not all of the features are necessary for the diagnosis. Often, the diagnosis is made in the late first or second trimester.

Prenatal diagnosis: It is based on ultrasound findings. Diagnosis may be challenging due to late onset or very subtle defects.

Prognosis: The outcome depends on the number and severity of the defects. CHD, anorectal and tracheoesophageal defects may require an early surgical approach. Vertebral anomalies and limb defects may pose significant functional impairment. Intelligence is usually normal in VACTERL.

Recurrence risk: VACTERL association is a sporadic anomaly thus the recurrence risk is extremely low.

Other Associations with Normal Karyotype

Defects commonly associated with CHD in the absence of genetic abnormalities are detailed below and shown in Fig. 14.19. The reported incidences of specific ECAs in association with CHD are variable across studies. Such defects are usually detected at the routine anomaly scan but may become apparent in the third trimester due to an associated finding, such as polyhydramnios. The detection of an ECA should always prompt a detailed fetal anatomy and cardiac survey.

Brain

- *Ventriculomegaly*: CHD more common when atrium of lateral ventricles measures 10–15 mm, less common >15 mm
- *Dandy Walker Malformation:* complete or partial agenesis of the cerebellar vermis with cystic dilation of posterior fossa. Defects more common in complete agenesis.
- *Holoprosencephaly:* various causes including genetic, teratogens and maternal diabetes
- *Agenesis of Corpus Callosum:* may be complete or partial. Cardiac defects very common in complete but also found in partial agenesis.
- *Microcephaly*: has a wide variety of causes including genetic, viral and environmental and cardiac defects are common.

Face

- *Cleft Lip and Palate:* commonly associated with structural anomalies. The incidence of cardiac abnormality is estimated to be about 7%.

Thorax

- *Oesophageal Atresia:* prenatal diagnosis is made from the finding of no visible stomach or a collapsed stomach and polyhydramnios. Cardiac defects are the most common non-syndromic structural abnormalities found. Also found as part of VACTERL.
- *Congenital Diaphragmatic Hernia:* can be left (90%) or right sided (10%). Often associated

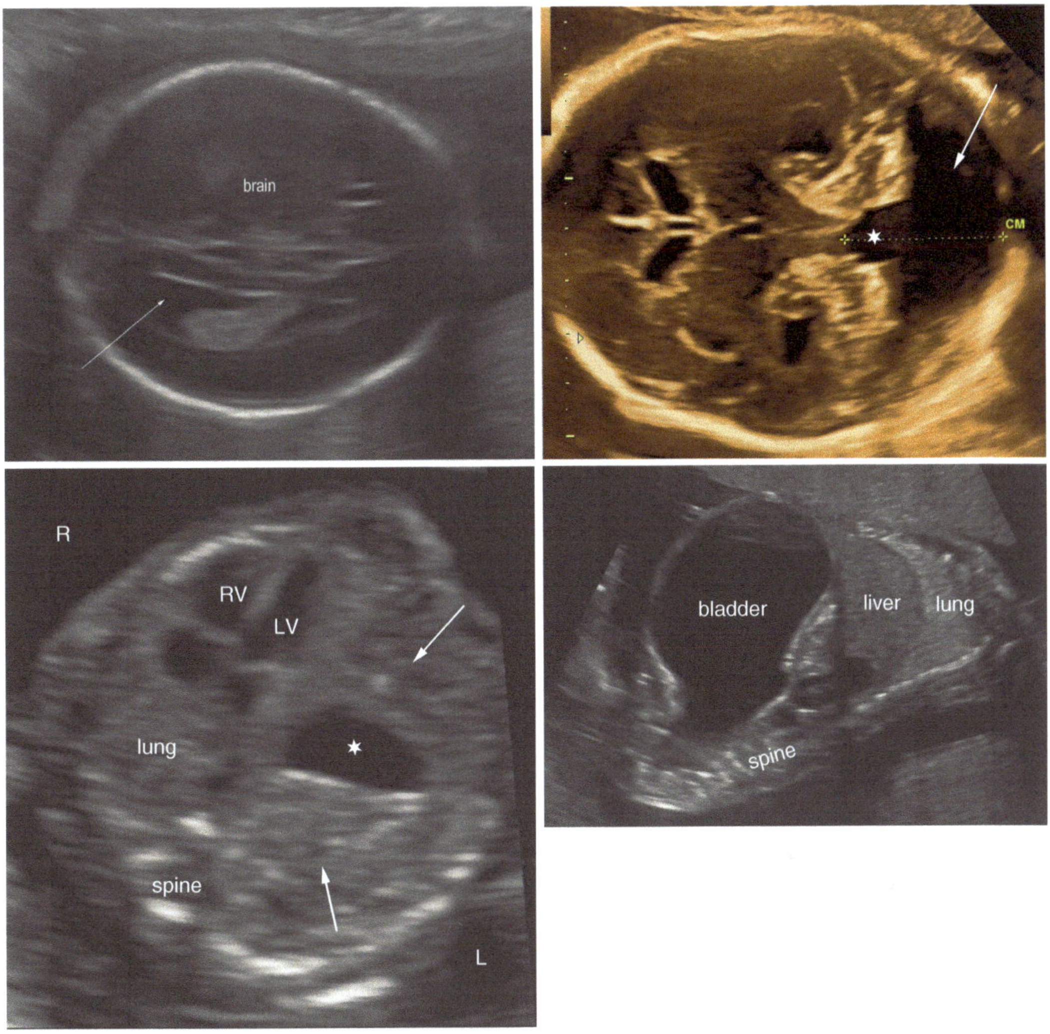

Fig. 14.19 (**a**) Axial, trans-ventricular section of head and brain in a fetus at 20 weeks with complete ACC. The trans-ventricular view shows absence of the cavum septum pellucidi, high-riding third ventricle between widely separated, parallel lateral ventricles and tear-drop dilatation (colpocephaly) of the posterior horns of the lateral ventricles (*white arrow*). (**b**) Axial, transcerebellar view of the head demonstrating vermian agenesis (*asterisk*) and cystic cisterna magna (*yellow arrow*) in a fetus at 24 weeks of gestation with Dandy Walker malformation. (**c**) Transverse section of the thorax in a fetus at 21 weeks of gestation affected by left-sided CDH. The stomach (*asterisk*) and loops of small bowel (*white arrow*) are displaced in the left hemithorax. There is mediastinal shift and a very small amount of lung tissue is seen behind the heart (*arrowhead*). (**d**) Mid-sagittal view of trunk at 18 weeks of gestation in a fetus diagnosed with posterior urethral valves. The bladder is severely dilated and occupies the whole abdomen. The white arrow shows splinting of the diaphragm with marked accentuation of its natural lower concavity. Note the increased echogenicity of the lung tissue as compared to the liver

with chromosome abnormality and genetic syndromes but isolated cardiac defects are found in about 10% of cases.

- *Pleural Effusion*: CHD is found in 5–10% of cases

Abdominal Wall

- *Exomphalos:* CHD is found in 30% of euploid cases
- *Pentalogy of Cantrell:* is a rare condition. Features are epigastric exomphalos, sternal

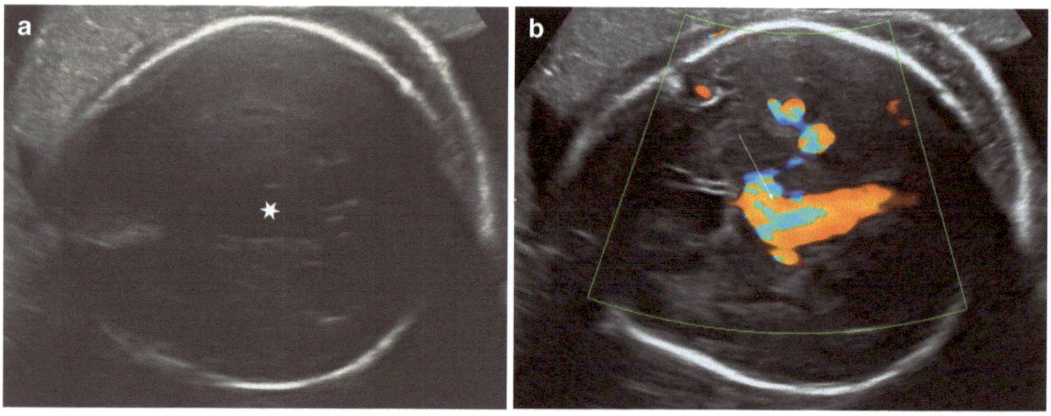

Fig. 14.20 (**a**) Axial views of head and brain in a fetus at 31 weeks of gestation with Vein of Galen malformation. The asterisk demonstrates an anechoic tubular structure situated supratentorially in the midline. (**b**) Axial views of head and brain in a fetus at 31 weeks of gestation with Vein of Galen malformation. With the aid of Colour Doppler investigation, it is evident the vascular nature of this structure and the flow turbulence (*white arrow*)

cleft, anterior diaphragmatic hernia, ectopia cordis and CHD (VSD and complex right-heart anomalies).

Gastro-intestinal Tract

- *Bowel Atresia:* duodenal atresia—CHD is found in about 20% of euploid cases. Jejunal and ileal atresia have a low incidence of CHD

Genito-urinary

- *Bilateral Renal Agenesis*: Cardiac defects are found in 25%, but some of these will be part of a more complex syndrome. Hypertrophic cardiomyopathy and pericardial effusion are commonly seen.
- *Horseshoe Kidney*
- *Bilateral Dysplastic Kidneys*
- *Bilateral Hydronephrosis*
- *Posterior Urethral Valves*

Vascular

- *Single Umbilical Artery*: CHD in 6% of cases
- *Intrahepatic Persistent Right Umbilical Vein*: CHD in 8% of cases
- *Agenesis of the Ductus Venosus*: Association with isolated CHD in 15% of cases. Where there is extra-hepatic drainage of umbilical vein there is a risk of congestive cardiac failure.
- *Vein of Galen Malformation:* this is a rare arteriovenous brain malformation. On ultrasound it appears as a cystic structure with turbulent flow on Colour Doppler investigation, located supratentorially in the midline above the cerebellum (Fig. 14.20). The diagnosis is rarely made before the third trimester as the lesion becomes larger and more evident due to increasing flow and shunting as gestation advances. Fetal brain MRI is a useful adjunct for diagnosis. As the vascular shunt becomes haemodynamically significant, the fetus may show signs of high-output cardiac failure with hepatic venous congestion as well as FH. The prognosis, traditionally dismal, has greatly improved in recent years due to reliable prenatal diagnosis and postnatal interventional neuroradiology with intravascular embolization techniques. However, hydrops and brain abnormalities related to hypoxaemia remain poor prognostic indicators.

Maternal Causes of Fetal Defects

It has been estimated that at least 10% of congenital abnormalities arise from environmental exposures including maternal medical conditions, infections, substance abuse and medications. Therefore, it is of paramount importance that the diagnostic work-up of a fetus with multiple abnormalities includes a thorough maternal history including past or present medical illnesses, drug history, information regarding occupational/environmental risk factors.

Metabolic disorders

Diabetes Mellitus

Epidemiology: Maternal diabetes mellitus (DM) is a leading cause of birth defects with the prevalence of congenital anomalies in this population ranging from 3 to 20% across studies. Although the risk is mostly related to pre-existing DM, a significant association with gestational diabetes (GDM) has also been reported. This is likely to be due to a significant overlapping with type 2 DM first diagnosed in pregnancy.

Pathogenesis: The mechanisms through which maternal hyperglycaemia leads to teratogenicity are complex and not fully understood. Animal studies have suggested an association with decreased cell proliferation/increase cell apoptosis due to high oxidative stress as well as altered gene expression.

Risk factors: There appears to be a strong, almost linear relation between glycaemic control at conception and risk of birth defects with HbA1c values >7% being associated with substantial risk of fetal defects.

Ultrasound features: Although virtually any birth defect can be associated with DM, more abnormalities are seen in the cardiovascular, central nervous and skeletal systems (Table 14.15). Caudal regression syndrome, a rare malformative cluster including sacral agenesis, lower limb and genito-urinary abnormalities is almost exclusively associated with maternal DM (Fig. 14.21). Fetal growth may be excessive (fetal macrosomia) in poorly controlled DM or reduced (FGR) in cases of DM with vascular complications.

Prognosis: Variable. Depending on type and severity of defects.

Table 14.15 Fetal defects in pre-existing maternal Diabetes Mellitus

• CHD: VSD, CoA, HLHS
• Caudal regression syndrome, sirenomelia, VATER/VACTERL
• CNS: NTDs (anencephaly, encephalocele, spina bifida), hydrocephaly, microcephaly
• Facial: cleft lip/cleft lip-palate
• GI tract: duodenal and anorectal atresia, hypoplastic left colon
• Skeletal abnormalities: limb reduction, talipes
• Genito-urinary: renal agenesis, cystic kidneys, hydronephrosis, hypospadias
• Fetal growth: macrosomia, FGR

CoA coarctation of the aorta, *CNS* central nervous system, *FGR* fetal growth restriction, *HLHS* hypoplastic left heart syndrome, *NTDs* neural tube defects, *TGA* transposition of the great arteries, *VSD* ventricular septal defect

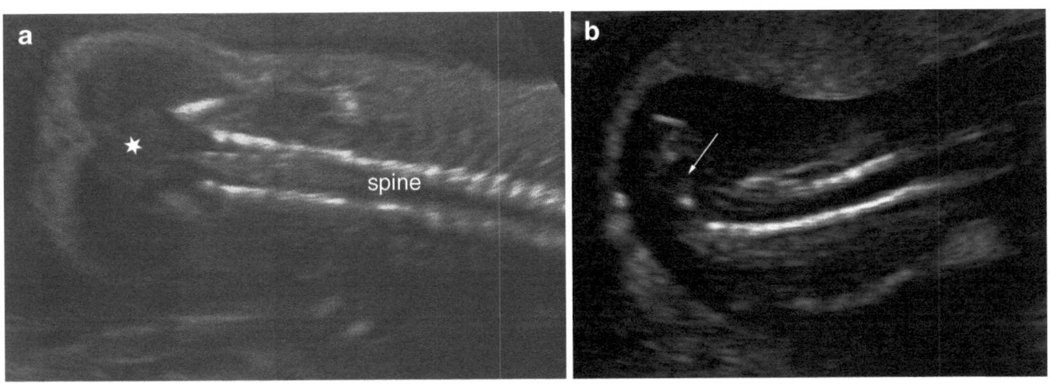

Fig. 14.21 (**a**) Coronal view of the lower spine demonstrating absence of the sacral vertebrae (*asterisk*) below the level of the pelvic bones (*white arrows*) in a fetus of a diabetic mother at 20 weeks of gestation (sacral agenesis). (**b**) Coronal view of the lower spine demonstrating absence of the sacral vertebrae (*arrowheads*) and unusual spinal curvature in a fetus of a diabetic mother at 15 weeks of gestation. In this fetus there was also total fusion of the lower limbs with single femur, tibia and foot (sirenomelia)

Recurrence risk: Optimising glycaemic control before conception and particularly during the first trimester of pregnancy has been shown to significantly reduce the risk of fetal defects without lowering it down to the background risk of the non-diabetic population. This is likely to be due to high rate (40%) of unplanned pregnancies in the women with DM.

Phenylketonuria

Definition: Phenylketonuria (PKU) is an autosomal recessive disorder caused by impaired enzymatic conversion of the essential amino-acid phenylalanine to tyrosine with subsequent hyperphenylalaninemia. High phenylalanine levels damage the developing brain and, without treatment, the classical presentation is of microcephaly and progressive, severe mental retardation. The UK national neonatal screening program for PKU and effective dietary treatment have greatly altered the prognosis of this disorder. Most affected individuals are treated with phenylalanine-free diet from an early age and have normal intellectual development. Uncontrolled maternal PKU with elevated levels of phenylalanine may cause teratogenicity in the fetus leading to a distinct syndrome (maternal PKU, mPKU) characterized by facial dysmorphism, microcephaly, significant neurocognitive impairment and CHD.

Epidemiology and risk factors: PKU is one of the most common inherited metabolic disorders with a prevalence of 1 in 10,000 in Europe. mPKU is rare.

Pathogenesis: Phenylalanine crosses the placenta by active transport, reaching higher concentrations in the fetal compartment. There is a linear relationship between maternal levels of phenylalanine and severity of birth defects. While the critical period for phenylalanine mediated brain and cardiac teratogenicity in the fetus is the first trimester of pregnancy, neurological abnormalities may result from exposure at any gestational age.

Ultrasound features: Congenital anomalies associated with mPKU are usually diagnosed in the mid (CHD including CoA, ToF, HLHS, VSD), or late (microcephaly, FGR), second trimester.

Prenatal diagnosis: Not usually indicated but can be performed in at risk families by molecular studies on chorionic villi, amniotic fluid or fetal blood.

Prognosis: Variable, depending on the severity of the phenotype.

Recurrence risk: Strict peri-conceptional and gestational dietary control have been shown to significantly decrease the risk of birth defects and improve growth and neurodevelopmental outcome in the offspring of women with PKU.

Infectious Disorders

Prenatal ultrasound can demonstrate a number of abnormalities associated with *in utero* infection involving multiple organ systems. These include intracranial abnormalities and parenchymal calcifications of the brain and the liver, cardiac abnormalities, anomalies of growth, placenta and amniotic fluid (Fig. 14.22). Ultrasound evidence of features consistent with fetal infection usually indicates a poor prognosis.

Being able to suspect and confirm a diagnosis of congenital infection prenatally is essential for counselling and perinatal management of affected pregnancies. There are wide differences in the teratogenic effects and options for treatment in fetuses with in utero infections.

Cytomegalovirus

Definition: Congenital cytomegalovirus (CMV) is the most common intrauterine infection and the leading infectious cause of sensorineural hearing loss and mental retardation.

Epidemiology: Congenital CMV occurs in 0.7% of live births worldwide. Primary and secondary maternal infections (reactivation of the endogen CMV strain or reinfection with a different strain) are thought to contribute equally to the burden of the disease. Primary maternal infections can be accurately confirmed and timed by IgG, IgM and IgG avidity serology. In contrast, there are still no validated methods for confirming secondary infections (Leurez-Ville and Ville 2017).

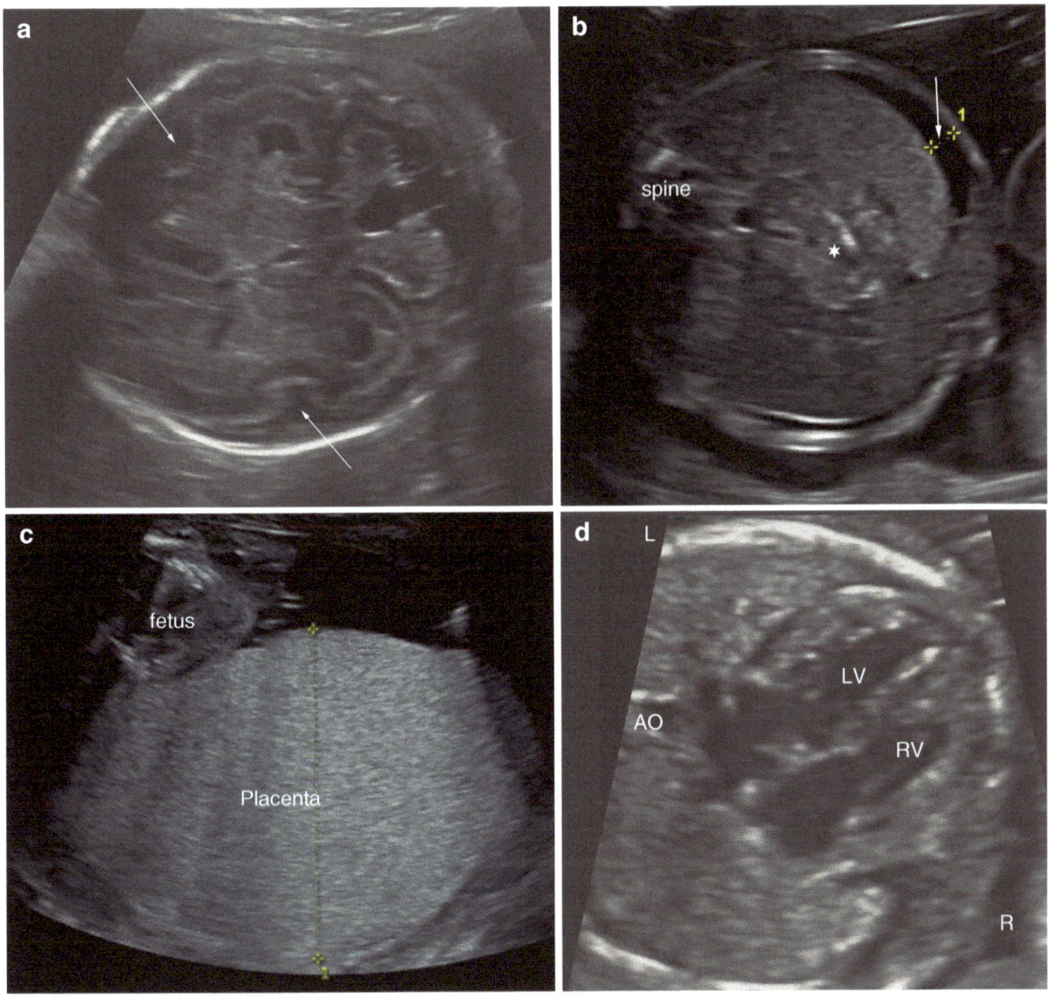

Fig. 14.22 (**a**) Axial, trans-cerebellar view of the brain in a fetus at 24 weeks' gestation with confirmed congenital cytomegalovirus infection. Note the very typical echogenic rim to the ventricular system and the "walnut aspect" (white arrows) of the brain, due to abnormal gyration and sulcation with consequent increased pericerebral spaces. (**b**) Axial view of the fetal abdomen in a fetus at 24 weeks' gestation with confirmed congenital cytomegalovirus infection. The yellow calipers highlight a rim of ascites. The stomach bubble is not visible due to compression by the enlarged liver. Note the echogenicity of the bowel mass (asterisk). (**c**) Placentitis appears as a thick and heterogeneous placenta with diffuse hyperechogenicity. Note the thickness of the placenta as compared to the fetus (F). (**d**) Transverse section of the thorax at the 4-chamber view in a fetus at 24 weeks' gestation with confirmed congenital cytomegalovirus infection. Note the enlarged, globular appearances of the heart and the diffuse myocardial hyperechogenicity

Screening: It is not universally recommended in the UK.

Natural history: Approximately 10% of infected newborns are symptomatic at birth (petechia, microcephaly, hepatosplenomegaly, FGR, chorioretinitis, thrombocytopenia, hepatitis). Among symptomatic neonates, mortality is as high as 30% and long-term sequelae (mental retardation, motor handicap and hearing loss) develop in 40–60% of cases. In the asymptomatic group, the risk of neurological morbidity including hearing loss is about 15%.

Ultrasound findings: Ultrasound features of fetal CMV infection may be progressive and sometimes only subtle or transient (Table 14.16).

- *Cardiac anomalies:* CMV cardiomyopathy is a rare finding, often associated with hydrops.

Table 14.16 Ultrasound features of congenital Cytomegalovirus infection

• Brain abnormalities: ventriculomegaly, intracranial calcifications, microcephaly, brain atrophy
• CHD: cardiomegaly, thickened hyperechogenic myocardium
• Abdominal abnormalities: hyperechogenic bowel, intra-epathic calcifications, hepatosplenomegaly, ascites
• Anomalies of growth: FGR with relatively larger abdomen (due to hepatosplenomegaly)
• Anomalies of fetal adnexa: Placentitis (thickened placenta), oligohydramnios or polyhydramnios

FGR fetal growth restriction

This typically presents as cardiomegaly with a thick myocardium often containing punctate calcifications manifestating as bright echogenity of the myocardium.

- *Extra-cardiac anomalies:* A thickened and inhomogeneous placenta (placentitis) may be an early sign of vertical transmission as the placenta is where the virus initially replicates. Once the virus reaches the fetal circulation, the fetal kidneys are usually the preferred target and therefore renal hyperechogenicity and more often oligohydramnios may be seen. Polyhydramnios may be less frequently seen as a result of stomach compression from liver enlargement. Involvement of the bowel (perforation, peritonitis or ileus) may present as hyperechogenicity. Brain lesions may be late-onset, progressive and challenging without the aid of fetal brain MRI. Features of overt systemic disease may include hepato-splenomegaly, liver and spleen calcifications, ascites and less often HF. FGR may develop as a result of either fetal infection or placental infection or both.

Prenatal diagnosis: Evidence of maternal seroconversion in the presence of compatible ultrasound fetal signs suggests a diagnosis of primary CMV infection. Diagnostic confirmation can be achieved by QF-PCR for CMV DNA in the amniotic fluid. This test has almost 100% sensitivity when the timing is appropriate (at least 6–8 weeks after seroconversion and always after 20 weeks' gestation).

Prognosis: Severe cerebral lesions are associated with a dismal prognosis thus termination of pregnancy should be discussed. In cases of proven maternal infection with non-severe or no ultrasound signs on serial examinations, the addition of fetal cerebral MRI is useful to refine the prognosis allowing negative predictive values of around 90%. In selected cases, FBS may also be considered as high viral load and thrombocytopenia (<10,000/mm^3) in fetal blood are predictors of poor prognosis.

Treatment: Antiviral treatment with valaciclovir has been shown to improve outcomes in infected fetuses with moderate or no signs of infection. However, the efficacy and safety of this treatment need confirmation in a RCT.

Recurrence risk: unknown.

Rubella

Definition: Rubella infection in utero causes a pattern of abnormalities known as "Congenital Rubella syndrome" including CHD, deafness, learning disability and ocular defects.

Epidemiology: The rate of infection has reduced significantly following effective vaccination programs. Outbreaks of infection are still seen due to migrants from areas without such programs or, more recently, due to fear of adverse effects of the MMR vaccine.

Natural history: Vertical transmission may happen during maternal viraemia, which occurs 5–7 days after exposure. Risk of transmission depends on gestational age and follows a bimodal distribution with peaks prior to 11 weeks (about 90%) and in the late third trimester (70%) and an average 45% risk between 12 and 30 weeks' gestation. The risk of fetal damage due to infection approaches 100% before 12 weeks, drops to 20% between 12–16 weeks and becomes negligible thereafter. There is no risk of deafness after 20 weeks.

Pathogenesis: Rubella is highly teratogenic and may lead to fetal damage through a direct cytopathic effect (eye, heart) and vascular damage (brain, growth).

Ultrasound features: A wide range of CHD has been described in fetuses with confirmed Rubella infection. Ocular abnormalities may be

Table 14.17 Ultrasound features of congenital Rubella syndrome

• CHD: PS, Ebstein's anomaly of the tricuspid valve, CoA, VSD
• CNS: Microcephaly, intracranial calcifications, ventriculomegaly, subependymal pseudocysts
• Eye defects: cataracts, microphthalmia
• Gastro-intestinal tract: Hepatosplenomegaly, echogenic bowel, meconium peritonitis
• Anomalies of growth: FGR with relatively larger abdomen (due to hepatosplenomegaly)
• Anomalies of fetal adnexa: Placentitis (thickened placenta), oligohydramnios or polyhydramnios

CoA coarctation of the aorta, *FGR* fetal growth restriction, *PS* pulmonary stenosis, *VSD* ventricular septal defect

difficult to diagnose. Other aspecific signs of congenital infection including brain abnormalities, hepatosplenomegaly and fetal growth restriction may also be present (Table 14.17).

Prenatal diagnosis: Fetal infection can be proven by direct isolation of the virus or genome on amniotic fluid samples obtained at least 6–8 weeks after maternal infection to avoid false-negative results. The need for prenatal diagnosis is usually determined by the gestational age at which the infection is likely to have occurred.

Treatment: Not available.

Prognosis: Prognosis depends on the timing of maternal infection, virological diagnosis (if available) and associated ultrasound findings.

Recurrence risk: Reinfection can occur and is more likely after prolonged or intense exposure and with vaccine-induced, rather than natural, immunity. However, it is usually subclinical and the risk to the fetus is thought to be <5%.

Exposure to Drugs

Anti-epileptics

Anti-epileptic drugs broadly fall into two categories: folic acid antagonists, such as carbamazepine, phenobarbital, and phenytoin and other anticonvulsants including sodium valproate and newer drugs such as topiramate and levetiracetam.

Exposure to anti-epileptic drugs *in utero* has been shown to cause a typical embryopathy characterized by fetal defects, growth restriction and hypoplasia of the midface and fingers. The risk of fetal defects is highest with sodium valproate. It is higher when exposure occurs in the first trimester, and also higher with polytherapy than monotherapy.

Numerous malformations are described in the literature in association with maternal epilepsy on treatment. However, most defects involve the central nervous and cardiovascular systems. Oral clefts are also common.

It is therefore recommended that both sodium valproate and polytherapy should be avoided in the first trimester of pregnancy to decrease the risk of major congenital malformations.

Anti-hypertensives

Angiotensin converting enzyme (ACE) inhibitors have long been known to have adverse fetal effects. Exposure in the second and third trimester of pregnancy has been shown to cause oligohydramnios, pulmonary hypoplasia, contractures, and long-lasting neonatal anuria. First-trimester exposure leads to a threefold increase in the risk of fetal defects involving the cardiovascular (VSD, PS), genito-urinary (renal dysplasia) and cranio-facial system (microcephaly, coloboma, spina bifida) (Cooper et al. 2006).

Recent case-control studies (Van Gelder et al. 2015) have reported an association between fetal defects (oesophageal atresia, hypospadias, VSDs and left heart defects) and pregnancy-induced hypertensive disease (rather than anti-hypertensives use) suggesting a possible underlying etiology in placental ischaemia.

Exposure to Teratogens

Alcohol

Definition: Elevated alcohol consumption in pregnancy may lead to a syndromic cluster (Fetal alcohol syndrome disorder, FASD) including characteristic facial features, birth defects and significant neurodevelopmental impairment. It may also contribute to increased risk of preterm delivery, fetal death, and stillbirth.

Epidemiology and risk factors: Prenatal alcohol exposure continues to be the leading preventable cause of birth defects and neurocognitive impairment with an estimated prevalence of 1–3 in 1000 affected live births worldwide. Risk and severity of birth defects are strictly related to the number of units of alcohol per day.

Pathogenesis: The mechanisms of alcohol-mediated teratogenicity may be heterogeneous. While the risk of fetal defects and FGR appears to be highest (>4-fold that of general population) during the first trimester, facial dysmorphism and neurocognitive impairments may result from heavy alcohol exposure both periconceptionally or at any gestational age. There is some evidence that maternal characteristics (black racial origin, low birth weight and gestational weight gain, low socio-economic status) may increase susceptibility to alcohol teratogenicity.

Ultrasound features: The most common findings on prenatal ultrasound include mild to moderate microcephaly and early onset FGR. Subtle facial features are not detectable antenatally (Table 14.18).

Prognosis: While the ultimate prognosis depends on type and severity of fetal defects, the most serious consequences of prenatal alcohol exposure are the effect on brain structure and function.

Table 14.18 Prenatal ultrasound features of Fetal alcohol syndrome disorder (FASD)

Common	Occasional
– *Growth*: FGR – *Cranio-facial*: Microcephaly, maxillary hypoplasia, short nose, smooth philtrum, thin upper lip – *Skeletal*: Joint anomalies (positional, functional), small distal phalanges – *Cardiac*: VSD	– *Cranio-facial*: Hydrocephalus, meningomyelocele, callosal anomalies, microphthalmia, cleft lip palate, ear abnormalities – *Skeletal*: Webbed neck, short femur, contractures – *Cardiac*: ToF, CoA

ASD atrial septal defect, *CoA* coarctation of the aorta, *FGR* fetal growth restriction, *ToF* tetralogy of fallot, *VSD* ventricular septal defect

Recurrence risk: A woman with chronic alcohol misuse has a risk of significant alcohol-related anomalies ranging from 30 to 50%, with the greatest risk being for intellectual disability.

Retinoids

Vitamin A is a necessary nutrient for growth, tissue differentiation, reproduction and vision. However, excessive oral intake by pregnant women through supplements (>5000 IU/day) or retinoid-based drugs used for skin conditions (acne, psoriasis) may result in teratogenesis.

Exposure *in utero* to retinoids may lead to a cranial-neural-crest tissue embryopathy (cranio-facial, CNS excluding NTDs, cardiac and thymic defects) thus resulting in a 22q11.2 deletion-like phenotype (Table 14.19).

These medications are contraindicated during pregnancy and periconceptionally (FDA category X). Of note, topical treatments with retinoids usually achieve low concentrations in maternal circulation and have not been associated with increased risk of fetal defects.

Lithium

Lithium is used to treat bipolar disorder and has been associated with CHD in the fetus due to effects on developing vasculature. The risk of fetal defects is thought to be relatively small and has to be balanced against maintaining maternal mental health when there is no alternative drug. It is recommended to avoid the drug in the first trimester if possible and use the lowest effective dose.

Table 14.19 Retinoid-related teratogenicity

• CNS: hydrocephalus, cerebellar hypoplasia, vermian agenesis, cortical anomalies
• Cranio-facial anomalies: micrognathia, cleft palate, eye anomalies
• CHD: VSD, PS, other
• Thymus hypoplasia/aplasia

ASD atrial septal defect, *CNS* central nervous system, *CoA* coarctation of the aorta, *FGR* fetal growth restriction, *PS* pulmonary stenosis, *VSD* ventricular septal defect

Approach to Investigation and Diagnosis

The approach to diagnosis and management relies on firstly, identifying fetuses at increased risk of abnormalities and secondly, understanding the type/pattern of fetal anomalies which increase the risk of CHD.

Upon investigation of any fetus with multiple abnormalities including CHD it is important to follow a step-by-step approach including the following:

Maternal Factors

- Diabetes
- Phenylketonuria
- Anti Rho and La antibodies
- Teratogens—Alcohol/Anticonvulsants/Anti-hypertensive/Lithium
- Maternal infection—Rubella/Parvovirus/CMV

Genetic Factors

- Parental genetic disorder—22q11.2 deletion/Williams/Noonan syndrome

First Trimester Scan Findings

- NT >3.5 mm
- Hydrops
- Fetal biometry (early onset FGR in triploidy and T18)
- Fetal defects: exomphalos, CDH, holoprosencephaly, oral cleft, skeletal dysplasia, megacystis >16 mm
- Vascular anomalies—absent ductus venosus
- Assessment of chorionicity in multiple pregnancies and detection of conjoined twins

Detailed Anatomy Survey (18–22 Weeks' Gestation)

- Detailed examination of all organ systems: CNS, chest, abdominal wall, renal, skeleton
- Hydrops
- Fetal biometry (early onset FGR)
- Uterine artery Dopplers

Third Trimester Scan

- Fetal biometry (diagnosis and follow-up of late onset FGR) and fetal Dopplers
- Third trimester anomalies: polyhydramnios, oligohydramnios, duodenal atresia, vein of Galen malformation
- Assessment of MCDA twins post laser, particularly ex-recipient
- Hydrops

References

Agathokleous M, Chaveeva P, Poon LC, et al. Meta-analysis of second-trimester marers for trisomy 21. Ultrasound Obstet Gynecol. 2013;41:247–61. https://doi.org/10.1002/uog.12364.

Atzei A, Gajewska K, Huggon IC, et al. Relationship between nuchal translucency thickness and prevalence of major cardiac defects in fetuses with a normal karyotype. Ultrasound Obstet Gynecol. 2005;26:154–47. https://doi.org/10.1002/uog.1936.

Bassett AS, Costain G, Marshall CR. Neuropsychiatric aspects of 22q11.2 deletion syndrome: considerations in the prenatal setting. Prenat Diagn. 2017;37:61–9. https://doi.org/10.1002/pd.4935.

Bataeva R, Bellsham-Revell H, Zidere V, et al. Reliability of fetal thymus measurement in prediction of 22q11.2 deletion: a retrospective study using four-dimensional spatiotemporal image correlation volumes. Ultrasound Obstet Gynecol. 2013;41:172–6. https://doi.org/10.1002/uog.11194.

Chaoui R, Heling K, Zhao Y, et al. Dilated cavum septi pellucidi in fetuses with microdeletion 22q11. Prenat Diagn. 2016;36:911–5. https://doi.org/10.1002/pd.4911.

Cooper WO, Hernandez-Diaz S, Argobast PG, et al. Major congenital malformations after first-trimester exposure to ACE inhibitors. N Engl J Med. 2006;354:2443–51.

Gil MM, Quezada MS, Revello R, et al. Analysis of cell-free DNA in maternal blood in screening for fetal aneuploidies: updated meta-analysis. Ultrasound Obstet Gynecol. 2015;45(3):249–66. https://doi.org/10.1002/uog.14791.

Gross SJ, Stosic M, McDonald-McGinn DM, et al. Clinical experience with single-nucleotide polymorphism-based non-invasive prenatal screening for 22q11.2 deletion syndrome. Ultrasound Obstet Gynecol. 2016;47:177–83. https://doi.org/10.1002/uog.15754.

Herberg U, Gross W, Bartmann P, et al. Long term cardiac follow up of severe twin to twin transfusion syndrome after intrauterine laser coagulation. Heart. 2006;92:95–100. https://doi.org/10.1136/hrt.2004.057497.

Leurez-Ville M, Ville Y. Fetal cytomegalovirus infection. Best Prac Res Clin Obstet Gynaecol. 2017;38:97–107. https://doi.org/10.1016/j.bpobgyn.2016.10.005.

Mogra R, Zidere V, Allan LD. Prenatally detectable congenital heart defects in fetuses with Down syndrome. Ultrasound Obstet Gynecol. 2011;38:320–4. https://doi.org/10.1002/uog.8977.

Nicolaides KH, Syngelaki A, Gil MM, et al. Prenatal detection of fetal triploidy from cell-free DNA testing in maternal blood. Fetal Diagn Ther. 2014;35:212–7. https://doi.org/10.1159/000355655.

Oepkes D, Haak M. Extracardiac malformations: associations and importance: consequences for perinatal management of fetal cardiac patients. Cardiol Young. 2014;24:55–9. https://doi.org/10.1017/S1047951114001425.

Pettit KE, Merchant M, Machin GA, et al. Congenital heart defects in a large unselected cohort of monochorionic twins. J Perinatol. 2013;33:457–61. https://doi.org/10.1038/jp.2012.

Rodríguez-López M, Cruz-Lemini M, Valenzuela-Alcaraz B, et al. Descriptive analysis of different phenotypes of cardiac remodeling in fetal growth restriction. Ultrasound Obstet Gynecol. 2016;50(2):207–14. https://doi.org/10.1002/uog.17365.

Ruiz A, Ferrer Q, Sánchez O, et al. Placenta-related complications in women carrying a foetus with congenital heart disease. J Mat Fet Neonat Med. 2015;29:3271–5. https://doi.org/10.3109/14767058.2015.1121480.

Song MS, Hu A, Dyhamenahali U, et al. Extracardiac lesions and chromosomal abnormalities associated with major fetal heart defects: comparison of intrauterine, postnatal and post-mortem diagnoses. Ultrasound Obstet Gynecol. 2009;33:552–9. https://doi.org/10.1002/uog.6309.

Sotiriadis A, Papatheodorou S, Eleftheriades M, et al. Nuchal translucency and major congenital heart defects in fetuses with normal karyotype: a meta-analysis. Ultrasound Obstet Gynecol. 2013;42:383–9. https://doi.org/10.1002/uog.12488.

Sperling L, Kiil C, Larsen LU, et al. Detection of chromosomal abnormalities, congenital abnormalities and transfusion syndrome in twins. Ultrasound Obstet Gynecol. 2007;29:517–26. https://doi.org/10.1002/uog.3918.

Springer S, Mlczoch E, Krampl-Bettelheim E, et al. Congenital heart disease in monochorionic twins with and without twin-to-twin transfusion syndrome. Prenat Diagn. 2014;34:994–9. https://doi.org/10.1002/pd.4411.

Springett A, Wellesley D, Greenlees R, et al. Congenital anomalies associated with Trisomy 18 and Trisomy 13: a registry-based study in 16 European Countries, 2000-2011. Am J Med Genet. 2015;167A:3062–9. https://doi.org/10.1002/ajmg.a.37355.

Stoll C, Dott B, Alembik Y, et al. Associated congenital anomalies among cases with Down syndrome. Eur J Med Genet. 2015a;58:674–80. https://doi.org/10.1016/j.ejmg.2015.11.003.

Stoll C, Dott B, Alembik Y, et al. Associated non-cardiac congenital anomalies among cases with congenital heart defects. Eur J Med Genet. 2015b. https://doi.org/10.1016/j.ejmg.2014.12.002.

Syngelaki A, Chelemen T, Dagklis T, et al. Challenges in the diagnosis of fetal non-chromosomal abnormalities at 11-13 weeks. Prenat Diagn. 2011;31:90–102. https://doi.org/10.1002/pd.2642.

Tegnander E, Williams W, Johansen OJ, et al. Prenatal detection of heart defects in a non-selected population of 30,149 fetuses: detection rates and outcome. Ultrasound Obstet Gynecol. 2006;27:252–65.

Van Mieghem T, Lewi L, Gucciardo L, et al. The fetal heart in twin-to-twin transfusion syndrome. Int J Paediatr. 2010. https://doi.org/10.1155/2010/379792.

Van Gelder MM, Van Bennekom CM, Louik C. Maternal hypertensive disorders, anti-hypertensive medication use, and the risk of birth defects: a case-control study. BJOG. 2015;122:1002–9. https://doi.org/10.1111/1471-0528.13138.

Vigneswaran TV, Homfray T, Allan LD, et al. Persistently elevated nuchal translucency and the fetal heart. J Matern Fetal Neonatal Med. 2017;4:1–5. https://doi.org/10.1080/14767058.2017.1342804.

Genetics of Congenital Heart Disease

15

Sahar Mansour

Abstract

Congenital heart disease (CHD) is the most common congenital malformation accounting for one-third of all congenital abnormalities with an incidence of 7–10 per 1000 live births. Congenital heart disease may be associated with chromosomal aneuploidy and single gene disorders. However, an underlying chromosomal or genetic abnormality is found in less than 20% of patients with CHD. However, there is probably a genetic contribution to CHD even it has not been identified. The genetics of congenital heart disease is highly complex. Mutations in different genes can cause an identical malformation, whilst identical mutations in the same gene can result in a spectrum of cardiac malformations. Environmental factors play a major role in the development of cardiac malformations.

Electronic Supplementary Material The online version of this chapter (https://doi.org/10.1007/978-3-319-77461-9_15) contains supplementary material, which is available to authorized users.

S. Mansour
St George's University Hospitals NHS Foundation Trust, London, UK
e-mail: smansour@sgul.ac.uk

Keywords

Genetics · Congenital heart disease · Recurrence risk · Non-invasive Prenatal Testing · Array CGH · Syndrome · Tuberous sclerosis

Introduction

Congenital heart disease (CHD) is the most common congenital malformation accounting for one-third of all congenital abnormalities with an incidence of 7–10 per 1000 live births and almost 3%, when including patients with bicuspid aortic valve (Gelb and Chung 2014).

Congenital heart disease may be associated with chromosomal aneuploidy (e.g. Down Syndrome (trisomy 21) and Turner syndrome (45,X0), common segmental chromosomal aneuploidies (e.g. 22q11 microdeletion) and single gene disorders (e.g. Noonan syndrome). An underlying chromosomal or genetic abnormality is found in less than 20% of patients with CHD (Gelb and Chung 2014).

However, there is probably a genetic contribution to CHD even it has not been identified. A large population study in Denmark (Øyen et al. 2009), demonstrated that there is a 4.2% risk of CHD if there is a family history of CHD (if chromosomal abnormalities were excluded). Parental consanguinity carries a two to threefold increased

© Springer International Publishing AG, part of Springer Nature 2018

J. Simpson et al. (eds.), *Fetal Cardiology*, https://doi.org/10.1007/978-3-319-77461-9_15

risk to the offspring and left sided lesions, e.g. bicuspid aortic valves and hypoplastic left heart, have a high heritability (Hinton et al. 2007).

The genetics of congenital heart disease is highly complex. Mutations in different genes can cause an identical malformation, whilst identical mutations in the same gene can result in a spectrum of cardiac malformations.

Environmental factors play a major role in the development of cardiac malformations. Common environmental factors include environmental teratogens, maternal exposures and infectious agents. Maternal factors such as smoking, alcohol, or maternal diabetes are known to increase the risk. Ingestion of drugs during the pregnancy, such as anti-seizure medications (e.g. sodium valproate) or congenital infections, such as Rubella can result in congenital heart disease in the fetus.

Seventy percent of CHD is isolated and non-syndromic. In this group, only 3–5% have a family history of CHD. Non-syndromic congenital heart disease is highly likely to be multifactorial in origin, with a genetic susceptibility interplaying with environmental factors (Ferencz et al. 1993).

Genomic Variation and How to Test for It

In humans, there are usually 23 pairs of chromosomes, thread like structures, in almost every cell's nucleus. There are 22 pairs of autosomes and a pair of sex chromosomes. Males have an X and a Y chromosome, females have two X chromosomes.

The chromosomes are made up of deoxyribonucleic acid (DNA). Less than 2% of human DNA codes for specific genes which transcribes into RNA and many are then translated into amino acids and proteins.

The human genome is made up of approximately 20,000–25,000 genes packaged into these 46 chromosomes. All humans have variation or variants in their genome which may be normal or pathogenic.

Large scale variants: include whole or partial chromosome duplications (e.g. trisomy 18, Edwards syndrome) or deletions (e.g. Monosomy X (Turner syndrome, or chromosome 4p-)).

Medium scale variants: include microdeletions or microduplications (e.g. 22q11 microdeletion).

Small scale variants: include single point variants within the gene with a change in just one or two base pairs (e.g. Noonan syndrome)—These are single gene disorders.

Congenital heart disease can occur with any of these forms of genomic variation.

Large Scale Variants: Chromosomal Abnormalities

Chromosomal imbalances result in multiple abnormalities which may include congenital heart disease.

Chromosome Analysis: Karyotyping

Until recently, traditional karyotyping by G-banding was the main method for looking at the chromosomes (*in many centres this has now been replaced by array CGH for both prenatal and postnatal diagnosis (see below)*). The lymphocytes from a blood sample, chorionic villous sample or amniocentesis are cultured. The cells are arrested in metaphase. The nucleus is burst to release the chromosomes and the chromosomes are stained with a Giemsa stain to demonstrate the bands on the chromosomes.

This method has a low resolution but is the preferred method to look for aneuploidies, triploidies, structural rearrangements (e.g. ring or marker chromosomes) and translocations. It will also detect large imbalances, deletions or duplications (usually more than 4 MB = 4,000,000 base pairs).

It is not the method of choice to detect small deletions/duplications and will not detect single gene disorders.

Quantitative Fluorescent Polymerase Chain Reaction (QFPCR)

QFPCR is a rapid and reliable test for the common aneuploidies. It is designed to look at the comparative number (or dosage) of the chromosomes to detect the common trisomies i.e. 13, 18 and 21. It relies simply on dosage so does not provide information about the structure of the chromosomes. A Robertsonian chromosomal translocation resulting in trisomy will not be detected using QFPCR. It can also detect monosomy X (Turner syndrome) and other sex aneuploidies, but is less reliable. If an abnormality is identified by QFPCR, a traditional karyotype is still required to look at the underlying mechanism.

Medium Scale Variants: Microdeletions/Duplications

Array Comparative Genomic Hybridisation (Array CGH)

The array CGH (also known as Microarray CGH or Comparative Microarray (CMA)) is a relatively new technique for looking at chromosomes. It compares reference DNA with patient/fetal DNA. It has a much higher resolution than traditional karyotyping, and will therefore detect microdeletions and microduplications which are too small to see under the microscope. The analysis is based on chromosomal dosage, so it is not an appropriate test for the detection of balanced rearrangements or triploidy.

Most centres in the UK will offer an array CGH on a Chorionic Villus Sample (CVS) or amniocentesis if the nuchal translucency is >3.5 mm or if there are structural abnormalities, including congenital heart disease.

The array CGH will detect very small copy number variants (CNV) (deletions and duplications <30 KB). These may be pathogenic (e.g. 22q11 microdeletion), benign (therefore frequently not reported) or a variant of unknown significance (VUS). There may also be incidental findings which may not be the explanation of the baby's structural abnormalities but may have implications for the fetus or other members of the family (for example the deletion of a gene causing an increased susceptibility to cancer). Prenatal array CGH has resulted in an increase of 6% of the detection of smaller chromosomal imbalances (Wapner et al. 2012).

Small-Scale Variants: Single Gene Disorders

A mistake within a gene will result in the development of a faulty amino acid/protein or transcription factor (a gene that controls the expression of other genes) leading to a genetic disorder. The problem may be due to a lack of protein (haplo-insufficiency) or interference of a faulty protein (dominant negative) or even gain of function of a protein (e.g. Noonan syndrome).

These small-scale variants cannot be detected by normal karyotyping or even array CGH. The testing is targeted to the gene (or genes) of interest. To date, the most common technique for identification of these variants is Sanger sequencing of the specific gene(s). Sanger sequencing is a technique for DNA sequencing based upon the selective incorporation of chain-terminating dideoxynucleotides by DNA polymerase during in vitro DNA replication. Although it is fairly rapid, only one gene can be sequenced at a time. However, massive parallel sequencing (next generation sequencing (NGS)) of the whole genome is becoming cheaper and more reliable. Next Generation Sequencing is a high-throughput approach to DNA sequencing using the concept of massively parallel processing. Many thousands or millions of sequencing reactions are performed in parallel rather than just one at a time, in contrast to conventional sequencing machines.

Modes of Inheritance (Mendelian)

There are two copies of every gene on the 22 pairs of autosomal chromosomes. A female has two copies of every gene on X chromosome but a male will only have one copy of the genes on the X chromosome.

Autosomal Dominant

In some conditions, a mistake (or point mutation) in only one copy of an autosomal gene is sufficient to cause an autosomal dominant condition. An autosomal dominant condition affects males and females equally. If a parent is affected, the offspring has a 50% chance (1 in 2) of being affected. However, mutations can occur as a new event (*de novo*) in the egg or sperm i.e. neither parent is affected.

Autosomal Recessive

In an autosomal recessive condition, there is a mistake (mutation) in both copies of the gene (bi-allelic). Usually the parents are both carriers but not affected.

If both parents are carriers, the offspring risk is 25% or 1 in 4. Autosomal recessive conditions are more frequent if the parents are consanguineous as they have shared ancestry and are therefore more likely to carry mutations in the same gene. First degree cousins have a 3% increased risk of having a child with an autosomal recessive genetic disorder.

X Linked Inheritance

In an X-linked recessive condition, a female may carry a mutation in one copy of a gene on the X chromosome but is not usually affected as she has a healthy copy of the same gene. Males with one faulty copy will have an X-linked recessive condition.

If a woman is a carrier, 50% of her sons will be affected. If a man is affected by an X-linked disorder e.g. haemophilia, all his daughters will be carriers (they will inherit his only X chromosome) but all his sons will be unaffected as they will inherit his Y chromosome. The mother is not always a carrier of an X-linked condition as the mutation may occur as a new event in the egg.

Prenatal Diagnosis: Approach to Investigation

Congenital Heart Disease Detected by Routine Screening

Any fetus with a nuchal translucency of more than 3.5 mm should be offered fetal echocardiography. This may be performed as early as 13 or 14 weeks gestation, which may detect the more severe forms of CHD. Repeat echocardiography is recommended later in the pregnancy. Any fetus with a structural abnormality that is known to be associated with CHD should also be offered echocardiography. This same cohort of pregnancies, i.e. with increased nuchal translucency or structural abnormalities should be offered an invasive test to test the fetus for chromosomal abnormalities. In most centres this is by QFPCR, for the common trisomies, followed by a karyotype or array CGH.

Invasive testing may be performed by chorionic villous sampling (CVS) (>11 weeks) or amniocentesis (>15 weeks).

The CVS is effectively a placental biopsy. The placenta usually has the same chromosomal configuration as the fetus, however, sometimes the chromosomal abnormality may be confined to the placenta and not affecting the fetus—confined placental mosaicism (CPM). If CPM is suspected (i.e. it appears to be mosaic in CVS or there are no structural abnormalities in the fetus), it is advisable to offer an amniocentesis. The amniocentesis is a much better representative of the fetus' chromosomes—as the fetus sheds cells from the bladder and skin into the amniotic fluid.

Family History of Congenital Heart Disease

Targeted prenatal diagnosis can be offered in the following situations:

1. Where there is a known genetic problem in the family or a previously affected child, if the genetic mutation has been identified.
2. Where there is a known familial chromosomal translocation in one of the parents (balanced reciprocal or Robertsonian)

Non-invasive Prenatal Testing

Non-invasive prenatal testing (NIPT) has been introduced over the past few years. It is a screening test but not a definitive test for the common trisomies. It is recommended that an invasive procedure is undertaken to confirm the chromosomal abnormality in the fetus.

Fragments of DNA from the placenta (cell free DNA) is present in the maternal circulation from as early as 5 weeks gestation. The common trisomies can be screened for by taking maternal blood and looking for an increase of one chromosome in comparison to the others. The accuracy of the test is reliant on how much of the fetal DNA is present in the mother's circulation (the fetal fraction). If the fetal fraction is low, the test is unreliable. It is also less accurate in women with a high BMI. If the fetal fraction is over 5–10%, it is highly reliable for trisomy 21 (>98%) but slightly less accurate for trisomy 18, trisomy 13 and even less accurate for the sex aneuploidies e.g. XO, Turner syndrome. This test can be offered to women from 9 or 10 weeks gestation (the fetal fraction is often too low before 9 weeks).

There is a false positive result in 1 in 300 pregnancies. This may be due to one of three reasons.

1. In early pregnancy, there may be a 'vanishing twin'—the placenta may still be shedding DNA fragments.
2. The DNA fragments come from the placenta and it may be that the chromosomal abnormality is confined to the placenta and is not affecting the baby.
3. Very occasionally, it can detect a problem that is in the mother but not in the fetus, such as a malignancy associated with an aneuploidy.

Preimplantation Genetic Diagnosis (PGD)

PGD is now available for single gene disorders, parents with a balanced chromosomal translocation with an increased risk of a chromosomal imbalance in the fetus, and fetal sexing for X-linked disorders. It involves the process of *in-vitro* fertilisation. The embryos are tested by removal of one or two cells at a few days post-conception. Only unaffected embryos are implanted. The limitations are that it is expensive, a licence is required for each new genetic condition and currently there is only a 33% success rate.

Indications for Referral to a Clinical Geneticist

Chromosomal and Mendelian syndromes account for approximately 20% of CHD (Gelb and Chung 2014). The genetic mechanisms involved in the remaining 80% are poorly understood. At present, if the fetus is found to have an isolated CHD with no other structural extracardiac abnormalities, a normal array CGH and no family history—it is very unlikely that a specific genetic defect will be identified.

If the fetus has a chromosomal abnormality (other than the common trisomies), the couple may benefit from meeting the geneticist to explain the abnormality and the likely prognosis for the baby. It is also essential to test the parents as some may carry a re-arrangement/translocation of the chromosomes which has given rise to the fetus' chromosomal imbalance. This will have implications for the assessment of the recurrence risk in future offspring.

If the fetus has normal chromosomes/array CGH but has extra-cardiac structural abnormalities, it may be possible to identify or consider other single gene disorders that may be suggested by the pattern of malformations. In the near future, it will be possible to do rapid clinical exome sequencing in this cohort to identify point mutations in any of the genes known to be associated with genetic disorders.

Families with a strong family history of congenital heart disease, even if the malformation is not identical, are likely to have an underlying genetic cause and may wish to be investigated further.

Recurrence Risks

Many parents wish to understand the risk of having another baby with congenital heart disease. If the fetus/child has a syndromic form of CHD, the recurrence risk is that of the syndrome.

If the fetus has a chromosomal abnormality which has not been inherited from either parent and the parents do not have a chromosomal translocation—then the recurrence risk is very low (<1%). There is a small recurrence risk as it is possible for one parent to carry the same abnormality in more than one egg or sperm (gonadal mosaicism).

If a *de novo* mutation is identified in a single gene (i.e. it has arisen for the first time in the fetus and neither parent carries the mutation), the risk is again very low at <1% (but not 0% as there is still the risk of gonadal mosaicism). *De novo* mutations have been identified in 10% of all patients with severe CHD and 20% of patients with CHD with extracardiac malformations (Zaidi and Brueckner 2017).

If there is an autosomal dominant condition and one of the parents is affected, the recurrence risk is 50% regardless of the sex of the baby. However, there is frequently variation in the type and severity of the malformation. Over the past 50 years with improved surgical treatment, the number of parents with CHD has increased. The risk of CHD in the offspring was found to be 4.1% by Burn et al. in 1998. This compared to a lower sibling risk of 2.1% (Burn et al. 1998).

If there is an autosomal recessive condition, and both parents are carriers, any future children have a 1 in 4 or 25% risk of being affected. The mode of inheritance in some types of CHD, for example CHD associated with laterality defects or Generalised arterial calcification of infancy, are often autosomal recessive. Therefore, the risk of recurrence in these groups are higher. Parental consanguinity confers an increased risk of an autosomal recessive condition in the offspring.

If the mother is a carrier of an X-linked recessive condition, 50% of her sons will be affected and 50% of her daughters will also be carriers.

In isolated CHD where no chromosomal or genetic syndrome has been identified (and there is no family history of CHD), there is an empirical recurrence risk based on the type of CHD. This risk is usually approximately 3% but ranges from just under 2% for some lesions e.g. transposition of the great arteries to 8% e.g. hypoplastic left heart. The genetics and recurrence risk of the specific heart lesions are described below. A recent paper by Brodwall et al. (2017) looked at the recurrence risk in siblings over a 16-year period. CHD in the first-born child of each sibling pair was associated with increased risk of CHD in the subsequent child, with adjusted Relative Risk Ratio (RRR) of 14.0 for same-sex twins, 11.9 for opposite-sex twins, 3.6 for full siblings, and 1.5 for half-siblings. Approximately half of the recurrent CHD were of the same or a similar type as the CHD in the sibling.

The possible explanations for the increased risk include shared genes, shared environmental factors, or a combination. Interestingly the RRR were higher in dizygotic twins than in full siblings, even though both groups share the same proportion of genes. Indicating that maternal factors and/or pregnancy factors may play a role. These numbers had been adjusted for maternal age and maternal diabetes. The recurrence risk in siblings was 4% with one previous child with CHD, and 10% with two previous children with CHD.

Syndromes Associated with CHD

Most chromosomal and genetic disorders can be associated with CHD, some more frequently than others. The characteristic facial features of patients with Turner syndrome and Noonan syndrome are shown in Figs. 15.1 and 15.2. The most frequent genetic disorders associates with CHD are listed in Tables 15.1 and 15.2 (adapted from Muntean et al. 2017) but more details can be found in Chap. 14.

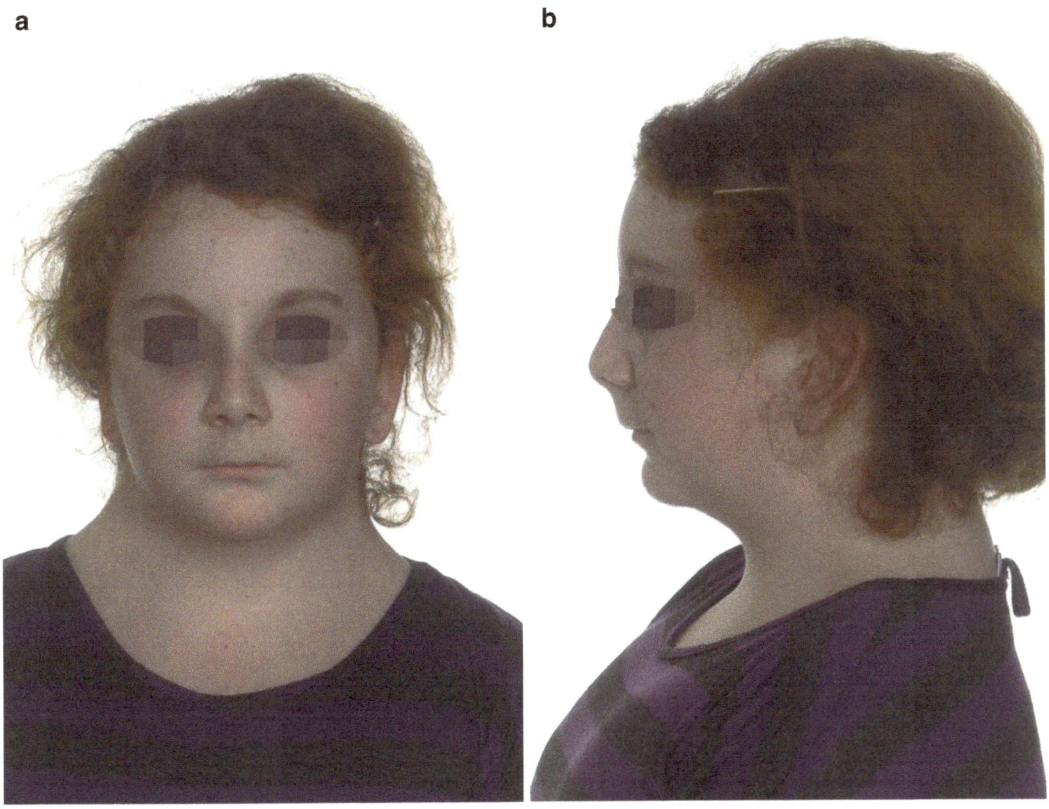

Fig. 15.1 (**a**, **b**) Turner syndrome (chromosomes 45,X0) demonstrating webbed neck and low set ears

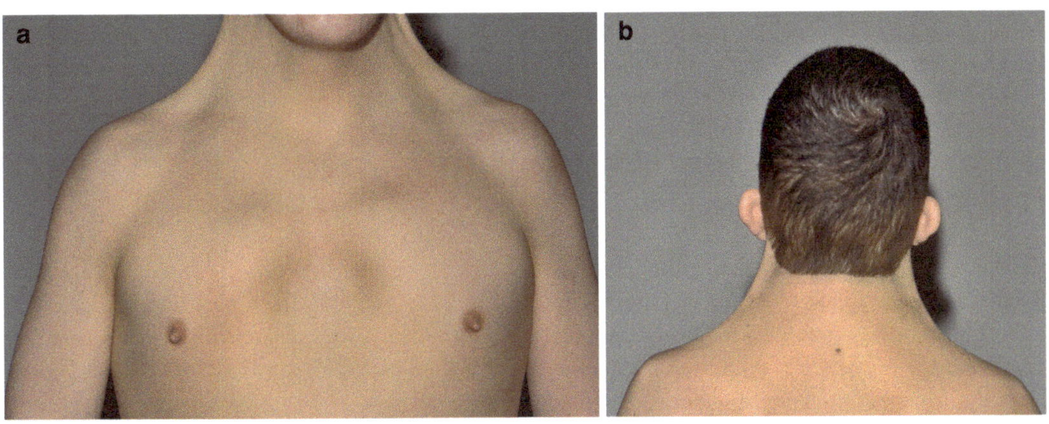

Fig. 15.2 (**a**, **b**) Noonan syndrome demonstrating webbed neck, low hairline, low set ears, broad chest, widely spaced nipples and pectus excavatum

Table 15.1 Common chromosomal disorders associated with CHD

Chromosomal abnormality	Prevalence of CHD (%)	Type of CHD
Trisomy 21	44	AVSD (39%) ASD secundum type (42%) VSD(43%) TOF
Trisomy 18	80	TOF, DORV, septal defects (VSD or AVSD) or CoA
Trisomy 13	>50	TOF, DORV, septal defects (VSD, ASD or AVSD) or valvular lesions
Turner syndrome (45,X0) Mosaic Turner syndrome	38 11	Left-sided cardiac malformations including BAV, CoA and HLHS
22q11 microdeletion	75–80	Outflow tract abnormalities especially interrupted aortic arch, common arterial trunk, TOF, RAA. Other defects e.g. VSD, AVSD
Williams syndrome (7q11.23 microdeletion)	80	SVAS (45%) peripheral pulmonary stenosis (37%) SVPS
1p36 deletion	70	Non-compaction of the myocardium (23%), VSD, ASD, TOF, CoA, PDA.

Table 15.2 Common genetic disorders associated with CHD

Single gene disorder	Genes	Prevalence of CHD	Type of CHD
Noonan syndrome spectrum (includes cardiofaciocutaneous syndrome)	Rasopathy genes >23 including *PTPN11, RIT1, KRAS*	80%	PS, ASD, VSD, TOF, CoA hypertrophic cardiomyopathy (20%)
Holt Oram syndrome	*TBX5*	75%	ASD, VSD, atrioventricular conduction delay/complete heart block Rare: HLHS, TAPVD, common arterial trunk
Alagille syndrome	*JAG1* *NOTCH2*		peripheral or valvular PS TOF, CoA
CHARGE syndrome	*CHD7*		TOF, DORV. aortic arch anomalies

AVSD atrioventricular septal defect, *ASD* atrial septal defect, *VSD* ventricular septal defect, *TOF* tetralogy of fallot, *DORV* double outlet right ventricle, *CoA* coarctation of the aorta, *BAV* bicuspid aortic valve, *AS* aortic stenosis, *HLHS* hypoplastic left heart syndrome, *RAA* right aortic arch, *SVAS* supra-valvular aortic stenosis, *SVPS* supra-valvular pulmonary stenosis, *PDA* patent ductus arteriosus, *PS* pulmonary valve stenosis, *TAPVD* total anomalous pulmonary venous drainage

Specific Heart Lesions

CHD is often considered in broad groupings, outlined here. Recurrence of CHD in families are often, but not always confined to these groupings. The aetiology of the CHD within each grouping is often the same but expressing variably within individuals. The groupings are predominantly geographical (within the heart) rather than related to the underlying embryology or genetics. They may change as more is learned about the underlying mechanism leading to the malformation. Selected groups of congenital heart disease are discussed below.

Left Heart Defects: HLHS/CoA/AS/BAV

Left-sided outflow tract obstruction (LVOTO) represents the most severe cardiac malformation, including bicuspid aortic valve (BAV), aortic valve stenosis (AS), coarctation of the aorta (CoA) and hypoplastic left heart syndrome (HLHS). LVOTO defects account for 15–20% of all CHDs and have wide clinical and anatomic heterogeneity.

When LVOTO defects are identified in a proband, the likelihood of finding LVOTO spectrum defects, including BAV, in family members is high, and recurrence risk of the same cardiovascular malformation or other LVOTO defects (including BAV) ranges from 8 to 22%, depending on the lesion present in the proband (Hinton et al. 2007; McBride et al. 2005).

Hypoplastic Left Heart Syndrome

Hypoplastic left heart syndrome (HLHS; MIM#241550) is a severe congenital heart defect (CHD) which accounts for approximately 4–8% of all CHD. Hypoplasia of the left ventricle (LV) and aorta are cardinal features. The ventricular septum is intact and the great arteries are normally related. HLHS accounts for approximately 25% of deaths associated with CHD. Overall, approximately 30% of fetuses with HLHS have a chromosomal imbalance (e.g. Turner syndrome (monosomy X), trisomy 18, 22q11.21-2 deletion, Jacobsen syndrome (chromosome 11q deletion) and microdeletions in 1q21.1) or genetic syndrome (e.g. Smith-Lemli-Opitz syndrome, Rubinstein-Taybi syndrome, and Holt-Oram syndrome) and/or the presence of extra-cardiac structural abnormalities.

A genetic origin in HLHS is also suggested by strong familial clustering of left heart defects including bicuspid aortic valves, aortic valve stenosis and coarctation of the aorta (Benson et al. 2016). A number of genes have been implicated in HLHS including *NKX2.5, GJA1* (connexion 43) and *ERBB4*, bi-allelic variants (i.e. both copies of the gene) in *MYH6* and *NOTCH1* and somatic mutations in *HAND1*. However, the genetics is complex and does not follow a simple Mendelian pattern and what appeared to be simple inheritance is complex due to variable expressivity, genetic heterogeneity (different genes causing the same cardiac defect), and reduced penetrance (inheritance of the familial mutation but no congenital heart disease). Variable expressivity is demonstrated by different types of heart defect in the same family, e.g. HLHS and BAV. Causes of this variable expressivity may include interactions with environmental risk factors or genetic modifiers—these are not yet understood.

Fetuses and neonates with HLHS should be carefully evaluated for extracardiac abnormalities which may indicate a specific chromosomal or genetic disorder. Genetic testing is not indicated in non-syndromic HLHS at the current time. First degree relatives should probably be screened by echocardiography as some type of CHD is found in 18.3%, particularly bicuspid aortic valve. Twenty two percent of siblings of HLHS probands will have some form of CHD, and up to 8% will have HLHS (Hinton et al. 2007).

Coarctation of the Aorta

Coarctation of the aorta accounts for between 5 and 8% of all CHD. Only 1–2% shows clear Mendelian inheritance with a family history. More than 90% of coarctation of the aorta is sporadic and non-syndromic. Syndromes with a high incidence of coarctation of the aorta include Turner syndrome (45,X0) with an incidence of 7–18%. Other associations of coarctation of the aorta include bicuspid aortic valve (30–50%) and VSD (25%) (Moosmann et al. 2015). There is a male dominance with a male-to-female ratio of 2.6 to 1.

Bicuspid Aortic Valve

Bicuspid aortic valve (BAV) is the most common congenital heart defect with a prevalence of 0.5–2%. BAV describes an aortic valve with two leaflets instead of the normal three but with a high degree of variability. Very often two of the three coronary leaflets are fused, most commonly the left and right coronary leaflets. It may occur in isolation or with other forms of CHD, 50% of patients with coarctation of the aorta have BAV. The most common genetic association is Turner syndrome. BAV is extremely difficult to visualise during fetal life, but may be feasible from the late second trimester onwards in experienced hands.

BAV is often identified in healthy individuals, but may be associated with serious long-term complications (approximately 35%) including progressive aortic valve disease (stenosis or regurgitation due to calcification), dilation of the aortic root and ascending aorta with a 6% lifetime risk of aortic dissection. When BAV is identified in a proband, it may also be identified in between 1 and 10% of first-degree relatives

(Hales and Mahle 2014). In some units, screening of first degree relatives is undertaken. Several genes have been implicated in association with BAV including *NOTCH1, FBN1, NKX2-5, ACTA2, TGFB2, SMAD6,* and *GATA5*. *NOTCH1* mutations have been found in 7% of familial left-sided heart defects compared to 1% of sporadic cases (Kerstjens-Frederikse et al. 2016). However, BAV development is still not fully understood and genetic testing for isolated (non-syndromic) BAV does not have a high yield (even in familial cases) and is not indicated (Freeze et al. 2016).

Aortic Stenosis (Congenital)

There is considerable overlap between the genetics of BAV and AS. AS is often associated with bi-leaflet or even uni-leaflet aortic valves.

Outflow Tract Defects

Tetralogy of Fallot (Including Pulmonary Atresia with VSD)

Tetralogy of Fallot (TOF) (OMIM #187500), the association of pulmonary stenosis with an overriding aorta, ventricular septal defect and right ventricular hypertrophy is one of the most common forms of cyanotic CHD accounting for 7–10% of all CHD with an incidence of 3 per 10,000. TOF can be diagnosed antenatally as early as 12 weeks of gestation. Pulmonary Atresia with VSD is considered to be a more severe form of TOF and has a similar aetiology.

The causes are highly heterogenous. Rauch et al. (2010) identified pathogenic genetic aberrations in 18% of patients. The chromosomal and genetic disorders include Trisomy 21, (5.2% of all TOF patients), trisomy 13, trisomy 18, 22q11 microdeletion (7.4%). Other chromosomal abnormalities are found in 3% of patients with TOF. Several genetic syndromes are associated with TOF including Noonan syndrome, Alagille syndrome (1.3%), VACTERL association and lymphoedema-distichiasis syndrome. There is also an increased risk with maternal diabetes and fetal alcohol syndrome. Variants in several genes and microdeletions/microduplications are implicated for an increased susceptibility to developing isolated TOF. In view of the high incidence of chromosomal aberrations including 22q11 microdeletion, a detailed chromosomal analysis (array CGH) is indicated for all cases of TOF, especially when detected antenatally. If a genetic syndrome is likely, the testing should be targeted for that condition. At present, there is no indication to do further genetic testing on non-familial isolated/non-syndromic TOF postnatally. If non-syndromic (i.e. isolated) and not familial, the recurrence risk is 3%.

Abnormalities of the Outflow Tracts (Conotruncal Abnormalities) Including Common Arterial Trunk/Interrupted Aortic Arch/Double Outlet Right Ventricle

This group of conditions carry a higher recurrence risk suggesting that some forms have monogenic inheritance. Microdeletions of chromosome 22q11.2 may account for up to 30% of conotruncal anomalies (Emanuel et al. 1992). Other genes implicated include *TBX1* (a gene located in the 22q11 region), *NKX2-5, GDF1, NKX2–6* (biallelic), *GATA6, ZFPM2* (in DORV) but the majority are single case reports.

Transposition of the Great Arteries TGA

TGA has a prevalence of 3.5 per 10,000 and accounts for 5% of all CHD. TGA is very rarely syndromic and extracardiac defects are far less common (10% compared with 35% in TOF). It is rarely associated with 22q11 microdeletion (1%). TGA may be associated with heterotaxy/laterality defects, predominantly right atrial isomerism but usually in combination with other abnormalities such as an AVSD rather than an isolated lesion. The only animal model for TGA is by treating pregnant mice with retinoic acid or with retinoic acid inhibitors, who may also develop heterotaxy (disturbance in laterality). There are a few familial cases of TGA in whom the first-degree relatives present with "congenitally corrected" TGA. Mutations in laterality genes including *Nodal, CFC1* and *ZIC3* have been identified in some of these families, confirming a pathogenetic relationship between TGA and laterality defects. In fact, some authors (Unolt et al. 2013) suggest that TGA and CCTGA should be included in the pathogenetic group of laterality defects rather than outflow tract defects. There appears to be an increased risk of TGA with maternal diabetes, maternal infection (such as influenza), intake of ibuprofen or ionizing radiation and possibly in vitro fertilization (Unolt et al. 2013). The recurrence risk in siblings with TGA is very low compared to other forms of CHD, approximately 1.8% (Digilio et al. 2001).

Septal Defects: ASD/VSD/AVSD

Septal defects account for approximately 40% of all CHD, with the commonest being VSDs (30% of CHD).

Atrial Septal Defect (ASD)

ASDs are one of the most common forms of CHD accounting for around 11%. During prenatal life, the foramen ovale is open to perform its physiological role, diverting more oxygenated blood from the right atrium to the left atrium. A "primum" atrial septal defect is a form of atrioventricular septal defect which will be considered in that category. Superior sinus venosus ASDs are located superiorly in the atrial septum and associated with anomalous drainage of some, or all, of the right pulmonary veins. This is exceedingly difficult to detect during fetal life, even in expert hands.

There are a multitude of syndromes associated with ASDs, including Holt Oram, Noonan, Ellis Van Creveld syndrome and most chromosomal disorders. If the ASD is non-syndromic, and isolated, a detailed family history should be taken. There are a few autosomal dominant families. If there is no family history of CHD, the recurrence risk is 3%. Genes implicated in the formation of non-syndromic ASD include *NKX2-5* often with atrio-ventricular conduction block and *GATA4*, with a family history of VSDs. Patients with an ASD should be carefully evaluated for a syndromic cause. Genetic testing is not indicated in non-syndromic forms with no family history.

Ventricular Septal Defects (VSDs)

VSDs are the single most common form of CHD accounting for approximately 30% of all CHD and a prevalence of approximately 4 per 1000. The causes are highly heterogenous, may occur in isolation or as part of a more complex CHD e.g. TOF. Several CNVs have been strongly associated with VSDs, the most common being 22q11 microdeletion (includes the *TBX1* gene) and 8p23.1 (includes *GATA4*). Between 5 to 8% of newborns with a VSD have an underlying chromosomal disorder.

Single genes associated with non-syndromic VSDs include *GATA4, NKX2-5, ZIC3, NF1, MYH7, TBX1, TNN13* and *PITX2*, but genetic testing is not indicated in isolated, non-familial VSD.

Atrioventricular Septal Defects AVSDs

AVSDs account for only 3% of all CHD, with a prevalence of 2 in 10,000. It is most commonly associated with Trisomy 21, which accounts for approximately 65% of all cases of complete AVSD (Maslen 2004). AVSDs occur in approximately 25% of children with trisomy 21. AVSDs may occur in other genetic syndromes particularly those associated with a laterality defect.

Occasionally the AVSD may be familial, some families have been reported with autosomal dominant AVSD with incomplete penetrance. However, the majority of non-syndromic AVSDs are sporadic with no family history (Maslen 2004). The sporadic cases, like other forms of CHD, are probably multifactorial with variants in some critical genes increasing the susceptibility to CHD. These include the *CRELD1* gene on chromosome 3p25 which may account for 6% of non-syndromic AVSD but with reduced penetrance. AVSD is a rare presentation in families with CHD due to mutations in *GATA4*.

Total Anomalous Pulmonary Venous Drainage (TAPVD)

TAPVD is a rare cyanotic congenital heart defect (CHD) affecting only 7.1 per 100,000 live births. The pulmonary veins fail to drain to the left atrium, leading to respiratory distress, circulatory collapse and hypoxia. Less than 2% are detected antenatally (Seale et al. 2012), but may present with increased nuchal translucency or bilateral pleural effusions.

TAPVD usually occurs in isolation but can occasionally be associated with a syndrome (approx. 4%). The most frequent associated syndromes are cat eye syndrome (due to an extra marker chromosome derived from chromosome 22), Holt-Oram syndrome, and defects of laterality, particularly right atrial isomerism. Approximately 14% are associated with other congenital heart malformations, usually small VSDs (Seale et al. 2010). A family history of CHD reported in 4% of cases, but only 1.4% had a sibling recurrence of isolated TAPVD (excluding cases with isomerism/heterotaxy) (Seale et al. 2012). The overall recurrence risk is not readily available but is considered to be much lower than other forms of CHD.

Laterality Disorders

Situs solitus describes the normal orientation of the visceral organs including the heart. During early embryonic life, different organs develop in the appropriate place, for example, the liver on the right, the spleen on the left and the bowel needs to take up its normal position. This process of "lateralization" may not proceed normally, leading to problems in multiple organs including the heart. Situs inversus is the mirror image of the usual arrangement. However, in some cases, the disturbance is more complex. The features of fetuses with different forms of laterality disturbance are outlined in Chap. 10. Heterotaxy, situs ambiguous, Ivemark syndrome or polysplenia/asplenia syndrome are all terms which have been used in the literature to describe this constellation of abnormalities. Affected fetuses typically have major structural and cardiovascular malformations. Disorders of laterality account for approximately 3% of all CHD with a prevalence of 1–2 in 10,000. This group of conditions is highly genetic but several genes are involved in the process of laterality. (Sutherland and Ware 2009).

The most frequent are genes in the NODAL signaling pathway including the ligand, *NODAL* (5–10%, autosomal dominant), the ligand co-factor, *CFC1* (6–21%, autosomal dominant) and an X-linked gene, *ZIC3* (>75% if there is an X-linked family history but only approx. 1% in sporadic cases). Often the dominant mutations have been inherited from asymptomatic parents suggesting reduced penetrance.

Some of the syndromes due to an underlying disorder of the cilia, may also present with laterality defects, e.g. Bardet-Biedl syndrome and Jeune Syndrome. Primary ciliary dyskinesia is an abnormality affecting the structure or function of the cilia which are crucial for normal laterality. This group of conditions is usually autosomal recessive but again, highly heterogenous. The most common is *DNAH5*. There is an increased risk of CHD in this condition. Many common and rare chromosomal abnormalities can (rarely) present with laterality defects including trisomy 13, 18 and 22q11 microdeletion. Maternal diabetes, maternal cocaine abuse and monozygotic twinning have all been associated with heterotaxy.

If a fetus is identified as having a laterality defect associated with CHD, an array CGH should be offered and the mother tested for diabetes (especially if the fetus has left atrial isomerism). If there is a family history of heterotaxy, further genetic testing may be considered. However, if there is no family history and the abnormality is isolated, genetic testing is unlikely to be fruitful. The recurrence risk for this group of disorders is slightly higher than for other forms of CHD at >5% (Oliverio et al. 2010).

Fetal Cardiomyopathy

Cardiomyopathy (CMO) is rarely diagnosed antenatally and is usually seen between 20 and 36 weeks gestation. The prognosis is poor with 38% of the fetuses dying in utero and a high mortality after birth (>33%). Most studies have adopted the standard World Health Organisation categorisation of cases and have subdivided into hypertrophic, dilated and unclassified forms of

CMO. During fetal life, although echocardiography is feasible to characterise the cardiomyopathy, other forms of testing may be more difficult, for example, magnetic resonance imaging. In addition, obtaining blood or other tissue samples for testing is more difficult than after birth.

Hypertrophic Cardiomyopathy

The most common causes of hypertrophic cardiomyopathy in the fetus (76%) is maternal diabetes or twin-to-twin transfusion. Both are usually reversible after birth (Pedra et al. 2002). Weber et al. 2014, reported on 21 fetuses with hypertrophic cardiomyopathy (HCM). The causes were mainly genetic or metabolic including Noonan syndrome, Hurler syndrome and congenital disorders of glycosylation (Weber et al. 2014).

Noonan syndrome is probably one of the most frequent genetic causes of HCM but the myocardial hypertrophy may only become evident in the third trimester. Other clues to this diagnosis would be an increased nuchal translucency in the first trimester and polyhydramnios.

Dilated Cardiomyopathy

Dilated cardiomyopathy is suspected when the ventricles become dilated with reduced ventricular function, in the absence of an obstructive lesion or abnormal loading conditions to explain the dilation and dysfunction. In this regard, it is important to exclude cardiac conditions including pulmonary stenosis, aortic stenosis, constriction of the arterial duct or post-ductal coarctation of the aorta. Features of dilated CMO may be absent in early gestation so that sequential review is necessary where there is a family history.

Dilated CMO may be primary (22%), including familial, mitochondrial and other metabolic disease (e.g. sialic acid storage disease). It may also be secondary to fetal anaemia, *in-utero* infection (including parvovirus, HIV, coxsackie and toxoplasma) or more rarely secondary to maternal anti-Ro antibodies even in the absence of rhythm disturbance. Intermittent fetal arrhythmias need to be excluded because myocardial dysfunction may persist even when the arrhythmia is not observed. The aetiology is unknown in approximately 25%, and of the whole group there was a recurrence of CMO in a subsequent pregnancy in 10% of cases. (Sivasankaran et al. 2005). Idiopathic medial calcification is an autosomal recessive condition with characteristic echogenicity of major arteries which causes its effects through a combination of systemic arterial hypertension and myocardial ischaemia, and may present with dilated CMO. This condition is discussed in more detail later in this chapter.

Whatever the underlying cause, Sivasankaran et al. (2005) reported that two thirds became hydropic at some stage in the pregnancy. Sixty-two percent survived the pregnancy (excluding termination of pregnancy) but only 37.5% survived to the age of 1 year. Fetal hydrops was a poor prognostic indicator.

Investigations for a primary cardiomyopathy should include virology (TORCH screen, coxsackie, parvovirus), metabolic screening and array CGH/karyotype. Testing for metabolic abnormalities before birth is extremely difficult both because of the invasive nature of sampling and whether interpretation of results will be meaningful in the context of a fetus where the placental circulation may remove toxic metabolites. Many different cardiomyopathy gene-panels are available but frequently take several weeks to complete so are, at present, often not useful during the pregnancy. Echocardiograms should be performed on first-degree relatives if a familial CMO is suspected. Fetal echocardiography in future pregnancies should be offered for all cases of CMO diagnosed in fetal life or early infancy.

Non-compaction of the Myocardium

In early fetal life, the blood supply to the myocardium of the primitive heart tube is derived from the blood pool itself. The heart muscle becomes more "compacted" as the coronary circulation develops to supply blood to the myocardium. *Non-compaction of the myocardium* (also known as non-compaction cardiomyopathy) probably results from a failure of this myocardial compaction process.

Non-compaction of the myocardium is rare, with an incidence in infants of 0.80 per 100,000 per year and accounts for around 9% of all the primary cardiomyopathies.

It may occur in isolation or may be associated with another CHD in 12%, particularly left ventricular outflow tract abnormalities (54%), Ebstein anomaly (25%), ventricular septal defects or laterality disturbance. It may be asymptomatic or present with heart failure, arrhythmias, conduction defects, or thrombo-embolism. Mortality in children with non-compaction ranges from 13 to 23% due to ventricular arrhythmias and heart failure.

There are multiple causes of non-compaction but it is commonly associated with a variety of chromosomal defects, particularly chromosome 1p36 deletion, and neuromuscular disorders. Neuromuscular causes include mitochondrial disorders, Barth syndrome (X-linked), myotonic dystrophy type 1, distal myopathy (MYH7) and Emery–Dreyfuss muscular dystrophy.

Non-compaction of the myocardium can occasionally be diagnosed *in-utero* (Fig. 15.3a, b, Videos 15.1 and 15.2). When detected, invasive testing by array CGH should be considered. Many cases are familial, autosomal dominant forms of non-compaction have been reported in 13–50%. It is recommended that relatives of patients should be scanned and, if familial, further genetic testing can be considered. Several genes associated with isolated non-compaction have been identified, including *CASQ2, HCN4, KCNQ1, MIB1, NKX2-5, NNT, PKP2, RYR2, SCN5A, TNNI3, TTN, YWHAE.*

Perinatal Arrhythmias

The diagnosis and management of fetal arrhythmias are covered in Chap. 11. Only arrhythmias with a familial or genetic basis will be covered in this section.

Long QT syndrome (LQTS)

The usual fetal presentation is sustained sinus bradycardia, typically between 90–110 beats per minute. LQTS can also be associated with ventricular tachycardia and/or second-degree AV block.

If LQTS is confirmed or suspected in the fetus (or in the mother), close observation is recommended. Any electrolyte or vitamin D deficiency should be corrected and drugs that lengthen QT interval should be avoided (www.torsades.org). Maternal administration of beta blockers has been used to prevent torsade des pointes with a variable degree of success. A family history should be obtained and family screening is warranted. Delivery of the fetus in a specialist centre is rec-

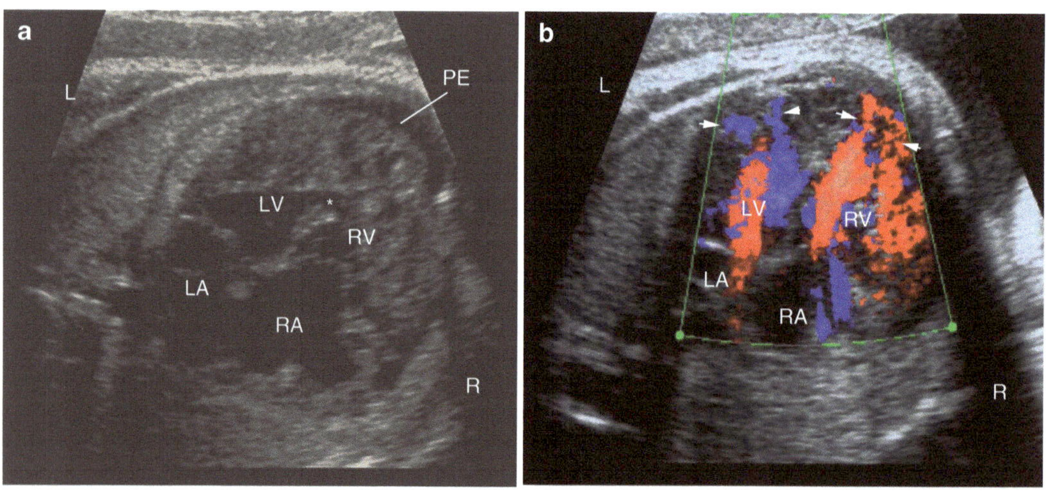

Fig. 15.3 (**a**, **b**) Four chamber view of non-compaction of the myocardium. (**a**) The heart is enlarged with a small pericardial effusion (PE) at the apex. There is a ventricular septal defect indicated by the asterisk. The apical portion of both the right and left ventricles is heavily trabelculated. (**b**) Four chamber view of the same fetus as pane A with the addition of colour flow Doppler. Deep crypts (*arrows*) are seen within the myocardium as the colour fills the deep resesses between the trabeculations

ommended (Wacker-Gussmann et al. 2014). The QT interval may be physiologically prolonged in the immediate neonatal period so will need to be repeated later in infancy in cases of doubt.

Supraventricular Tachycardia (SVT)

Fetal SVT accounts 70% of fetal tachycardias. In a minority of cases, a Wolff-Parkinson-White (WPW) pattern may be observed on the fetal ECG. Parental ECGs should be obtained if there is a family history of tachycardia as in a minority of cases WPW may be familial. It may be due to alcohol, or nicotine consumption.

Ventricular Tachycardia (VT)

VT is very rare in fetuses. The most frequent association is long QT syndrome but non-compaction of the myocardium of cardiac tumours may also be associated with VT.

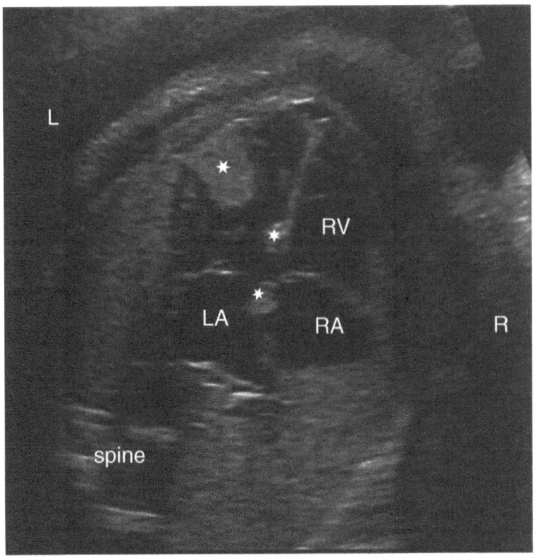

Fig. 15.4 Rhabdomyomas: Four chamber view of the fetal heart showing three rhabdomyomas (shown by *asterisks*). The rhabdomyomas have a rounded contour with uniform echogenicity and are located within the myocardium itself

Cardiac Tumours

Perinatal cardiac tumours are rare and predominantly benign. Rhabdomyoma is the most common (>75%) (Fig. 15.4), followed by teratoma (Fig. 15.5, Videos 15.3 and 15.4), fibroma, vascular tumours, and myxoma (Isaacs 2004). Intracardiac teratomas and fibromas usually present in the first year of life. Cardiac tumours may lead to a diagnosis of a specific genetic disorder depending on the type of tumour. These include tuberous sclerosis, familial myxoma syndrome (skin and mucous membrane lesions, cardiac myxoma, mammary myxofibroadenomas, and endocrine lesions of the adrenal, pituitary, and testis), Neurofibromatosis type 1, Gorlin syndrome (naevoid basal cell carcinoma syndrome), and, rarely, the Beckwith–Wiedemann syndrome (macrosomia, macroglossia, and omphalocele). Depending on the size and location, cardiac tumours may cause obstruction and interfere with myocardial function or cause arrhythmias, leading to a stillbirth, or sudden death.

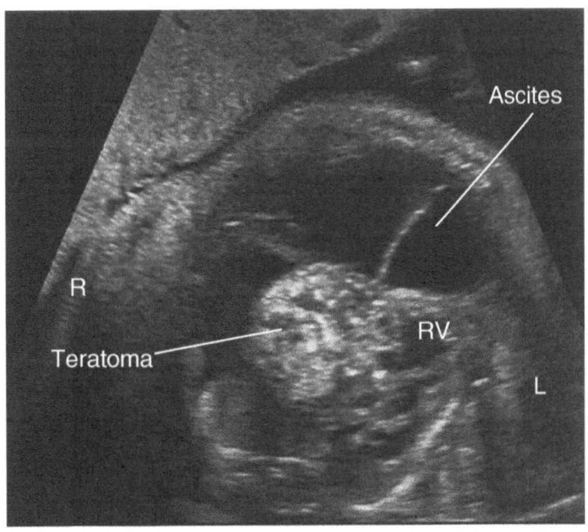

Fig. 15.5 Intrapericardial teratoma. This fetus has a large intrapericardial teratoma associated with fetal hydrops. Note that the teratoma is almost circular but has a non-uniform echogenicity with dark cystic areas

Cardiac Rhabdomyomas

Rhabdomyomas are examples of hamartomas (overgrowths of normal tissue) and are highly indicative of an underlying diagnosis of Tuberous Sclerosis (TS) (Fig. 15.4). Multiple rhabdomyomas are nearly always caused by a mutation in one of the two Tuberous Sclerosis genes *TSC1* (chromosome 9q34) or *TSC2* (chromosome 16p13.3). Single rhabdomyomas often become multiple at a later gestation or at post mortem, so there is still a high risk of TS. TS is confirmed in 50–80% of fetuses with cardiac rhabdomyomas.

Tuberous sclerosis is an autosomal dominant condition. In 50% of the cases, one of the parents will be a carrier of the mutation but, because of variable expression, may have minimal symptoms. There is significant intra-familial variation. TS is frequently associated with seizures, autism and moderate to severe intellectual disability (50%). If the mutation has occurred as a new event in the fetus (*de novo*) there is still a small risk that more than one egg or sperm carry the same mutation (germline mosaicism) with a sibling recurrence risk of 2–4%.

If a cardiac rhabdomyoma is suspected during the pregnancy, it is important to do a careful examination of the parents for signs of Tuberous Sclerosis (ash leaf macules, subungual fibromas, shagreen patch, facial angiofibromas). Genetic testing of the fetus and fetal MRI of the brain to look for cortical and subependymal tubers (usually present after 26 weeks gestation), can provide further confirmatory evidence of a diagnosis of TS. If the differential diagnosis of the cardiac tumour is in doubt, fetal cardiac MRI at a specialist centre may assist in tumour differentiation. If the cardiac rhabdomyoma does not cause obstruction, it will frequently regress in the first year of life and rarely requires surgery.

Intracardiac Pericardial Teratomas

These tumours are very rare and usually detected antenatally on routine ultrasound scanning. They may present with bilateral pleural effusions or fetal hydrops, possibly resulting in a stillbirth or perinatal death (Fig. 15.5, Videos 15.3 and 15.4).

Generalised Arterial Calcification of Infancy (GACI)/Idiopathic Medial Calcification

Generalised Arterial Calcification of Infancy is an extremely rare autosomal recessive condition but it is included here as the findings on the antenatal scan are very distinctive and can lead to an accurate prenatal diagnosis (Fig. 15.6a, b, Video 15.5). It is characterized by antenatal widespread arterial calcification with narrowing of the large and medium sized vessels. This may result in heart failure with a dilated cardiomegaly and fetal hydrops or respiratory distress, edema, cyanosis and hypertension in the neonate. Infant

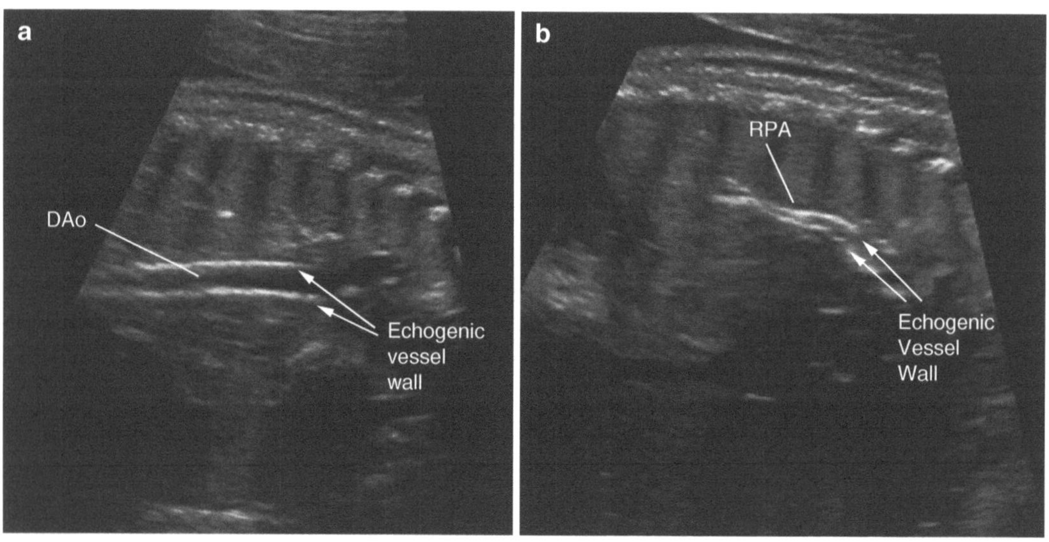

Fig. 15.6 (**a**, **b**) Idiopathic medial calcification. The arterial walls are intensely echogenic, matching the echogenicity of the surrounding ribs. In figure **a**, the descending aorta (DAo) is illustrated and in figure **b**, the echogenicity of the right pulmonary artery (RPA) is evident

mortality is very high in this conditions with a few exceptions surviving into the second and third decade.

Fetal echocardiography or the detailed fetal anomaly scan may detect echo, linear brightness of the main arteries near the heart (Fig. 15.6a, b, Video 15.5). The disease process may affect the coronary arteries leading to myocardial ischaemia and ventricular dysfunction as well as the renal arteries causing systemic arterial hypertension. Consequently, there may be left ventricular hypertrophy, a dilated CMO and/or pericardial effusion and oedema.

It is caused by bi-allelic mutations in the *ENPP1* or *ABCC6* gene. Mutations in *ENPP1* can also cause Autosomal recessive hypophosphataemic rickets. Infants with GACI who survive into childhood may develop hypophosphataemic rickets. ENPP1 usually converts extracellular ATP into AMP and pyrophosphate (PPi). PPi is considered the principal negative regulator of calcification and mineralization. When ENPP1 is defective, there is less extracellular PPi and more calcification.

Mutations in the ABCC6 gene also cause Pseudoxanthoma Elasticum (PXE), a genetic condition which affects the elasticity of the skin, arteries, eyes and gastrointestinal system. Many survivors of GACI present later with features of PXE, e.g. angioid streaks on fundoscopy or skin changes (Ferreira et al. 2014).

Genetic Susceptibility to Congenital Heart Defects

Copy Number Variants (Microdeletions/Microduplications)

Multiple studies have confirmed that there are an excess number of copy number variants (CNV) in patients with syndromic and non-syndromic CHD compared with controls. Array CGH testing of fetuses with CHD identifies CNVs in approximately 14%, 4% are 22q11 deletions, 7% other pathogenic CNV and 3% variants of unknown significance (Costain et al. 2016).

Soemedi et al. (2012) detected rare, *de novo* CNVs in about 5% of CHD trios (proband and their unaffected parents). These CNVs show incomplete penetrance and variable expression.

1q21.1 deletions and duplications are identified in approximately 1% of all TOF. The intra-familial family history of CHD is highly variable. The best candidate gene in the 1q21.1 region is *GJA5* gene that encodes connexin 40, a cardiac gap junction protein expressed in the right ventricular outflow tract.

8p23.1 deletions (and duplications) are associated particularly with septal defects, but again show high intra-familial variability. The transcription factor, *GATA4* is located at 8p23.1 and is highly likely to be causative.

15q11.2 deletions are now considered to be susceptibility loci for neurodevelopmental and neuropsychiatric disorders. Many studies have shown an increased susceptibility to a broad spectrum of CHD. However, no clear candidate genes have been identified in the 15q11.2 region.

Genes Associated with an Increased Susceptibility to CHD

Single gene mutations have been identified by investigating families with a high incidence of isolated CHD. Interestingly, several of these genes may cause the same type of CHD and conversely, the same mutation in the same gene may cause several different subtypes of CHD, even within the same family (Su et al. 2017).

De novo mutations contribute to approximately 10% of CHD, in approximately 400 genes, many involved in chromatin remodelling or histone modification. There are a number of well recognised syndromes associated with CHD caused by chromatin remodelling gene mutations, such as CHARGE and Kabuki syndrome. The chromatin remodelling genes are important for epigenetic regulation. It has been found that chromatin remodelling and histone modification are essential in heart development (Edwards and Gelb 2016).

The pathways include chromatin remodelling, Notch signalling, Nodal signalling, transcription factors, cilia function, sarcomere structure and function, and RAS signalling.

Transcription Factor Genes

A transcription factor is a protein that binds to DNA and regulates gene expression by promoting or suppressing transcription from DNA to RNA i.e. genes that control the expression of other genes. They are characterised by containing at least one DNA binding site. Variants in several transcription factors have be implicated in conferring an increased susceptibility to CHD, including NKX2-5, GATA4, 5, 6, and T-box factors (TBX1, TBX2, TBX3, TBX5, TBX18, and TBX20). *GATA4*, *NKX2.5*, and *TBX5* are all transcription factors and may form a complex that is necessary for cardiac septation.

GATA4

The transcription factor *GATA4* plays a crucial role in cardiomyocyte differentiation and heart development. *GATA4*-deficient mice die at an early stage of severe CHD. Mutations in the *GATA4* gene result in many types of congenital heart failure, particularly septal defects (Zhang et al. 2017).

TBX5

Mutations in *TBX5* cause Holt-Oram syndrome characterised by upper limb defects associated with CHD, typically septal and/or conduction defects.

NKX2-5

The characteristic CHD lesion associated with *NKX2.5* mutations are atrial septal defects and/or conduction defects. However, it may cause a broad range of CHD including heterotaxy and TOF (Zaidi and Brueckner 2017).

Nodal Signalling Genes

NODAL, FOXH1, GDF1, CFC1

The Nodal signalling pathway functions through the transforming growth factor-β receptors and is essential for left-right patterning.

Loss-of-function mutations in genes involved in Nodal signalling e.g. Nodal, Cripto, Cryptic, and FoxH1, have been identified in patients with heart defects and may cause two subtypes of CHD.

1. CHD associated with isomerism or heterotaxy
2. isolated congenital heart defects. e.g. transposition of the great arteries, double outlet right ventricle (DORV), tetralogy of Fallot, and isolated ventricular septal defects (Barnes et al. 2016).

Notch Signalling Genes

NOTCH1, NOTCH2, JAG1

The Notch signalling genes, Notch 1, Notch 2, and Delta-like 1 are required for the determination of the embryonic left-right axis and proper looping of the heart tube. Heterozygous *NOTCH1* mutations may result in a variety of abnormalities of the aortic valve, from a bicuspid aortic valve to a severe aortic valve stenosis, and subsequent left ventricular hypoplasia. It may account for approximately 5% of bicuspid aortic valve (Zaidi and Brueckner 2017). A recent paper by Kerstjens-Frederikse et al. (2016) described pathogenic mutations in *NOTCH1* in 7% of familial and 1% of sporadic Left Sided CHD. CHD was identified in 75% of NOTCH1 mutation carriers, confirming a high penetrance. Although Left-sided CHD were the most frequent malformations, right sided-CHD and conotruncal defects occurred in 18%, and 10% had thoracic aortic aneurysms. Mutations in Jagged 1 (JAG1) are causative of Alagille syndrome (see Table 15.2) but may also cause isolated CHD, particularly TOF and pulmonary stenosis.

References

Benson DW, Martin LJ, Lo CW. Genetics of hypoplastic left heart syndrome. J Pediatr. 2016;173:25–31.

Brodwall K, Greve G, Leirgul E, Tell GS, Vollset SE, Øyen N. Recurrence of congenital heart defects among siblings—a nationwide study. Am J Med Genet. 2017;173(6):1575–85.

Burn J, Brennan P, Little J, Holloway S, Coffey R, Somerville J, Dennis NR, Allan L, Arnold R, Deanfield JE, Godman M, Houston A, Keeton B, Oakley C, Scott O, Silove E, Wilkinson J, Pembrey M, Hunter

AS. Recurrence risks in offspring of adults with major heart defects: results from first cohort of British collaborative study. Lancet. 1998;351(9099):311–6.

Costain G, Silversides CK, Bassett AS. The importance of copy number variation in congenital heart disease. NPJ Genom Med. 2016;1:16031.

Digilio MC, Casey B, Toscano A, Calabrò R, Pacileo G, Marasini M, Banaudi E, Giannotti A, Dallapiccola B, Marino B. Complete transposition of the great arteries: patterns of congenital heart disease in familial precurrence. Circulation. 2001;104(23):2809–14.

Edwards JJ, Gelb BD. Genetics of congenital heart disease. Curr Opin Cardiol. 2016;31(3):235–41.

Emanuel BS, Budarf ML, Sellinger B, Goldmuntz E, Driscoll DA. Detection of microdeletions of 22q11.2 with fluorescence in situ hybridization (FISH): diagnosis of DiGeorge syndrome (DGS), velo-cardio-facial (VCF) syndrome, CHARGE association and conotruncal cardiac malformations. (Abstract). Am J Hum Genet. 1992;51(suppl):A3.

Ferencz C, Rubin JD, Loffredo CA, Magee CA. Epidemiology of congenital heart disease: the Baltimore-Washington Infant Study, 1981–1989. New York: Futura Publishing Company; 1993.

Ferreira C, Ziegler S, Gahl W. Generalized Arterial Calcification of Infancy. 2014. In: Pagon RA, Adam MP, Ardinger HH, et al., editors. GeneReviews® [Internet]. Seattle, WA: University of Washington, Seattle; 1993–2017. https://www.ncbi.nlm.nih.gov/books/NBK253403/.

Freeze SL, Landis BJ, Ware SM, Helm BM. Bicuspid aortic valve: a review with recommendations for genetic counseling. J Genet Couns. 2016;25(6):1171–8.

Gelb BD, Chung WK. Complex genetics and the etiology of human congenital heart disease. Cold Spring Harb Perspect Med. 2014;4(7):a013953.

Hales AR, Mahle WT. Echocardiography screening of siblings of children with bicuspid aortic valve. Pediatrics. 2014;133(5):e1212–7.

Hinton RB Jr, Martin LJ, Tabangin ME, Mazwi ML, Cripe LH, Benson DW. Hypoplastic left heart syndrome is heritable. J Am Coll Cardiol. 2007;50:1590–5.

Isaacs H. Fetal and neonatal cardiac tumors. Pediatr Cardiol. 2004;25(3):252–73.

Kerstjens-Frederikse WS, van de Laar IM, Vos YJ, Verhagen JM, Berger RM, Lichtenbelt KD, Klein Wassink-Ruiter JS, van der Zwaag PA, du Marchie Sarvaas GJ, Bergman KA, Bilardo CM, Roos-Hesselink JW, Janssen JH, Frohn-Mulder IM, van Spaendonck-Zwarts KY, van Melle JP, Hofstra RM, Wessels MW. Cardiovascular malformations caused by NOTCH1 mutations do not keep left: data on 428 probands with left-sided CHD and their families. Genet Med. 2016;18(9):914–23.

Maslen CL. Molecular genetics of atrioventricular septal defects. Curr Opin Cardiol. 2004;19(3):205–10.

McBride KL, Pignatelli R, Lewin M, Ho T, Fernbach S, Menesses A, Lam W, Leal SM, Kaplan N, Schliekelman P, Towbin JA, Belmont JW. Inheritance analysis of congenital left ventricular outflow tract obstruction malformations: segregation, multiplex relative risk, and heritability. Am J Med Genet A. 2005;134A(2):180–6.

Moosmann J, Uebe S, Dittrich S, Rüffer A, Ekici AB, Toka O. Novel loci for non-syndromic coarctation of the aorta in sporadic and familial cases. PLoS One. 2015;10(5):e0126873.

Muntean I, Togănel R, Benedek T. Genetics of congenital heart disease: past and present. Biochem Genet. 2017;55(2):105–23.

Oliverio M, Digilio MC, Versacci P, Dallapiccola B, Marino B. Shells and heart: are human laterality and chirality of snails controlled by the same maternal genes? Am J Med Genet A. 2010;152A(10):2419–25.

Øyen N, Poulsen G, Boyd HA, Wohlfahrt J, Jensen PK, Melbye M. Recurrence of congenital heart defects in families. Circulation. 2009;120(4):295–301.

Pedra SR, Smallhorn JF, Ryan G, Chitayat D, Taylor GP, Khan R, Abdolell M, Hornberger LK. Fetal cardiomyopathies: pathogenic mechanisms, hemodynamic findings, and clinical outcome. Circulation. 2002;106(5):585–91.

Barnes RM, Brian L, Black T. Nodal signaling and congenital heart defects. In: Nakanishi T, et al., editors. Etiology and morphogenesis of congenital heart disease. Tokyo, Japan: Springer; 2016.

Rauch R, Hofbeck M, Zweier C, Koch A, Zink S, Trautmann U, Hoyer J, Kaulitz R, Singer H, Rauch A. Comprehensive genotype-phenotype analysis in 230 patients with tetralogy of Fallot. J Med Genet. 2010;47(5):321–31.

Seale AN, Uemura H, Webber SA, Partridge J, Roughton M, Ho SY, McCarthy KP, Jones S, Shaughnessy L, Sunnegardh J, Hanseus K, Berggren H, Johansson S, Rigby ML, Keeton BR, Daubeney PE, British Congenital Cardiac Association. Total anomalous pulmonary venous connection: morphology and outcome from an international population-based study. Circulation. 2010;122(25):2718–26.

Seale AN, Carvalho JS, Gardiner HM, Mellander M, Roughton M, Simpson J, Tometzki A, Uzun O, Webber SA, Daubeney PE, British Congenital Cardiac Association. Total anomalous pulmonary venous connection: impact of prenatal diagnosis. Ultrasound Obstet Gynecol. 2012;40(3):310–8.

Sivasankaran S, Sharland GK, Simpson JM. Dilated cardiomyopathy presenting during fetal life. Cardiol Young. 2005;15(4):409–16.

Soemedi R, Wilson IJ, Bentham J, Darlay R, Töpf A, Zelenika D, Cosgrove C, Setchfield K, Thornborough C, Granados-Riveron J, Blue GM, Breckpot J, Hellens S, Zwolinkski S, Glen E, Mamasoula C, Rahman TJ, Hall D, Rauch A, Devriendt K, Gewillig M, O'Sullivan J, Winlaw DS, Bu'Lock F, Brook JD, Bhattacharya S, Lathrop M, Santibanez-Koref M, Cordell HJ, Goodship JA, Keavney BD. Contribution of global rare copy-number variants to the risk of sporadic congenital heart disease. Am J Hum Genet. 2012;91(3):489–501.

Su W, Zhu P, Wang R, Wu Q, Wang M, Zhang X, Mei L, Tang J, Kumar M, Wang X, Su L, Dong N. Congenital heart diseases and their association with the variant distribution features on susceptibility genes. Clin Genet. 2017;91(3):349–54.

Sutherland MJ, Ware SM. Disorders of left-right asymmetry: heterotaxy and situs inversus. Am J Med Genet C Semin Med Genet. 2009;151C(4):307–17.

Unolt M, Putotto C, Silvestri LM, Marino D, Scarabotti A, Massaccesi V, Caiaro A, Versacci P, Marino B. Transposition of great arteries: new insights into the pathogenesis. Front Pediatr. 2013;1:11.

Wacker-Gussmann A, Strasburger JF, Cuneo BF, Wakai RT. Diagnosis and treatment of fetal arrhythmia. Am J Perinatol. 2014;31(7):617–28.

Wapner RJ, Martin CL, Levy B, Ballif BC, Eng CM, Zachary JM, Savage M, Platt LD, Saltzman D, Grobman WA, Klugman S, Scholl T, Simpson JL, McCall K, Aggarwal VS, Bunke B, Nahum O, Patel A, Lamb AN, Thom EA, Beaudet AL, Ledbetter DH, Shaffer LG, Jackson L. Chromosomal microarray versus karyotyping for prenatal diagnosis. N Engl J Med. 2012;367(23):2175–84.

Weber R, Kantor P, Chitayat D, Friedberg MK, Golding F, Mertens L, Nield LE, Ryan G, Seed M, Yoo SJ, Manlhiot C, Jaeggi E. Spectrum and outcome of primary cardiomyopathies diagnosed during fetal life. JACC Heart Fail. 2014;2(4):403–11.

Zaidi S, Brueckner M. Genetics and genomics of congenital heart disease. Circ Res. 2017;120(6):923–40.

Zhang Y, Ai F, Zheng J, Peng B. Associations of GATA4 genetic mutations with the risk of congenital heart disease: A meta-analysis. Medicine (Baltimore). 2017;96(18):e6857.

Useful Websites

The Unique rare chromosomal disorders support group provide a number of helpful, informative and accurate leaflets. http://www.rarechromo.co.uk/html/home.asp

Array CGH leaflet. http://www.rarechromo.org/information/Other/Array%20CGH%20FTNW.pdf

FutureLearn run a MOOC (Massive Online Open Course) on 'The Genomics Era: The future of genetics in medicine. https://www.futurelearn.com/courses/the-genomics-era/3/register

Impact of Prenatal Diagnosis of Congenital Heart Disease on Outcome

16

Lindsey E. Hunter

Abstract

Prenatal diagnosis of congenital heart disease has been shown to have a positive impact on postnatal morbidity and mortality for some, but not all cardiac lesions. Overall, prenatal diagnosis has a positive impact on lesions with duct-dependent systemic or pulmonary circulation and where there is failure of mixing in transposition of the great arteries. The impact on other lesions such as septal defects, tetralogy of Fallot or total anomalous pulmonary venous drainage does not show improvement of outcome based on current evidence.

Keywords

Congenital heart disease · Prenatal diagnosis · Outcome · Mortality · Morbidity

Electronic Supplementary Material The online version of this chapter (https://doi.org/10.1007/978-3-319-77461-9_16) contains supplementary material, which is available to authorized users.

L. E. Hunter
Royal Hospital for Children, Glasgow, UK
e-mail: lindsey.hunter@ggc.scot.nhs.uk

Introduction

Prenatal detection of congenital heart disease (CHD) has been evolving since the early 1980s and in developed countries is a well-established subspecialty of paediatric cardiology. The main objective of prenatal diagnosis is to identify severe or critical congenital heart defects early in pregnancy. However, with developing expertise and understanding of CHD, prenatal diagnosis has an increasing role which includes risk stratification, identification of extra-cardiac or chromosomal abnormalities, optimal timing and location of delivery and the development of a tailored neonatal management plan. Such information also supports parental choices and truly informed consent for postnatal intervention. Individualised stratification of risk has assumed great importance in recent years due to the resurgence of interest in prenatal cardiac intervention which aims to alter the natural history of selected cardiac lesions. A fundamental question is whether prenatal diagnosis has a positive impact on postnatal outcome with respect to morbidity, mortality or quality of outcome (Table 16.1).

© Springer International Publishing AG, part of Springer Nature 2018

J. Simpson et al. (eds.), *Fetal Cardiology*, https://doi.org/10.1007/978-3-319-77461-9_16

Table 16.1 Cardiovascular benefit of prenatal diagnosis

Cardiac lesion	Prenatal intervention	Postnatal intervention
Transposition of the Great Arteries	–	• Prostaglandin E • Balloon atrial septostomy (BAS)
Coarctation of the aorta	–	• Prostaglandin E
Total Anomalous Pulmonary Venous Drainage (obstructed)	–	• Emergency surgical repair
Hypoplastic left heart syndrome	Stenting of restrictive atrial septum	• Prostaglandin E • Delivery onto cardio-pulmonary bypass or ECLS • Emergency BAS or septectomy
Critical aortic stenosis	Balloon aortic valvuloplasty	• Prostaglandin E • Aortic valvuloplasty • Surgical intervention
Pulmonary Atresia intact ventricular septum	Balloon pulmonary valvuloplasty	• Prostaglandin E • Pulmonary valvuloplasty • Surgical intervention
Tachyarrythmia (SVT/atrial flutter)	Trans-placental therapy	• Optimal timing of delivery • Cardioversion
Congenital complete heart block	Maternal steroids	• Isoprenaline • Temporary and permanent pacing

Cardiovascular Benefit After Prenatal Diagnosis

Critical congenital heart disease (CHD) has been defined as cardiac defects '*requiring intervention or treatment within the first 24 hours of life to prevent death*' (Slodki et al. 2016). Each individual diagnosis of congenital heart disease is heterogeneous, comprising a wide spectrum of severity. Thus, prenatal detection allows individual risk stratification and emphasises the importance of accurate diagnostic information for parental counselling. The approach to counselling after a prenatal diagnosis of CHD is covered in Chap. 13.

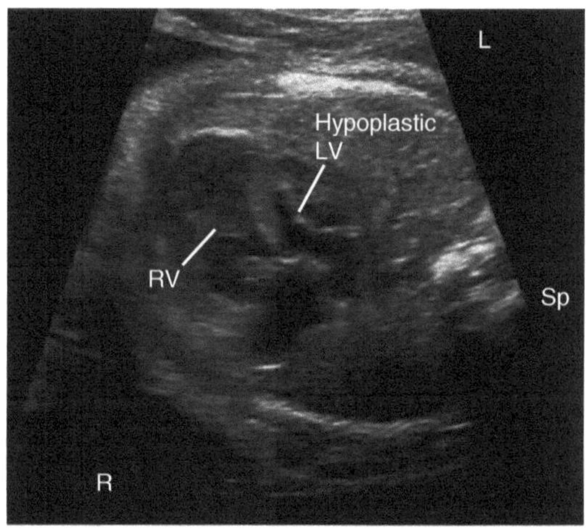

Fig. 16.1 Four chamber view demonstrating a well-developed right atrium and ventricle, but a hypoplastic left ventricle. *Sp* spine, *RV* right ventricle, *LV* left ventricle

Hypoplastic Left Heart Syndrome

HLHS is a classic lesion where blood flow to the systemic circulation is dependent on patency of the arterial duct (Fig. 16.1, Video 16.1). Without institution of prostaglandin E the vast majority of babies will die within a week of delivery. Within the spectrum of HLHS, specific phenotypes have been identified which are associated with worse early and long term outcomes including restrictive or intact atrial septum, the presence of left ventricular coronary sinusoids and significant tricuspid regurgitation. Those infants who are not diagnosed during fetal life may present in severe congestive cardiac failure with associated hypoxia, metabolic acidosis and end-organ damage. Initial studies reported improved surgical mortality following prenatal diagnosis (Tworetzky et al. 2001) but a recent meta-analysis has shown better haemodynamic status in infants diagnosed prenatally but no difference in mortality following initial Norwood surgery (Thakur et al. 2016). An important limitation is that all of the studies were from tertiary centres and none was population based so that infants who might not have survived to reach the tertiary centre were not included.

Coarctation of the Aorta

Coarctation of the aorta is normally suspected when there is asymmetry of ventricular and great arterial size with dominance of the right heart structures (Fig. 16.2a, b, Video 16.2). Hypoplasia of the transverse aortic arch and abnormal morphology of the aortic arch assist in prenatal assessment. The patency of the arterial duct and parallel nature of the fetal circulation mean that high Doppler gradients around the aortic arch and other evidence of frank obstruction of the aortic arch are rarely observed.

In the majority of cases, coarctation of the aorta is a duct dependent lesion and is classified as critical CHD, therefore requiring intervention to maintain ductal patency by administration of prostaglandin E. Failure to do so will result in closure of the arterial duct, obstruction of the aortic arch leading to a reduction in systemic tissue perfusion, increasing metabolic and lactic acidosis, with subsequent myocardial dysfunction and cardiovascular collapse. There is evidence that prenatal suspicion of coarctation is associated with improved outcomes after birth, with a reduction in preoperative morbidity and mortality and improved ventricular function at presentation (Matsui et al. 2008).

The aetiology of cardiac asymmetry in the context of coarctation of the aorta has not been explained by traditional imaging methods. Reduced left ventricular (LV) global systolic longitudinal strain and diastolic strain rate has been observed in fetuses with coarctation of the aorta (Miranda et al. 2016). Fetal cardiac MRI is being explored to improve assessment of the aortic arch (Lloyd et al. 2016). A potential intervention being studied is maternal administration of oxygen with the aim of reducing the fetal pulmonary vascular resistance thereby increasing pulmonary venous return to the left atrium. This would have the potential effect of increasing preload to the left ventricle and increasing antegrade flow around the aortic arch which, it is hypothesised, would increase the size of left heart structures including the aortic arch and impact on the natural history of the lesion. Initial studies were uncontrolled or single observer reports. Currently, acute or chronic administration of maternal oxygen is done on a research basis with some reports demonstrating improved growth of the aorta (Zeng et al. 2016).

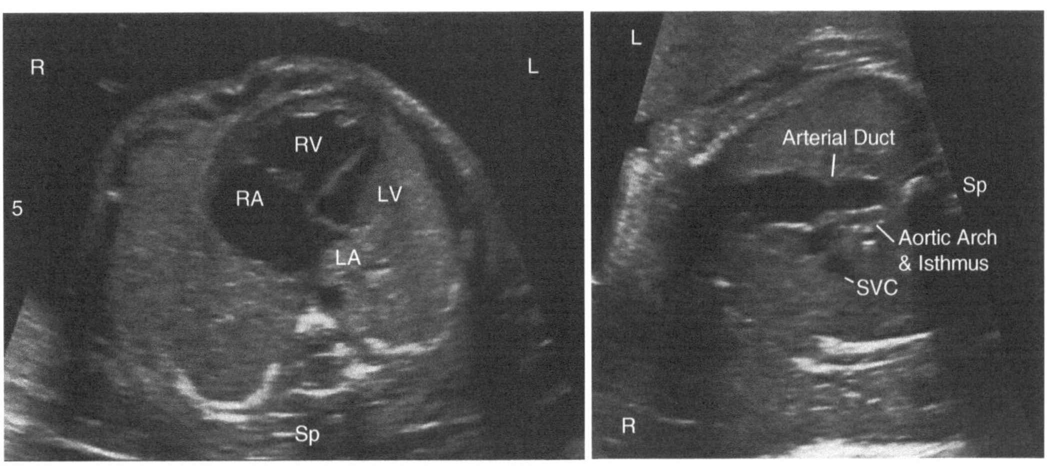

Fig. 16.2 Mid second trimester fetus with coarctation of the aorta (**a**) ventricular imbalance (**b**) great artery imbalance, transverse arch and aortic isthmus are significantly smaller than the ductal arch. *LA* left atrium, *LV* left ventricle, *RA* right atrium, *RV* right ventricle, *SVC* superior vena cava, *Sp* spine

Transposition of the Great Arteries

The most convincing evidence of benefit for prenatal detection of congenital heart disease is the reduction of preoperative and postoperative mortality in neonates with transposition of the great arteries (Fig. 16.3, Video 16.3). In addition to reducing mortality, prenatal detection reduces the incidence of preoperative metabolic acidosis; reduces length of hospital stay and reduces the incidence of neurological insult (Jouannic et al. 2004). Recent work, using MRI scanning, has demonstrated a reduced incidence of brain injury in infants with prenatally diagnosed TGA compared to the postnatally diagnosed cohort. The impact of these findings on later neurodevelopmental outcome is under investigation (Peyvandi et al. 2016). Thus, delivery is planned in a tertiary cardiac centre with early administration of neonatal prostaglandin E to maintain ductal patency. However, even in the prenatally detected cohort, the failure of mixing at the level of the atrial septum/arterial duct can be unpredictable. Despite early prostaglandin therapy, studies suggest a 4% mortality due to inadequate mixing at atrial level. This emphasises the need for delivery at a site where an emergency balloon atrial septostomy can be undertaken. Recent work has used the ratio of the size of the foramen ovale to the septal length to predict need for early septostomy (Vigneswaran et al. 2017). Although useful these markers are not sensitive enough to detect all high risk fetuses and there will always be a cohort of infants presenting with profound cyanosis despite an unrestrictive arterial duct.

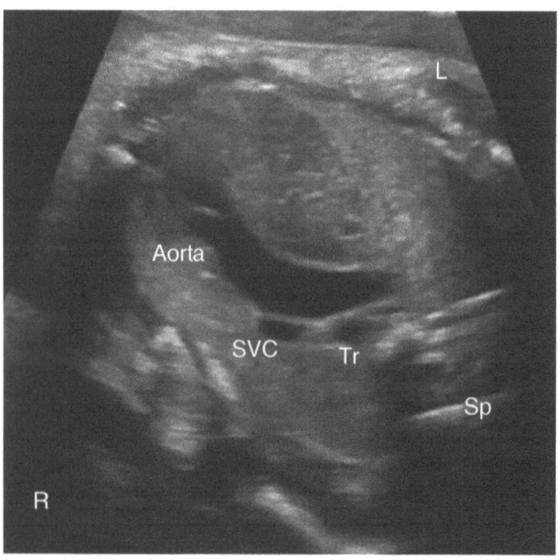

Fig. 16.3 Transverse view of transposition of the great arteries, aorta arising anteriorly from the right ventricle, only two vessels visualised in the normal three vessel view as the great arteries arise in parallel. *Tr* trachea, *SVC* superior vena cava, *Sp* spine

Total Anomalous Pulmonary Venous Drainage

Total anomalous venous drainage (TAPVD) is a rare congenital heart defect in which all the pulmonary veins drain to the right atrium, systemic veins or the coronary sinus. Isolated TAPVD remains a challenging prenatal diagnosis even in the hands of an experienced paediatric/fetal cardiologist with less than 5% of cases diagnosed before birth. Some patients present with obstruction to the pulmonary venous confluence which manifests itself with severe hypoxaemia, respiratory distress and metabolic acidosis requiring emergent cardiac surgery after delivery. However, the benefits of prenatal diagnosis remain controversial, this may allow for early investigation and surgical intervention in the presence of obstruction, but, a multicentre, international study did not report a significant difference in mortality between the cohort diagnosed prenatally versus those only diagnosed after birth (Seale et al. 2012).

Pulmonary Atresia

Pulmonary atresia, presents in two very different morphologies, pulmonary atresia ventricular septal defect (VSD) or pulmonary atresia with intact ventricular septum (Fig. 16.4, Video 16.4). Both morphologies have differing extra-cardiac and karyotypic associations, thus prenatal diagnosis is important to provide accurate parental counselling. Despite different morphologies and prognoses, both conditions are neonatal duct dependent lesions which benefit from early intervention to prevent profound cyanosis and cardiovascular

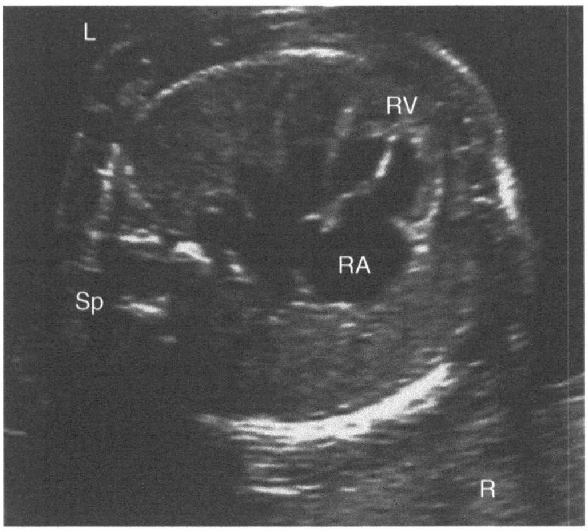

Fig. 16.4 Four chamber view of pulmonary atresia and intact ventricular septum, dilated right atria and ventricle, with bright papillary muscles and tethered tricuspid valve. *RV* right ventricle, *RA* right atrium, *LA* left atrium, *LV* left ventricle, *Sp* spine

compromise. Published data has demonstrated improved condition at presentation in the prenatally diagnosed group but without a significant difference in early mortality.

Prenatal Intervention Following Prenatal Diagnosis

There is evidence that certain congenital cardiac defects may benefit from prenatal intervention by potentially halting the physiological and anatomical progression of the disease, for example, critical aortic stenosis; pulmonary atresia intact ventricular septum or HLHS with restrictive atrial septum. However the strongest evidence to support prenatal intervention relates to the management of fetal tachyarrhythmias.

Tachyarrhythmias

Fetal tachycardias, usually due to supraventricular tachycardia or atrial flutter, are a clear example of benefit of prenatal diagnosis in terms of outcome. Untreated tachycardias increase the risk of heart failure, fetal hydrops and the incidence of intrauterine demise. Prenatal therapy is usually administered transplacentally and reversion to sinus rhythm is associated with improved outcome. The optimal drug choice for prenatal therapy remains controversial (Jaeggi et al. 2011).

Management of fetal tachycardias is covered more extensively in Chap. 12.

Congenital Complete Heart Block

Congenital complete atrioventricular (AV) block occurs in approximately 1 in 20,000 live births and is associated with a risk of intrauterine and postnatal demise. Congenital complete AV block may be associated with underlying structural congenital heart disease or in association with a multifactorial, autoimmune process, related to the trans-placental transfer of maternal autoantibodies anti-Ro/SSA or Anti-La/SSB, which attach to and damage cardiac myocytes and conduction tissue of susceptible fetuses (Fig. 16.5).

The optimal therapy for immune-mediated complete heart block remains controversial. There is large institutional variation in practice and no large randomised trials. For fetuses with complete heart block maternal β stimulation (using salbutamol) to increase the fetal ventricular escape rate and maternal dexamethasone have been used most frequently but without consensus as to the optimal treatment strategy. Management of fetuses with heart block is discussed further in Chap. 12 (Hunter et al. 2015).

Critical Pulmonary Stenosis/ Pulmonary Atresia

Pulmonary atresia intact ventricular septum exhibits parallels to the progressive nature of prenatal critical aortic stenosis, encompassing a wide spectrum of pathology, with evidence of progressive right ventricular hypoplasia. Fetal balloon pulmonary valvuloplasty may be undertaken with technical success. There remains considerable debate with respect to selection criteria for suitable candidates. In practice, cases are referred to subspecialist centres for consideration

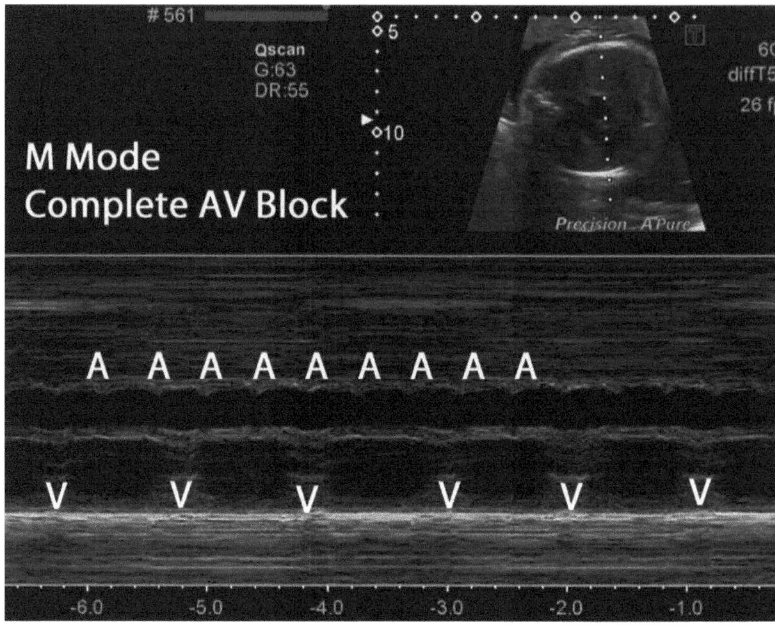

Fig. 16.5 M mode representation of complete atrioventricular block. *A* atrial, *V* ventricular

of intervention and decisions made on a case by case basis. Although demonstrated to be technically successful in this carefully selected cohort, this early intervention does not obviate the need for catheter or surgical intervention postnatally. An international registry has been set up to analyse technical success and patient outcome (Moon-Grady et al. 2015).

HLHS/Restrictive Atrial Septum

In utero atrial septal restriction of HLHS prevents adequate blood from exiting the left atrium into the well-developed right heart structures, creating a significant pressure gradient and resultant left atrial hypertension. Prolonged exposure to left atrial hypertension during prenatal development results in permanent vascular remodelling within the pulmonary venous vessels and the development of pulmonary lymphangiectasia. In the immediate neonatal period, atrial septal restriction prevents adequate oxygenated blood from exiting the left atrium and entering the systemic circulation. In the absence of urgent atrial decompression or immediate bypass support the neonate will become profoundly hypoxic and acidotic. Despite immediate neonatal intervention, study data reports survival in this cohort to be less than 50%, attributable to the irreversible damage within the lung parenchyma and the ineffectiveness of the Fontan circulation. Most recently, the adverse effects of this abnormal physiology have been investigated by fetal MRI. A specific pattern called "nutmeg lung" has been identified which has been associated with uniformly poor outcome (Saul et al. 2016).

Pulmonary venous inflow Doppler waveform assessment is an important indicator of atrial restriction in prenatal HLHS. In the most severe presentation of atrial restriction or an intact atrial septum, a 'to fro' pattern representing absent diastolic forward flow, is evident in the pulmonary venous waveform (Fig. 16.6a, b). Recent work has used the ratio of the velocity-time integrals of antegrade flow into the left atrium against retrograde flow out of the left atrium to predict the need for urgent decompression of the left atrium with a cut-off value of 3:1 being adopted by most centres (Divanović et al. 2011).

Prenatal intervention, in the form of in utero balloon atrial septostomy or interatrial stenting, has been attempted in a highly selected cohort of fetuses with evidence of a restrictive or intact atrial septum, in a bid to prevent the development of irreversible pathological changes within the

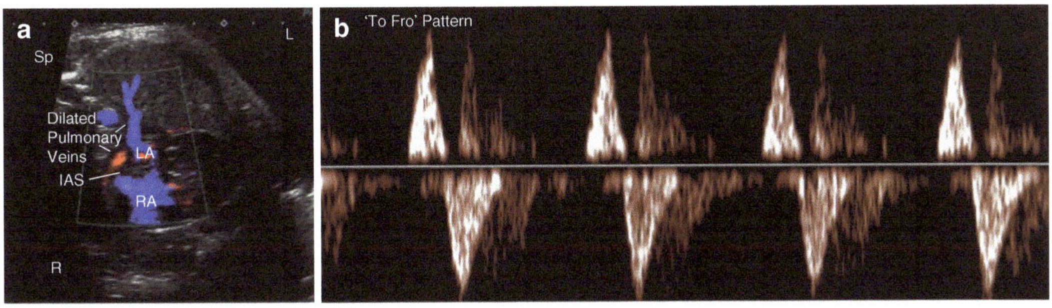

Fig. 16.6 Four chamber view of the pulmonary venous return (red/blue) to the left atrium in HLHS. (**a**) The pulmonary veins are dilated and there is absence of flow across the intact atrial septum. (**b**) 'To fro' pattern of severe atrial septal restriction. *RA* right atrium, *LA* left atrium, *IAS* intact atrial septum, *Sp* spine

pulmonary vasculature. The management of such cases remains controversial. Data on outcome is being collected as part of an international registry (Moon-Grady et al. 2015). In some centres delivery is undertaken in cardiac theatre and the neonate placed immediately on to Extra Corporeal Life Support (ECLS) or cardiopulmonary bypass. The option of compassionate care may also be discussed in this high risk group.

Critical Aortic Stenosis

Aortic valve stenosis may become progressively more severe with advancing gestation. At the severe end of the spectrum, critical aortic stenosis (AS) is a progressive lesion characterised by suboptimal growth of left heart structures—the natural history is the development of a morphology akin to hypoplastic left heart by term. This challenging diagnosis can go undetected at the second trimester screening scan as the four chamber view may appear 'near normal'. The postnatal management of critical AS depends on the size, function and other features of the left heart such as endocardial fibroelastosis. In some cases postnatal management is directed towards a two ventricle circulation but in others the management is similar to classical HLHS. Early administration of prostaglandin E and access to catheter or surgical intervention is essential to reduce morbidity and mortality associated with a duct dependent circulation and univentricular palliation. As the natural history of prenatal critical AS is to develop into HLHS by term, specific criteria have been determined to assess which fetuses may benefit from prenatal balloon dilation of the aortic valve in an attempt to promote growth of the left heart structures and allow a biventricular surgical repair in childhood. Intervention in the form prenatal aortic balloon valvuloplasty is an area of great interest and the long term success is under intense international scrutiny. The evolving hypoplastic left heart syndrome (eHLHS) score was developed to predict which fetuses with critical AS, in the absence of fetal intervention, would progress to HLHS by term. The score incorporates four components: (1) the presence of L-R shunting at atrial level; (2) retrograde filling of the aortic arch from the arterial duct; (3) LV dysfunction and (4) monophasic pattern of the mitral valve inflow. Selection of suitable candidates for intervention is further refined using the 'Threshold Scoring' system which examines the 'z scores' of the left heart structures and the gradient across the aortic or mitral valve. The challenges of fetal intervention not only include technical success but timely patient detection and selection before irreversible vascular damage has occurred. Although intervention may increase the probability of a biventricular pathway, childhood is not free from further surgical intervention, left ventricular diastolic dysfunction and the potential need for cardiac transplantation (Hunter et al. 2015). An international registry is recording the prenatal echocardiographic data, results of intervention and outcome of prenatal intervention for critical aortic stenosis (Moon-Grady et al. 2015).

Limited Cardiovascular Benefit After Prenatal Diagnosis

Some congenital heart defects are not commonly associated with haemodynamic instability in the neonatal period, therefore prenatal detection does not infer cardiovascular benefit. These defects include 'pink'/well balanced Tetralogy of Fallot; atrioventricular septal defect (AVSD) and ventricular septal defect (VSD). Although not a direct cardiac benefit, the benefits of prenatal diagnosis in terms of parental preparation and investigation for associated malformations still apply.

Tetralogy of Fallot

Tetralogy of Fallot (ToF) is an abnormality of the outflow tracts commonly detected in the prenatal period by examining the outflow tract views and three vessel view in the upper mediastinum (Fig. 16.7a, b, Video 16.5). Many infants diagnosed with ToF have adequate pulmonary blood flow with minimal or no cyanosis in the early neonatal period therefore delivery in a tertiary cardiac centre is not indicated. Equally, prenatal suspicion of inadequate pulmonary blood flow may indicate earlier neonatal intervention, and assessment using specific prenatal prognostic parameters may guide location of delivery. These prognostic parameters include: aortic: pulmonary artery ratio; main pulmonary artery/branch pulmonary artery diameters in the third trimester and peak systolic pulmonary valve velocity in the mid second trimester. Complete prenatal assessment must also include acknowledgment of the potential associated chromosomal abnormalities, in particular 22q11.2 deletion, a multisystem disorder which may affect the cardiovascular system, immune function, neurodevelopment and psychiatric health in later life.

Atrioventricular Septal Defect

In the presence of a balanced atrioventricular septal defect (AVSD) neonates are anticipated to be haemodynamically stable in the immediate postnatal period, and therefore delivery may arranged out with the tertiary cardiac centre (Fig. 16.8, Video 16.6).

Although prenatal detection does not influence the prenatal cardiac or early cardiovascular

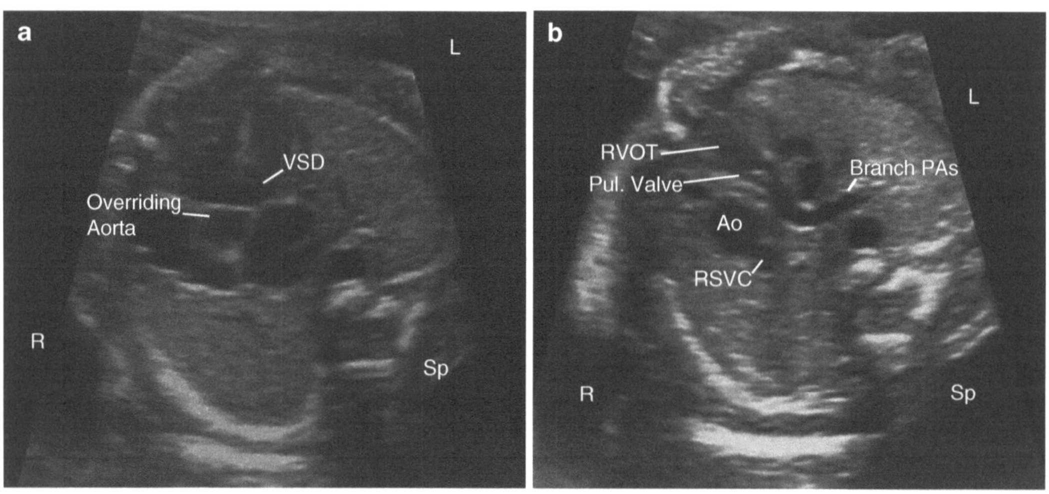

Fig. 16.7 Tetralogy of fallot (**a**) ventricular septal defect and an overriding aorta (**b**) great artery disproportion, smaller pulmonary valve, main pulmonary artery and branch pulmonary arteries. *LA* left atrium, *RA* right atrium, *LV* left ventricle, *LA* left atrium, *VSD* ventricular septal defect, *Pul* pulmonary, *Desc Ao* descending aorta, *PA* pulmonary artery, *Ao* aorta, *RAA* right aortic arch, *RSVC* right superior vena cava, *RVOT* right ventricular outflow tract, *Sp* spine

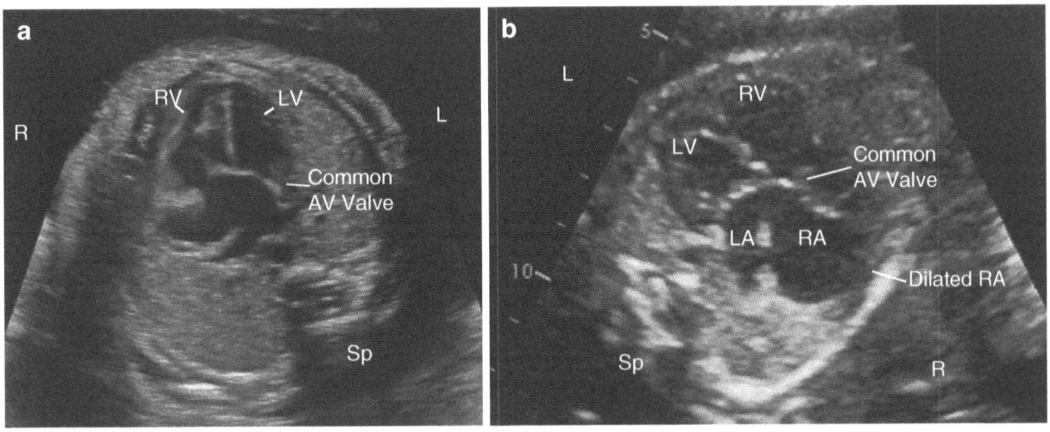

Fig. 16.8 Atrioventricular septal defect (**a**) common AV valve with balanced ventricular and atrial dimensions (**b**) common AV valve with marked cardiomegaly and dilated right atrium, secondary to significant AV valve regurgitation. *RV* right ventricle, *LV* left ventricle, *AV* atrioventricular, *RA* right atrium, *Sp* spine

management, there is a recognised association between the lesion and karyotypic abnormalities, particularly trisomy 21. Atrioventricular septal defects may also be unbalanced with marked ventricular or great artery disproportion, altering the suitability for biventricular surgical septation, which must be reflected in the parental counselling, particularly in the context of other fetal abnormalities. In addition, varying degrees of atrioventricular valve regurgitation may be observed and should be monitored throughout gestation. In the presence of severe atrioventricular valve regurgitation, cardiomegaly, cardiac failure and intrauterine death are known to occur. Conversely, atrioventricular septal defects may present in association with more complex congenital cardiac defects, for example isomerism/disorders of laterality, encompassing abnormal systemic or pulmonary venous return; outflow tract abnormalities; conduction disorders and extra cardiac abnormalities. Determining the cardiac situs in the presence of an AVSD is essential as the incidence of karyotypic abnormalities in the context of isomerism of the atrial appendages is extremely low (Morlandoa et al. 2017).

Ventricular Septal Defects

Small ventricular septal defects (VSD) are often challenging to detect in the fetus due to the almost equal pressure within the left and right ventricle. The normal postnatal pattern of shunting demonstrated by colour flow Doppler is absent. Neonates with isolated muscular VSDs are haemodynamically stable in the initial neonatal period due to elevated pulmonary vascular resistance and small muscular defects may close spontaneously by term. Detection of a perimembranous or maligned VSD are significant both because of the extra-cardiac associations and because VSDs can co-exist with more severe forms of CHD which should be excluded.

Prenatal Diagnosis and Neurodevelopmental Outcomes

The vast majority of data on the impact of prenatal diagnosis of CHD on outcome is from major tertiary centres in developed countries. Most studies report outcome in terms of mortality, length of stay in hospital and obvious short term morbidity. Few studies are population based to gauge how patients fare out with the cardiac centre. As surgical outcomes improve and PICU care advances the emphasis is rapidly switching towards quality of outcome, particularly with respect to neurodevelopmental outcome in infancy and throughout childhood. Recent data suggests a positive impact of prenatal diagnosis on early brain development and brain injury but this needs to be further evaluated in terms of neurodevelopmental and behavioural abnormalities which are becoming increasingly recognised in CHD survivors (Peyvandi et al. 2016).

References

Beaton AZ, Pike JI, Stallings C, Donofrio MT. Predictors of repair and outcome in prenatally diagnosed atrioventricular septal defects. JASE. 2013;26:208–16.

Divanović A, Hor K, Cnota J, Hirsch R, Kinsel-Ziter M, Michelfelder E. Prediction and perinatal management of severely restrictive atrial septum in fetuses with critical left heart obstruction: clinical experience using pulmonary venous Doppler analysis. J Thorac Cardiovasc Surg. 2011;141(4):988–94.

Hunter LE, Simpson JM. Atrioventricular block during fetal life. J Saudi Heart Assoc. 2015;27(3):164–78.

Hunter LE, Chubb H, Miller O, Sharland G, Simpson JM. Fetal aortic valve stenosis: a critique of case selection criteria for fetal intervention. Prenat Diagn. 2015;35(12):1176–81.

Jaeggi ET, Carvalho JS, De Groot E, Api O, Clur SB, Rammeloo L, McCrindle BW, Ryan G, Manlhiot C, Blom NA. Comparison of transplacental treatment of fetal supraventricular tachyarrhythmias with digoxin, flecainide, and sotalol results of a nonrandomized multicenter study. Circulation. 2011;124:1747–54.

Jouannic JM, Gavard L, Fermont L, Le Bidois J, Parat S, Vouhe PR, Dumez Y, Sidi D, Bonnet D. Sensitivity and specificity of prenatal features of physiological shunts to predict neonatal clinical status in transposition of the great arteries. Circulation. 2004;110:1743–6.

Lloyd DF, van Amerom JF, Pushparajah K, Simpson JM, Zidere V, Miller O, et al. An exploration of the potential utility of fetal cardiovascular MRI as an adjunct to fetal echocardiography. Pren Diagn. 2016;36(10):916–25.

Matsui H, Mellander M, Roughton M, Jicinska H, Gardiner HM. Morphological and physiological predictors of fetal aortic coarctation. Circulation. 2008;118(18):1793–801.

Miranda JO, Hunter LE, Tibby S, Sharland G, Miller O, Simpson JM. Myocardial deformation in fetuses with coarctation of the aorta: a case controlled study. Ultrasound Obstet Gynecol. 2016. https://doi.org/10.1002/uog.15939.

Moon-Grady AJ, Morris SA, Belfort M, Chmait R, Dangel J, Devlieger R, Emery S, Frommelt M, Galindo A, Gelehrter S, Gembruch U, Grinenco S, Habli M, Herberg U, Jaeggi E, Kilby M, Kontopoulos E, Marantz P, Miller O, Otaño L, Pedra C, Pedra S, Pruetz J, Quintero R, Ryan G, Sharland G, Simpson J, Vlastos E, Tworetzky W, Wilkins-Haug L, Oepkes D, International Fetal Cardiac Intervention Registry. International fetal cardiac intervention registry: a worldwide collaborative description and preliminary outcomes. J Am Coll Cardiol. 2015;66(4):388–99.

Morlandoa M, Bhidea A, Familiaria A, Khalila A, Morales-Rosellóa J, Papageorghioua AT, Carvalho JS. The association between prenatal atrioventricular septal defects and chromosomal abnormalities. Eur J Obstet Gynecol Reprod Biol. 2017;208:31–5.

Peyvandi S, De Santiago V, Chakkarapani E, Chau V, Campbell A, Poskitt KJ, Duan X, Barkovich AJ, Miller S, McQuillen P. Association of prenatal diagnosis of critical congenital heart disease with postnatal brain development and the risk of brain injury. JAMA Pediatr. 2016;170(4):e154450.

Saul D, Degenhardt K, Iyoob SD, Surrey LF, Johnson AM, Johnson MP, Rychik J, Victoria T. Hypoplastic left heart syndrome and the nutmeg lung pattern in utero: a cause and effect relationship or prognostic indicator? Pediatr Radiol. 2016;46(4):483–9.

Schidlow DN, Tworetzky W, Wilkins-Haug LE. Percutaneous fetal cardiac interventions for structural heart disease. Am J Perinatol. 2014;31(07):629–36.

Seale AN, Carvalho JS, Gardiner HM, Mellander M, Roughton M, Simpson J, Tometzki A, Uzun O, Webber SA, Daubeney PE, British Congenital Cardiac Association. Total anomalous pulmonary venous connection: impact of prenatal diagnosis. Ultrasound Obstet Gynecol. 2012;40:310–8.

Slodki M, Respondek-Liberska M, Pruetz JD, Donofrio MT. Fetal cardiology: changing the definition of critical heart disease in the newborn. J Perinatol. 2016;36(8):575–80.

Thakur V, Munk N, Mertens L, Nield L. Does prenatal diagnosis of hypoplastic left heart syndrome make a difference?—a systematic review. Prenat Diagn. 2016;36:854–63.

Tworetzky W, McElhinney D, Reddy V, Brook M, Hanley F, Silverman N. Improved surgical outcome after fetal diagnosis of hypoplastic left heart syndrome. Circulation. 2001;103(9):1269–73.

Vigneswaran TV, Zidere V, Miller OI, Simpson JM, Sharland GK. Usefulness of the prenatal echocardiogram in fetuses with isolated transposition of the great arteries to predict the need for balloon atrial septostomy. Am J Cardiol. 2017;119(9):1463–7.

Zeng S, Zhou J, Peng Q, Deng W, Zhang M, Zhao Y, et al. Sustained maternal hyperoxygenation improves aortic arch dimensions in fetuses with coarctation. Sci Rep. 2016;6:39304.

17 Obstetric and Fetal Medicine Management of the Fetus with Congenital Heart Disease

Fergus P. McCarthy, Pippa Kyle, and Owen I. Miller

Abstract

The Obstetric and Fetal Medicine management of the fetus with congenital heart disease is challenging and requires multidisciplinary care involving obstetric, midwifery and neonatology input in addition to the clinical care provided by paediatric cardiology services. This chapter discusses the principles of management for pregnant women following the diagnosis of congenital heart disease. Clear care pathways, good multi-disciplinary team work and frequent clear communication are required to optimise care and outcomes.

Keywords

Obstetrics · Multidisciplinary care · Fetal medicine · Karyotype · Communication · Congenital heart disease

F. P. McCarthy (✉)
Women's Health Academic Centre, King's College London, London, UK
e-mail: Fergus.mccarthy@ucc.ie

P. Kyle
Guys & St Thomas' NHS Foundation Trust, London, UK
e-mail: Pippa.Kyle@gstt.nhs.uk

O. I. Miller
Evelina London Children's Hospital, Guy's and St Thomas' NHS Foundation Trust, London, UK
e-mail: owen.miller@gstt.nhs.uk

Introduction

Fetal congenital heart disease requires multidisciplinary care involving obstetric, midwifery and neonatology input in addition to the clinical care provided by paediatric cardiology services. Accurate diagnosis, with clear pathways of care and communication are essential to ensure the best outcomes and parent experience. Evidence to support different pathways of management of pregnant women whose fetuses have congenital heart disease is limited. One ideal model includes a combined maternity and children's hospital on the same site as a paediatric cardiac surgical centre. Although, this option is not available in many centres, the principles of management we feel are relevant to most units.

Antenatal Care and Fetal Medicine Consultation

Screening and Diagnosis

Approximately 90% of fetal heart abnormalities occur in low-risk women. This provides the rationale for incorporation of cardiac views into midtrimester anomaly scans (see Chap. 1) to identify cardiac abnormalities in the absence of other risk factors. Other candidates for fetal cardiac assessment include high-risk women, selected by family history, or when extracardiac fetal abnormalities are diagnosed within the

© Springer International Publishing AG, part of Springer Nature 2018
J. Simpson et al. (eds.), *Fetal Cardiology*, https://doi.org/10.1007/978-3-319-77461-9_17

current pregnancy. The degree of involvement by fetal medicine, fetal cardiac and obstetric teams will depend on whether the fetal heart abnormality is isolated or associated with other fetal co-morbidity or other maternal co-morbidity. The indications for detailed fetal echocardiography are broadly accepted by international bodies and are discussed in detail in Chap. 1.

Initial Fetal Medicine and Fetal Cardiac Consultation

Following the diagnosis of a suspected or confirmed fetal heart abnormality, the pregnant woman should be referred to a tertiary-level fetal medicine centre for consultation both with a fetal medicine specialist and with a fetal cardiologist. In some centres this may occur in a combined multidisciplinary clinic; in other centres the two services may run in parallel.

The fetal medicine component of the consultation will include;

- Full detailed anomaly scan. Up to 50% of cases may have extracardiac anomalies.
- Consideration of additional investigations looking at aetiology (fetal karyotyping) or more specialised imaging in selected cases e.g. MRI of the fetal brain in suspected tuberous sclerosis.
- Explanation of significance of sonographic findings.
- Involvement of other subspecialists as necessary e.g. clinical geneticists, paediatric neurologists.

The fetal cardiology component will include:

- A comprehensive fetal echocardiogram by a cardiologist or sonographer with experience and knowledge of congenital heart disease
- Explanation of the cardiac lesion and its implications

Once all initial information is available, counselling is undertaken with the fetal medicine specialist covering the overall fetal status and prognosis and the fetal cardiologist covering the cardiac lesion, the treatment options including prenatal intervention, postnatal surgery and long term cardiac prognosis. In cases with an isolated fetal heart abnormality, the counselling may be led predominantly by the fetal cardiologist. In contrast, those cases with multiple abnormalities, including chromosomal abnormalities may have a poorer outcome that is more dependent on the underlying cause of the multiple defects and the interaction between the different affected organ systems. This discussion and counselling is usually led by the fetal medicine specialist.

Management options for the parents will vary by country and culture but may include:

- continuation of the pregnancy aiming for a live birth and post-natal management as required.
- planned palliative care without cardiac intervention after birth for severe cardiac lesions
- termination of pregnancy, where this is lawful and requested by parents. Depending on the gestational age, termination of pregnancy may involve a feticide procedure. The option of post-mortem examination following termination of pregnancy is also discussed with the parents.

For continuing pregnancies, regular antenatal monitoring of the fetus is recommended, to check fetal and maternal well-being. The ongoing counselling and support for parents expecting a fetus with CHD is covered in detail in Chap. 12. In brief, continuing support is crucial with ongoing contact and high-quality written information where possible. Most centres will provide a specialist fetal cardiac liaison nursing service (Bratt et al. 2015).

Fetal heart abnormalities are associated with an increased risk of an underlying chromosomal disorder. The risk varies depending on the lesion but parents should have the option to consider fetal chromosomal testing before they are booked for delivery in the tertiary unit. The identification of an additional structural anomaly significantly increases the possibility of an underlying chromosomal disorder. Fetal abnormalities associated with CHD are addressed in depth in Chap. 14.

The timing of the initial fetal medicine appointment will depend on indication:

- If there is a suspicion of CHD, the fetus should be seen as soon as possible
- If based on other risk factors, then review can be scheduled at a gestational age when the couple will have time to reflect on all the information, be able to opt for invasive testing if required, and allow enough time to obtain karyotype results in a timely manner to be able to decide between all options discussed above.

Ongoing Pregnancy Management

If no concerns apart from the fetal CHD are raised during the initial fetal medicine consultation then the patient may continue their routine obstetric care locally rather than in a tertiary centre. This is judged on a case-by-case basis and depends on local expertise and policy. Surveillance of the fetal heart abnormality will continue with the fetal cardiologist, usually at intervals of around 6–8 weeks. This allows time for ongoing discussion and assessment for disease progression. Fetal medicine review may be indicated to check fetal growth and well-being. At any time, new obstetric or other fetal concerns should prompt re-referral to fetal medicine. One of the fundamental decisions relates to site of delivery. This will be guided either by the presence of a duct dependent cardiac lesion or other materno-fetal indications for delivery in a specialist centre.

For those cases where a decision has been made for delivery in a tertiary centre (see Table 17.1), careful co-ordination involving fetal medicine, midwifery, neonatology and paediatric cardiology is required. At our own centre, this involves joint meetings to discuss the care plan tailored to the specific case. Late assessment by fetal medicine is important to confirm the mode and timing of delivery. The development of maternal complications such as pre-eclampsia or gestational diabetes which may alter timing of delivery is also assessed at this point.

For cases with multiple abnormalities in addition to a fetal cardiac condition, continued surveillance will be undertaken by the fetal medicine team, as there is a higher risk for both fetal and obstetric complications in this patient group.

Midwifery Care

Highly skilled midwifery care is an essential component of care for the expectant mother and fetus with a cardiac abnormality. There is significant anxiety and stress associated with this diagnosis, notwithstanding some of the practical issues related to being transferred to a tertiary hospital for delivery. The antenatal booking should allow sufficient time to cover all administrative and supportive needs. At our centre, this booking visit includes full history, relevant blood tests, liaison midwifery contacts and a plan for labour and delivery is agreed taking account of the individual circumstance. This is complemented by the offer of

- specific antenatal classes for parents expecting a child with CHD. Prospective parents can be given a tour of the hospital birth centre and newborn care unit including intensive care.
- For referrals with a complex social history, appropriate contact is made with local services, including social and mental health services.
- Where there is concomitant maternal medical comorbidity (e.g. diabetes, rheumatology, adult congenital heart), appropriate specialty medical teams are also involved and kept informed at each stage of pregnancy.

Communication

By necessity, comprehensive management following the fetal diagnosis of a cardiac abnormality involves multiple specialist teams, hence timely, careful communication is critical. It is essential that communications are punctual and comprehensive, both within the tertiary unit and with local services. In our practice, all reports are copied to the mother who holds a comprehensive hand-held record. The use of standardised reports is encouraged to facilitate transmission of key

Table 17.1 Cardiac lesion and recommended level of care for delivery

	Recommended delivery in tertiary unit with paediatric cardiology services	For discussion at MDT[a] at 30 weeks' gestation and consideration of delivery at tertiary unit	May deliver locally
Structural	1. Duct dependent or potentially duct dependent systemic circulation (a) Hypoplastic left heart (b) Critical aortic stenosis (c) Severe coarctation of the aorta (Very high suspicion of coarctation of the aorta) 2. Duct dependent or potentially duct-dependent pulmonary circulation (a) Pulmonary atresia with intact ventricular septum (b) Critical pulmonary stenosis (c) Pulmonary atresia with ventricular septal defect ± collaterals (d) Severe tetralogy of Fallot (hypoplastic pulmonary arteries ± retrograde pulmonary artery flow 3. Transposition of the great arteries ± other associated lesions 4. Total anomalous pulmonary venous drainage 5. Severe Ebstein's anomaly (increased Cardio-Thoracic Ratio ± reversed flow in duct ± hypoplastic Pulmonary arteries ± hydrops) 6. Complex anatomy with potential pulmonary or systemic blood flow obstruction e.g. isomerism, double inlet ventricle, discordant atrioventricular connection 7. Cardiorespiratory interaction—respiratory compromise highly likely. e.g. Absent pulmonary valve syndrome	1. Coarctation of the aorta – "Medium suspicion" e.g. hypoplastic aortic arch, antegrade flow 2. Tetralogy of Fallot with some/moderate Right Ventricular outflow tract obstruction 3. Mild/Moderate aortic valve stenosis 4. Mild/moderate pulmonary valve stenosis 5. Mild Ebstein's: heart not enlarged, antegrade PA flow	1. Lesions with postnatal left to right shunt physiology (a) Isolated Ventricular septal defect (b) Atrioventricular septal defect without associated cardiac lesions 2. Coarctation of the aorta with LOW suspicion/cannot exclude (may still need postnatal echo) 3. Tetralogy of Fallot with no/minimal pulmonary obstruction (good sized Pulmonary arteries, antegrade duct flow) 4. Family history of cardiomyopathy with no abnormal fetal echocardiographic findings
Arrhythmia	1. Uncontrolled fetal tachycardia 2. Uncontrolled fetal bradycardia		1. Tachycardias which have been effectively treated prenatally 2. Irregular fetal heart rhythms due to atrial/ventricular ectopic beats
Functional	1. Cardiomyopathy—with significant impairment of cardiac function		

[a]MDT multidisciplinary meeting with Fetal medicine/Obstetrics/Midwifery/Neonatal/Fetal cardiology/Genetics input present

information to health professionals involved in the care of the woman.

A system should also be in place to allow clear communication with the local fetal medicine unit, the local paediatric team and the local midwifery team who will continue to support the woman through her pregnancy.

Within our centre, a unifying patient list is available to the whole multi-disciplinary team involved in the care of the mother and baby. This means that the details of all deliveries being planned is available to clinical teams who may be planning surgical and intensive care activity. The anticipated intensity of care required postnatally is outlined to facilitate activity planning and planned delivery scheduling. Our current practice is to discuss cases imminently due for delivery at our cardiac surgical conference the week prior to delivery so that staff are familiar with cases.

Antenatal Education Day

We have found antenatal education days to be helpful for expectant parents. They have the option to attend group antenatal study days, where an opportunity exists to meet with other parents facing the same challenges of caring for a child with a congenital heart abnormality as well as meeting the involved clinical teams. Practical issues such as transport to the centre, accommodation after delivery, are discussed. Other facets of care can be discussed including normal labour physiology, pain relief options, induction of labour (where indicated), specific intrapartum care considerations and expectations for immediate management of their baby by neonatologists.

Timing of Delivery

The timing of delivery for those that progressed normally during the pregnancy is balanced between maximising gestational age and reducing possible fetal mortality and morbidity. One US cohort of several hundred infants born with CHD demonstrated that for every week increase in gestational age and 100 g increase in birth weight, length of stay decreased by 12.3 ± 2.7% ($p < 0.001$) and 3.9 ± 0.9% ($p < 0.001$) (Peyvandi et al. 2017).

- For women who live distant from the planned site of delivery (>1 h), and have a fetus with a significant cardiac abnormality who will require immediate attention, we advocate delivery by 39 weeks' gestation.
- For mothers who live locally we advocate allowing spontaneous onset of labour unless there is an alternative indication for delivery.
  - For local patients with no indication for early delivery, antenatal care can continue normally and women only see the specialist (cardiac) midwifery/obstetric team at around 39–40 weeks. A fetus with a major anomaly has a higher risk for stillbirth and therefore delivery is planned by 41 weeks' gestation for all of these pregnancies.

Mode of Delivery

Vaginal delivery rates are approximately 50–60% in our series and women should be encouraged to deliver vaginally (Jowett et al. 2014). Benefits include:

- improved respiratory adaptation for the fetus by being exposed to maternal labour
- a faster recovery for the mother, which is critical to assist her in mobilising and visiting her baby in the NICU/PICU, and
- reduced complexity with subsequent pregnancies.

Elective Caesarean section is arranged for predominantly obstetric indications only. The exceptions include fetal arrhythmias in which intrapartum fetal monitoring cannot be performed, as well as selected high risk cases identified by fetal cardiology as needing emergency cardiac intervention; such as HLHS with a restrictive atrial septum. Fortunately, these cases are rare. Emergency Caesarean section is more likely to occur in fetuses with heart failure, low birth weight, and primiparous mothers (Miyoshi et al. 2017).

Location of Delivery

Careful consideration must be paid during antenatal consultations to location of delivery. Factors to consider include: cardiac lesion, local services, distance from tertiary unit, local expertise, and parental preferences. Table 17.1 provides suggested guidelines on when delivery may occur locally versus delivery in the tertiary referral unit. The most important factor that determines place of delivery (i.e. local hospital versus tertiary unit) is timing for first cardiac surgical intervention. Certain conditions require early cardiac intervention (TGA, HLHS), whereas others may not require early intervention. Even if delivery is planned at the tertiary centre, close liaison with local neonatologists, obstetricians and paediatricians is essential in case of unplanned local delivery. For those planning to deliver locally, a clear neonatal management plan should be agreed with the local neonatal/paediatric team.

Complex Cases Associated with Fetal Growth Restriction, Maternal Pre-eclampsia or Preterm Labour

Cases that require early delivery for non-cardiac indications, should have multi-disciplinary team input to plan optimal delivery. Complex fetal cardiac conditions delivered <36 weeks' gestation and with low birth weight tend to have a poorer outcome with mortality of approximately 70% (Andrews et al. 2006). Moreover if there are multiple fetal abnormalities in addition to a fetal cardiac abnormality, prognosis is very guarded if the fetus delivers preterm.

Antenatal Steroids

Antenatal corticosteroids are advised <35 weeks' gestation to avoid respiratory distress syndrome after birth. Practice will vary by institution and region but we offer antenatal steroids up to 34 + 6 weeks' gestation according to Royal College of Obstetricians and Gynaecologists guidelines (NICE 2015). In some cases with a high risk for cardiorespiratory dysfunction, including those with severe structural CHD, antenatal corticosteroid administration may be extended up to 38 + 0 weeks' gestation. This is decided on an individual basis.

Fetal Growth Restriction and Pre-eclampsia

It has been shown that babies born with congenital heart disease are smaller when compared to controls; 25% of such neonates are small for gestational age (SGA) (Story et al. 2015). However, it does appear that the prognosis in these cases with less severe growth restriction but deliver near term, is dependent more on the type of CHD rather than whether growth restriction is present or not. For example, babies with HLHS are usually around the 50th centile but have high mortality due to the lesion itself. Coarctation of the aorta is associated with an increased incidence of growth restriction but short term outcome no different between SGA and non-SGA foetuses (Story et al. 2015).

Women carrying a fetus with congenital heart disease have also been shown to have a higher incidence of pre-eclampsia compared with pregnant controls (5.7% vs. 1.2%) (Ruiz et al. 2016). As a result regular monitoring for this complication is advocated.

Intrapartum Care

Care in labour occurs in the hospital birth centre and where possible a member of the specialist midwifery team who has met the woman antenatally provides one-to-one care in labour with specialist medical oversight. Normal labour monitoring and electronic fetal monitoring are advocated although mobilisation in labour is acceptable. Maternal pain relief by routine methods as required.

Postnatal Care

Where possible, for babies on the NICU, postnatal accommodation for the parents should be as close as possible to the NICU to allow optimal access to the newborn. Postnatally, the mother should be reviewed regularly by the specialist midwifery/obstetric team and discharge planning and ongoing routine postnatal review planned before handover to local teams.

Compassionate Care and Bereavement

For the majority of fetuses with CHD, the emphasis will be on planning surgery and other interventions after birth. However, in a minority of cases either the CHD and/or associated abnormalities may be so severe that the option of non-intervention after birth is discussed with parents. These cases with a high risk for fetal and neonatal death and/or significant morbidity may not be operable or indeed survive long enough for paediatric cardiac surgery. In this situation, careful consultation with all relevant subspecialties, including palliative care, is vital so that a postnatal management plan taking account of all relevant information can be agreed between subspecialists and the parents. The fetal medicine team has a key role in this, not only with respect to care of the baby after birth but agreeing an appropriate birth plan with the parents including bereavement support.

If intra-uterine or neonatal death occurs, postmortem examination may be considered and discussed with parents. Specialist perinatal pathology is recommended.

Local pathways for notification and review of all neonatal and infant deaths should be followed. Bereavement follow-up in such cases would normally be with the paediatric cardiology or neonatal teams unless there were specific obstetric or fetal medicine concerns additional to the fetal cardiac abnormality. In-utero death should be followed up by either the fetal medicine team or the local obstetric team depending on the circumstances and timing of fetal loss.

Future Pregnancies

The risk of recurrence is important information for parents who have had an infant with congenital heart disease. The genetics of CHD, including recurrence risks are discussed in Chap. 14. Parents need to be given an estimate of the recurrence risk tailored to their particular situation, involving clinical geneticists where necessary. In future pregnancies, detailed fetal echocardiography should be offered. The exact timing will vary by institution. At our own centre, early fetal echocardiography is offered at 13–14 weeks' gestational age where a previous pregnancy has been affected by significant CHD. Such early scans are repeated in the midtrimester at around 19–21 weeks' gestational age, even if the early scan is reported as normal.

If there were other fetal anomalies in the index pregnancy, a detailed fetal medicine review, ultrasound and discussion is recommended either around the time of the 1st trimester scan, or 16–20 weeks' gestation.

Challenges

Key challenges for tertiary referral units include accurate diagnosis, triage of antenatal care between local and tertiary hospitals, rapid access, coordination of appointments for patients particularly when living long distances away, planning for optimal site and mode of delivery, and providing support for parents. Clear communication both locally and at the tertiary unit is essential.

Conclusion

Caring for pregnant women affected by congenital heart disease is challenging but rewarding and requires clear pathways, good multi-disciplinary team work and frequent clear communication to optimise care and outcomes.

References

Andrews RE, Simpson JM, Sharland GK, Sullivan ID, Yates RW. Outcome after preterm delivery of infants antenatally diagnosed with congenital heart disease. J Pediatr. 2006;148(2):213–6.

Bratt EL, Jarvholm S, Ekman-Joelsson BM, Mattson LA, Mellander M. Parent's experiences of counselling and their need for support following a prenatal diagnosis of congenital heart disease—a qualitative study in a Swedish context. BMC Pregnancy Childbirth. 2015;15:171.

Jowett VC, Sankaran S, Rollings SL, Hall R, Kyle PM, Sharland GK. Foetal congenital heart disease: obstetric management and time to first cardiac intervention in babies delivered at a tertiary centre. Cardiol Young. 2014;24(3):494–502.

Miyoshi T, Katsuragi S, Neki R, Kurosaki KI, Shiraishi I, Nakai M, Nishimura K, Yoshimatsu J, Ikeda T. Cardiovascular profile score as a predictor of acute intrapartum non-reassuring fetal status in infants with congenital heart defects. J Matern Fetal Neonatal Med. 2017;30(23):2831–7. https://doi.org/10.1080/14767058.2016.1265930.

National Institute for Clinical Excellence (NICE). 2015. https://www.nice.org.uk/guidance/ng25/evidence/fullguideline-pdf-2176838029

Peyvandi S, Nguyen TA, Almeida-Jones M, Boe N, Rhee L, Anton T, Sklansky M, Tarsa M, Satou G, Moon-Grady AJ, et al. Timing and mode of delivery in prenatally diagnosed congenital heart disease—an analysis of practices within the University of California Fetal Consortium (UCfC). Pediatr Cardiol. 2017;38(3):588–95.

Ruiz A, Ferrer Q, Sanchez O, Ribera I, Arevalo S, Alomar O, Mendoza M, Cabero L, Carrerras E, Llurba E. Placenta-related complications in women carrying a foetus with congenital heart disease. J Matern Fetal Neonatal Med. 2016;29(20):3271–5.

Story L, Pasupathy D, Sankaran S, Sharland G, Kyle P. Influence of birthweight on perinatal outcome in fetuses with antenatal diagnosis of congenital heart disease. J Obstet Gynaecol Res. 2015;41(6):896–903.

Post-Natal Cardiac Management of the Fetus with Congenital Heart Disease

18

Marietta Charakida and Owen I. Miller

Abstract

Prenatal detection of congenital heart disease (CHD) has improved over the past decade. Antenatal diagnosis of CHD allows parental counselling regarding fetal intervention, post-natal surgical options, more intensive pregnancy surveillance, delivery planning and immediate post-natal management. Accurate risk stratification can be performed for fetuses with CHD aiming to reduce perinatal and postnatal morbidity and mortality. For the baby with CHD who is likely to need cardiac intervention in the neonatal period, multidisciplinary coordination involving fetal medicine specialists, obstetricians, neonatologists and fetal/paediatric cardiologists is facilitated. In this chapter, the risk stratification for delivery of fetuses with CHD and the long-term considerations about postnatal cardiac management of CHD are discussed.

Electronic Supplementary Material The online version of this chapter (https://doi.org/10.1007/978-3-319-77461-9_18) contains supplementary material, which is available to authorized users.

M. Charakida · O. I. Miller (✉)
Evelina London Children's Hospital, Guy's and St Thomas' NHS Foundation Trust, London, UK
e-mail: owen.miller@gstt.nhs.uk

Keywords

Postnatal management · Risk stratification · Congenital heart disease · Fontan · Transposition

Introduction

Over the last years, there have been significant advances in fetal cardiac imaging and this has led to an increased number of newborns diagnosed prenatally with congenital heart disease (CHD) (Donofrio et al. 2014). Accurate fetal diagnosis allows assessment of disease severity, monitoring of progression, prediction of clinical course and provides an opportunity for comprehensive prenatal counselling and family support. Individualised planning for specialised delivery in selected cases has the goal of improved fetal and postnatal outcomes. Pre-natal risk assessment (Table 18.1) and clinical experience allows fetal CHD to be divided into three major risk categories (Donofrio et al. 2013; Sanapo et al. 2016):

1. **Critical** CHD lesions, where postnatal instability and urgent cardiac intervention is anticipated
2. **Severe** CHD lesions, where postnatal instability is possible and cardiac intervention in the neonatal period is anticipated
3. **Non-urgent CHD lesions**, where postnatal stability is anticipated and no change in the delivery plan is needed.

© Springer International Publishing AG, part of Springer Nature 2018

J. Simpson et al. (eds.), *Fetal Cardiology*, https://doi.org/10.1007/978-3-319-77461-9_18

Table 18.1 Risk stratification for delivery of fetuses with CHD

Risk	Definition	Example congenital	MDT needed	Delivery plan
Critical	Instability expected at delivery Immediate cardiac intervention soon after birth	HLHS with IAS TGA with IAS Obstructed TAPVD	Yes	• Planned delivery in perinatal cardiac centre (planned induction) • Cardiology on site
Severe	Stability expected at delivery Cardiac intervention planned in neonatal period	Severe outflow tract obstruction with duct dependence Severe Ebstein's anomaly CHD with intracardiac mixing Sustained tachyarrhythmia Complete heart block	Yes	• Consider planned delivery in perinatal cardiac centre • Early cardiology assessment ± intervention available
Non-urgent	Stability expected during first weeks of life	Isolated septal defects VSD, AVSD Benign arrhythmias Other CHD i.e. ToF with mild/moderate PS	No	• Routine delivery plan • Elective cardiology assessment in neonatal period

Abbreviations: *CHD* congenital heart disease, *MDT* multi-disciplinary team, *HLHS* hypoplastic left heart, *IAS* intact atrial septum, *TGA* transposition of great arteries, *TAPVD* total anomalous pulmonary venous drainage, *VSD* ventricular septal defect, *AVSD* atrioventricular septal defect, *ToF* tetralogy of Fallot, *PS* pulmonary stenosis

Critical CHD Lesions

Some CHD lesions will predictably need immediate post-natal cardiac intervention:

Table 18.2 Predictors of atrial septal restriction in HLHS

Fetal predictors of a severely restrictive atrial septum in HLHS
• Atrial Septum—thick or not freely mobile • Interatrial communication—small or absent • Abnormal pulmonary venous Doppler—forward/reversed VTI ratio ≤ 3

Hypoplastic Left Heart with Intact Atrial Septum

Hypoplastic left heart syndrome (HLHS) is characterized by underdevelopment of the left ventricle associated with stenosis or atresia of the mitral and/or aortic valve, thus pulmonary venous blood must cross the interatrial septum to the right atrium. The presence of a relatively unrestricted communication at the atrial level is necessary for oxygenated blood to be delivered to the body and to prevent pulmonary venous congestion. It has been estimated that 6% of patients with HLHS will have an intact atrial septum and up to 22% have some degree of restriction of left to right flow (see Table 18.2) through the atrial septal defect (Video 18.1, Fig. 18.1). Significant restriction at the atrial level in these patients results in haemodynamic instability postnatally with severe cyanosis, acidosis and pulmonary venous congestion. Therefore, an urgent intervention to create or enlarge the atrial communication is needed. In some patients with HLHS, a levoatrial cardinal vein or other channel between left atrial and systemic circulation may provide left atrial decompression but such a communication is rarely sufficient.

Management

Prenatal diagnosis of a restrictive atrial septum in HLHS allows consideration of prenatal fetal cardiac intervention (available in selected centres) or for a planned delivery in a perinatal cardiac centre with immediate postnatal intervention (Sathanandam et al. 2016). In some centres, delivery is performed by planned Caesarean section at term with either an immediate catheter intervention (balloon atrial septostomy ± stenting of atrial septum) or immediate surgical atrial septectomy. The interventional strategy will be determined by the clinical status of the

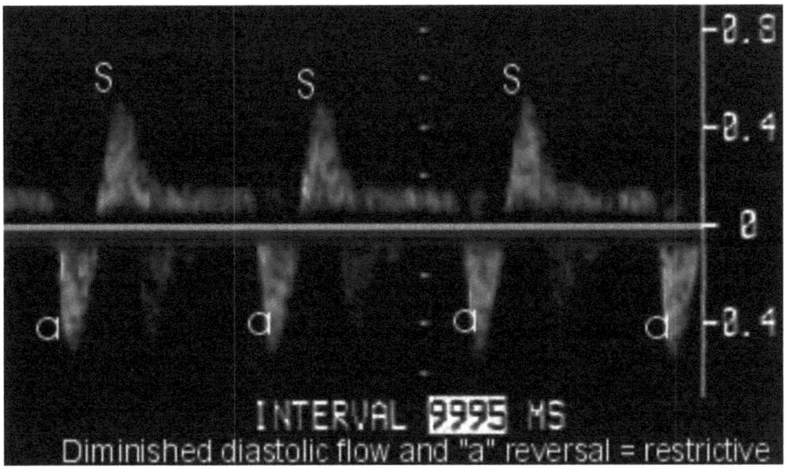

Fig. 18.1 Pulmonary venous Doppler in a fetal case of hypoplastic left heart. The diminished diastolic flow and significant A wave reversal in the pulmonary venous Doppler is indicative of restriction at the atrial level

neonate and the available expertise in the tertiary centre. Surgical atrial septectomy requires cardiopulmonary bypass, which may add an additional risk to a critically ill neonate.

Outcome

The outcomes among patients with HLHS and a restrictive or intact atrial septum remain poor despite aggressive early management strategies. These neonates may already have established pulmonary vascular abnormalities and/or pulmonary lymphangiectasia, associated with intrauterine left atrial hypertension. This may preclude the possibility of single ventricle repair. These patients remain at increased risk even after surgical palliation and/or orthotopic heart transplantation.

Transposition of Great Arteries with Intact Atrial Septum

Prenatal detection of transposition of great arteries (TGA) is well established and most neonates with TGA will have an uncomplicated preoperative course. A prostaglandin E infusion is routinely commenced soon after birth to maintain patency of the arterial duct, and thus haemodynamic stability while an initial cardiac assessment is made.

In fetal life, there is normally preferential streaming of more oxygenated blood across the foramen to the left ventricle. In the fetus with TGA the systemic venous blood is directed into the pulmonary artery rather than the aorta. Thus, in the fetus with TGA, the aortic blood perfusing the brain will have a lower oxygen saturation compared to normal. The impact of this on neurodevelopment is the subject of ongoing research.

After birth, the systemic and pulmonary circulations in TGA function in parallel and therefore mixing of oxygenated and deoxygenated blood at the level of the atrial septum and the arterial duct is essential for adequate oxygen delivery to vital tissues. The most important mixing is at the atrial level and in up to 25% of neonates the atrial septal communication can become small and "restrictive". In about 5% of cases, a combination of a constricted arterial duct and a severely restrictive foramen will lead to severe hypoxia, acidosis and sometimes death in the first hours after birth if an urgent balloon atrial septostomy is not performed. This procedure involves passing a balloon catheter via the systemic veins or umbilical vein through the right atrium to the left atrium. The balloon is inflated in the left atrium and then pulled sharply back across the atrial septum to increase the size of the communication (foramen ovale) between the atriums (Videos 18.2a and 18.2b).

Prediction of which fetuses with TGA will develop severe restriction of the foramen ovale is difficult during fetal life. Specific echocardiographic features have been proposed (Vigneswaran et al. 2017) but there is no consensus in the literature as to which are the best markers (see Table 18.3).

Table 18.3 Fetal Predictors of inadequate circulatory mixing in fetus with Transposition of the Great Arteries

At atrial level
• Hypermobile atrial septum (primum septum oscillates between the left and right atrium)
• Redundant atrial septum (primum septum herniates more than 50% beyond the plane of the septum secundum across the length of the left atrium
• Restrictive atrial septum: A small orifice with colour flow aliasing across the atrial septum
• Fixed atrial septum: The angle between the primum and secundum septums is < 30°
• Flat atrial septum: No mobility of the atrial septum
• Foramen ovale/total atrial septal length < 0.5
At ductal level (ductal restriction)
• Small size of the ductus arteriosus as measured against reference standards for gestational age (z score)
• Left to right diastolic shunt at arterial duct

Management

Delivery of the fetus with TGA is recommended in a tertiary perinatal cardiac centre where immediate commencement of a prostaglandin infusion to maintain ductal patency and urgent postnatal cardiac review can occur. For fetuses with high suspicion of a restrictive foramen ovale, a cardiac interventionist should be available for emergency balloon atrial septostomy.

Outcome

The prenatal diagnosis of TGA has aided the perinatal management and delivery planning of these infants, lowering preoperative morbidity and mortality and preventing delivery room compromise. Early and late results of the Arterial Switch Operation have dramatically improved in the past 20 years (Tobler et al. 2010).

Obstructed Total Anomalous Pulmonary Venous Connection

Total anomalous pulmonary venous connection (TAPVC) is another critical CHD lesion. In this condition, the pulmonary veins connect directly to the systemic venous circulation and do not return to the left atrium (see Chap. 10). Obstructed TAPVC occurs most commonly when the pulmonary veins drain below the diaphragm into the liver and subsequently to inferior vena cava. Pulmonary venous drainage is impaired leading to pulmonary venous congestion and severe hypoxemia in the neonate.

Management

Prenatal diagnosis of isolated TAPVC is difficult, but recognition allows planned delivery in a perinatal cardiac centre. Obstructed TAPVC is a surgical emergency. Immediate newborn intensive care support is essential to stabilise the neonate, optimise the ventilation and support the circulation. Urgent corrective cardiac surgery is indicated to reconnect the pulmonary venous return to the left atrium.

Outcome

Surgical correction of TAPVC can be achieved with low mortality and good long-term outcome. However, if complicated by pulmonary vein stenosis either at presentation or secondary to the repair, the long-term outcome is guarded.

Severe CHD Lesions

This group of congenital heart defects will involve

Duct Dependent Lesions (see Table 18.4)

- Duct dependent systemic circulation (left sided obstructed lesions)
- Duct dependent pulmonary circulation (right sided obstructed lesions and its variants)
- Poor mixing lesions (transposition physiology)

Other Lesions

- Right to left shunt with intracardiac mixing lesions (i.e. common arterial trunk)
- Sustained tachyarrhythmias
- Complete heart block

Duct Dependent Systemic Circulation

This group of cardiac abnormalities includes severe aortic valve stenosis, aortic coarctation, interrupted aortic arch and hypoplastic left heart syndrome. Systemic perfusion relies on patency of the arterial duct with flow predominantly right to left from pulmonary artery to descending aorta.

Management

Delivery should be planned in a tertiary perinatal centre with specialised cardiac facilities on site or in a tertiary neonatal centre with a plan for early transfer to a specialised cardiac centre. Initiation of a prostaglandin infusion may avoid neonatal collapse by maintaining patency of the arterial duct. Early cardiology review is essential to coordinate further management.

Outcome

Medium and long-term outcome in this group of congenital heart defects will depend on the underlying anatomy (see below).

Critical Aortic Stenosis

In critical aortic valve stenosis, balloon aortic valvuloplasty or surgical valvotomy can be performed in the first days after birth but only if the size of the mitral valve (MV) and left ventricle (LV) is judged to be adequate to sustain the systemic circulation. If the MV or LV are inadequate then management is similar to hypoplastic left heart syndrome.

Medium term concerns include aortic regurgitation and recurrent aortic valve stenosis with the need for repeat interventions (Brown et al. 2010). Life-long follow up is required for all patients who have undergone such neonatal intervention.

In the longer term, the aortic valve may need to be replaced with a prosthetic valve, which will require anticoagulation. Prosthetic valves are unsuitable for very young patients, as even the smallest available prosthetic valves may be too large and the risks of anticoagulation are higher. In this situation, the patient's own pulmonary valve may be moved to the aortic position and a donor pulmonary valve inserted into the pulmonary position. This is known as a Ross operation.

Coarctation of the Aorta

In cases where there is aortic coarctation, early surgery, either with end-to-end anastomosis via a lateral thoracotomy or extended arch repair via a median sternotomy will be needed. The type of operation will be determined by the degree of hypoplasia of the aortic arch and the presence of other associated lesions.

Table 18.4 Duct dependent congenital heart defects

Duct dependent lesions	CHD lesions	Pathophysiology
Duct dependent systemic circulation	• Severe aortic valve stenosis • Aortic coarctation • Interrupted aortic arch • Hypoplastic left heart syndrome	Duct dependent systemic circulation, hence need to maintain ductal patency with postnatal prostaglandin administration
Duct dependent pulmonary circulation	• Critical/severe PS/PA • Tetralogy of Fallot with severe PS • Tricuspid atresia with PS/PA • Univentricular heart with PA/PS • Functional pulmonary atresia in severe Ebstein's anomaly	Duct dependent pulmonary circulation, hence need to maintain ductal patency with postnatal prostaglandin administration
Poor mixing lesions	• Transposition of great arteries	Patency of arterial duct with prostaglandin is employed to achieve adequate mixing of blood and adequate oxygenation

Abbreviations: *PS* pulmonary stenosis, *PA* pulmonary atresia

Patients with aortic coarctation have 90% survival at 60 years. Long-term concerns involve the risk of recoarctation of the aorta, aortic root dilatation, aortic aneurysm formation and systemic hypertension. In recent years, surgeons have tended to perform more extensive repairs of the aortic arch than previously, to reduce the risk of recoarctation.

All patients with repaired coarctation require life-long follow up to check for the associated complications listed above. The development of hypertension is multifactorial and is the most important contributor to increased cardiovascular risk after aortic coarctation repair (Choudhary et al. 2015). Aggressive control of blood pressure is therefore essential and the incidence of hypertension is lower in patients operated in the early neonatal period compared to those undergoing later surgery.

Hypoplastic Left Heart Syndrome

Hypoplastic left heart syndrome is discussed in detail in Chap. 7, it represents the most severe form of left heart obstruction and requires extensive multistage surgery to eventually achieve a single ventricle palliation (see below).

Duct Dependent Pulmonary Circulation

Right Heart Obstruction

This group includes abnormalities such as severe pulmonary valve stenosis, tetralogy of Fallot with severe pulmonary stenosis or atresia, or severe Ebstein's anomaly of tricuspid valve or tricuspid dysplasia and functional pulmonary atresia. In obstructive right heart lesions, there is reduced forward flow into the main pulmonary artery and lung perfusion and hence neonatal oxygenation relies on patency of the arterial duct with flow predominantly left to right from the aorta to the pulmonary artery.

Management

Delivery should be planned to occur in a tertiary perinatal centre with specialised cardiac facilities or in a tertiary neonatal centre with a plan for early transfer to a cardiac centre. Following delivery, prostaglandin infusion is indicated to maintain ductal patency.

Depending on the underlying anatomy and the clinical status of the neonate, an interventional or surgical approach will be planned. For neonates with critical pulmonary stenosis/pulmonary atresia with an adequate tricuspid valve and right ventricle, radiofrequency perforation of the atretic pulmonary valve or balloon dilation of the right ventricular outflow tract and/or stenosed pulmonary valve can be performed. Alternatively, a surgical systemic to pulmonary artery shunt (i.e. modified Blalock-Taussig shunt) might be undertaken. Catheter intervention with stenting of the arterial duct or stenting of the right ventricular outflow tract can also be performed to ensure adequate pulmonary blood flow and to support the growth of anatomically small pulmonary arteries, thus providing a better substrate for subsequent surgical repair. The choice of approach is dictated by the individual anatomy and institutional preference.

In cases of severe Ebstein's anomaly of the tricuspid valve (Fig. 18.2, Video 18.3) or severe tricuspid dysplasia with functional pulmonary atresia, pulmonary vasodilators such as oxygen and inhaled nitric oxide can be administered to reduce pulmonary vascular resistance and promote forward flow to the pulmonary arteries. If adequate oxygenation cannot be achieved, then opening of the arterial duct or a systemic to pulmonary artery may become necessary.

Outcome

Short term neonatal outcome will depend on establishing a reliable source of pulmonary blood flow; initially by maintaining patency of the arterial duct and then by establishing either forward flow e.g. outflow tract balloon or stent or by placing a systemic to pulmonary artery synthetic shunt.

Medium and long-term outcome will depend on the underlying anatomy. In the most severe cases with severe hypoplasia of the right ventricle, a single ventricle (Fontan) palliation (see below) may be required.

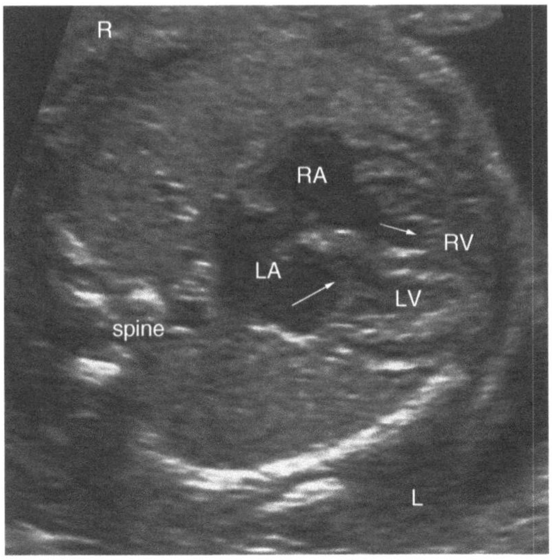

Fig. 18.2 This is a transverse view at the level of four chamber which demonstrates the apical displacement of the tricuspid valve in comparison to the mitral valve. This appearance is typical of Ebstein's anomaly

For less severe RV hypoplasia, the results of catheter or surgical intervention for pulmonary atresia or critical pulmonary valve stenosis are good although later re-intervention may be required. Pulmonary regurgitation and residual or recurrent pulmonary valve stenosis are the main concerns. Long-term follow up is indicated with careful attention to pulmonary valve and right ventricular haemodynamics (Voet et al. 2012; Roos-Hesselink et al. 2006).

The long-term outcome of Ebstein's anomaly is variable. Symptomatic neonates with Ebstein's anomaly who require no intervention have good long-term survival (Shinkawa et al. 2010). However, the worst affected infants can present with massive cardiac enlargement, compression, associated lung hypoplasia and severe hypoxaemia. Surgical repair of the tricuspid valve is usually reserved for patients beyond infancy and more typically of school age. For patients needing intervention on the tricuspid valve, overall survival is lower. A high incidence of arrhythmias is one of the main long-term concerns in patients with Ebstein's anomaly. Regular functional testing is helpful as symptoms are difficult to assess.

Transposition of the Great Arteries

Transposition of the great arteries, is a term usually used to describe discordant ventricular-arterial connections, where the left ventricle gives rise to the pulmonary artery and the right ventricle gives rise to the aorta. Mixing of oxygenated and deoxygenated blood occurs at different levels i.e. atrial level, arterial duct and at ventricular level if a ventricular septal defect is present.

Management

Delivery can be planned in a tertiary perinatal centre with specialised cardiac facilities or in a tertiary neonatal centre with a plan for early transfer to a cardiac centre. A prostaglandin infusion should be commenced to maintain patency of the arterial duct. Cardiology review with detailed echocardiography will be needed to assess the site(s) and adequacy of intracardiac mixing. Balloon atrial septostomy in the first days of life might be needed to improve intracardiac mixing until the primary surgical repair is undertaken. In the current era, the arterial switch operation (ASO) is the preferred surgical approach for suitable anatomy and is usually undertaken within the first 1–3 weeks of life. Coronary arteries anatomy is highly variable in this condition and their aortic origins and epicardial course will need to be clarified by echocardiography after birth. Some coronary variations such as when the coronary passes through the myocardium or through the wall of great vessels "intramural course" make the arterial switch operation more difficult and increase the risk of the surgery. If a ventricular septal defect is present, then this is usually closed at the same time as the arterial switch operation.

Outcome

Early surgical mortality is low and medium term morbidity includes branch pulmonary artery stenosis and neo-aortic root dilatation. Late complications may include coronary stenosis following the coronary artery transfer at the original neonatal ASO. The long-term results from the ASO are excellent with long-term survival reaching 96% at 25 years (Tobler et al. 2010).

Complex Transposition

The term "transposition of the great arteries" is also used to describe various other malpositions of the aorta or pulmonary artery. Although used commonly to describe non-standard great artery arrangements, we advise describing the actual morphology based on ventricle of origin and position of the great arteries. This caters for complex morphologies where one of the other great artery may be stenosed or actually atretic. It also caters for double outlet arrangements (see Chap. 8).

In more complex forms of transposition, particularly when there are other associated cardiac abnormalities i.e. pulmonary stenosis, the ASO may not be possible and other surgical approaches i.e. Rastelli (Fig. 18.3) repair may be required.

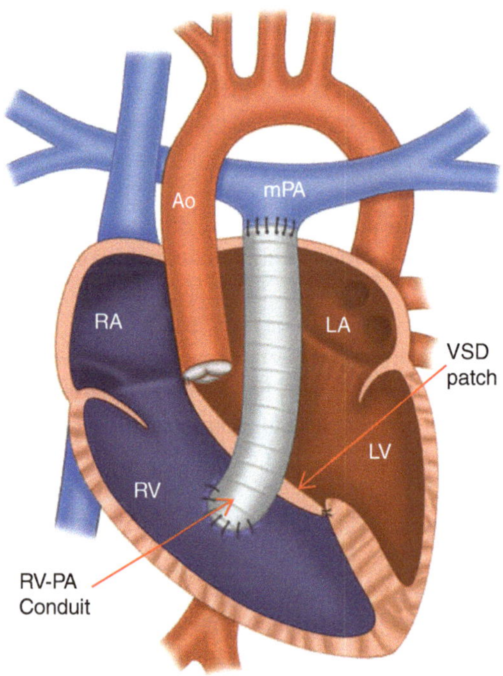

Fig. 18.3 In the Rastelli operation the pulmonary artery is divided from the left ventricle. The left ventricle is tunnelled to the aorta and the ventricular septal defect is closed with a patch. A valved conduit or a homograft is used to connect the right ventricle to the pulmonary artery

The prognosis is less favorable in the context of other associated cardiac abnormalities. Some forms of complex transposition are not suitable for corrective surgery and may need to follow a single ventricle (Fontan) palliative surgical pathway (see below).

Other Lesions

Common Arterial Trunk

Common Arterial Trunk (CAT) is characterised by the presence of a single outlet arising from the heart, which gives rise to the aorta, pulmonary and coronary arteries (see Chap. 8). The truncal valve may be thickened and dysplastic and usually overrides a large ventricular septal defect. This condition is often associated with genetic abnormalities, most commonly 22q11 deletion (Allan et al. 2000).

Management

For fetuses with CAT plus truncal valve insufficiency or other cardiac associated lesions, delivery in a tertiary perinatal cardiac centre is advised. In the presence of aortic arch interruption or obstruction, maintaining patency of arterial duct with a prostaglandin infusion is needed to ensure adequate perfusion of the lower body. For a fetus with otherwise uncomplicated CAT, delivery in a cardiac centre is not mandatory but early cardiology review is advised.

The postnatal course of neonates with CAT will depend on the presence of other associated lesions i.e. aortic arch abnormalities and the degree of abnormality of the truncal valve. In the absence of any other major cardiac abnormalities, these babies will develop symptoms of heart failure as the pulmonary vascular resistance falls. In some cases when there is significant truncal valve insufficiency and coronary steal, signs of heart failure may develop shortly after birth. One stage repair early in the neonatal period is preferred to minimise the development of pulmonary vascular obstructive disease, which may preclude repair later in life. The repair consists of closure of the ventricular septal defect and restoration of a connection between the right ventricle and pulmonary arteries. In selected cases, repair of the truncal valve is undertaken if this is stenotic or regurgitant. There is variation as to the preferred surgical technique.

Outcome

Following primary neonatal repair, the RV-PA conduit will ultimately stenose and need replacing during later childhood. This may involve surgical replacement or catheter intervention with balloon dilatation or stent implantation. Although the surgical outcomes have improved with long term survival up to 83% at 15 years in uncomplicated patients with CAT, there is significant comorbidity during childhood with significant burden of operative and catheter based intervention and deficits in exercise performance and quality of life.

In the presence of other associated lesions such as interrupted aortic arch or when there is moderate to severe truncal valve insufficiency the prognosis is worse than in simple CAT.

Rhythm Abnormalities

Fetal rhythm abnormalities that will require cardiac review in early neonatal period involve fetal tachyarrhythmias or complete heart block (Strasburger et al. 2007). These are discussed in greater detail in Chap. 11.

Fetal Tachyarrhythmia

The most common type of an abnormality is supraventricular tachycardia (Simpson 2006). In cases of fetal tachycardia with late presentation (near term), delivery of the fetus may be advocated to allow direct administration of antiarrhythmic therapy to the neonate. As there is a risk of recurrence of tachycardia after birth, early neonatal cardiology review is advocated.

Management

In most cases, we advise initiation of antiarrhythmic therapy in the neonatal period, however some centres only initiate therapy if a postnatal tachycardia is demonstrated.

Outcome

Overall the outcome for fetal and neonatal tachyarrhythmias is favorable with complete resolution in most cases by the end of the first year of life. Late recurrence of some arrhythmias is, however, recognised.

Complete Heart Block

Complete heart block manifests as complete interruption of the electrical communication between the atriums and ventricles. It is an uncommon arrhythmia and most cases are congenital and can be detected antenatally. Congenital complete heart block can occur as an isolated anomaly and can be associated with maternal connective tissue disease and the presence of autoantibodies to Ro and La antigens, but in some patients, is associated with structural heart disease (Eliason et al. 2011).

In fetal life, the diagnosis of complete heart block is suspected when a slow heart rate is detected and fetal echocardiography is used to establish the diagnosis using M-mode and spectral Doppler techniques to demonstrate the faster atrial rate and the dissociated slower ventricular rate.

Management

Although most newborns with isolated complete heart block are haemodynamically stable, the postnatal management varies between centres. Isoprenaline can be used in symptomatic neonates until temporary pacing is secured. Permanent pacing is required for neonates who develop symptoms of heart failure or failure to thrive. The threshold for pacing is lower in the presence of structural heart disease (Strasburger et al. 2007; Gregoratos et al. 2002).

Outcome

Complete heart block associated with fetal hydrops carries a much worse prognosis. The vast majority of live-born infants will require pacing by the time they reach adolescence. Our recent experience has reported almost 80% survival at 30 years for liveborn infants (Ho et al. 2015).

Long term follow-up of cardiac rhythm, pacing and cardiomyopathy is indicated.

Non-urgent CHD

Left to Right Shunt Lesions

The commonest CHD lesions with potential for a postnatal "left to right" shunt include ventricular septal defects (VSD) or atrioventricular septal defects (AVSD). These fetuses are at minimal risk during pregnancy, delivery and in the immediate postnatal period. The symptoms of breathlessness, poor feeding and poor weight gain commonly present at 4–6 weeks of life, due to the expected post-natal fall in pulmonary vascular resistance leading to an increased pulmonary blood flow when compared to systemic blood flow.

Cardiac surgery is usually undertaken at 3–6 months of age and involves complete correction on cardiopulmonary bypass. VSDs are repaired using synthetic patches or occasionally by direct suture closure. In AVSD, the atrioventricular valves and septal defects are repaired during single stage surgery in most cases. For AVSDs around 15–20% of patients will require further surgery on their inlet valves later in life.

Long term cardiology follow up will be needed. Depending on the presence of residual lesions or other associated cardiac defects; repeat cardiac interventions or surgery might be needed later in life.

Valvar Abnormalities

Fetuses with mild valve abnormalities i.e. mild pulmonary valve stenosis or mild aortic stenosis with normal cardiac function are also unlikely to become symptomatic immediately after birth. However, these CHD lesions may be progressive in infancy, hence regular postnatal cardiology follow up is advised. The need and timing for an intervention will be determined by the severity of the valvar disease and cardiac function.

Benign Fetal Arrhythmia

Benign fetal arrhythmias i.e. atrial or ventricular ectopics with normal cardiac function usually resolve soon after birth. Neonatal evaluation and a postnatal electrocardiogram (ECG) will suffice to confirm normal electrical activity. If ECG is normal, these babies do not require long term cardiology follow up.

Long Term Considerations

Pre-natal counseling following a fetal diagnosis of CHD must involve multiple aspects aside from the primary cardiac diagnosis. These include any associated genetic or extracardiac malformations, the potential evolution of the cardiac defect during fetal life and the effect of multiple postnatal interventions/operations, particularly on the long-term neurodevelopmental outcome and quality of life. This discussion is particularly important when considering a biventricular correction compared to a univentricular palliation.

Biventricular vs. Univentricular Surgery

Biventricular Outcome

Where possible, the aim is to recreate a circulation with separation of the pulmonary and systemic blood flows. Ideally with the right heart pumping blood to the lungs, and the left heart pumping blood to the systemic circulation (brain and other vital organs). This "biventricular" outcome is possible in many congenital heart lesions, essentially in cases where there are two good sized ventricles and two good sized arteries. For example, septal defects and outflow tract stenoses are often amenable to surgical correction. Even in relatively complex lesions (TGA, DORV etc.), this biventricular outcome is possible where there are two good ventricles and two good great arteries. Intracardiac baffles and or switching of the great artery positions may be necessary but is achievable at low risk.

Single Ventricle Palliation

Unfortunately, in many severe heart abnormalities, these basic requirements are not met, usually with imbalance of the ventricular or great artery size, or absence of either inlet, outlet or both; for example, Tricuspid Atresia has a single inlet and a hypoplastic RV; Double Inlet Left Ventricle has a dominant LV and rudimentary RV; and Hypoplastic Left Heart Syndrome has a dominant RV, rudimentary LV and a hypoplastic aorta. In such cases, it is not possible to achieve separate pulmonary and systemic circulations and therefore a multi-stage surgical programme is required to create a functional single ventricle circulation.

This "Single Ventricle Strategy" can be achieved by a variety of surgical techniques depending on the initial morphology. In principle, when there is only a single dominant ventricle, this ventricle must be surgically connected to the aorta, which requires a ventricular pump to circulate blood at systemic pressure throughout the body.

The initial single ventricle palliation was introduced by Fontan to deal with tricuspid atresia and right heart hypoplasia (Fontan and Baudet 1971). As the LV was already in continuity with the aorta ensuring adequate pulmonary blood flow was the main surgical requirement. This was achieved by creating an anastomosis between the systemic venous return to the pulmonary arteries. There have been numerous modifications to the original technique over the last decades but the principle remains the same. The inferior and superior caval venous return is channeled into the right pulmonary artery either via an intracardiac tunnel or an extracardiac conduit (Fig. 18.4). The end result is a total cavo-pulmonary connection (TCPC) where all systemic venous return bypasses the heart and is delivered directly to the pulmonary circulation. As there is no "pump" in the TCPC circuit, a good functional result requires that the lungs are healthy, the pulmonary arteries are of adequate calibre and the pulmonary vascular resistance is not elevated.

Systemic Outflow Obstruction

For left heart hypoplasia (mitral atresia, aortic atresia, HLHS), a single ventricle strategy is also required, but the dominant ventricle supplying the

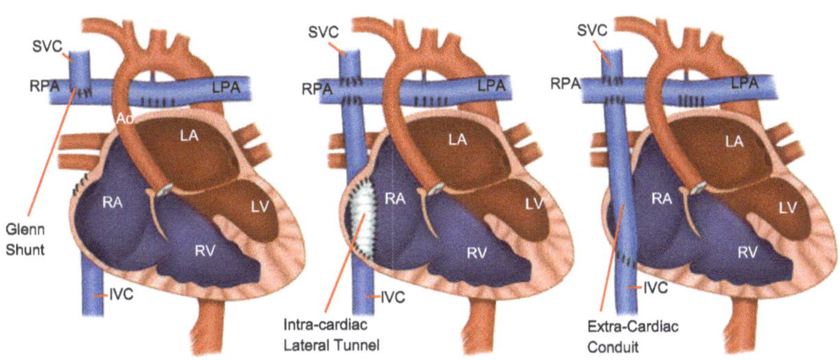

Fig. 18.4 The first diagram on the left demonstrates the Glenn shunt. At this operation the SVC is disconnected from the right atrium and the blood is directed to the right pulmonary artery. A variation of the Glenn operation is the Hemi-Fontan where the continuity of the SVC to the right atrium is maintained when the blood from SVC is directed to the right pulmonary artery. The last stage of Fontan completion will involve redirecting the blood from the IVC to the right pulmonary artery. This can be achieved by maintaining the continuity to the right atrium (lateral tunnel) or can be performed by creating an extracardiac tunnel (extracardiac Fontan). *IVC* inferior caval vein, *SVC* superior caval vein

aorta is the RV. The initial surgical requirement is to create a "neo-aorta" from the RV using the native main pulmonary artery and augmenting the aortic arch (usually using homograft material) and incorporates the small native aorta to carry blood retrograde to the coronary arteries. This procedure was pioneered by Norwood et al. (1981) and is commonly called the Norwood 1 procedure (Fig. 18.5). The branch pulmonary arteries are transected and connected to the systemic circulation by a surgically created shunt. This can either be a modified Blalock-Taussig type shunt where a Gore-Tex graft is placed between the subclavian artery and the branch pulmonary artery; or by a restrictive RV to PA conduit using a small Gore-Tex tube (Sano modification).

Hybrid Operation

To avoid cardio-pulmonary bypass in small, premature or unstable neonates an off bypass "hybrid" palliation is undertaken is some centers. This combines surgical and catheter techniques with surgical placement of bilateral pulmonary artery bands through a midline sternotomy, and by stenting of the arterial duct by direct catheter intervention, and finally a percutaneous atrial septostomy if needed. The hybrid is a temporising measure and will need conversion to a Norwood-type repair once the infant is more resilient.

Once the systemic outlet is created, the subsequent surgical pathway is similar to the Fontan strategy with the later creation of a TCPC in two separate operations:

- At 4–6 months of age, the second stage of univentricular palliation (hemi-Fontan or Glenn) directs blood from superior vena cava to the pulmonary arteries bypassing the heart.
- At 2–4 years of age, the third stage connects the inferior caval vein to the pulmonary arteries, converting a "parallel" to a "series" circulation (Gewillig 2005). The TCPC can be

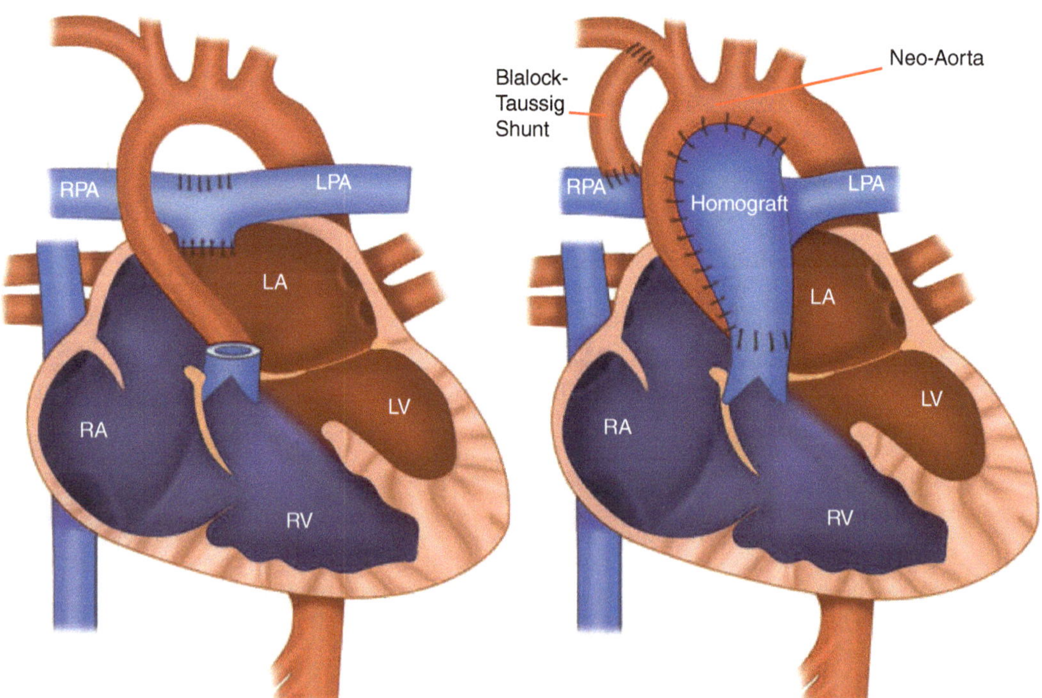

Fig. 18.5 The Norwood 1 operation involves the following steps: The main pulmonary artery is transected and is anastomosed to the ascending aorta (Damus-Kaye-Stansel operation). To augment the pulmonary artery blood flow a Gore-Tex shunt is usually created a systemic to pulmonary artery communication between the right subclavian artery and the right pulmonary artery (modified Blalock-Taussig shunt)

performed using either an extra cardiac conduit between the IVC to pulmonary artery or an intracardiac baffle. Improvements in surgical techniques have translated in improved outcomes with survival up to 91% reported at 10 years (Downing et al. 2017).

Thus, the final common pathway for either right or left heart hypoplasia is the TCPC.

Unrestricted Pulmonary Blood Flow

Single ventricle circulations with unrestricted pulmonary blood flow but adequate systemic outflow will need an initial procedure to restrict excessive pulmonary blood flow, as leaving an infant with high pulmonary blood flow for a prolonged period risks the development of irreversible pulmonary vascular disease which may preclude a later TCPC. This flow restriction is usually achieved by placing a restrictive band around the main pulmonary artery (PA Band).

Long Term Outcome

Even the "perfect" Fontan/TCPC has a recognized attrition rate over time as a result of complications related to the circulatory physiology. With time the compliance of the single ventricle decreases, resulting in increasing filling pressure and diastolic dysfunction. When the Fontan circulation fails, a typical manifestation is venous congestion, low cardiac output and a large hypocontractile dyskinetic ventricle.

The failing Fontan patient may have many symptoms and signs:

- Decreased exercise tolerance with a limited ability to increase cardiac output
- Cardiac rhythm disturbances with a further adverse haemodynamic effect
- Elevated central venous pressure, low cardiac output and lymphatic congestion may result with time in lymphoid fluid leaking into the interstitium of the gut or the bronchi resulting in protein losing enteropathy, plastic bronchitis, venous thrombosis with pulmonary embolism.
  - Protein losing enteropathy is a rare complication, occurring in 1–5% of Fontan patients. High protein chyle with lymphocytes leaks into the gut, resulting in hypoalbuminemia, oedema, abdominal distension, diarrhoea, lymphocytopaenia and progressive cardiac cachexia.
  - Plastic bronchitis results in bronchial casts with life-threatening airway obstruction.
- Thromboembolic complications are commonly reported and relate to circulatory stasis and alterations in the coagulation system.
- Liver fibrosis and cirrhosis can also occur as a result of abnormal chronic elevation of the pressure in the inferior caval vein.

The use of heart transplantation has also been proposed as an alternative form of palliation for these patients, which may be associated with a better quality of life (Razzouk et al. 1996). However due to limitation in donor availability this approach is often limited.

Conclusion

Fetal echocardiography can successfully predict postnatal risk and improve perinatal care for newborns diagnosed in utero with congenital heart defect. Planning for postnatal care of critical or severe congenital heart defect involves good communication between fetal cardiologists, fetal medicine specialists, obstetricians and neonatologists. Site of delivery for fetuses with CHD should be decided based on diagnosis, the need for early cardiac intervention, the presence of major extracardiac abnormalities and the level of care that is available locally. Early identification and careful planning of fetuses at increased risk has the potential to reduce neonatal complications and early adverse outcome.

Although many lesions can be corrected towards a more normal biventricular circulation, a significant number must follow a single ventricle surgical pathway where the longer term prognosis remains guarded despite advances in surgical techniques.

References

Allan L, Hornberger L, Sharland G. Textbook of fetal cardiology. London: Greenwich Medical Media; 2000. p. 261.

Brown DW, et al. Aortic valve reinterventions after balloon aortic valvuloplasty for congenital aortic stenosis: intermediate and late follow up. J Am Coll Cardiol. 2010;56:1740–9.

Choudhary P, et al. Late outcomes in adults with coarctation of the aorta. Heart. 2015;101:1190–5.

Donofrio MT, et al. Diagnosis and treatment of fetal cardiac disease. A scientific statement from the American Heart Association. Circulation. 2014;129:2183–242.

Donofrio MT, et al. Risk stratified postnatal care of newborns with critical congenital heart disease. Am J Cardiol. 2013;111:737–47.

Downing TE, et al. Long-term survival after the Fontan operation: twenty years of experience at a single center. J Thorac Cardiovasc Surg. 2017;154(1):243–253.e2.

Eliason H, et al. Isolated atrioventricular block in the fetus: a retrospective multinational, multicentre study of 175 patients. Circulation. 2011;124(18):1919–26.

Fontan F, Baudet E. Surgical repair of tricuspid atresia. Thorax. 1971;26(3):240–8.

Gewillig M. The Fontan circulation. Heart. 2005;91:839–46.

Gregoratos G, et al. ACC/AHA/NASPE 2002 guideline update for implantation of cardiac pacemakers and antiarrhythmia devices—summary article: a report of the American College of Cardiology/American Heart Association Task Force on Practice Guidelines (ACC/AHA/NASPE Committee to Update the 1998 Pacemaker Guidelines). J Am Coll Cardiol. 2002;40:1703–19.

Ho A, et al. Isolated complete heart block in fetus. Am J Cardiol. 2015;116(1):142–7.

Norwood WI, Lang P, Castenada AR, Campbell DN. Experience with operations for hypoplastic left heart syndrome. J Thorac Cardiovasc Surg. 1981;82(4):511–9.

Razzouk AJ, et al. Transplantation as a primary treatment for hypoplastic left heart syndrome: intermediate results. Ann Thorac Surg. 1996;62:1–7.

Roos-Hesselink JW, et al. Long term outcome after surgery for pulmonary stenosis (a longitudinal study of 22-33 years). Eur Heart J. 2006;27(4):482–8.

Sathanandam SK, et al. Management of hypoplastic left heart syndrome with intact atrial septum: a two-centre experience. Cardiol Young. 2016;26(6):1072–81.

Sanapo L, Moon-Grady AJ, Donofrio MT. Perinatal and delivery management of infants with congenital heart disease. Clin Perinatol. 2016;43:55–71.

Shinkawa T, et al. Management and long-term outcome of neonatal Ebstein anomaly. J Thorac Cardiovasc Surg. 2010;139(2):354–8.

Simpson JM. Fetal arrhythmias. Ultrasound Obstet Gynecol. 2006;27(6):599–606.

Strasburger JF, et al. Perinatal arrhythmias. Diagnosis and management. Clin Perinatol. 2007;34(4):627–52.

Tobler D, et al. Cardiac outcomes in young adult survivors of the arterial switch operation for transposition of the great arteries. J Am Coll Cardiol. 2010;56:58.

Vigneswaran TV, et al. Usefulness of the Prenatal Echocardiogram in foetuses with isolated transposition of great arteries to predict the need for balloon atrial septostomy. Am J Cardiol. 2017;119(9):1463–7.

Voet A, et al. Long-term outcome after treatment of isolated pulmonary valve stenosis. Int J Cardiol. 2012;156(1):11–5.

Index

© Springer International Publishing AG, part of Springer Nature 2018
J. Simpson et al. (eds.), *Fetal Cardiology*, https://doi.org/10.1007/978-3-319-77461-9

G

MIX
Papier | Fördert gute Waldnutzung
FSC® C083411

Kolibri 360 GmbH
Ferdinand-Jühlke-Straße 7
99095 Erfurt, Deutschland
produktsicherheit@kolibri360.de